Clinical Immunology

and

Serology

A Laboratory Perspective

second edition

CHRISTINE DORRESTEYN STEVENS,
EdD, MT(ASCP)

*Professor of Clinical Laboratory Sciences and
Head, Department of Health Sciences
Western Carolina University
Cullowhee, North Carolina*

F. A. DAVIS COMPANY • Philadelphia

F. A. Davis Company
1915 Arch Street
Philadelphia, PA 19103
www.fadavis.com

Printed in the United States of America

Last digit indicates print number: 10 9 8 7 6 5 4 3

Acquisitions Editor: Christa Fratantoro
Developmental Editor: Michelle L. Clarke
Cover Designer: Louis J. Forgione

As new scientific information becomes available through basic and clinical research, recommended treatments and drug therapies undergo changes. The author(s) and publisher have done everything possible to make this book accurate, up to date, and in accord with accepted standards at the time of publication. The author(s), editors, and publisher are not responsible for errors or omissions or for consequences from application of the book, and make no warranty, expressed or implied, in regard to the contents of the book. Any practice described in this book should be applied by the reader in accordance with professional standards of care used in regard to the unique circumstances that may apply in each situation. The reader is advised always to check product information (package inserts) for changes and new information regarding dose and contraindications before administering any drug. Caution is especially urged when using new or infrequently ordered drugs.

Library of Congress Cataloging-in-Publication Data

Stevens, Christine Dorresteyn.
    Clinical immunology and serology : a laboratory perspective/Christine Dorresteyn
Stevens.–2nd ed.
        p. ; cm.
    Includes bibliographical references and index.
    ISBN 0-8036-1095-5 (alk. paper)
        1. Immunodiagnosis–Laboratory manuals. 2. Serodiagnosis–Laboratory manuals. 3. Clinical immunology. I. Title.
    [DNLM: 1. Immunity–physiology. 2. Immunologic Diseases–diagnosis. 3. Immunologic Techniques. 4. Immunologic
Tests. 5. Serologic Tests. QW 540 S844c 2003]
    RB46.5.S73 2003
    616.07'56–dc21

                                                                                    2003043928

To my wonderful children:
Eric and Kathy, and Kevin and Melissa;
and in loving memory of Charles,
my husband of 33 years and my best friend.

Preface

*T*he second edition of *Clinical Immunology and Serology: A Laboratory Perspective* is built on the success of the first edition. All the features that readers enjoyed have been retained and strengthened, and some new features have been added. The number of illustrations has increased, and case studies have been devised for most of the chapters. New chapters include: an overview of safety in the clinical immunology lab, an explanation of molecular techniques, the role of cytokines in the immune response, and an expansion of immunoproliferative and immunodeficiency diseases. The book remains a practical introduction to the field of clinical immunology that combines essential theoretic principles with serologic techniques commonly used in the clinical laboratory. It is written primarily for clinical laboratory science students at the 2- and 4-year levels, but it may also serve as a valuable reference for practicing laboratorians and other allied health professionals. The theory is comprehensive but concise, and the emphasis is on direct application to the clinical laboratory. The text is readable and user-friendly, with learning objectives, chapter outlines, and a glossary of all key terms. Each chapter is a complete learning module that contains theoretic principles, illustrations, definitions of relevant terminology, procedures for simulated clinical testing, and questions and case studies that help to evaluate learning.

The basic four-part organization of the book has been retained. Part I describes the nature of the immune system, with an emphasis on constituents of the lymphoid system, characteristics of T and B cells, the nature of antigens, the structure of antibodies, contributions of cytokines, and the role of complement in amplification of the immune response. Part II concentrates on basic immunologic procedures and gives the theoretic and practical considerations involved in precipitation reactions, agglutination reactions, labeled immunoassays, and molecular techniques. Immune disorders are the focus of Part III, including discussions of hypersensitivity, autoimmune diseases, transplantation, tumor immunology, and immunoproliferative and immunodeficiency diseases. Part IV describes serologic testing for diseases such as syphilis, Lyme disease, streptococcal infections, viral diseases, human immunodeficiency virus (HIV), fungal infections, and parasitic diseases.

The organization of the chapters is based on the experience of many years of teaching immunology to clinical laboratory science students. This book has been designed to provide the necessary balance of theory with practical application because it is essential for the practitioner to have a thorough understanding of the theoretic basis for testing methodologies. Because the field of immunology is expanding so rapidly, the challenge in writing this book has been to ensure adequate coverage but to keep it on an introductory level. Every chapter has been revised and updated to include current practices as of the time of writing. It is hoped that this book will kindle an interest in both students and laboratory professionals in this exciting and dynamic field.

Acknowledgements

I am grateful for the assistance I received from a number of sources during the preparation of this second edition. I would like to thank the following reviewers for their helpful suggestions with newly added chapters: Donna Broderick, Linda Dezern, Karen Long, Marguerite Neita, and Diane Wyatt.

A special word of appreciation is due to my contributors, Russell Cheadle, Norma Cook, Eugene Heise, Maureane Hoffman, Linda Miller, Kate Rittenhouse-Olson, Susan Strasinger, and Diane Wyatt, who shared their expertise to enrich the manuscript.

I would also like to thank the administration at Western Carolina University for granting me a Scholarly Development Assignment, which allowed me to begin the revision of the text and to complete the manuscript in a more timely fashion that otherwise would not have been possible with a full teaching load. Special thanks to my acquisitions editor, Christa Fratantoro, for her patience and helpful suggestions, and for knowing when I needed a lift to keep me going. I also appreciate the efforts of Michelle Clarke, Developmental Editor, and Susan Rhyner, Manager of Creative Development, who have become my good friends during this revision. As always, Ona Kosmos has helped to keep all of us straight. My immunology students, past, present, and future, are the inspiration and reason for writing this book. I learn as much or more from your curiosity and your questioning as you do from me.

My husband Charles supported and encouraged me even during his final illness. To my two wonderful sons Eric and Kevin, and their wives Kathy and Melissa, you are a continued blessing and my source of strength.

Contributors

RUSSELL F. CHEADLE, MS, MT(ASCP)
Associate Professor and Program Director
Medical Laboratory Technology
University of Rio Grande
Rio Grande, Ohio

NORMA B. COOK, MA, MT(ASCP)
Retired Associate Professor
Clinical Laboratory Sciences
Western Carolina University
Cullowhee, North Carolina

EUGENE R. HEISE, PhD, DIPLO. (ABHI)
Department of Microbiology and Immunology
Wake Forest University School of Medicine
Winston-Salem, North Carolina

MAUREANE HOFFMANN, MD, PhD
Professor of Pathology and Immunology
Duke University and Durham VA Medical Centers
Durham, North Carolina

LINDA E. MILLER, PhD, SI(ASCP)
Professor
Department of Clinical Laboratory Sciences
Upstate Medical University
Syracuse, New York

KATE RITTENHOUSE-OLSON, PhD, SI(ASCP)
Associate Professor and Director
Biotechnology Program
Department of Clinical Laboratory Science
The University at Buffalo
Buffalo, New York

SUSAN KING STRASINGER, DA, MT(ASCP)
Medical Technology
University of Florida
Pensacola, Florida

DIANE WYATT, MS, MT(ASCP), CLS(NCA)
Associate Professor
Clinical Laboratory Science Program
University of Tennessee Health Science Center
Memphis, Tennessee

Consultants

DONNA BRODERICK, MS, MT
Harcum Junior College
Program Director
Medical Lab Technology
Bryn Mawr, Pennsylvania

LINDA DEZERN, MS, MT(ASCP)
Thomas Nelson Community College
Program Director
Medical Lab Technology
Hampton, Virginia

KAREN S. LONG, MS, CLS(NCA), MT(ASCP)
West Virginia University
Associate Professor
School of Medicine
Medical Tech Program
Morgantown, West Virginia

MARGUERITE NEITA, PhD, MT
Howard University
Associate Professor
College of Pharmacy, Nursing, and Allied Health Sciences
Washington, D.C.

DIANE WYATT, MS, MT(ASCP), CLS(NCA)
University of Tennessee—Memphis
Associate Professor
Clinical Laboratory Science Program
Memphis, Tennessee

Contents

Color Plates follow p. xvi.

Part II Basic Immunologic Procedures   *113*

Chapter 16   Immunodeficiency Diseases 248

Maureane Hoffman, MD, PhD and Christine Stevens

Chapter 17   Transplantation Immunology 262

Eugene R. Heise, PhD, Diplo. (ABHI)

Chapter 18   Tumor Immunology 278

Kate Rittenhouse-Olson, PhD, SI(ASCP)

Part IV Serologic Diagnosis of Infectious Diseases   **293**

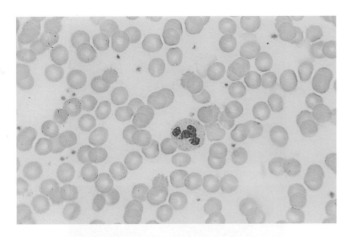

Color Plate 1. Photo of a neutrophil. (*From Harr, R: Clinical Laboratory Science Review, ed. 2. FA Davis, Philadelphia, 2000. Color Plate 30.*) See Fig. 2–1 in the text.

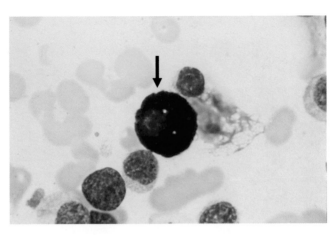

Color Plate 4. Photo of a mast cell. (*From Harmening, D: Clinical Hematology and Fundamentals of Hemostasis, ed. 4. FA Davis, Philadelphia, 2002. Color Plate 42.*) See Fig. 2–4 in the text.

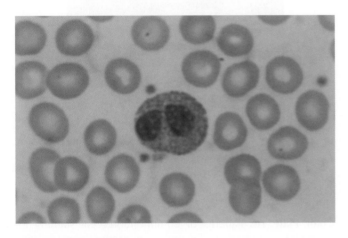

Color Plate 2. Photo of a eosinophil. (*From Harmening, D: Clinical Hematology and Fundamentals of Hemostasis, ed. 4. FA Davis, Philadelphia, 2002. Color Plate 12.*) See Fig. 2–2 in the text.

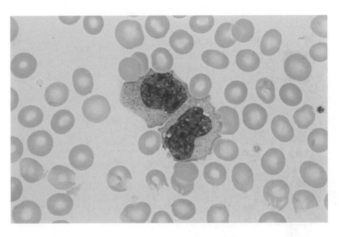

Color Plate 5. Photo of a monocyte. (*From Harmening, D: Clinical Hematology and Fundamentals of Hemostasis, ed. 4. FA Davis, Philadelphia, 2002. Color Plate 15.*) See Fig. 2–5 in the text.

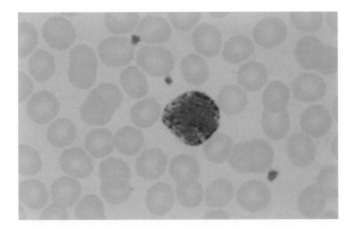

Color Plate 3. Photo of a basophil. (*From Harmening, D: Clinical Hematology and Fundamentals of Hemostasis, ed. 4. FA Davis, Philadelphia, 2002. Color Plate 13.*) See Fig. 2–3 in the text.

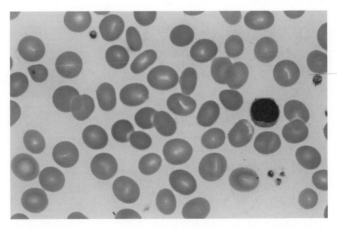

Color Plate 6. Typical lymphocyte found in peripheral blood. (*From Harr, R: Clinical Laboratory Science Review, ed. 2. FA Davis, Philadelphia, 2000. Color Plate 31.*) See Fig. 3–1 in the text.

Color Plates

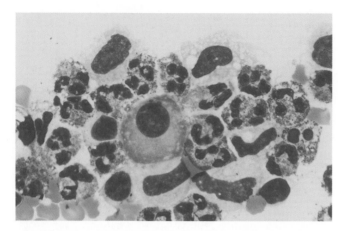

Color Plate 7. A typical plasma cell. (*From Harr, R: Clinical Laboratory Science Review, ed. 2. FA Davis, Philadelphia, 2000. Color Plate 28.*) See Fig. 3–7 in the text.

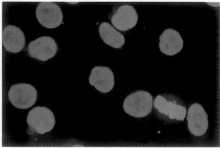

homogeneous pattern

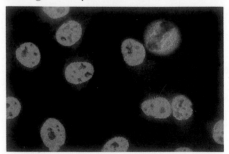

speckled pattern

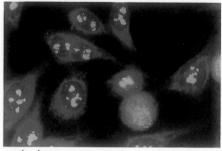

nucleolar pattern

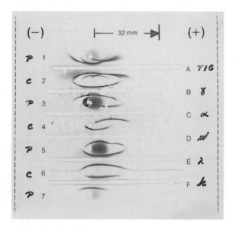

Color Plate 8. Immunoelectrophoresis film showing normal controls (odd-numbered wells) and patient serum (even-numbered wells). Reactions in wells 1 and 5 indicate an IgM monoclonal gammopathy with lambda light chains. (*From Harr, R: Clinical Laboratory Science Review, ed. 2. FA Davis, Philadelphia, 2000. Color Plate 4, with permission.*) See Fig. 9–7 in the text.

Color Plate 10. Patterns of immunofluorescent staining for antinuclear antibodies. Examples of predominant staining patterns obtsained are homogeneous–staining of the entire nucleus, speckled pattern–staining throughout the nucleus, and nucleolar pattern–staining of the nucleolus. (*Courtesy of DiaSorin, Inc., with permission.*) See Fig. 14–2 in the text.

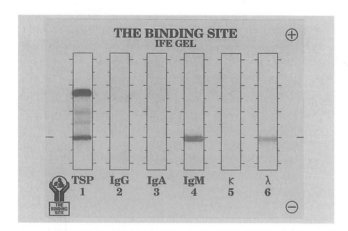

Color Plate 9. Immunofixation electrophoresis. (*Courtesy of The Binding Site Ltd., Birmingham, UK.*) See Fig. 9–8 in the text.

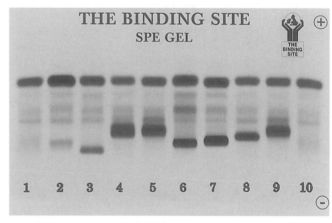

Color Plate 11. Agarose gel electrophoresis of serum samples on an SPE gel. (*Courtesy of The Binding Site Ltd., Birmingham, UK.*) See Fig. 15–2 in the text.

Part I

Nature of the Immune System

chapter 1

Historical Concepts and Introduction to Serologic Testing

Learning Objectives

After finishing this chapter, the reader will be able to:
1. Define immunity and describe Jenner's role in the development of immunity to smallpox.
2. Discuss Pasteur's work with attenuated vaccines.
3. Explain how the controversy over humoral versus cellular immunity contributed to expanding knowledge in the field of immunology.
4. Distinguish a hapten from an antigen.
5. Explain what an antibody is.
6. Describe the effect of Landsteiner's discoveries on both immunochemistry and transfusion medicine.
7. Discuss Koch's contribution to the elucidation of cell-mediated immunity.
8. Define the following: serology, agglutination, and precipitation.

Key Terms

Antibodies	Delayed hypersensitivity	Passive immunity
Antigens	Hapten	Phagocytosis
Attenuated vaccine	Humoral immunity	Serology
Cellular immunity	Immunity	Vaccination
Cross-immunity	Immunology	Variolation

All scientific knowledge is advancing at a rapid pace, but nowhere are the changes more rapid than in the field of immunology. Virtually the entire history of immunology has been recorded within the last 100 years, and it is only in the recent past that the most significant part of this history has been written. It was not until the 1960s that the cells responsible for the immune response were identified and characterized. At the same time, pioneering techniques to measure small amounts of substances using antibodies with radioactive or enzyme tags were developed. These discoveries have affected testing in every area of the laboratory and have played a significant role in the diagnosis and treatment of disease.

Immunology can be defined as the study of the reactions of a host when foreign substances are introduced into the body. Foreign substances that induce such an immune response are called **antigens.** Antigens are usually thought of as harmful infectious agents, but they may also be harmless environmental substances, such as pollen, which can trigger a response in some individuals.

Early studies in immunology concentrated on the body's ability to protect itself and combat these various agents, or antigens, without producing harm to the tissues involved. As knowledge of the field accumulated, the scope of immunology was significantly broadened to include the study of the molecular mechanisms for the immune response, the development of testing for disease states in the laboratory, the recognition that the body can respond to self-antigens in what is known as autoimmune diseases, and the manipulation of the immune system for treatment of disease. All of these topics are covered in later chapters.

Immunity and Immunization

Immunology as a science had its beginnings in the study of **immunity,** the condition of being resistant to infection. The first written records of experimentation date back to the 1500s, when the Chinese developed a practice of inhaling powder made from smallpox scabs to produce protection against this dreaded disease. This practice of deliberately exposing an individual to material from smallpox lesions was known as **variolation.** The theory was that if an individual was exposed in a healthy state as a child or young adult, the effects of the disease would be minimized. This was not always the case, however.

Further refinements did not occur until the late 1700s, when an English country doctor by the name of Edward Jenner discovered a remarkable relationship between exposure to cowpox and immunity to smallpox. Injecting individuals with material from a cowpox lesion provided protection against smallpox.[1] This procedure of injecting cellular material became known as **vaccination,** from *vacca,* the Latin word for cow. The phenomenon in which exposure to one agent produces protection against another agent is known as **cross-immunity.** Within 50 years of this discovery, most of the European countries had initiated a compulsory vaccination program.[2]

In working with the bacteria that caused chicken cholera, Louis Pasteur, a key figure in the development of both microbiology and immunology, accidentally found that old cultures would not cause disease in chickens.[3] Subsequent injections of more virulent organisms had no effect on the birds that had been previously exposed to the older cultures. In this manner, the first **attenuated vaccine** was discovered. Attenuation, or change, may occur through heat, aging, or chemical means, and it remains the basis for many of the immunizations that are used today.

Pasteur applied the principle of attenuation to the prevention of rabies. Although he did not know the causative agent, he recognized that the central nervous system was affected, and thus he studied spinal cords from rabid animals. He noted that spinal cords left to dry for a few days were less infectious to laboratory animals than fresh spinal cords. In 1885, when a boy who was bitten severely by a rabid dog was brought to his home, Pasteur tried out his new procedure. The boy received a series of 12 injections beginning with material from the least infectious cords and progressing to the fresher, more infectious material. Miraculously, he survived, and a modification of this procedure is the standard treatment for rabies today.

Cellular Versus Humoral Immunity

In the late 1800s, scientists turned to identification of the actual mechanisms producing immunity in a host.[3] Elie Metchnikoff, a Russian scientist, observed that foreign objects introduced into transparent starfish larvae became surrounded by motile cells that attempted to destroy these invaders. He called this process **phagocytosis,** meaning cells that eat cells.[3] He hypothesized that immunity to disease was based on the action of these scavenger cells.

Other researchers contended that noncellular elements in the blood were responsible for protection from microorganisms. Emil von Behring demonstrated that diphtheria and tetanus toxin, produced by the microorganisms as they grow, could be neutralized by the noncellular portion of the blood of animals previously exposed to the microorganisms. This method of conferring resistance is known today as **passive immunity.** The theory of **humoral immunity** was thus born, and this sparked a long lasting dispute over the relative importance of cellular versus humoral immunity.

In 1903 an English physician named Almoth Wright linked the two theories by showing that the immune response involved both cellular and humoral elements. He observed that certain humoral, or circulating, factors called *opsonins* acted to coat bacteria so that they became more susceptible to ingestion by phagocytic cells.[4] This was the first expression of the notion that serum factors in the blood were formed in response to exposure to foreign substances. These serum factors are known as **antibodies.**

Long before antibodies were actually isolated, Paul Ehrlich theorized that specialized cells carried antibodies and that the molecular structure of these molecules contained unique receptor sites for the antigens that triggered their formation.[2] The lock and key concept of the fit between antigen and antibody was substantiated by later research on the structure of antibody molecules. It was not until 1948, however, that plasma cells were discovered to be the source of antibodies.[1] During the 1950s and 1960s, researchers identified two types of lymphocytes, namely T cells and B cells, and determined that plasma cells were derived from B cells. Presence of both T cells and B cells were found to be necessary for a normal immune response.

Antigens and Haptens

Exploring the mechanisms of immunity in the host naturally led to examination of the substances that would trigger this response, namely antigens. Karl Landsteiner, a famous researcher in immunology, made a number of significant contributions in this area with his painstaking research on chemical groups that add or change the specificity of antigens. He coined the term **hapten** to refer to simple chemical groups that could bind to antibody but which were incapable of stimulating antibody formation unless tied to a larger carrier molecule. His book *The Specificity of Serological Reactions* established the immunochemical basis for immunologic reactions.

Landsteiner, however, is perhaps best remembered for his discovery of the ABO blood groups and the naturally occurring ABO antibodies or agglutinins found in serum. As a result of his work, the use of blood transfusions became an accepted therapeutic practice, and he was awarded the Nobel Prize in 1930.

Cell-Mediated Immunity

The search for the cells that actually produced antibodies led to a re-emphasis on the nature of **cellular immunity.** In attempting to discover a cure for tuberculosis (TB), Robert Koch injected guinea pigs with an extract of tubercle bacilli, expecting to produce antibodies. Instead, skin lesions, which were characterized by a hard red lump with a necrotic center, developed slowly over a period of days after exposure to the antigen.[5] This was called **delayed hypersensitivity.** Later, it became clear that this phenomenon was caused by the blood cells known as T lymphocytes.

Experiments in the 1970s showed that T lymphocytes play a major role in the immune response. T cells produce a number of soluble factors responsible for the cellular cooperation necessary for antibody production and recruitment of other white blood cells. These soluble factors, called *cytokines,* are the focus of extensive research today. They are beginning to be used as therapeutic agents in the treatment of cancer, anemia, and a number of other diseases, and their role will likely be expanded in the future. In addition, certain T cells called cytotoxic T cells are now known to provide an important means of defense against tumor cells or normal cells that harbor intracellular parasites such as viruses or mycobacteria.

The Age of Serology

The history of laboratory testing closely follows developments in the field of immunology in general. Serologic investigations were a natural outgrowth of the study of immunity, and the time period from 1900 to 1950 has been called the era of international serology.[5] **Serology** is the study of the noncellular components in the blood. At this time, attention was turned to research on the production and use of serum to control disease, and a number of scientific institutes were created for this purpose. The Institut Pasteur was established in France in 1888, following the success of Pasteur's rabies immunization.[5] In London, the Lister

Institute was created, and a number of other institutions in Europe appeared at this time.

Bacterial agglutination was first described by Gruber and Durham in 1896.[3] Shortly thereafter, Widal developed an agglutination test for the diagnosis of typhoid fever, a test which still bears his name today. *Agglutination* is the process by which particulate antigens, such as cells, aggregate to form larger complexes when a specific antibody is present. *Precipitation,* the combination of soluble antigen with soluble antibody, was discovered by Kraus when he combined filtrates of bacterial cultures with specific antisera.[3] Many of the tests performed in today's clinical laboratory fall into the category of serologic tests, which use either precipitation or agglutination as an endpoint.

Other Historical Developments

Many other outstanding scientists have made important contributions to the field of immunology. A list of the Nobel prizewinners for immunologic investigations is given in Table 1–1, and more details are presented in individual chapters. Through the actions of these individuals, the scope of immunology has broadened greatly from the original focus on immunity to the study of the mechanisms of the immune response and to the development of testing that plays a major role in today's clinical laboratory.

TABLE 1–1. Nobel Prize Winners in Immunology		
Year	**Scientist**	**Research**
1901	Emil von Behring	Serum antitoxins
1905	Robert Koch	Cellular immunity in TB
1908	Elie Metchnikoff, Paul Ehrlich	Phagocytosis Immunity
1913	Charles Richet	Anaphylaxis
1919	Jules Bordet	Complement
1930	Karl Landsteiner	Human blood group antigens
1960	Macfarlane Burnet, Peter Medawar	Discovery of immunologic tolerance
1972	Gerald Edelman, Rodney Porter	Structure of antibodies
1977	Rosalyn Yalow	Radioimmunoassay
1980	George Snell, Jean Dausset, Baruj Benacerraf	Major histocompatibility complex
1984	Niels Jerne, Georges Koehler, Cesar Milstein	Immunoregulation Monoclonal antibody
1987	Susumu Tonegawa	Antibody diversity
1991	E. Donnall Thomas, Joseph Murray	Transplantation
1996	Peter Doherty, Rolf Zinkernagel	Cytotoxic T cell recognition of virally infected cells

SUMMARY

The study of immunology began as an interest in achieving immunity, or resistance to disease. Edward Jenner, an Englishman, performed the first successful vaccination against smallpox and ushered in the age of immunologic investigation. Another well-known name in the early history of immunology is Louis Pasteur, whose discovery of attenuated vaccines formed the basis of modern vaccination programs used today. The controversy over cellular versus humoral immunity was responsible for spawning much important research in the early years. Elie Metchnikoff identified phagocytic cells as an instrument of cellular immunity, and Emil von Behring showed that a humoral, or noncellular, factor in the blood could neutralize tetanus and diph-

theria toxins. Both of these theories were brought together by Wright, an English physician who observed that both circulating and cellular factors are necessary to produce immunity.

Karl Landsteiner investigated the nature of antigens, the substances that trigger the immune response. In addition, he is credited with the discovery of the ABO blood groups, the identification of which led to the ability to transfuse blood more safely on a scientific basis.

Many other significant contributions have broadened the field of immunology so that it now includes the genetic basis for the immune response, the phenomenon of hypersensitivity, the nature of cell cooperation, and the manipulation of the immune system to suppress graft rejection and increase immune surveillance against cancerous cells.

Exercise: Landsteiner's Lab

BACKGROUND

In 1901 Karl Landsteiner mixed serum and cells from himself and five lab associates. He discovered so-called naturally occurring antibodies to red blood cells, meaning that individuals have antibodies present without prior exposure to foreign red blood cells. These naturally occurring antibodies demonstrated specificity because they caused agglutination of only certain red cells. The agglutination patterns found were called A and B and zero (later changed to O). Each pattern indicated the presence or absence of a particular antigen on that red cell. Using blood obtained from the class or random samples, Landsteiner's discovery will be re-created. A matrix will be used to record results. Each student will test his or her serum against his or her own cells and the cells of classmates or the other specimens. The composite matrix will be recorded and interpreted to determine the blood types found.

PRINCIPLE

Two drops of serum from one specimen will be placed in a test tube with two drops of a 3-percent solution of red cells. If agglutination occurs, the red cells have an antigen present that is reacting with antibodies naturally present in the serum of individuals with a different red cell type. This procedure is followed with one student using his or her own serum to test all other red cell suspensions in the class. Positive and negative reactions will be recorded.

REAGENTS, MATERIALS, AND EQUIPMENT

Test tubes, 12 × 75 mm
Saline (0.85 percent)
Disposable pipettes
Blood bank centrifuge

SPECIMEN COLLECTION

Collect blood aseptically by venipuncture into two sterile tubes, one with ethylenediaminetetra-acetic acid (EDTA), and the other with no anticoagulant. Allow the plain tube to clot. Separate the serum without transferring any cellular elements. Do not use grossly hemolyzed, excessively lipemic, or bacterially contaminated specimens. Fresh non-heat inactivated serum is recommended for the test. However, if the test cannot be performed immediately, serum may be stored between 2°C and 8°C for up to 72 hours. If there is any additional delay, freeze the serum at −18°C or below.

PROCEDURE

1. Take 5 drops of EDTA whole blood collected or 3 drops of packed red cells and place in a 12- × 75-mm disposable glass test tube using a disposable blood bank pipette.
2. Fill the tube almost to the top with saline, and mix well.
3. Centrifuge in a blood bank centrifuge for approximately 45 seconds.
4. Decant the supernate, and fill the tube almost to the top with saline. Spin again.
5. Repeat this procedure until the cells have been washed three times.
6. After the final wash, fill the tube about three-fourths full with saline. This will be the 3- to 5-percent solution that will be used for testing.
7. Put your number and initials on the cell suspension tube. (Compare with reagent red cells to be sure that the right concentration has been achieved.)
8. Label 12- × 75-mm blood bank tubes with your initials and the numbers for every member of the class.
9. Put two drops of your own serum in each of the tubes.
10. Place two drops of cell suspension in the tube with your number.
11. Pass your cell suspension on to all classmates, so they can put your cells in a tube with their serum.
12. When all tubes have serum and cells, spin for 30 seconds in a blood bank centrifuge and observe for agglutination by gently shaking the red blood cell button loose from the side of each test tube. Use a magnifying lamp to see the reaction. Cells that remain clumped together after shaking indicate a positive reaction.
13. Construct a matrix similar to the following sample. Record all the results on the matrix.
14. Record + if cells clump in any of the tubes. Record 0 if they do not clump.
15. Interpret the results as a class.

RESULTS: SAMPLE LANDSTEINER MATRIX

Serum (Across) Versus Cells (Down)

	1	2	3	4	5	6	7	8	9	10
1	0	0	0	0	0	0	0	0	0	0
2	0	0	0	0	0	0	0	0	0	0
3	+	+	0	0	+	0	+	+	0	+
4	+	+	0	0	+	0	+	+	0	+
5	0	0	0	0	0	0	0	0	0	0
6	+	+	0	0	+	0	+	+	0	+
7	0	0	0	0	0	0	0	0	0	0
8	+	+	+	+	+	+	+	0	+	+
9	+	+	0	0	+	0	+	+	0	+
10	0	0	0	0	0	0	0	0	0	0

INTERPRETATION OF RESULTS

By looking at the sample table shown previously, it is possible to distinguish three distinct patterns. Cells that are numbered 1, 2, 5, 7, and 10 did not react with any other sera. Landsteiner called these zero or O. The two other patterns present were randomly designated A and B. One of these is represented by the cells numbered 3, 4, 6, and 9, and they could be called type A. Number 8 cells display a third agglutination pattern, and they could be labeled type B. Note that sera from individuals designated as type O contain antibodies to the two other cell types. In Landsteiner's original group, there were no AB individuals. If blood from an AB individual was selected, then an additional pattern would emerge. Cells from an AB individual would agglutinate with the sera from all others, and the serum would not agglutinate any other cells.

Review Questions

1. Jenner's work with cowpox, which provided immunity against smallpox, demonstrates which phenomenon?
   a. Natural immunity
   b. Cross-immunity
   c. Attenuation of vaccines
   d. Reactivity of haptens

2. Metchnikoff first described which of the following?
   a. Phagocytosis
   b. Variolation
   c. Humoral immunity
   d. Opsonization

3. Which of the following can be attributed to Pasteur?
   a. Discovery of opsonins
   b. Research on haptens
   c. First attenuated vaccines
   d. Discovery of the ABO blood groups

4. If cells from an individual are not agglutinated by serum from anyone else, this represents which Landsteiner blood type?
   a. Type A
   b. Type B
   c. Type O
   d. Type AB

5. Which of the following is an example of humoral immunity?
   a. Phagocytic cells attacking bacteria
   b. Delayed hypersensitivity reaction
   c. Neutralization of toxin by serum
   d. T cells destroying tumor cells

6. The study of the noncellular components in the blood is known as:
   a. Immunity
   b. Serology
   c. Variolation
   d. Delayed hypersensitivity

7. Serum factors in the blood that are formed in response to foreign substances are known as:
   a. Antibodies
   b. Antigens
   c. Haptens
   d. Cytotoxic T cells

8. In searching for a cure for TB, Koch was the first to observe which phenomenon?
   a. Bacterial agglutination
   b. Precipitation
   c. Phagocytosis
   d. Delayed hypersensitivity

References

1. Talmage, DW: History of immunology. In Stites, DP, Terr, AI, and Parslow, TG (eds): Medical Immunology, ed. 9. Appleton & Lange, Stamford, Conn., 1997, pp 1–7.

2. http://www.keratin.com/am/am003.shtml, accessed March 18, 2002.

3. Silverstein, AM: The history of immunology. In Paul, WE (ed): Fundamental Immunology, ed. 4. Lippincott Williams & Wilkins, Philadelphia, 1999, pp 19–35.

4. Clark, WR: The Experimental Foundations of Modern Immunology, ed 4. John Wiley & Sons, New York, 1991.

5. Kiple, KF (ed): The Cambridge World History of Human Disease. Cambridge University Press, Cambridge, 1993, pp 126–140.

Natural Immunity

Learning Objectives

After finishing this chapter, the reader will be able to:
1. Differentiate between the external and the internal defense systems.
2. Distinguish natural from acquired immunity.
3. List the steps in the process of phagocytosis.
4. Explain the importance of phagocytosis in both natural and acquired immunity.
5. Describe the types of white blood cells capable of phagocytosis.
6. Discuss the intracellular mechanism for destruction of foreign particles during the process of phagocytosis.
7. Discuss the role of acute phase proteins.
8. Describe the process of inflammation.
9. Recognize false-positive and false-negative reactions in the latex agglutination test for C-reactive protein.
10. Determine the significance of abnormal levels of acute phase reactants.

Key Terms

Acquired immunity	Diapedesis	Opsonins
Acute phase reactants	External defense system	Phagocytosis
C-reactive protein	Inflammation	Phagolysosome
Chemotaxin	Internal defense system	Phagosome
Complement	Natural immunity	Respiratory burst

Natural (or innate) **immunity** is the ability of the individual to resist infection by means of normally present body functions. These are considered nonadaptive or nonspecific and are the same for all pathogens or foreign substances to which one is exposed. No prior exposure is required, and the response does not change with subsequent exposures. Many of these mechanisms are subject to influence by such factors as nutrition, age, fatigue, stress, and genetic determinants. **Acquired immunity,** in contrast, is a type of resistance that is characterized by specificity for each individual pathogen and the ability to remember a prior exposure, which results in an increased response upon repeated exposure. Both systems are essential to maintain good health, and in fact, they operate in concert and are dependent upon one another for maximal effectiveness. Natural immunity is considered first, and the rest of the book addresses acquired immunity.

The natural defense system can be considered as being composed of two parts: the external defense system and the internal defense system. The external defense system is designed to keep microorganisms from entering the body. If these defenses are overcome, then it is the job of the internal defense system to clear invaders as quickly as possible. Internal defenses can be categorized into cellular mechanisms and humoral factors. Both of these work together to promote phagocytosis, which destroys foreign cells and organisms. The process of inflammation brings cells and humoral factors to the area where they are needed to promote healing. If the healing process is begun and resolved as quickly as possible, this lessens the chance that damage to the tissues may occur.

External Defense System

The **external defense system** is composed of structural barriers that prevent most infectious agents from entering the body. First and foremost is the unbroken skin and the mucosal membrane surfaces. To understand how important a role these play, one has only to look at victims of severe burns and see how vulnerable they are to infection. Not only does the skin serve as a major structural barrier, but the presence of several secretions discourages the growth of microorganisms. Lactic acid in sweat, for instance, and fatty acids from sebaceous glands maintain the skin at a pH of approximately 5.6. This acid pH keeps most microorganisms from growing.

Additionally, each of the various organ systems in the body has its own unique mechanisms. In the respiratory tract, mucous secretions and the motion of cilia lining the nasopharyngeal passages clear away almost 90 percent of the deposited material. The flushing action of urine plus its slight acidity help to remove many potential pathogens from the genitourinary tract. Lactic acid production in the female genital tract keeps the vagina at a pH of about 5, another means of preventing invasion of pathogens. In the digestive tract, acidity of the stomach, which is caused by production of hydrochloric acid, keeps the pH as low as 1 and serves to halt microbial growth. Lysozyme is an enzyme found in many secretions such as tears and saliva, and it attacks the cell walls of microorganisms, especially those that are gram-positive.

In many locations of the body there is a normal flora that often keeps pathogens from being able to establish themselves in these areas. The significance of the presence of normal flora is readily demonstrated by looking at the side effects of antibiotic therapy. Frequently, yeast infections caused by *Candida albicans* arise; this is the result of wiping out normal flora that would ordinarily compete with such opportunists.

Internal Defense System

The second part of natural immunity is the **internal defense system,** in which both cells and soluble factors play essential parts. The internal defense system is designed to recognize molecules that are unique to infectious organisms.[1] This typically involves recognition of a carbohydrate such as mannose that is found in microorganisms and is not evident on human cells. By activation of certain white blood cells, natural immunity also helps to initiate the acquired immune response. There are five principle types of leukocytes or white cells in peripheral blood. These are neutrophils, eosinophils, basophils, monocytes, and lymphocytes. Certain of these white blood cells participate in a process known as phagocytosis, the most important function of the internal defense system. **Phagocytosis** is the engulfment of cells or particulate matter by leukocytes, macrophages, and other cells. This process destroys most of the foreign invaders that enter the body. Furthermore, phagocytosis is a necessary first step in the initiation of the specific immune response. The white blood cells that are capable of phagocytosis are known as the myeloid line and arise from a common precursor in the marrow. These can be further divided into granulocytes and monocytes or mononuclear cells. Those considered granulocytes are the neutrophils, basophils, and eosinophils. Each of these cell types is described in this chapter. Lymphocytes form the basis of the acquired immune response, and these are discussed in Chapter 3. Several cell lines that are found in the tissues, namely macrophages, mast cells, and dendritic cells, are also discussed here because they all contribute to the process of natural immunity.

Cellular Defense Mechanisms

Neutrophils

The neutrophil or polymorphonuclear neutrophilic leukocyte (PMN) represents approximately 50 to 70 percent of the total peripheral white blood cells.[2] These are around 10 to 15 μm in diameter, with a nucleus that has between two and five segments (Fig. 2–1, Color Plate 1). They contain a large number of neutral staining granules, which are classified as primary and secondary granules. Primary granules contain enzymes such as myeloperoxidase, acid phosphatase, neutral proteinases, lysozyme, acid hydrolases, β-glucuronidase, and elastase.[3,4] Secondary granules are characterized by the presence of collagenase, lysozyme, lactoferrin, plasminogen activators, and alkaline phosphatase.[4] Normally, half of the total neutrophil population is found in a marginating pool on the walls of blood vessels, while the rest circulate freely for approximately 6 to 10 hours. There is a continuous interchange, however, between the marginating and the circulating pools.

Neutrophils are capable of moving from the circulating blood to the tissues through a process known as **diapedesis,** or movement through blood vessel walls. This begins with margination and adherence to the vessel wall. Then neutrophils form pseudopods, which squeeze through junctions of the endothelial cells. They may wander randomly through the tissue or be attracted to a specific area by chemotactic factors. **Chemotaxins** are chemical messengers that cause migration of cells in a particular direction. Factors that are chemotactic for neutrophils include complement components; proteins from the coagulation cascade; products from bacteria and viruses; and secretions from mast cells, lymphocytes, macrophages, and other

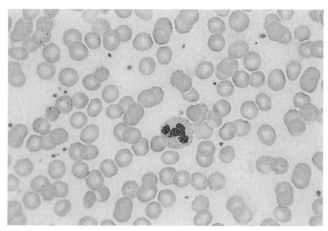

FIG. 2–1. Photo of a neutrophil. (From Harr, R: Clinical Laboratory Science Review, ed. 2. FA Davis, Philadelphia, 2000. Color Plate 30.) See Color Plate 1.

neutrophils.[3] Once in the tissues, neutrophils have a life span of about 5 days.[5]

Eosinophils

Eosinophils are approximately 12 to 16 μm in diameter, and they normally make up 1 to 3 percent of the circulating white blood cells in a nonallergic person. Their number increases in an allergic reaction or in response to many parasitic infections. The nucleus is usually bilobed or ellipsoidal and is often eccentrically located (Fig. 2–2, Color Plate 2). Eosinophils take up the acid eosin dye, and the cytoplasm is filled with large orange to reddish-orange granules. These granules contain enzymes such as acid phosphatase, β-glucuronidase, arylsulfatase, phospholipase, peroxidase, histaminase, aminopeptidase, and ribonuclease.[3] These cells are capable of phagocytosis but are much less efficient than neutrophils because of the smaller numbers present and their lack of digestive enzymes.[5] Their most important role lies in neutralizing basophil and mast cell products and in the killing of certain parasites,[6] as discussed in Chapter 23.

Basophils

Basophils are found in very small numbers, representing less than 1 percent of all circulating white blood cells. The smallest of the granulocytes, they are 10 to 14 μm in diameter and contain coarse densely staining deep-bluish-purple granules that often obscure the nucleus[5] (Fig. 2–3, Color Plate 3). Constituents of these granules are histamine, eosinophil chemotactic factor of anaphylaxis, and a small amount of heparin—all of which have an important function in inducing and maintaining immediate hypersensitivity reactions.[3,6] Histamine is a

vasoactive amine that contracts smooth muscle, and heparin is an anticoagulant. The granules lack hydrolytic enzymes, although peroxidase is present. They are very delicate and can be easily disrupted, releasing the contents to the surrounding tissue and the bloodstream. Basophils are thought to be capable of phagocytosis, but this occurs to a much lesser extent than occurs with neutrophils or eosinophils. They are only present for a few hours in the bloodstream.

Mast Cells

Tissue mast cells resemble basophils and may share a common stem cell precursor, although this has never been definitively proven.[3,5] Mast cells are larger with a small round nucleus and more granules than the basophil (Fig. 2–4, Color Plate 4). They are found in connective tissue, especially around blood and

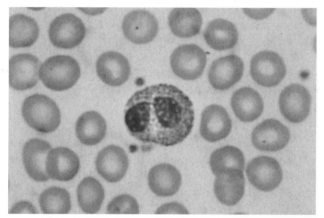

FIG. 2–2. Photo of an eosinophil. (From Harmening, D: Clinical Hematology and Fundamentals of Hemostasis, ed. 4. FA Davis, Philadelphia, 2002. Color Plate 12.) See Color Plate 2.

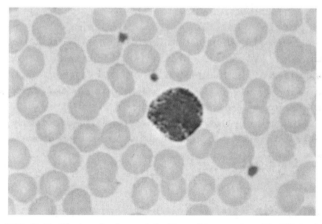

FIG. 2–3. Photo of a basophil. (From Harmening, D: Clinical Hematology and Fundamentals of Hemostasis, ed. 4. FA Davis, Philadelphia, 2002. Color Plate 13.) See Color Plate 3.

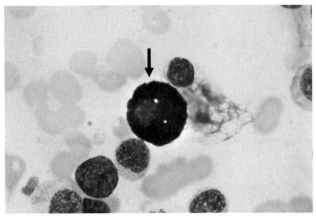

FIG. 2–4. Photo of a mast cell. (From Harmening, D: Clinical Hematology and Fundamentals of Hemostasis, ed. 4. FA Davis, Philadelphia, 2002. Color Plate 42.) See Color Plate 4.

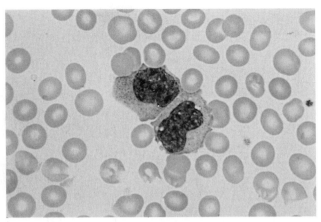

FIG. 2–5. Photo of two monocytes. (From Harmening, D: Clinical Hematology and Fundamentals of Hemostasis, ed. 4. FA Davis, Philadelphia, 2002. Color Plate 15.) See Color Plate 5.

lymphatic vessels. They have a long life span and may be capable of proliferation in the tissues.[5] The enzyme content of the granules helps to distinguish them from basophils because they contain acid phosphatase, alkaline phosphatase, and protease.[3] The mast cell, like the basophil, plays a role in hypersensitivity reactions.

Monocytes

Monocytes or mononuclear cells are the largest cells in the peripheral blood, with a diameter that can vary from 12 to 22 μm and an average size of 18 μm. One distinguishing feature is an irregularly folded or horseshoe-shaped nucleus that occupies almost one-half of the entire cell's volume (Fig. 2–5, Color Plate 5). The abundant cytoplasm stains a dull grayish-blue and has a ground-glass appearance caused by the presence of fine granules. These granules are actually of two types, one of which contains peroxidase, acid phosphatase, and arylsulfatase, indicating that these granules are similar to the lysosomes of neutrophils.[3] The other type of granule may contain β-glucuronidase, lysozyme, and lipase, but no alkaline phosphatase. Digestive vacuoles may also be observed in the cytoplasm. These make up 4 to 10 percent of total circulating white blood cells; however, they do not remain in the circulation for long. They stay in peripheral blood for up to 70 hours, and then they migrate to the tissues and become known as macrophages.

Tissue Macrophages

All tissue macrophages arise from monocytes. These can be thought of as macrophage precursors because additional differentiation and cell division takes place in the tissues. The transition from monocyte to macrophage is characterized by progressive cellular enlargement to

between 25 and 50 μm. As the monocyte matures into a macrophage, there is an increase in endoplasmic reticulum, lysosomes, and mitochondria. Unlike monocytes, macrophages contain no peroxidase at all.[3,5] There are no conclusive data to indicate that monocytes are predestined for any particular tissue, so tissue distribution appears to be a random phenomenon.[7]

Macrophages have specific names according to their particular tissue location. Some are immobile, but others progress through the tissues by means of ameboid action. Macrophages in the lung are alveolar macrophages; in the liver, Kupffer cells; in the brain, microglial cells; and in connective tissue, histiocytes. Macrophages may not be as efficient as neutrophils in phagocytosis because their motility is slow compared with that of the neutrophils. However, their life span appears to be in the range of months rather than days. The monocyte-macrophage system plays an important role in initiating and regulating the immune response.[6] Their functions include microbial killing, tumoricidal activity, killing of intracellular parasites, phagocytosis, secretion of cell mediators, and antigen presentation.[7] Killing activity is enhanced when macrophages become "activated" by contact with microorganisms or with chemical messengers called cytokines, which are released by T lymphocytes during the immune response (see Chapter 6).

Dendritic Cells

Dendritic cells are so named because they are covered with long membranous extensions that make them resemble nerve cell dendrites. Their main function is to phagocytize antigen and present it to helper T lymphocytes. Although their actual developmental lineage is not known, they are believed to be descendents of the myeloid line.[2] They are classified according to their tissue location, in a similar manner to macrophages. Langerhans' cells are found on skin and mucous membranes; interstitial dendritic cells populate the major organs such as the heart, lungs, liver, kidney, and the gastrointestinal tract; and interdigitating dendritic cells are present in the T lymphocyte areas of secondary lymphoid tissue and the thymus.[2] After capturing antigen in the tissue by phagocytosis or endocytosis, dendritic cells migrate to the blood and to lymphoid organs where they present antigen to T lymphocytes to initiate the acquired immune response. They are the most potent phagocytic cell in the tissue.

Phagocytosis

The process of phagocytosis itself consists of four main steps: (1) physical contact between the white cell and the foreign particle, (2) formation of a phagosome, (3) fusion with cytoplasmic granules to form a phagolysosome, and (4) digestion and release of debris to the outside (Fig. 2–6). Physical contact is a random association, aided by chemotaxis, whereby cells are attracted to the site of inflammation by chemical substances such as soluble bacterial factors, complement components, or C-reactive protein (CRP). Receptors on the cell surface come into contact with the foreign particle surface by a continuous "zippering" process that occurs as increasing numbers of receptors on the cell surface come in contact with the particle surface.[8] Attachment

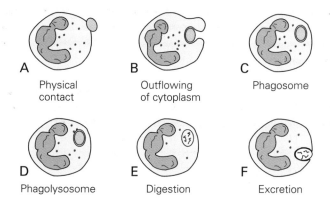

FIG. 2–6. Steps involved in phagocytosis. *(A)* Adherence: Physical contact between the phagocytic cell and the microorganism occurs, aided by opsonins. *(B)* Outflowing of cytoplasm to surround the microorganism. *(C)* Formation of phagosome: Microorganism is completely surrounded by a part of the cell membrane. *(D)* Formation of the phagolysome: Cytoplasmic granules fuse with membrane of phagosome, emptying contents into this membrane-bound space. *(E)* Digestion of the microorganism by hydrolytic enzymes. *(F)* Excretion of contents of phagolysosome to the outside by exocytosis.

of microorganisms to cell receptors is enhanced by **opsonins,** a term derived from the Greek word meaning to prepare for eating. Opsonins are serum proteins that attach to a foreign substance and help prepare it for phagocytosis. CRP, complement components, and antibodies are important opsonins. Phagocytic cells have receptors for immunoglobulins and for complement components, which aid in contact and in initiating ingestion.[9] Opsonins may act by neutralizing the surface charge on the foreign particle, making it easier for the cells to approach one another.

Once attachment has occurred, the cellular cytoplasm flows around the particle and eventually fuses with it. An increase in oxygen consumption, known as the **respiratory burst,** occurs within the cell as the pseudopodia enclose the particle within a vacuole. The structure formed is known as a **phagosome.** The phagosome is gradually moved toward the center of the cell. Next, contact with cytoplasmic granules takes place, and fusion between granules and the phagosome occurs. At this point, the fused elements are known as a **phagolysosome.** The granules then release their enzymes, and digestion occurs. Any undigested material is excreted from the cells by exocytosis. The actual process of killing is oxygen-dependent and results from the generation of bactericidal metabolites.

Resting cells derive their energy from anaerobic glycolysis; however, when the process of phagocytosis is triggered, the respiratory burst produces greater energy via oxidative metabolism. The hexose monophosphate shunt is used to reduce nicotine adenine dinucleotide phosphate (NADP) to reduced nicotinamide adenine dinucleotide (NADPH). NADPH then donates an electron to oxygen in the presence of NADPH oxidase, a membrane-bound enzyme, and O_2^- (superoxide) is formed. Superoxide is highly toxic but can be rapidly converted to more lethal products. The enzyme superoxide dismutase (SOD) converts superoxide to hydrogen peroxide or the hydroxyl radical (OH) by adding hydrogen ions. Hydrogen peroxide has long been considered an important bactericidal agent, and it is more stable than any of the free radicals. Its effect is potentiated by the formation of hypochlorite ions. This is accomplished through the action of the enzyme myeloperoxidase in the presence of chloride ions. Hypochlorite ions are powerful oxidizing agents. All of these substances contribute to killing within the phagocyte (Fig. 2–7).

A second pathway for killing of microorganisms also exists. Nitric oxide synthetase is induced when the phagocytic cell comes in contact with a microorganism. This enzyme forms nitric oxide from the amino acid arginine and molecular oxygen. Nitric oxide is a soluble, highly labile, free radical gas that is capable of

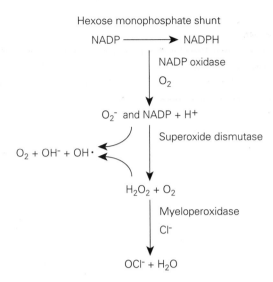

Hexose monophosphate shunt

$$NADP \longrightarrow NADPH$$

NADP oxidase

O_2

$$O_2^- \text{ and } NADP + H^+$$

Superoxide dismutase

$$O_2 + OH^- + OH \cdot$$

$$H_2O_2 + O_2$$

Myeloperoxidase

Cl^-

$$OCl^- + H_2O$$

FIG. 2–7. Creation of oxygen radicals in the phagocytic cell. The hexose monophosphate shunt is used to reduce NADP to NADPH. NADPH can reduce oxygen in the presence of NADPH oxidase to O_2^-, known as superoxide. Superoxide is converted to hydrogen peroxide through the action of the enzyme SOD. Myeloperoxidase catalyzes formation of the hypochlorite radical, a very powerful oxydizing agent. OHs, other powerful oxidizing agents, may also be formed.

operating against organisms that invade the cytosol. In the presence of other reactive oxygen species within the phagosome, nitric oxide is converted to peroxynitrite and other products, which are highly toxic to bacteria, yeast, and viruses.[6,8]

Acute Phase Reactants

Soluble factors known as acute phase proteins are also an important part of the internal defense system. **Acute phase reactants** are normal serum constituents that increase rapidly by at least 25 percent due to infection, injury, or trauma to the tissues.[10] Some of the most important ones are CRP, serum amyloid A, complement components, mannose-binding protein, alpha-1

antitrypsin (AAT), haptoglobin, fibrinogen, ceruloplasmin, and alpha-1 acid glycoprotein.[10–13] They are produced primarily by hepatocytes (liver parenchymal cells) within 12 to 24 hours in response to an increase in certain intercellular signaling polypeptides called cytokines (see Chapter 6 for a complete discussion of cytokines). These cell messengers, notably interleukin-1 (IL-1), interleukin-6 (IL-6), and tumor necrosis factor alpha (TNF–α) are mainly produced by monocytes and macrophages at the sites of inflammation.[10] Table 2–1 summarizes characteristics of the main acute phase reactants.

C-Reactive Protein

C-reactive protein (CRP) is a trace constituent of serum originally thought to be an antibody to the c-polysaccharide of pneumococci. It increases rapidly within 4 to 6 hours following infection, surgery, or other trauma to the body. Levels increase dramatically as much as 100- to 1000-fold, reaching a peak value within 24 to 72 hours.[12] They also decline rapidly with cessation of the stimulus. Elevated levels are found in conditions such as bacterial infections, rheumatic fever, viral infections, malignant diseases, tuberculosis, and after a heart attack.[12]

CRP is a homogeneous molecule with a molecular weight of 118,000 and a structure that consists of five identical subunits held together by noncovalent bonds. It is a member of the family known as the pentraxins, all of which are proteins with five subunits. It acts much like an antibody because it is capable of opsonization (or coating of foreign particles), agglutination, precipitation, and activation of complement by the classical pathway. However, binding is calcium-dependent, and the main substrate is phosphocholine, a common constituent of microbial membranes. It also binds to specific receptors found on monocytes, macrophages, and neutrophils, thus promoting phagocytosis. In addition, CRP binds to small ribonuclear proteins, which may help to limit a possible autoimmune response.[14]

Protein	Half-Life	Response Time (hr)	Normal Concentration (mg/dL)	Increase
CRP	24 hr	6–10	0.5	20–1000×
Serum amyloid A			0.03	1000×
AAT	4 days	24	200–400	2–5×
Fibrinogen	2 days	24	110–400	2–5×
Haptoglobin	2 days	24	40–200	2–5×
Ceruloplasmin	4 days	48–72	20–45	2×
C3	?	48–72	60–140	30%–60%
Alpha-1 acid glycoprotein	5 days	?	40–105	2–5×

TABLE 2–1. Characteristics of Acute Phase Reactants

CRP=C-reactive protein; AAT=alpha-1 antitrypsin.

Thus, CRP can be thought of as a primitive nonspecific form of antibody molecule, which is able to act as a defense against microorganisms or foreign cells until specific antibody can be produced.

Because the levels rise and then decline so rapidly, CRP is the most widely used indicator of acute inflammation. Although it is a nonspecific indicator of disease or trauma, monitoring of the levels can be useful clinically to follow a disease process. Following CRP levels in surgery, for instance, can indicate whether healing is proceeding normally. It is also a noninvasive means of following the course of malignancy and organ transplantation because a rise in the level may mean a return of the malignancy, or in the case of transplantation, the beginning of organ rejection.[12]

In accord with the finding that atherosclerosis, or coronary artery disease, is the result of a chronic inflammatory process,[15] recent research indicates that an increased level of CRP is a significant risk factor for myocardial infarction and ischemic stroke.[16–21] The results of randomized prospective studies have shown that healthy men with an increased CRP greater than 3.0 mg/L had three times the risk of experiencing a heart attack in the next 8 to 10 years, independent of cholesterol levels.[20] Postmenopausal healthy women had an even greater risk factor, a sixfold increase in the possibility of a heart attack or stroke compared with their counterparts with lower CRP levels.[22] Thus, monitoring CRP may be as important a preventative measure as following cholesterol levels, although only high-sensitivity tests for CRP are useful for this purpose.[16]

Serum Amyloid A

Serum amyloid A is the other major protein, the concentration of which can increase almost 1000-fold, as is the case in CRP. It is an apolipoprotein that is synthesized in the liver, and normal circulating levels are approximately 30 μg/mL. It is a precursor to amyloid deposition. Although the exact function is not known, serum amyloid A is reported to cause adhesion and chemotaxis of phagocytic cells and lymphocytes.[10] It may also be able to bind lysosomal enzymes released during inflammation, thus contributing to the mopping up of the area.[6] Increased levels have also been found to be a risk factor for heart attack in women.[23]

Complement

Complement is the name given to a series of serum proteins that are normally present and the overall function of which is mediation of inflammation. There are nine such proteins that are activated by bound antibody in a sequence known as the classical cascade; an additional number are involved in the alternate pathway that is triggered by microorganisms themselves. The major functions of complement are opsonization, chemotaxis, and lysis of cells. Complement is discussed more fully in Chapter 7.

Mannose-Binding Protein

Mannose-binding protein is a trimer that acts as an opsonin that is calcium-dependent. It is able to recognize foreign carbohydrates such as mannose and a number of other sugars found primarily on bacteria, some yeasts, viruses, and several parasites.[6] It is widely distributed on mucosal surfaces throughout the body. Binding activates the complement cascade and helps to promote phagocytosis.[1] Normal concentrations are up to 10 μg/mL.

Alpha-1 Antitrypsin

PROTEASE - any enzyme that aid in the breakdown of proteins

AAT is the major component of the alpha band when serum is electrophoresed. Although the name implies that it acts against trypsin, it is a general plasma inhibitor of proteases released from leukocytes, especially elastase.[11,24] Elastase is an endogenous enzyme that can degrade elastin and collagen. In chronic pulmonary inflammation, lung tissue is damaged because of its activity. Thus, AAT acts to "mop up" or counteract the effects of neutrophil invasion during an inflammatory response.

AAT deficiency can result in premature emphysema, especially in individuals who smoke or who are exposed to a noxious occupational environment.[25] In such a deficiency, uninhibited proteases remain in the lower respiratory tract, leading to destruction of parenchymal cells in the lungs and to emphysema or idiopathic pulmonary fibrosis.[26] It has been estimated that as many as 100,000 Americans suffer from this deficiency.[27] There are at least 17 alleles of the gene coding for AAT that are associated with low production of the enzyme.[11] One particular variant gene for AAT is associated with lack of its secretion from the liver, and such individuals are at risk of developing liver disease in addition to emphysema.[28] Homozygous inheritance of this most severe variant gene may lead to development of cirrhosis in early childhood.[25]

AAT can also react with any serine protease, such as those generated by triggering of the complement cascade or fibrinolysis.[12] Once bound to AAT, the protease is completely inactivated; subsequently it is removed from the area of tissue damage and catabolized.

Haptoglobin

Haptoglobin is an alpha-2 globulin with a molecular weight of 100,000; its primary function is to bind irreversibly to free hemoglobin released by intravascular hemolysis. Once bound, the complex is cleared rapidly by Kupffer and parenchymal cells in the liver, thus preventing loss of free hemoglobin.[3] The rise in plasma haptoglobin is the result of de novo synthesis by the liver and does not represent release of previously formed haptoglobin from other sites.[11] A 2- to 10-fold increase in haptoglobin can be seen following inflammation. Early in the inflammatory response, however, haptoglobin levels may drop because of intravascular hemolysis and consequently mask the protein's behavior as an acute phase reactant. Thus, plasma levels must be interpreted in the light of other acute phase reactants. Normal plasma concentrations range from 50 to 200 mg/dL.[3] Haptoglobin plays an important role in protecting the kidney from damage and in preventing the loss of iron by urinary excretion.[12] In addition, it may provide protection against reactive oxygen species, which are generated in the process of phagocytosis.[10]

Fibrinogen

Fibrinogen is the most abundant of the coagulation factors in the plasma, and it forms the fibrin clot.[11] The molecule is a dimer with a molecular weight of 340,000. A small portion is cleaved by thrombin to form fibrils that make up a fibrin clot. This increases the strength of a wound and stimulates endothelial cell adhesion and proliferation, which are critical to the healing process.[10] Formation of a clot also serves as a barrier to help prevent the spread of microorganisms further into the body. Normal levels range from 110 to 400 mg/dL.[11] Fibrinogen also serves to promote aggregation of red blood cells, and if levels are increased, this contributes to an increased risk for developing coronary artery disease, especially in women.[23,29]

Ceruloplasmin

Ceruloplasmin consists of a single polypeptide chain with a molecular weight of 132,000.[11] It is the principal copper-transporting protein in human plasma. It binds 90 to 95 percent of the copper found in plasma by attaching six cupric ions per molecule.[12] Ceruloplasmin functions as the primary transport protein in the transfer of copper to cytochrome C oxidase. Cytochrome C oxidase is essential to aerobic energy production, which increases in phagocytosis and wound healing. Ceruloplasm also serves as a scavenger of superoxide radicals generated by phagocytes in the process of clearing tissue debris or micro-organisms.[12] Additionally, ceruloplasmin appears to be involved in iron transport and helps to increase uptake in iron-deficient cells. It oxidizes Fe^{2+} to Fe^{3+}, which may serve as a means of releasing iron from ferritin.[11]

A depletion of ceruloplasmin is found in Wilson's disease, which is characterized by a massive increase of copper in the tissues. Renal tubular reabsorption defects result in excess excretion of proteins, glucose, and other elements.[11]

Alpha-1 Acid Glycoprotein

Alpha-1 acid glycoprotein has a high carbohydrate content and a molecular weight of 44,000.[11] Although considered an acute phase reactant, its exact function is not known. Normal levels are between 40 and 105 mg/dL. Alpha-1 acid glycoprotein binds progesterone and may be important in its transport or metabolism. It is also able to bind to drugs such as lidocaine, keeping them in an inactive circulating pool.[11]

Inflammation

The overall reaction of the body to injury or invasion by an infectious agent is known as **inflammation.** Both cellular and humoral mechanisms are involved in this complex, highly orchestrated process. Each individual reactant plays a role in initiating, amplifying, or sustaining the reaction, and a delicate balance must be maintained for the process to be speedily resolved. The four cardinal signs or clinical symptoms are redness, swelling, heat, and pain. Major events associated with the process of inflammation are: (1) increased blood supply to the infected area; (2) increased capillary permeability caused by retraction of endothelial cells lining in the vessels; (3) migration of white blood cells, mainly neutrophils, from the capillaries to the surrounding tissue; and (4) migration of macrophages to the injured area (Fig. 2–8).[3,6]

Chemical mediators, such as histamine, which are released from injured mast cells, cause dilation of the blood vessels, and bring additional blood flow to the affected area, resulting in redness and heat. The increased permeability of the vessels allows fluids in the plasma to leak to the tissues. This produces the swelling and pain associated with inflammation. Soluble mediators, including acute phase reactants, initiate and control the response. Amplification occurs through formation of clots by the coagulation system and then the triggering of the fibrinolytic system.

As the endothelial cells of the vessels contract, neutrophils move through the endothelial cells of the vessel and out into the tissues. They are attracted to the site of injury or infection by the chemotaxins mentioned previously. Neutrophils, which are mobilized within 30 to 60 minutes after the injury, are the major type of cell present in *acute inflammation.*[12] Neutrophil emigration may last 24 to 48 hours and is proportional to the level of chemotactic factors present in the area.

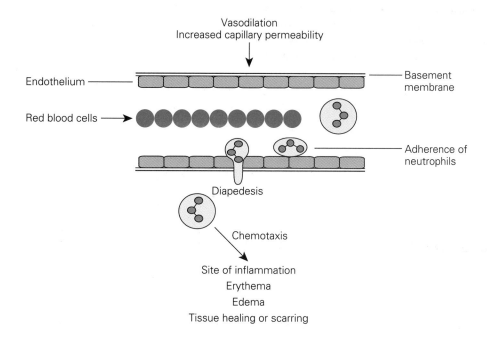

FIG. 2–8. Events in the inflammatory response. Increased blood supply to the affected area is followed by increased capillary permeability and migration of neutrophils to the tissues. Clinical signs at the site of inflammation include edema and erythema. Tissue healing, with or without scarring, eventually results.

Migration of macrophages from surrounding tissue and from blood monocytes occurs several hours later and peaks at 16 to 48 hours.[12] Macrophages attempt to clear the area through phagocytosis, and in most cases the healing process is completed with a return of normal tissue structure.[12] However, when the inflammatory process becomes prolonged, it is said to be *chronic,* and tissue damage and loss of function may result. Specific immunity with infiltration of lymphocytes may contribute to the damage. Thus, a failure to remove microorganisms or injured tissue may result in continued tissue damage.

SUMMARY

Natural immunity encompasses all the body's defense mechanisms for resisting disease. These are always present and the response is nonspecific in that it is the same for any infectious agent encountered. External defenses are structural barriers such as skin, mucous membranes, and cilia that keep microorganisms from entering the body. Internal defenses are centered on the process of phagocytosis, which is the engulfment of cells or particulate matter by leukocytes, macrophages, and other cells. This process destroys most of the foreign cells that have penetrated the external defenses.

Cells that are most active in phagocytosis include neutrophils, monocytes, and macrophages. Physical contact between the phagocytic cell and the foreign particle is aided by chemotaxis, whereby cells are attracted to the area, and opsonization, or coating of the foreign particle by serum proteins such as complement and antibody. Once contact has been made, cytoplasm flows around the foreign particle to form a phagosome. Fusion of the phagosome with lysosomal granules creates a phagolysosome. Inside this structure, enzymes are released, and the foreign particle is digested. The process is oxygen-dependent, and killing results from the creation of hypochlorite and hydroxyl ions, which damage protein irreversibly.

Acute phase reactants are serum constituents that increase rapidly in response to infection or injury to the tissues. They enhance the process of phagocytosis by attracting leukocytes to the area of injury and by coating the foreign material so that it can be ingested more easily. Other functions of the acute-phase reactants include neutralization of mediators and proteolytic enzymes generated during the process of responding to pathogens. CRP is the most widely monitored of the acute phase reactants and is the best indicator of acute inflammation.

Inflammation is the body's response to injury or invasion by a pathogen, and it is characterized by increased blood supply to the affected area, increased capillary permeability, migration of neutrophils to the surrounding tissue, and migration of macrophages to the injured area. Inflammation and the process of phagocytosis are considered natural immunity in that the response to any injury or pathogen is nonspecific. Phagocytosis, however, must occur before the specific immune response can be initiated, and thus this process is essential to both natural and acquired immunity.

Case Studies

1. A 45-year-old male named Rick went to his physician for an annual checkup. Although he was slightly overweight, his laboratory results indicated that both his total cholesterol and his high-density lipoprotein cholesterol were within normal limits. His fibrinogen level was 450 mg/dL and his CRP level was 3.5 mg/dL. His physical examination was perfectly normal. The physician cautioned Rick that he might be at risk for a future heart attack, and he counseled him to be sure to exercise and eat a healthy low-fat diet. Rick's wife told him that as long as his cholesterol level was normal, he didn't have anything to worry about. Who is correct? Explain your answer.

2. A 20-year-old female college student went to the infirmary with symptoms of malaise, fatigue, sore throat, and a slight fever. A complete blood count was performed, and both the red blood cell count and white blood cell count were within normal limits. A rapid strep test was performed, and the results were negative. A slide agglutination test for infectious mononucleosis was indeterminate, although results of a slide agglutination test for CRP were positive. Results of a semiquantitative CRP determination indicated an increased level of approximately 20 mg/dL. The student was advised to return in a few days for a repeat mononucleosis test. How does a test result showing an increase in CRP help in a presumptive diagnosis of infectious mononucleosis?

Exercise: In Vitro Phagocytosis

PRINCIPLE

A drop of whole blood is mixed with a drop of a bacterial culture and incubated at room temperature to demonstrate engulfment of bacteria by leukocytes.

REAGENTS, MATERIALS, AND EQUIPMENT

Test tubes, 12 × 75 mm
Broth culture of *Staphylococcus epidermidis*
Lancets for finger puncture
Heparinized microhematocrit tubes
Microscope slides
Wright-Giemsa Sure Stain (Fisher Scientific, Fairlawn, NJ)

PROCEDURE

1. Take two 12- × 75-mm test tubes, and label one 0 minutes and the other 5 minutes.
2. Do a finger puncture and fill a heparinized microhematocrit tube about three-quarters full of blood. Note that blood drawn in an ethylenediaminetetra-acetic acid tube within the last 10 minutes can also be used.
3. Using a black rubber bulb, expel one drop of blood into each labeled test tube.
4. Add one drop of *Staphylococcus epidermidis* culture to each tube, using a disposable Pasteur pipette.
5. Shake the tubes to mix, and make a blood film of the 0 tube immediately. Let the other tube incubate for 5 minutes at room temperature before making a blood film.

Method for Making Blood Smears

1. Obtain two clean glass slides, one of which will be used as a spreader slide.
2. With a Pasteur pipette, carefully place a small drop of blood at one end of a microscope slide.
3. Holding the spreader slide with the thumb and forefinger, place the spreader slide slightly in front of the drop of blood on the other slide, maintaining a 30-degree angle between the slides.
4. Move the spreader slide back toward the drop of blood. As soon as the slide comes in contact with the drop of blood, the blood will start to spread along the edge of the slide.
5. Keeping the spreader slide at a 30-degree angle, push the spreader slide rapidly over the length of the slide. There should be a feathered edge on the end of the smear.

Wright-Giemsa Sure Stain (Fisher Scientific, Fairlawn, NJ)

1. Allow the blood smear to air dry.
2. Dip the slides in stain for 10 to 15 seconds.
3. Dip the slides in distilled or deionized water for 15 to 30 seconds.
4. Rinse the slides by dipping in fresh distilled or deionized water for a few seconds.
5. Blot the back of the slides to remove excess stain and let them air dry.
6. Use immersion oil and look for engulfment.

INTERPRETATION OF RESULTS

These blood smears will be more watery than usual because of the addition of the broth culture with bacteria; therefore, it may be difficult to get a blood smear with a feathered edge. The feathered edge is not essential, however, as long as the blood cells are spread out on the slide. There should be a noticeable difference between the 0- and the 5-minute slide. The 0-minute slide will probably not show much engulfment, but bacteria may be seen in contact with leukocytes. The 5-minute slide should show bacteria within the cell, as small purple dots. Neutrophils will be the predominant phagocytic cells, but an occasional monocyte may be seen. If lymphocytes are the only white blood cells seen, the bacterial suspension was too heavy, and the phagocytic cells destroyed themselves in attempting to engulf the bacteria present.

Exercise: Latex Agglutination Test for C-Reactive Protein

PRINCIPLE

CRP is an acute phase reactant that increases rapidly following infection or trauma to the tissues. It is used as an early and reliable indicator of acute inflammation. In this procedure, CRP is measured by reacting serum with latex particles coated with antibody to CRP. In this case, the CRP is acting as the antigen. If CRP is present above normal threshold levels, antigen–antibody combination will result in a visible agglutination reaction. An elevated CRP level is a sensitive, although nonspecific, indicator of inflammation.

REAGEANTS, MATERIALS, AND EQUIPMENT

(Kit from Wampole, Remel, or other manufacturers)
CRP latex reagent, which contains a 1-percent

suspension of polystyrene latex particles coated with antihuman CRP produced in goats or rabbits

Positive human serum control with a concentration of approximately 20 mg/dL of CRP

Negative human serum control

Glycine-saline buffer diluent with pH of 8.2

Disposable sampling pipettes

Glass slide with six ovals

Applicator sticks

Not in kit but needed: timer; serologic pipettes; test tubes, 12 × 75 mm

WARNING

Latex reagent controls and buffer contain 0.1-percent sodium azide as a preservative. Sodium azide may react with lead and copper plumbing to form highly explosive metal azides. On disposal, flush with a large volume of water to prevent azide buildup.

CAUTION

Each donor unit used in the preparation of controls is tested by Food and Drug Administration–approved method for the presence of antibodies to human immunodeficiency virus (HIV) and for hepatitis B surface antigen, and it was found to be negative. However, because no test method can offer complete assurance that HIV, hepatitis B virus, or other infectious agents are absent, the reagent should be handled with the same care as a clinical specimen.

SPECIMEN COLLECTION

Collect blood aseptically by venipuncture into a clean, dry, sterile tube, and allow it to clot. Separate the serum without transferring any cellular elements. Do not use grossly hemolyzed, excessively lipemic, or bacterially contaminated specimens. Fresh nonheat inactivated serum is recommended for the test. However, if the test cannot be performed immediately, serum may be stored between 2°C and 8°C for up to 72 hours. If there is any additional delay, freeze the serum at −18°C or below.

PROCEDURE★

Qualitative Slide Test:

1. Clean a glass slide with mild detergent. Rinse with water and dry thoroughly.
2. Be sure reagents and specimens are at room temperature. The sample is tested both undiluted and diluted 1:5. Prepare a 1:5 dilution by placing 0.1 mL of the sample into a 12 × 75-mm test tube and adding 0.4 mL of the glycine-saline buffer diluent. Mix thoroughly.
3. Using one of the capillary tubes provided, fill it about two-thirds full with undiluted serum. While holding the pipette perpendicular to the slide, deliver one free-falling drop to the center of one oval on the slide. Using a clean capillary pipette, repeat the procedure with the 1:5 dilution. If a calibrated pipetter is used instead of the capillary pipettes provided, adjust the pipetter to deliver 0.05 mL (50 μL).
4. Using the squeeze-dropper vials provided, add one drop of positive control and one drop of negative control to separate ovals on the slide. Note: A positive and a negative control should be run with each test.
5. Resuspend the latex reagent by gently mixing the vial until the suspension is homogeneous. Using the dropper provided, add one drop of CRP latex reagent to each serum specimen and to each control.
6. Using separate applicator sticks, mix each specimen and control until the entire area of each oval is filled.
7. Tilt the slide back and forth, slowly and evenly, for 2 minutes. Place the slide on a flat surface and observe for agglutination using a direct light source.

Semiquantitative Slide Test

1. If a positive reaction is obtained, the specimen may be serially diluted with glycine–saline buffer to obtain a semiquantitative estimate of the CRP level.
2. Begin with a 1:2 dilution of patient serum obtained by mixing equal parts of specimen and glycine–saline buffer. Blend the tube contents thoroughly.
3. Add 0.1 mL of buffer to the desired number of test tubes. Add 0.1 mL of 1:2 dilution to the first tube; mix and transfer 0.1 mL to the next additional tube. Continue until all tubes are diluted.
4. Perform a slide agglutination test on each dilution by repeating the procedure (steps 3 through 7) as listed previously, and look for agglutination.

RESULTS

1. A positive reaction is reported when either the undiluted specimen or the 1:5 dilution shows agglutination, indicating the presence of CRP in the serum at a level of 1.0± 0.2 mg/dL or more.
2. The strength of the reaction may be graded as follows:
   4+ large clumping with clear fluid in background
   3+ moderate clumping with fairly clear background
   2+ small clumping with slightly opaque fluid in background
   1+ very small clumping with fluid definitely opaque
3. The titer is represented by the last dilution that shows a positive reaction.
4. A negative reaction is characterized by a lack of visible agglutination in both the undiluted specimen and 1:5 dilution.

★ From Seradyne SeraTest CRP, manufactured for Remel, 12076 Santa Fe Drive, Lenexa, KS 66215.

INTERPRETATION OF RESULTS

The latex agglutination test for CRP is a screening test for elevated levels of CRP in serum. A level of 1 mg/dL or higher gives a positive result with the undiluted specimen, and a level of higher than 5 mg/dL is positive in the 1:5 dilution. Normal levels range from 0.1 mg/dL in newborns to 0.5 mg/dL in adults. Usually, with the onset of a substantial inflammatory stimulus, such as infection, myocardial infarction, or surgical procedures, the CRP level increases very significantly (10-fold or less) above the value reported for healthy individuals. Following surgery, CRP levels rise sharply and usually peak between 48 and 72 hours. Levels decrease after the third postoperative day and should return to near normal between the fifth and the seventh postoperative day. Thus, CRP levels can be used to monitor the outcome of surgery. CRP testing can also be used to monitor graft rejection, drug therapy with anti-inflammatory agents, and recurrence of malignancies. For patients with rheumatoid arthritis, elevated CRP can be used as an indicator of the active stage of the disease. In most situations, however, it is desirable to have more than one determination so that base levels can be established.

LIMITATIONS OF PROCEDURES

1. Reagent, controls, and test specimens should be brought to room temperature and gently mixed before using.
2. It is essential that the glass slide be thoroughly clean before performing the test. It should be washed in mild detergent and rinsed several times with distilled water.
3. Reagent and control should not be used after the expiration date indicated on the outside kit label.
4. Do not use the CRP reagent if there is evidence of freezing.
5. False-negative reactions may be caused by high levels of CRP in undiluted specimens. A 1:5 dilution should always be run for this reason. False-positive reactions may occur with a reaction time longer than 2 minutes, or with specimens that are lipemic, hemolyzed, or contaminated with bacteria. Therefore, any visibly contaminated, lipemic, or hemolyzed specimen should not be used.
6. Discard buffer if contaminated (evidence of cloudiness or particulate material in solution).

1. Enhancement of phagocytosis by coating of foreign particles with serum proteins is called:
   a. Opsonization
   b. Agglutination
   c. Solubilization
   d. Chemotaxis

2. Which of the following peripheral blood cells plays a key role in killing of parasites?
   a. Neutrophils
   b. Monocytes
   c. Lymphocytes
   d. Eosinophils

3. Which of the following plays an important role as an external defense mechanism?
   a. Phagocytosis
   b. CRP
   c. Lysozyme
   d. Complement

4. The process of inflammation is characterized by all of the following except:
   a. Increased blood supply to the area
   b. Migration of white blood cells
   c. Decreased capillary permeability
   d. Appearance of acute phase reactants

5. Skin, lactic acid secretions, stomach acidity, and the motion of cilia represent which type of immunity?
   a. Natural
   b. Acquired
   c. Adaptive
   d. Auto

6. The structure formed by the fusion of engulfed material and enzymatic granules within the phagocytic cell is called a:
   a. Phagosome
   b. Lysosome
   c. Vacuole
   d. Phagolysosome

7. Which of the following white blood cells is capable of further differentiation in the tissues?
   a. Neutrophil
   b. Eosinophil
   c. Basophil
   d. Monocyte

8. The presence of normal flora acts as a defense mechanism by which of the following means?
   a. Maintaining an acid environment
   b. Competing with pathogens for nutrients
   c. Keeping phagocytes in the area
   d. Coating mucosal surfaces

9. Measurement of CRP levels can be used for all of the following except:
   a. Monitoring drug therapy with anti-inflammatory agents
   b. Tracking the normal progress of surgery
   c. Diagnosis of a specific bacterial infection
   d. Determining active phases of rheumatoid arthritis

10. Which of the following is (are) characteristic(s) of acute phase reactants?
    a. Rapid increase following infection
    b. Enhancement of phagocytosis
    c. Nonspecific indicators of inflammation
    d. All of the above

11. A latex agglutination test for CRP is run on a 12-year-old girl who has been ill for the past 5 days with an undiagnosed disease. The results obtained are as follows: negative with the undiluted serum and positive with the 1:5 dilution. What should the technologist do next?
    a. Repeat the entire test.
    b. Report the results as indeterminate.
    c. Set up serial dilutions for a semiquantitative test.
    d. Obtain a new sample.

12. Which is the most significant agent formed in the phagolysosome for the killing of microorganisms?
    a. Proteolytic enzymes
    b. Hydroxyl radicals
    c. Hydrogen peroxide
    d. Superoxides

13. The action of CRP can be distinguished from that of antibody in which of the following ways:
    a. CRP acts before antibody appears.
    b. Only antibody triggers the complement cascade.
    c. Binding of antibody is calcium-dependent.
    d. Only CRP acts as an opsonin.

References

1. Fearon, DT, and Locksley, RM: The instructive role of innate immunity in the acquired response. Science 272:50, 1996.
2. Chapter 15. In Goldsby, RA, Kindt, TJ, and Osborne, BA: Kuby Immunology, ed. 4. WH Freeman, New York, 2000, pp 371–393.
3. The Leukocyte. In McKenzie, SB: Textbook of Hematology, ed. 2.
   Lippincott Williams and Wilkins, Baltimore, 1996, pp 55–89.
4. Strauss, RG: Cell biology and disorders of neutrophils. In Harmening, DM (ed): Clinical Hematology and Fundamentals of Hemostasis, ed. 2. FA Davis, Philadelphia, 1992.
5. Lawrence, LW: The phagocytic leukocytes-morphology, kinetics, and

function. In Steine-Martin EA, Lotspeich-Steininger, CA, and Koepke, JA (eds): Clinical Hematology: Principles, Procedures, and Correlations, ed. 2. Lippincott Williams & Wilkins, Philadelphia, 1998.

6. Roitt, I: Roitt's Essential Immunology, ed. 9. Blackwell Science, Oxford, 1997.

7. Johnston, RB Jr: Current concepts: Immunology. Monocytes and macrophages. N Engl J Med 318:747, 1988.

8. Parslow, TG, and Bainton, DF: Innate immunity. In Stites, DP, Terr, AI, and Parslow, TG (eds): Medical Immunology, ed. 8. Appleton and Lange, Stamford, Conn., 1997, pp 25–42.

9. Rotrosen, D, and Gallin, JI: Disorders of phagocyte function. Annu Rev Immunol 5:127, 1987.

10. Gabay, C, and Kushner, I: Acute-phase proteins and other systemic responses to inflammation. N Engl J Med 340:448, 1999.

11. McPherson, RA: Specific proteins. In Henry, JB (ed): Clinical Diagnosis and Management by Laboratory Methods, ed. 19. WB Saunders, Philadelphia, 1997.

12. Miller, LE, et al: Manual of Laboratory Immunology, ed. 2. Lea & Febiger, Philadelphia, 1991.

13. Hotaling, M: Amino acids and proteins. In Lehmann, CA, and Kaszczuk, S (eds): Saunders Manual of Clinical Laboratory Science. WB Saunders, Philadelphia, 1998, pp 17–43.

14. Westhuyzen, J, and Healy, H: Review: Biology and relevance of C-reactive protein in cardiovascular and renal disease. Ann Clin Lab Sci 30:133, 2000.

15. Ross, R: Atherosclerosis—An inflammatory disease. N Engl J Med 340:115–26, 1999.

16. Ridker, PM, Glynn, RJ, and Hennekens, CH: C-reactive protein adds to the predictive value of total and HDL cholesterol in determining risk of first myocardial infarction. Circulation 97:2007, 1998.

17. Whicher, J, Biasucci, L, and Rifai, N: Inflammation, the acute phase response and atherosclerosis. Clin Chem Lab Med 37:495–503, 1999.

18. Danesh, J, Collins, R, and Appleby, P, et al: Association of fibrinogen, C-reactive protein, albumin, or leukocyte count with coronary heart disease: Meta-analyses of prospective studies. JAMA 279:1477, 1998.

19. Ridker, PM: Evaluating novel cardiovascular risk factors: Can we better predict heart attacks? Ann Intern Med 130:933–937, 1999.

20. Ridker, PM, Cushman, M, and Stampfer, MJ, et al: Inflammation, aspirin, and the risk of cardiovascular disease in apparently healthy men. N Engl J Med 336:973, 1997.

21. Haverkate, F, Thompson, SG, and Pyke, SD, et al: Production of C-reactive protein and risk of coronary events in stable and unstable angina. European Concerted Action on Thrombosis and Disabilities Angina Pectoris Study Group. Lancet 349:462–466, 1997.

22. Marker of systemic inflammation can predict cardiovascular risk. Geriatrics 54:59, 1999.

23. Ridker, PM, Hennekens, CH, and Buring, JE, et al: C-reactive protein and other markers of inflammation in the prediction of cardiovascular disease in women. N Engl J Med 342:836, 2000.

24. Lomas, DA, Evans, DL, and Finch, JT, et al. The mechanism of Z alpha 1-antitrypsin accumulation in the liver. Nature 357:605, 1992.

25. Wulfsberg, EA, Hoffmann, DE, and Cohen, MM: Alpha 1-antitrypsin deficiency. Impact of genetic discovery on medicine and society. JAMA 271:217–222, 1994.

26. Kim, H, Lepler, L, and Daniels, A, et al: Alpha 1-antitrypsin deficiency and idiopathic pulmonary fibrosis in a family. South Med J 89:1008, 1996.

27. Key, S, DeNoon, DJ, and Boyles, S: A genetic disorder leading to emphysema is unexpectedly common. Disease Weekly Plus June 2:16, 1997.

28. Alpha 1-antitrypsin, Z, and the liver. Lancet 340:402–403, 1992.

29. Rose, VL, and Foody, JM: Elevated fibrinogen levels increase risk of heart disease in women. Am Fam Phys 59:3158, 1999.

The Lymphoid System

Learning Objectives

After finishing this chapter, the reader will be able to:

1. Differentiate between primary and secondary lymphoid organs.
2. Describe the function and architecture of a lymph node.
3. Compare a primary and a secondary follicle.
4. Discuss the role of the thymus in T cell maturation.
5. Describe maturation of a B cell from the pro-B cell to a plasma cell.
6. Explain what constitutes a cluster of differentiation.
7. Identify and discuss the function of the following key antigens on T cells: CD2, CD3, CD4, and CD8.
8. Compare and contrast the CD3 receptor on a T cell and surface immunoglobulin on a B cell.
9. Explain how CD2 can be used as a T cell marker.
10. Describe a cytokine.
11. Differentiate T cell subsets on the basis of antigenic structure and function.
12. Explain how natural killer (NK) cells recognize target cells.
13. Discuss the principles involved in separation of cells by flow cytometry.
14. Describe how fluorescent antibody staining is applied to detection of surface immunoglobulin on B cells.
15. Apply knowledge of T and B cell function to immunologically based disease states.

Key Terms

Antibody-dependent cell
  cytotoxicity
Apoptosis
Bone marrow
Cell flow cytometry
Clusters of
  differentiation(CD)
Cytokine

Germinal center
Lymph node
Memory cell
Negative selection
Periarteriolar lymphoid
  sheath
Plasma cell
Positive selection

Primary follicle
Rosetting
Secondary follicle
Spleen
Thymocyte
Thymus

The key cell involved in the immune response is the lymphocyte. Lymphocytes represent approximately 20 percent of the circulating white blood cells. The typical small lymphocyte is between 8 and 12 μm in diameter and has a large rounded nucleus that may be somewhat indented. The nuclear chromatin is dense and tends to stain deeply (Fig. 3–1, Color Plate 6). Cytoplasm is sparse, containing few organelles and no specific granules, and consists of a narrow ring surrounding the nucleus.[1] These cells are unique because they arise from a hematopoietic stem cell and then are further differentiated in the primary lymphoid organs. They can be separated into two main classes, depending on where this differentiation takes place. The primary lymphoid organs in humans are the bone marrow and the thymus.

Once lymphocytes mature in the primary organs, they are released and make their way to secondary organs. Secondary organs include the spleen, lymph nodes, appendix, tonsils, and other mucosal-associated lymphoid tissue. It is in the secondary organs that the main contact with foreign antigens takes place. The spleen serves as a filtering mechanism for antigens in the bloodstream, and lymph nodes filter fluid from the tissues. Mucosal surfaces in the respiratory and alimentary tracts are backed with lymphoid tissue as an additional means of contacting foreign antigens as they enter the body.

Lymphocytes are segregated within the secondary organs according to their particular functions. T lymphocytes are the effector cells that serve a regulatory role, and it is the B lymphocytes that actually produce antibody. Both types of cells recirculate continuously from the bloodstream to the secondary lymphoid organs and back, in an attempt to increase contact with foreign antigens.

This chapter describes the primary lymphoid organs and examines their role in the development of antigen-specific lymphocytes. Secondary organs are presented in terms of the climate produced for development of the immune response. Specific characteristics of the major types of lymphocytes are discussed, and ways to identify them in the laboratory are presented.

Primary Lymphoid Organs

Bone Marrow

All lymphocytes arise from pluripotential hematopoietic stem cells that appear initially in the yolk sac of the developing embryo and are later found in the fetal liver. The bone marrow assumes this role when the infant is born. **Bone marrow** can be considered the largest tissue of the body, with a total weight of 1300 to 1500 g in the adult.[2] Bone marrow fills the core of all long bones and is the main source of hematopoietic stem cells, which develop into erythrocytes, granulocytes, monocytes, platelets, and lymphocytes. Each of these lines has specific precursors that originate from the pluripotential stem cells. Although a lymphoid precursor has not been specifically isolated, there is evidence of a common progenitor for both T and B cells, the two main types of lymphocytes.[3,4] Lymphocyte precursors are further developed in the primary lymphoid organs.

The bone marrow thus functions as the center for antigen-independent lymphopoiesis. Lymphocyte stem cells are released from the marrow and travel to additional primary lymphoid organs where further maturation takes place. One subset goes to the thymus and develops into T cells. In humans, B cell maturation takes place within the bone marrow itself. Together, the thymus and bone marrow produce approximately 10^9 mature lymphocytes each day.[5]

Thymus

T cells, the second main type of lymphocyte, develop their identifying characteristics in the thymus. The **thymus** is a small, flat, bilobed organ found in the thorax or chest cavity right below the thyroid gland and overlying the heart (Fig. 3–2). In humans, it weighs an average of 22 g at birth, reaches about 35 g at puberty, and then gradually atrophies.[5] It was first

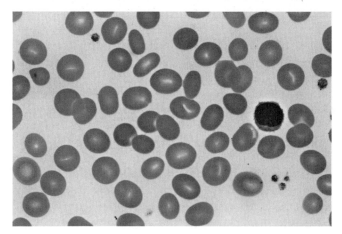

FIG. 3–1. Typical lymphocyte found in peripheral blood. (From Harr, R: Clinical Laboratory Science Review, FA Davis, Philadelphia, 2000, Color Plate 31.) See Color Plate 6.

presumed that early in life the thymus produces enough virgin T lymphocytes to seed the entire immune system, so it is no longer necessary later on. However, new evidence indicates that although the thymus diminishes in size, it is still capable of producing T lymphocytes throughout a person's lifespan.[6]

Each lobe of the thymus is divided into lobules filled with epithelial cells that play a central role in this differentiation process. Surface antigens are acquired as the lymphocytes travel from the cortex to the medulla over a period of 2 to 3 weeks.[7]

Mature T lymphocytes are then released from the medulla. Progenitors of T cells appear in the fetus as early as 8 weeks in the gestational period.[5] Thus,

differentiation of lymphocytes appears to take place very early in fetal development and is essential to acquisition of immunocompetence by the time the infant is born.

Secondary Lymphoid Organs

Once differentiation occurs, mature T and B lymphocytes are released from the bone marrow and the thymus. They migrate to secondary lymphoid organs and become part of a recirculating pool. Each individual lymphocyte spends most of its lifespan in solid tissue, entering the circulation only periodically to go from one secondary organ to another.[5] The *secondary lymphoid organs* include the spleen, lymph nodes, tonsils, appendix, Peyer's patches in the intestines, and other mucosal-associated lymphoid tissue (MALT) (see Fig. 3–2). Lymphocytes in these organs travel through the tissue and return to the bloodstream by way of the thoracic duct. Approximately 1 to 2 percent of the total lymphocyte pool recirculates every hour.[8] This continuous recirculation increases the likelihood of a lymphocyte coming into contact with its specific antigen. Lymphopoiesis, or reproduction of lymphocytes, occurs in the secondary tissue, but this is strictly dependent on antigenic stimulation, while formation of lymphocytes in the bone marrow is antigen-independent. Most naïve or resting lymphocytes die within a few days after leaving the primary lymphoid organs unless activated by the presence of a foreign antigen.[5] It is this second process that gives rise to long-lived memory cells and shorter-lived effector cells that are responsible for the generation of the immune response.

Spleen

The **spleen** is the largest secondary lymphoid organ, having a length of approximately 12 cm and weighing 150 g in the adult. It is located in the upper left quadrant of the abdomen, just below the diaphragm and surrounded by a thin connective tissue capsule. The organ can be characterized as a large discriminating filter because a major function is to filter out old and damaged cells and foreign antigens from the blood.

Splenic tissue can be divided into two main types: red pulp and white pulp. The red pulp makes up more than one-half of the total volume, and its function is the destruction of old red blood cells. Blood flows from the arterioles into the red pulp and then exits by way of the splenic vein. The white pulp contains the lymphoid tissue, and this is arranged around arterioles in a **periarteriolar lymphoid sheath** (Fig. 3–3). This sheath contains small lymphocytes, large lymphocytes, macrophages, plasma cells, and granulocytes.

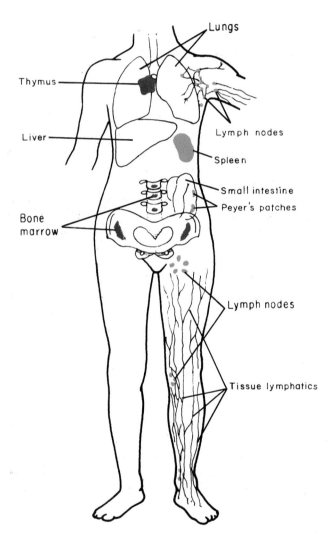

FIG. 3–2. Sites of lymphoreticular tissue. Primary organs include the bone marrow and the thymus. Secondary organs are distributed throughout the body and include the spleen, lymph nodes, and mucosal-associated lymphoid tissue. The spleen filters antigens in the blood, while the lymphatic system filters fluid from the tissues. (From Widmann, FK: An Introduction to Clinical Immunology, FA Davis, Philadelphia, 1989, with permission.)

Lymphocytes enter and leave this area by means of the many capillary branches that connect to the arterioles.

T cells are found close to the central arterioles, while the B cells are located beyond this zone. B cells are typically organized into clusters called follicles. **Primary follicles** contain B cells that are not yet stimulated by antigen. The white pulp comprises approximately 20 percent of the total weight of the spleen. Each day, approximately one-half of the blood volume passes through the spleen, where lymphocytes and macrophages can constantly survey for infectious agents or other foreign matter.[5]

Lymph Nodes

Lymph nodes are located along lymphatic ducts and serve as central collecting points for lymph fluid from adjacent tissues. Lymph fluid arises from passage of fluids and low-molecular-weight solutes out of blood vessel walls and into the interstitial spaces between cells. Some of this interstitial fluid returns to the bloodstream through venules, but a portion flows through the tissues and is eventually collected in thin-walled vessels known as lymphatic vessels.[5]

Lymph nodes are especially numerous near joints and where the arms and the legs join the body. Nodes range in size from 1 mm to about 25 mm in diameter.

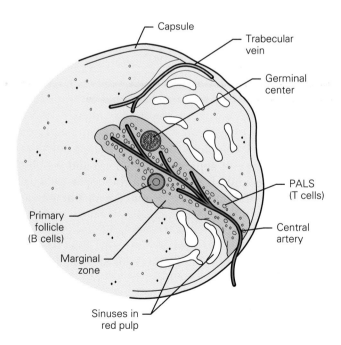

FIG. 3–3. Cross-section of the spleen showing organization of the lymphoid tissue. T cells surround arterioles in the PALS. B cells are just beyond in follicles. When stimulated by antigen, the B cells form germinal centers. All of the lymphoid tissue is referred to as the white pulp.

Filtration is a main function of these organs. The lymph fluid flows slowly through spaces called sinuses, which are lined with macrophages, creating an ideal location for phagocytosis to take place. The tissue is organized into an outer cortex and an inner medulla.

Lymphocytes and any foreign antigens present enter nodes via afferent lymphatic vessels. A small number of lymphocytes are also able to enter the nodes from the bloodstream by means of specialized venules called high endothelial venules located in paracortical areas.[8] Just underneath the outer capsule is an area called the subcapsular sinus, which is lined with macrophages (Fig. 3–4). Here phagocytosis and antigen processing take place. Below this is the cortex, which contains aggregations of B cells in primary follicles similar to those found in the spleen. These are the mature, resting B cells that have not yet been exposed to antigen. A small number of T cells and specialized cells called *follicular dendritic cells* are also located here. Follicular dendritic cells are only found in lymphoid follicles and have long cytoplasmic processes that radiate out like tentacles. These cells exhibit a large number of receptors for antibody and complement and are thought to be responsible for the regulation of activities of memory B cells.[9]

Secondary follicles consist of antigen-stimulated proliferating B cells. The interior of a secondary follicle is known as the **germinal center** because it is here that blast transformation of the B cells takes place. **Plasma cells,** which actively secrete antibody, and **memory cells,** which are just a step away from forming plasma cells, are present. Generation of B cell memory is a primary function of lymph nodes.[8]

T lymphocytes are mainly localized in the paracortex, the region between the follicles and the medulla. T lymphocytes are in close proximity to antigen-presenting cells called *interdigitating cells.* The medulla is less densely populated but contains some T cells (in addition to B cells), macrophages, and a small number of plasma cells.

Particulate antigens are removed as the fluid travels across the node from cortex to medulla. The transit time through a lymph node is approximately 18 hours. Fluid and lymphocytes exit by way of the efferent lymph vessels. Such vessels form a larger duct that eventually connects with the thoracic duct and the venous system. In this manner, lymphocytes are able to recirculate continuously between lymph nodes and the peripheral blood.

If contact with antigen takes place, lymphocyte traffic is shut down for about 24 hours in an attempt to immobilize the antigen.[8] Lymph nodes become enlarged, and within several days, germinal centers are visible. Enlargement of the nodes is known as

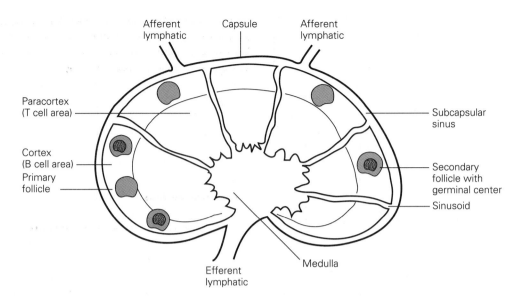

FIG. 3–4. Structure of a lymph node. A lymph node is surrounded by a tough outer capsule. Right underneath is the subcapsular sinus, where lymph fluid drains from afferent lymphatic vessels. The outer cortex contains collections of B cells in primary follicles. When stimulated by antigen, secondary follicles are formed. T cells are found in the paracortical area. Fluid drains slowly through sinusoids to the medullary region and out the efferent lymphatic vessel to the thoracic duct.

lymphadenopathy. Recirculation of expanded numbers of lymphocytes then occurs.

Other Secondary Organs

Additional areas of lymphoid tissue include the MALT, which is found in the gastrointestinal, respiratory, and urogenital tracts. Here macrophages and lymphocytes are localized at some of the main ports of entry for foreign organisms. Peyer's patches represent a specialized type of MALT, located at the lower ileum of the intestinal tract.

The tonsils are small masses of macrophages and lymphoid tissue found in the mucous membrane lining of the oral and pharyngeal cavities. Their function is to respond to pathogens entering the respiratory and alimentary tracts. Another location of lymphoid tissue is the appendix. All of these secondary organs function as potential sites for contact with foreign antigen, and they increase the probability of an immune response.

The epidermis contains a number of intraepidermal lymphocytes. Most of these are T cells, which are uniquely positioned to combat any antigens that enter through the skin. This association of lymphocytes is known as the cutaneous-associated lymphoid tissue.

Within each of these secondary organs, T and B cells are segregated and perform specialized functions. B cells differentiate into memory cells and plasma cells and are responsible for humoral immunity or antibody formation. T cells play a role in cell-mediated immunity, and as such, they produce sensitized lymphocytes that secrete cytokines. **Cytokines,** formerly known as lymphokines, are small polypeptides that regulate the functions of lymphocytes and other cells involved in the immune response. The characteristics and markers for each type of lymphocyte are considered separately.

Surface Markers on Lymphocytes

Proteins that appear on cell surfaces can be used as markers to differentiate T cells and B cells. Proteins can also be used to distinguish the developmental stages of the two types of cells according to when these proteins appear. Such proteins, or antigens, have been detected by monoclonal antibodies, extremely specific antibodies made by cloning a single antibody-producing cell. (Refer to Chapter 5 for a discussion of preparation of monoclonal antibodies.)

A number of laboratories have developed monoclonal antibodies, and each used its own nomenclature for the sets of antigens found. In an attempt to relate research findings and standardize the nomenclature, scientists set up the International Workshops on Human Leukocyte Antigens, beginning in 1982.[10] Panels of antibodies from different laboratories were used for analysis, and antibodies reacting similarly with standard cell lines were said to define **clusters of differentiation (CD).** As each antigen, or CD, was found, it was assigned a number. The name *cluster of differentiation* came about because the exact nature of the proteins identified by the various antibodies was not known. This CD classification now acts as a reference in standardizing names of membrane proteins found on all human white blood cells. The seventh Workshop and Conference on Human Leukocyte Differentiation Antigens was held in June 2000, and the list of CD designations currently numbers more than 150.[10] The antigens that are most important in characterizing T lymphocytes and B lymphocytes are shown in Table 3–1 and are referred to in the following discussion of T cell and B cell development.

Stages in B Cell Differentiation

Pro-B Cells

B cells are derived from a lymphoid-myeloid precursor that remains in the bone marrow for maturation. Here these cells go through a developmental process that will prepare them for their role in antibody production and, at the same time, restrict the types of antigens to which any one cell can respond. This part of B cell development is known as the antigen-independent phase. During this maturation process, there are rearrange-

ments of genes coding for the heavy and light chains of an antibody molecule and changes in expression of intracellular and surface-bound markers that help to distinguish each phase. The end result is a B lymphocyte programmed to produce a unique antibody molecule, which consists of two identical light chains and two identical heavy chains (see Chapter 5 for details). Although portions of each chain are identical for every antibody molecule, it is the so-called variable regions that make each antibody molecule specific for a certain antigen or group of antigens. Heavy chains are coded for on chromosome 14, and light chains are coded for on chromosomes 2 and 22.

The first recognizable cell in the B cell lineage is the *pro-B cell.* The distinctive markers on pro-B cells include surface antigens *CD19* and *CD45R,* and intracellular proteins *terminal deoxyribonucleotide transferase (TdT)* and *recombinase activating gene (RAG)-1 and RAG-2 enzymes* (Fig. 3–5A).[11,12] Gene rearrangement of the deoxyribonucleic acid (DNA) that codes for antibody production occurs in a strict developmental sequence.[13] Rearrangement of genes on chromosome 14, which code for the heavy chain part of the antibody molecule, takes place first in a random fashion (see Chapter 5 for

TABLE 3–1. Surface Markers on T and B Cells

Antigen	Molecular Weight (kd)	Cell Type	Function
CD2	45–58	Thymocytes, T cells, NK cells	Involved in T cell activation
CD3	20–28	Thymocytes, T cells	Associated with T cell antigen receptor; role in TCR signal transduction
CD4	55	Helper T cells, monocytes, macrophages	Co-receptor for MHC class II; receptor for HIV
CD5	58	Mature T cells, thymocytes, subset of B cells (B1)	Positive or negative modulation of T and B cell receptor signaling
CD8	60–76	Thymocyte subsets, cytotoxic T cells	Co-receptor for MHC class I
CD10	100	B and T cell precursors, bone marrow stromal cells	Protease; marker for pre-B CALLA
CD16	50–80	Macrophages, NK cells, neutrophils	Low affinity Fc receptor, mediates phagocytosis and ADCC
CD19	>120	B cells, follicular dendritic cells	Part of B cell coreceptor, signal transduction molecule that regulates B cell development and activation
CD21	145	B cells, follicular dendritic cells, subset of immature thymocytes	Receptor for complement component C3d; part of B cell coreceptor with CD 19
CD23	45	B cells, monocytes, follicular dendritic cells	Regulation of IgE synthesis; triggers release of Il-1, Il-6, and GM-CSF from monocytes
CD25	55	Activated T, B cells, monocytes	Receptor for IL-2
CD44	85	Most leukocytes	Adhesion molecule mediating homing to peripheral lymphoid organs
CD45R	180	Different forms on all hematopoietic cells	Essential in T and B cell antigen-stimulated activation
CD 56	175-220	NK cells, subsets of T cells	Not known
CD 94	70	NK cells, subsets of T cells	Subunit of NKG2-A complex involved in inhibition of NK cell cytotoxicity

NK = Natural killer; TCR = CD3-αβ receptor complex; MHC = major histocompatibility class; HIV = human immunodeficiency virus; CALLA = common acute lymphoblastic leukemia antigen; Fc = Fragment crystallizable; ADCC = antibody-dependent cell cytotoxicity; IgE = immunoglobulin E; GM-CSF = granulocyte-macrophage colony-stimulating factor.

details). Recombinase enzymes RAG-1 and RAG-2 cleave the DNA at certain possible recombination sites, and TdT helps to join the pieces back together by incorporating additional nucleotides in the joining areas.[14,15] If the rearrangement of one chromosome is successful and the cell is able to synthesize heavy chains, then no further rearrangement of the other chromosome 14 occurs.[13] If, however, the first try is not successful, then the second chromosome 14 goes through the same process. About 50 percent of all pro-B cells fail at both tries, and these cells die in the marrow.[13] Successful rearrangement commits a B cell to further development and ultimately to formation of a particular antibody against a specific antigen or group of antigens. CD19 acts as a coreceptor that helps to regulate B cell development and activation. CD45 is a membrane glycoprotein found on all hematopoietic cells, but the type found on B cells is the largest form, and it is designated CD45R. It is a tyrosine-specific phosphatase that is involved in signaling in B cell activation. These two B cell markers remain on the cell surface throughout subsequent developmental stages.

Differentiation of pro-B cells into pre-B cells requires the microenvironment provided by bone marrow stromal cells.[12] Stromal cells interact directly with pro-B and pre-B cells, and they secrete cytokines, chemical messengers that are necessary for the developmental process. The most important of these is IL-7, which regulates both proliferation and differentiation of B cell precursors.[14,16]

Pre-B Cells

When synthesis of the part of the antibody molecule known as a heavy chain occurs, this signals the beginning of the *pre-B stage*.[12,13] The first heavy chains synthesized are the μ chains, which belong to the class of immunoglobulins called IgM. The μ chains accumulate in the cytoplasm. Some pre-B cells express μ chains on the cell surface and these are accompanied by an unusual light chain molecule called a surrogate light chain.[12,17] Surrogate light chains consist of two short polypeptide chains that are noncovalently associated with one another (Fig. 3–5B). They are not immunoglobulin proteins but are thought to be essential for regulating B cell development. The combination of the two heavy chains with the surrogate light chains forms a receptor known as a pre-B cell receptor. This receptor adheres to bone marrow stromal cell membranes and transmits a signal to prevent rearrangement of any other heavy chain genes.[12,14,16] It appears that only pre-B cells expressing the μ heavy chains in association with surrogate light chains survive and proceed to further differentiation.[12,17,18] Pre-B cells typically divide several times before further differentiation occurs. This phase lasts for approximately 2 days.[13]

Immature B Cells

Immature B cells are recognized by the appearance of complete IgM molecules on the cell surface (Fig. 3–5C). This indicates that rearrangement of the genetic sequence coding for light chains on either chromosome 2 or 22 has taken place by this time. Completion of light chain rearrangement commits a cell to production of an antibody molecule with specificity for a particular antigen or group of related antigens. Regions on both the light and heavy chains known as variable regions determine this specificity. Once surface immunoglobulins appear, μ chains are no longer detectable in the cytoplasm.

Other surface proteins appearing on the immature B cell include receptors for complement components.

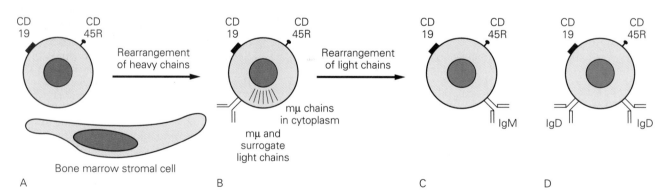

FIG. 3–5. B cell development in the bone marrow. Selected markers are shown for the various stages in the differentiation of B cells. Stages up to the formation of mature B cells occur in the bone marrow. *(A)* Pro-B cell. *(B)* Pre-B cell. *(C)* Immature B cell. *(D)* Mature B cell.

CD21 acts as a receptor for a breakdown product of C3, known as C3d. This is also the means by which the Epstein Barr virus gains entry into B cells, which occurs in infectious mononucleosis.[19] Such receptors enhance the likelihood of contact between B cells and antigen because antigen frequently becomes coated with complement fragments during the immune response.

At this stage, there is evidence that self-antigens give a negative signal to immature B cells, resulting in arrested maturation and cell death.[7] Immature B cells that tightly bind self-antigens through cross-linking of surface IgM molecules are eliminated or inactivated.[15,20] Thus, many B cells capable of producing antibody to self-antigens are deleted from the marrow by the process of programmed cell death, or **apoptosis.** It is estimated that more than 90 percent of B cells die in this manner without leaving the bone marrow.[12,21]

Mature B Cells

In addition to IgM, mature B cells exhibit IgD, another class of antibody molecule, on their surface. At the same time, surface IgM increases in density (Fig. 3–5D). Both IgM and IgD have the same specificity for a particular antigen or group of antigens. These surface immunoglobulins provide the primary activating signal to B cells when contact with antigen takes place.[19] Also associated with mature B cells are major histocompatibility class (MHC) II products (see Chapter 4 for a complete discussion of MHC antigens). These glycoproteins are embedded in the cell membrane and are recognized by a subset of T cells, the T helper cells, which aid in antibody production. Mature B cells are released from the marrow and seed peripheral lymphoid organs. Unless contact with antigen occurs, the life span of a mature B cell is only a few days.[12] If, however, a B cell is stimulated by antigen, it undergoes transformation to a blast stage, which eventually forms memory cells and antibody-secreting plasma cells. This process is known as the antigen-dependent phase of B cell development.

Small subpopulations of B cells, known as B-1 cells, have IgM but little or no IgD on their surface. They also express a surface marker known as CD5, which is normally found on T cells.[12] B-1 cells appear to arise before the major group of B cells, known as B-2 cells. These B cells appear to be capable of editing the gene coding for variable regions of both heavy and light chains, giving them the ability to respond to more than one antigen.[12] Most of these respond best to carbohydrate rather than protein antigens, and they tend to produce only antibody of the IgM class. They are formed during fetal life and are usually found in the peritoneal cavity.[13] They are the major source for antibody production in the infant and young child.

Activated B Cells

In primary follicles located in peripheral lymphoid tissue, when antigens act to crosslink surface immunoglobulins on B cells, a phenomenon known as lymphocyte capping can readily be detected (Fig. 3–6). This represents the migration of surface immunoglobulins to one pole of the cell where antigen contact has taken place. Visualization of this event is easily accomplished by using fluoresceine-tagged anti-immunoglobulin antibodies. This is the first step in antigen-dependent activation of B cells.

Activated B cells exhibit other identifying markers that include CD25. CD25 is found on both activated T and B cells, and it acts as a receptor for interleukin-2 (IL-2), a growth factor produced by T cells.[19] Additional receptors that appear at this time are specific for other growth factors produced by T cells and for other immunoglobulin classes.[2]

When B cells are activated in this manner, they transform to become blasts that will give rise to both plasma cells and so-called memory cells. Within these germinal centers, blasts can give rise to as many as 10^4 cells in 3 to 4 days.[8]

Plasma Cells

Plasma cells are large, spherical or ellipsoidal cells between 10 and 20 μm in size and are characterized by the presence of abundant cytoplasmic immunoglobulin and little to no surface immunoglobulin (Fig. 3–7, Color Plate 7).[22] The nucleus is eccentric or oval with heavily clumped chromatin that stains darkly. An abundant endoplasmic reticulum and a clear well-defined Golgi zone are present in the cytoplasm. This represents the most fully differentiated lymphocyte, and its main function is antibody production. Plasma cells are not normally found in the blood but are located in germinal centers in the peripheral lymphoid organs. After several days of antibody production, they die without further proliferation.[14]

Memory cells (see Fig. 3–6) are also found in germinal centers and have a much longer life span than a resting B cell.[11,12] These represent progeny of antigen-stimulated B cells that are capable of responding to antigen with increased speed and intensity. They are similar in appearance to unstimulated B cells, but they remain in an activated state for months or years, ready to respond to the initial antigen. Figure 3–5 summarizes the changes that take place as B cells mature from the pro-B stage to memory cells or plasma cells.

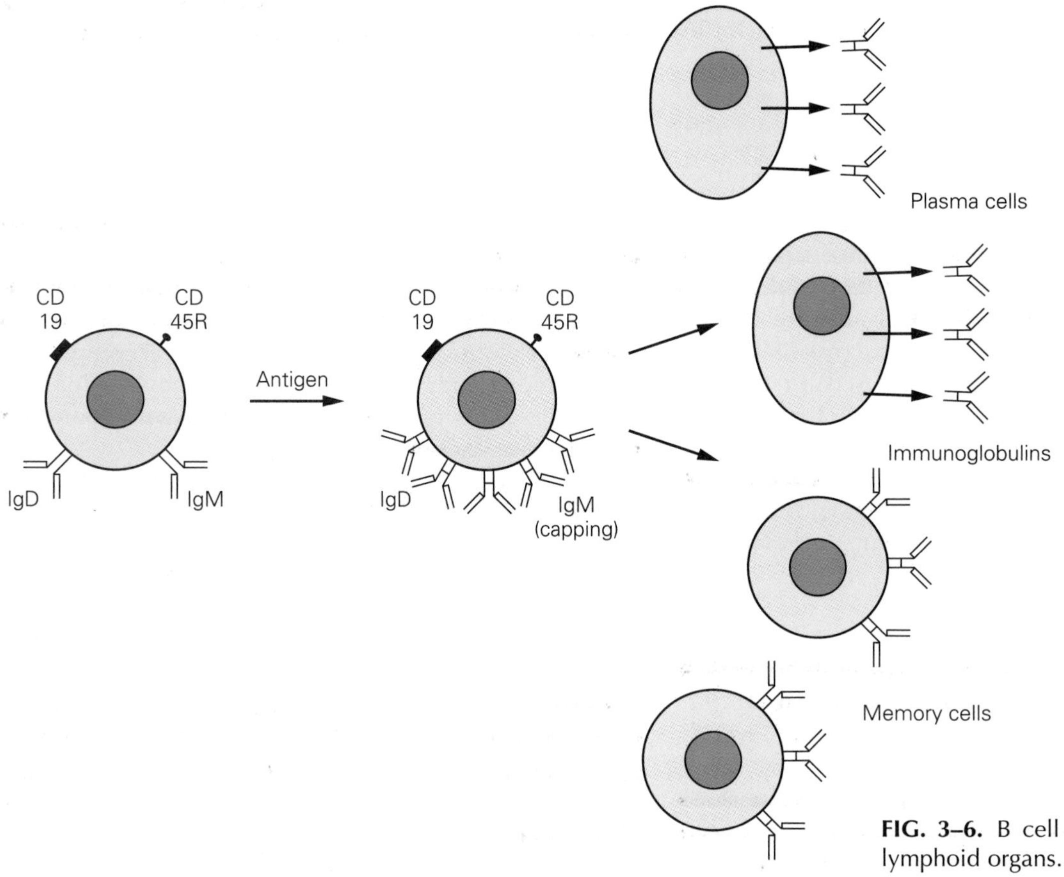

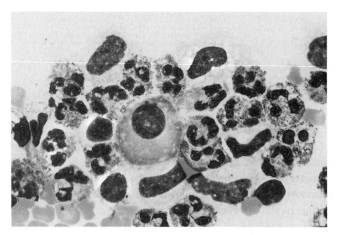

FIG. 3–6. B cell activation in peripheral lymphoid organs.

FIG. 3–7. A typical plasma cell. (From Harr, R: Clinical Laboratory Science Review, FA Davis, Philadelphia, 2000, Color Plate 28.) See Color Plate 7.

T Cell Differentiation

The majority of circulating lymphocytes in the peripheral blood (60 to 80 percent) are T cells, and these become differentiated in the thymus. Lymphocyte precursors called pro-thymocytes enter the thymus from the bone marrow. Although it is not absolutely clear, current research indicates that these precursors differ from the original hematopoietic stem cells in the bone marrow. However, they may still have the potential to become related cells, including B cells, macrophages, or dendritic cells, in addition to T lymphocytes.[4,23] Early surface markers on pro-thymocytes committed to becoming T cells include CD44 and TdT.[3,24,25]

Within the lobules of the thymus are two main zones, the outer cortex and the inner medulla. As pro-thymocytes travel through the thymus, they go through a process similar to that of B cells in the marrow, in that there is an orderly rearrangement of the genes coding for the antigen receptor, and at the same distinct surface markers appear that allow them to be recognized as specific T cell subsets. More than 85 percent of the lymphocytes are located in the cortex, and these are immature cells.[25] Maturation is an elaborate process that takes place over a 3-week period as cells filter through the cortex to the medulla.[7] Thymic stromal cells include epithelial cells, macrophages, and dendritic cells, all of which play a role in T cell development. Interaction with these cells under the influence of cytokines helps the T cells to mature and differenti-

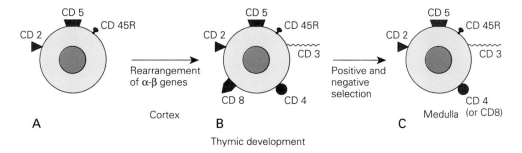

FIG. 3–8. Stages in T cell development. *(A)* Double-negative thymocyte—lymphocyte precursors enter the thymic cortex and develop CD2, CD5, and CD45R antigens. *(B)* Double-positive thymocyte—when rearrangement of *a* and *b* genes is complete, thymocytes express CD3, CD4, and CD8. *(C)* Mature T cell—positive and negative selection take place, and the T cell becomes single-positive; that is, either CD4+ or CD8+.

ate.[25] It is estimated that approximately 99 percent of the cortical cells die intrathymically, so a significant selection process occurs as maturation takes place.

Double-Negative Stage

Acquisition of surface antigens and the ability to recognize foreign antigens in association with self-MHC molecules takes place in three main stages. Early **thymocytes** lack CD4 and CD8 markers, hence they are known as double-negative thymocytes (Fig. 3–8*A*). Some early surface markers that develop are CD2, CD5, CD7, and CD45R.[2,5] The CD2 antigen was the original means of identifying T cells because it is a receptor for sheep red blood cells. T cells mixed with sheep red blood cells exhibit a phenomenon known as **rosetting,** in which sheep cells encircle the T cells, making a daisy pattern as they adhere to CD2 receptors (Fig. 3–9). These large double-negative thymocytes actively proliferate in the outer cortex under the influence of interleukin-7.[3,26]

Rearrangement of the genes that code for the antigen receptor begins at this stage (Fig. 3–8*B*).[5] CD3, the complex that serves as the T cell antigen receptor, consists of eight noncovalently associated chains, six of which are common to all T cells.[4,20] However, two chains, the alpha (α) and beta (β) chains, contain variable regions that recognize specific antigens (Fig. 3–10). These are coded for by selecting gene segments and deleting others, as is the case with B cells. This is also under the control of the RAG enzymes. There is a possibility of approximately 10^{15} combinations for rearrangement of these two variable regions.[27] Rearrangement of the β chain occurs first. The appearance of a functional β chain on the cell surface sends a signal to suppress any further β chain gene rearrangements. Signaling by the β chain also triggers the thymocyte to become CD4-positive (CD4+) as well as CD-8 positive.[27,28]

Early on, some thymocytes, representing 5 percent

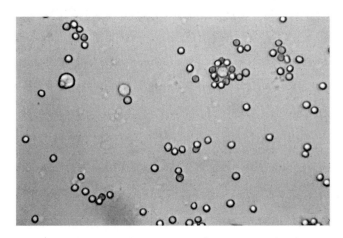

FIG. 3–9. T cell rosette. T cell surrounded by sheep red blood cells that attach to CD2 receptors on T cell.

or less of the total number, rearrange and express two other chains, gamma (γ) and delta (δ). It is not known how this process is controlled, but these cells proceed down a different developmental pathway. Cells expressing the γδ receptor typically remain negative for both CD4 and CD8. However, as mature T cells, they appear to represent the dominant T cell population in the skin, intestinal epithelium, and pulmonary epithelium. Although their function is not absolutely clear, new evidence indicates that they may act like natural killer (NK) cells to mediate tumor-cell lysis.[4,24,27] They are capable of recognizing stress proteins called MICA and MICB that are only found on tumor and virally-infected cells.[29] Any cells bearing these proteins are eliminated by the γδ T cells.

Double-Positive Stage

At this second stage, when thymocytes express both CD4 and CD8 antigens, they are called double-positive.[10,18] Double-positive thymocytes proliferate, and then begin to rearrange the genes coding for the

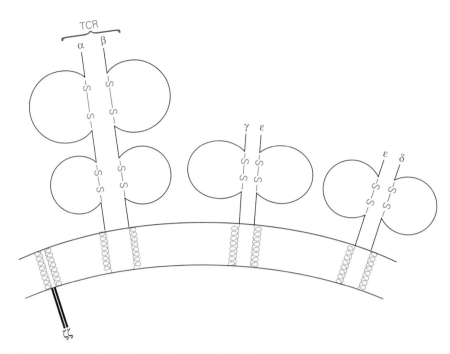

FIG. 3–10. The CD3:T cell receptor complex. The T cell receptor that recognizes antigen consists of two chains, α and β, which have constant and variable regions. Four other types of chains are collectively known as CD3. These are ε, γ, δ, and θ. They take part in signaling to the interior of the cell when antigen binding occurs.

alpha chain.[27,28] When the CD3-αβ receptor complex (TCR) is expressed on the cell surface, a process known as **positive selection** begins (Fig. 3–8C). Because T cells recognize foreign antigen only in association with class I or class II MHC molecules, this receptor must be able to recognize both foreign antigens and self-MHC antigens. Any thymocytes that are unable to recognize self-MHC antigens die without leaving the thymus. This selection process eliminates more than 90 percent of the double-positive thymocytes in the cortex.

Selection appears to be influenced by the number of TCR receptors expressed on the T cell. Most cells express very low levels of the TCR receptor, and these are the ones that do not survive. Those cells expressing moderate levels of TCR receptor bind by means of the αβ chains to MHC antigens on cells within the thymus.[17,30] In fact, this recognition of MHC protein associated with small peptides has been found to be essential for positive selection.[31] TCR binding apparently transmits a signal that results in survival.[27] Thymic epithelial cells that express high levels of MHC molecules are responsible for the positive selection.

A second selection process takes place among surviving double-positive T cells. There is evidence that those T cells capable of reacting with self-antigens are destroyed. This process is called **negative selection.** Antigen-presenting cells, rather than the thymic stromal cells, are responsible for negative selection. These include macrophages and dendritic cells. Research indicates that those T cells that bind with a high affinity to self-antigens undergo death by apoptosis. This process appears to take place in the cortico-medullary junction.[4,24]

Mature T Cells

Survivors of negative selection exhibit only one type of marker, either CD4 or CD8. It is not certain how one marker is selected over the other, but it may depend on with which MHC protein the cell interacts and exposure to certain cytokines.[16] CD4+ T cells recognize antigen along with MHC Class II protein, while CD8+ T cells interact with antigen and MHC Class I proteins. The two separate mature T cell populations thus created (Fig. 3–8D) differ greatly in function. T cells bearing the CD4 receptor are termed helper or inducer cells (Fig. 3–8D), while the CD8-positive (CD8+) population consists of cytotoxic T cells (Fig. 3–8E). Approximately two-thirds of peripheral T cells express CD4 antigen, while the remaining one-third express CD8 antigen. These mature T cells are released from the thymus and seed peripheral lymphoid organs. Resting T cells have a life span of up to several years in these peripheral organs.[4]

Antigen Activation

When antigen recognition occurs in secondary lymphoid tissue, T lymphocytes are transformed into large activated cells that are characterized by polyribosome-filled cytoplasm. Activated T lymphocytes express receptors for IL-2, just as activated B cells do (Fig. 3–11).[19] T lymphoblasts differentiate into functionally active small lymphocytes that produce cytokines. Activities of specific cytokines include assisting B cells in the commencement of antibody production, killing of tumor and other target cells, rejection of grafts, stimulation of hematopoiesis in the bone marrow, and initiation of delayed hypersensitivity allergic reactions. This type of immune response is known as cell-mediated immunity (see Chapter 6 for a full description of cell-mediated immunity). In addition to effector cells, T memory cells are generated also. In a similar manner to memory B cells, they are able to proliferate sooner than naïve T cells. They also express a broader array of cytokines and appear to persist for years.[4,24,32] Table 3–2 summarizes the differences between T cells and B cells in structure and function.

Third Population or Natural Killer Cells

A small percentage of lymphocytes do not express the markers of either T cells or B cells. These lymphocytes are approximately 15 μm in diameter, generally larger than T cells and B cells, and they contain kidney-shaped nuclei with condensed chromatin and prominent nucleoli.[22] They have a higher cytoplasmic-nuclear ratio, and the cytoplasm contains a number of azurophilic granules.[33] These large granular lymphocytes make up 5 to 15 percent of the circulating lymphoid pool[24,34] and are found mainly in the spleen and peripheral blood. They have been named NK cells because they have the ability to mediate cytolytic reactions and kill target cells without prior exposure to them. The response is directed nonspecifically against many types of target cells.

There are no surface antigens that are unique to NK cells, but they express a specific combination of antigens that can be used for identification. One such antigen is CD16, which is a receptor for the fragment

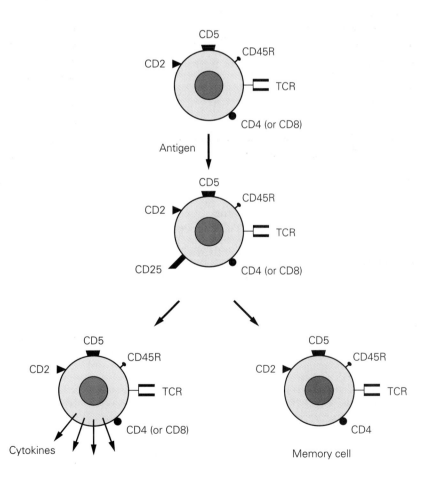

FIG. 3–11. Activated T cell—exposure to antigen causes production of CD25 receptor. Sensitized T cell—secretes cytokines.

TABLE 3–2. Comparison of T and B Cells

T Cells	B Cells
1. Develop in the thymus	1. Develop in the bone marrow
2. Found in blood (60%–80% of circulating lymphocytes), thoracic duct fluid, lymph nodes	2. Found in bone marrow, spleen, lymph nodes
3. Identified by rosette formation with SRBCs	3. Identified by surface immunoglobulin
4. End products of activation are cytokines	4. End product of activation is antibody
5. Antigens include CD2, CD3, CD4, CD8	5. Antigens include CD19, CD20, CD21, CD40, MHC class II
6. Locate in paracortical region of lymph nodes	6. Locate in cortical region of lymph nodes

SRBC = Sheep red blood cells.

crystallizable portion, or nonspecific end, of the immunoglobulin molecule IgG. Other surface antigens may include CD56 and CD94.[33,34] They are also identified by their lack of CD3, CD4, and CD8.

NK cells probably arise from a common progenitor of T cells because they have cytoplasmic CD3 components but no actual antigen receptors on the surface.[33] Recent evidence indicates that in the absence of a thymus, fetal thymocytes develop into NK cells instead of CD4 or CD8 lymphocytes. Therefore, it is believed that immature thymocytes give rise to T cells or NK cells depending on the microenvironment.[35]

NK cells are capable of recognizing any foreign cell and destroying it without regard to MHC restriction. They represent the first line of defense against virally infected and tumor cells.[34] They may play a complementary role to that of CD8 cytotoxic lymphocytes. If foreign cells escape the action of cytotoxic T cells, NK cells are able to step in and lyse the virally infected or tumor cell.[35]

Exposure to IL-2 causes NK cells to be more active in the killing of tumor cells. Their cytolytic effect is also increased.[35] When so activated, they are called lymphokine-activated killer (LAK) cells.[22,24,26] Extensive research is being conducted on the use of LAK cells in patients with cancer.

NK cells also have the ability to produce cytokines after stimulation with IL-2 or with the CD16 ligands, so NK cells may also play a regulatory role in addition to their cytolytic activity.[24] The cytokines produced include gamma interferon, tissue necrosis factor alpha, and granulocyte-macrophage colony stimulating factor.[24,33]

Mechanism of Cytotoxicity

For years it has been a mystery how NK cells tell the difference between normal and abnormal cells. However, the mechanism is now beginning to be uncovered. It appears that there is a balance between activating and inhibitory signals that enables NK cells to distinguish healthy cells from infected or cancerous ones.[36] The inhibitory signal is based on recognition of MHC class I protein, which is expressed on all healthy cells.[37] If NK cells react with MHC proteins, then inhibition of natural killing occurs. Specific receptors on NK cells responsible for this binding include killer cell inhibitory receptors (KIRs). There are a number of different types of KIRs expressed on NK cells.[37]

Diseased and cancerous cells, however, tend to lose their ability to produce MHC proteins. NK cells are thus triggered by a lack of MHC antigens, sometimes referred to as recognition of "missing self."[38] This lack of inhibition appears to be combined with an activating signal switched on by the presence of proteins produced by cells under stress, namely those cells that are infected or cancerous. These proteins are named MICA and MICB. A receptor called NKG2D on NK cells binds MICA or MICB and sends a signal to destroy the cell.[29,38–40] If an inhibitory signal is not received, then NK cells release substances called perforins and granzymes (Fig. 3–12). Perforins are pore-forming proteins that polymerize in the presence of Ca2+ and form channels in the target cell membrane.[36] Granzymes are packets of serine esterase enzymes that may enter through the channels and mediate cell lysis.[36,41]

Antibody-Dependent Cell Cytotoxicity

Another method of destroying target cells is available to NK cells. They recognize and lyse antibody-coated cells by means of a process called **antibody-dependent cell cytotoxicity.** Binding occurs through the CD16 receptor for IgG. Any target cell coated with IgG can be bound and destroyed. This method is not unique to NK cells because monocytes, macrophages, and neutrophils also exhibit such a receptor and act in a similar manner. Nonetheless, the overall importance of NK cells as a defense mechanism is demonstrated by the fact that patients found lacking these cells have recurring viral infections or pneumonia.[24]

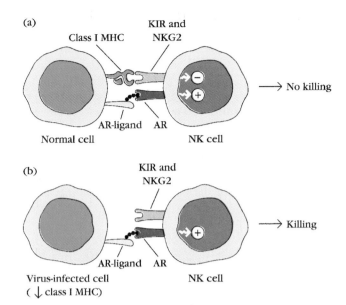

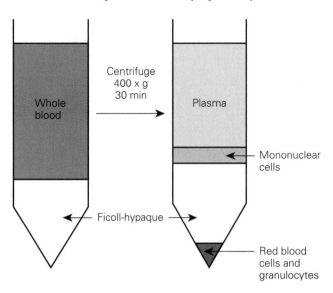

FIG. 3–12. Mechanism of NK cell cytotoxicity. (From Goldsby, RA, Kindt, TJ, and Osborne, BA: Kuby Immunology, ed.4. WH Freeman, New York, 2000, p.362, with permission.)

FIG. 3–13. Ficoll-Hypaque separation of cells in peripheral blood. Whole blood diluted with buffer is layered onto Ficoll-Hypaque medium in a plastic centrifuge tube. Tubes are spun at 4003 *g* for 30 minutes. Red blood cells and granulocytes settle to the bottom of the tube, while mononuclear cells (monocytes and lymphocytes) form a band at the interface of the Ficoll-Hypaque and plasma.

Laboratory Identification of Lymphocytes

Identification of lymphocytes as either T cells or B cells may be useful in diagnosis of any of the following states: lymphoproliferative malignancies, immunodeficiency diseases, unexplained infectious diseases, monitoring of transplants, and acquired immunologic abnormalities such as acquired immunodeficiency syndrome (AIDS). Most methods are based on separation of mononuclear cells from whole blood and detection of specific cell surface markers.

One of the most frequently used methods for obtaining lymphocytes is density gradient centrifugation with Ficoll-Hypaque. Ficoll-Hypaque is available commercially and has a specific gravity that varies between 1.077 and 1.114, depending on the manufacturer.[42] Diluted defibrinated or heparinized blood is carefully layered on top of the solution, and the tube is centrifuged. Centrifugation produces three distinct layers: plasma at the top of the tube, a mononuclear layer banding on top of the density gradient solution, and erythrocytes and granulocytes at the bottom of the tube (Fig. 3–13).

Once a lymphocyte population has been obtained, segregation into subsets can be accomplished by the use of fluorescence microscopy or flow cytometry. Both techniques rely on the use of labeled monoclonal antibodies against specific surface antigens. Some of the more common antigens tested for include CD2, CD3, CD4, CD7, and CD8 on T cells and CD19, CD20, CD22, and surface immunoglobulin on B cells.[24,43]

Fluorescence Microscopy

Staining of lymphocytes can be done in either a direct or an indirect manner. Direct immunofluorescence involves the use of monoclonal antibodies to which a fluorescent tag is attached. The most commonly used dyes are fluorescein and phycoerythrin, which produce color at a wavelength of 490 nm, and rhodamine, which is excited at a wavelength of 545 nm.

Indirect immunofluorescence uses an unlabeled antibody that first combines with the antigen by itself. Then an anti-immunoglobulin that is complexed to a dye is added. This will react only with cells previously coated with antibody (Fig. 3–14). Fluorescence is read manually with a fluorescence microscope. It takes experience to be able to read correctly and screen out extraneous background material (refer to Chapter 11 for additional details on immunofluorescence). Additionally, it is difficult to obtain quantitative data. For these reasons, flow cytometry has essentially replaced microscopic methods in the clinical laboratory.[44]

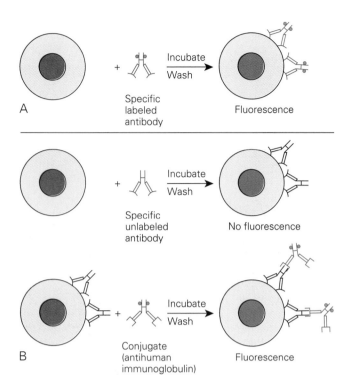

FIG. 3–14. Immunofluorescence. *(A)* Direct immunofluorescence. Fluorescent-labeled antibody directed against a specific CD marker is applied to a slide prepared with patient cells. The slide is washed, and if the marker is present, cells fluoresce under a fluorescent microscope. *(B)* Indirect immunofluorescence. Specific unlabeled antibody is applied to a slide with patient cells. The slide is washed, and a labeled antibody conjugate is added. This second antibody is directed against human immunoglobulin. If specific antibody is bound to patient cells, the second antibody will bind to the first antibody. The slide is washed again, and fluorescence indicates presence of the specific marker.

Cell Flow Cytometry

Cell flow cytometry is an automated system for identifying cells based on the scattering of light as cells flow in single file through a laser beam. Scattering is read in both a forward and a side direction. The amount of forward light scatter (LS) is a measure of cell size, while side scatter is a measure of granularity. Components of a flow cytometer, also known as a fluorescence-activated cell sorter, include a sample delivery system, a laser for cell illumination, photodetectors for signal detection, and a computer-based management system (Fig. 3–15).[44] A pressurized isotonic sheath fluid surrounds the flow cell. The sheath fluid and the sample both emerge from the flow chamber through a small opening. The difference in pressure between the sheath fluid and the sample keeps cells to

the center and creates a laminar flow, or stream of cells that flow in single file.

As a cell enters the laser beam, light is scattered in many directions. Optical detectors located at specific angles from the LS pick up the light scattering, and the scattered light is converted to electrical impulses by photomultiplier tubes.[44] These signals are converted to digital signals and displayed on a histogram that contains a number of channels or bins. Forward LS (angles from 2 to 10 degrees) relates to cell size. Light scattered at 90 degrees relates to the internal cell structure, especially granularity. Thus, the combination of these two values can be used to characterize different cell types (Fig. 3–16).

Parameters, or gates, can be chosen to analyze only lymphocytes. Gating means placing a cursor in a location so that a negative population appears on one side, and a positive population on the other side. This allows for screening out of debris and also localization of subpopulations of cells. Fluorescent antibodies are used to screen for subpopulations, such as B cells, T helper cells, and T cytotoxic cells. The antibodies used are monoclonal, and each has a different fluorescent tag. The percent of cells exhibiting fluorescence of a certain wavelength is determined. The absolute number and percent of lymphocytes is obtained by doing a complete blood count and a differential. This is a very sensitive and accurate technique.[44] Figure 3–17 gives some examples of how cell flow patterns are used to identify particular lymphocyte populations.

Applications of flow cytometry include actual physical separation of cells in addition to identification of specific populations. Enumeration of CD4+ T cells remains the highest volume test because this is used in classifying stages of human immunodeficiency virus infection.[42] Other uses include identification of leukemias and lymphomas.

Other Methods

The rosette technique using sheep red blood cells has been a historical method for enumeration of T lymphocytes. Lymphocytes are separated out from whole blood and then mixed with a suspension of sheep red blood cells. If three or more red blood cells are attached to a lymphocyte, this is considered a rosette. Using a counting chamber, 200 cells are counted and the percent forming rosettes is calculated. This technique is not as precise as those mentioned previously because rosetting can be influenced by cold-reacting antilymphocyte antibodies that are formed in diseases such as rheumatoid arthritis and infectious mononucleosis. Therefore, this method is no longer used in clinical laboratories.

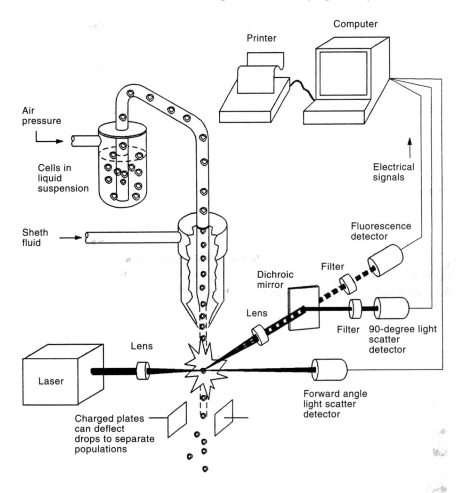

FIG. 3–15. Flow cytometry. Components of a laser-based flow cytometer include a fluid system for cell transportation, a laser for cell illumination, photodetectors for signal detection, and a computer-based management system. Both forward and 90-degree LS are measured, indicating cell size and type.

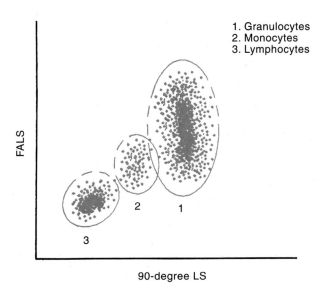

1. Granulocytes
2. Monocytes
3. Lymphocytes

FIG. 3–16. Peripheral blood leukocyte analysis by simultaneous evaluation of forward-angle light scatter (FALS) and 90-degree LS. (From Harmening, D: Clinical Hematology and Fundamentals of Hemostasis, ed. 3. FA Davis, Philadelphia, 1997, with permission.)

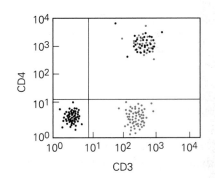

FIG. 3–17. Example of a flow pattern using two different markers. CD3 identifies the T cell population. CD4 identifies the percentage of the T cell population that are T helper cells (CD4$^+$). Three distinct populations are identified: CD3$^+$CD4$^+$ in the upper right quadrant; CD3$^+$CD4$^-$ in the lower right quadrant; and CD3$^-$CD4$^-$ in the lower left quadrant.

Monoclonal antibodies with an enzyme label are also available, and these do not require use of a fluorescence microscope to read. Enzyme-linked immunosorbent assay methods typically use antibodies to specific CD antigens, and these are reacted with the sample.

After washing, a second antibody with an enzyme tag is reacted with the specimen. A second wash step is performed, and then substrate is added. A color change will take place if the specific antigen is present. This technique is particularly useful in analysis of tissue sections.

SUMMARY

All undifferentiated lymphocytes arise in the bone marrow from hematopoietic stem cells. They mature in the primary lymphoid organs. For B cells this takes place in the bone marrow itself, while T cells acquire their specificity in the thymus. B and T cells can be recognized by the presence of surface antigens, or CDs, that are detected by monoclonal antibodies. B cell markers include CD19, MHC class II proteins, and surface immunoglobulins. The surface immunoglobulins act as receptors for antigen. MHC class II proteins allow B cells to interact with T helper cells in the production of antibody. When contact with specific antigen occurs, B cells differentiate into plasma cells, which produce antibody. In the process, memory cells are also created. These can rapidly respond the next time that same antigen is seen. Production of antibody is known as humoral immunity.

T cells are distinguished by the presence of CD3, CD2, and either CD4 or CD8. CD2 is the receptor that interacts with sheep red blood cells to form rosettes, a simple test for the enumeration of T cells. Cells that express CD4 belong to a T cell subset that includes helper/inducer cells, while CD8-carrying T cells are cytotoxic/suppressor cells. The CD3 marker serves as the receptor for antigen. The major portion of it is common to all T cells, but two chains, the alpha and beta chains, contain variable regions that are able to bind to only certain antigens. T cells go through a positive and then a negative selection process, whereby the surviving cells recognize MHC determinants along with foreign antigen. The T cells are responsible for cell-mediated immunity, which involves production of cytokines that serve as regulatory factors for the immune response.

A third class of lymphocytes, known as NK cells, are found in the peripheral blood and represent 5 to 15 percent of the total lymphocyte population. These are larger and contain more cytoplasm and granules than T cells or B cells. They are responsible for killing target cells, including virally infected and cancerous cells, without previous exposure or sensitization to them. They do this by recognizing missing self-MHC antigens, in addition to detecting the presence of stress proteins on infected and cancerous cells. This is an important first line of defense against invasion by such cells.

Laboratory determination of individual lymphocyte populations is essential in diagnosis of such conditions as lymphomas, immunodeficiency diseases, unexplained infections, or acquired immune diseases, including AIDS. Lymphocytes are identified using monoclonal antibodies directed against specific surface antigens. Reactions can be identified manually by employing a fluorescence microscope, by immunoenzyme staining methods, or through the use of cell flow cytometry, which categorizes cells on the basis of light scattering. Automated methods eliminate subjectivity and are more precise, although more costly.

Case Studies

1. A 3-year-old male child is sent for immunologic testing because of recurring respiratory infections, including several bouts of pneumonia. The results show decreased immunoglobulin levels, especially of IgG. Although his white blood cell count was within the normal range, the lymphocyte count was low. Flow cytometry was performed to determine if a particular subset of lymphocytes was low or missing. It was determined that he had a low number of CD3+ lymphocytes, although the CD19+ lymphocyte population was normal. How can this be interpreted? How can this account for his recurring infections?

2. A 33-year-old female with symptoms of fatigue and a low-grade fever sought medical attention. Although her red blood cell count was within the normal range, her white blood cell count was greatly elevated. The following flow cytometry pattern was obtained when white blood cells were separated and analyzed (Fig. 3–18). What type of white blood cells are present? Are they precursor cells or more highly differentiated?

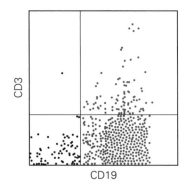

FIG. 3–18. Flow cytometry pattern for case study.

Exercise: Enumeration of T Cells

PRINCIPLE

Lymphocytes are separated from whole blood by using a ficoll density gradient, which causes erythrocytes and granulocytes to settle at the bottom of a conical centrifuge tube while mononuclear cells form a layer at the top of the gradient. Sheep red blood cells are used to identify the T cell population of lymphocytes because these spontaneously complex with T cells through the CD2 receptor. If three or more sheep cells surround a T cell, this is known as a rosette. Quantitation of T cells provides information about cell-mediated immunity, which plays an important role in regulation of the immune response and defense against virally infected or cancerous cells.

SPECIMEN COLLECTION

Collect blood by venipuncture using sterile technique. A freshly drawn heparinized blood specimen is needed for this procedure because use of ethylenediaminetetra-acetic acid (EDTA) will result in poor recovery of mononuclear cells. An additional EDTA tube may be drawn for a complete blood cell count and a differential.

REAGENTS, MATERIALS, AND EQUIPMENT

Centrifuge
Microscope slides
Coverslips, 22 × 22 mm
Pasteur pipettes
Disposable serologic pipettes: 1 mL, 5 mL, 10 mL
Conical plastic centrifuge tubes
Glass test tubes, 12 × 75 mm
Histopaque-1077 (Sigma Diagnostics, St. Louis, Missouri) or other Ficoll-Hypaque solution
Sheep red blood cells (Becton-Dickinson)
Sterile phosphate buffered saline (PBS)

PROCEDURE

1. Add 3 mL of Histopaque-1077 to a 15-mL plastic conical centrifuge tube.
2. Dilute 3 mL of heparinized blood with an equal amount of sterile phosphate buffered saline (PBS). Mix and carefully layer on top of the Histopaque-1077.
3. Centrifuge at 400 × g at room temperature for 30 minutes. Allow the centrifuge to coast to a stop. Do not use the brake. The opaque interface that develops is the mononuclear layer.
4. Aspirate and discard the upper layer to within 0.5 cm of the mononuclear layer.

5. Carefully remove the opaque interface with a capillary pipette and dispense into a 15-mL centrifuge tube. Do not exceed 1.5 mL total volume in the transfer. Add 10 mL of PBS, mix well, and centrifuge at 400 × g for 10 minutes.
6. Decant the supernatant, and drain the last drops by inverting the tube on top of a paper towel.
7. Add 1 mL of PBS, and resuspend the cells by aspirating carefully with a Pasteur pipette.
8. Obtain a final cell count of 6×10^6 cells/mL with a hemacytometer. Fill the counting chamber, and count the cells in the four corner squares of the chamber. Multiply by 20 to obtain the total number of mononuclear cells harvested. Add more buffer if further dilution is necessary.
   NOTE: The instructor can prepare the cell suspension before the laboratory begins if time is short.
9. Prepare sheep red blood cell suspension by placing about 3 mL of sheep red blood cells in a 15-mL centrifuge tube and filling with buffer. Centrifuge for 10 minutes at 400 × g. Resuspend 0.1 mL of packed cells in 19.9 mL buffer to achieve a concentration of 0.5 percent.
10. Pipette 0.5 mL of the lymphocyte suspension into a 12-× 75-mm test tube. Pipette 0.5 mL of sheep red blood cell suspension into the same tube, and mix well.
11. Centrifuge mix at 250 × g for 5 minutes. Remove the centrifuge tube carefully so the cells are not disturbed. Incubate at room temperature for 1.5 to 2 hours. Cells can also be incubated overnight at 4°C, if preferred.
12. After incubation, carefully resuspend the cells by holding the tube almost horizontal and carefully twisting around the long axis.
13. With a capillary pipette and no bulb, gently transfer the rosettes to a clean microscope slide and add a cover slip. Place the cover slip carefully so that no air bubbles are formed. Observe the rosettes using a 40 × objective.
14. Count only those lymphocytes that are surrounded by three or more sheep red cells. Count a total of 200 lymphocytes, including those that do not form rosettes. The percent of T lymphocytes can be obtained by dividing the number of lymphocytes in rosettes by the total number of lymphocytes counted.

INTERPRETATION OF RESULTS

In a normal adult T lymphocytes compose 52 to 81 percent of the total number of lymphocytes. A low percent of T lymphocytes may be an indicator of a T cell disorder. Some of these conditions include AIDS, Hodgkin's disease, chronic lymphocytic leukemia, and immunodeficiency diseases.

Care must be taken in the performance of this procedure. Rosettes can be disrupted, so resuspension after centrifugation must be done very gently, otherwise the percent of T lymphocytes will be falsely lowered. In addition, lymphocytes must be distinguished from sheep red blood cells because both cells are about the same size. Lymphocytes, however, are more refractile because of the presence of a nucleus.

The mononuclear layer also contains monocytes. These should not be counted as nonrosetting lymphocytes because this too will falsely lower the percent of T cells found. Monocytes are considerably larger than lymphocytes, and they contain more cytoplasm, which has a granular appearance.

This technique is not as accurate a detection of specific antigens with monoclonal antibody because of the fragile nature of the rosettes formed. It is, however, less expensive to perform and is of historic significance because this represents the first means of T cell identification.

Bibliography

Baseler, MW, et al: Immunologic evaluation of patients with human immunodeficiency virus infection. In Rose, NR, et al (eds): Manual of Clinical Immunology, ed. 5. American Society for Microbiology, Washington, D.C., 1997, p 764–772.

Myers, RL: Immunology: A Laboratory Manual. WC Brown, Dubuque, Iowa, 1989.

Review Questions

1. Which of the following is a primary lymphoid organ?
   a. Lymph node
   b. Spleen
   c. Thymus
   d. MALT

2. What type of cells would be found in a primary follicle?
   a. Unstimulated B cells
   b. Germinal centers ⎫
   c. Plasma cells   ⎬ secondary follicle
   d. Memory cells   ⎭

3. Which of the following is true of NK cells?
   a. They rely on memory for antigen recognition
   b. They share antigens with B cells
   c. They are found mainly in lymph nodes
   d. They recognize a lack of MHC proteins

4. Where are all undifferentiated lymphocytes made?
   a. Bone marrow
   b. Thymus
   c. Spleen
   d. Lymph nodes

5. In the thymus, positive selection of immature T cells is based upon recognition of which of the following?
   a. Self-antigens
   b. Stress proteins
   c. MHC antigens
   d. μ chains

6. Which of these are found on a mature B cell?
   a. IgG and IgD
   b. IgM and IgD
   c. Alpha and beta chains
   d. CD3

7. Which receptor on T cells is responsible for rosetting with sheep red blood cells?
   a. CD2
   b. CD3
   c. CD4
   d. CD8

8. Which of the following can be attributed to antigen-stimulated T cells?
   a. Humoral response
   b. Plasma cells
   c. Cytokines
   d. Antibody

9. Which is a distinguishing feature of a pre-B cell?
   a. μ chains in the cytoplasm
   b. Complete IgM on the surface
   c. Presence of CD21 antigen
   d. Presence of CD25 antigen

10. When does genetic rearrangement for coding of light chains take place?
    a. Before the pre-B cell stage
    b. As the cell becomes an immature B cell
    c. Not until the cell becomes a mature B cell
    d. When the B cell becomes a plasma cell

11. Which of the following antigens are found on the T cell subset known as helper/inducers?
    a. CD3
    b. CD4
    c. CD8
    d. CD11

12. Where does the major portion of antibody production occur?
    a. Peripheral blood
    b. Bone marrow
    c. Thymus
    d. Lymph nodes

13. Which of the following would represent a double-negative thymocyte?
    a. CD2−CD3+CD4-CD8+
    b. CD2+CD3−CD4−CD8−
    c. CD2-CD3+CD4+CD8−
    d. CD2+CD3+CD4+CD8−

14. Flow cytometry separates cells on the basis of which of the following?
    a. Forward and side LS of an interrupted beam of light
    b. Front angle scatter only of an interrupted light beam
    c. Absorbance of light by different types of cells
    d. Transmittance of light by cells in solution

References

1. Morris, MW, and Davey, FR: Basic examination of blood. In Henry, JB (ed): Clinical Diagnosis and Management by Laboratory Methods, ed. 19. WB Saunders, Philadelphia, 1996.
2. Hutchison, RE, and Davey, FR: Hematopoiesis. In Henry, JB (ed): Clinical Diagnosis and Management by Laboratory Method, ed. 19. WB Saunders, Philadelphia, 1996.
3. Shortman, K, and Wu, L: Early T lymphocyte progenitors. Annu Rev Immunol 14:29–47, 1996.
4. Benoist, C, and Mathis, D: T-lymphocyte differentiation and biology. In Paul, WE (ed): Fundamental Immunology, ed. 4. Lippincott Williams & Wilkins, Philadelphia, 1999, pp 367–405.
5. Parslow, TG: Lymphocytes and lymphoid tissue. In Stites, DP, Terr, AI,

and Parslow, TG (eds): Medical Immunology, ed. 9. Appleton & Lange, Stamford, Conn., 1997.

6. Weissman, IL, and Shizuru, JA: Immune reconstitution. N Engl J Med 341:1227, 1999.

7. Nossal, GJ: Negative selection of lymphocytes. Cell 76:229, 1994.

8. Lydyard, P, and Grossi, C: The lymphoid system. In Roitt, IM, Brostoff, J, and Male, DK (eds): Immunology, ed. 5. Mosby, St. Louis, 1996, pp 31–41.

9. Goldsby, RA, Kindt, TJ, and Osborne, BA: Cells and organs of the immune system. In Goldsby, RA, et al (eds): Kuby Immunology, ed. 4. WH Freeman, New York, 2000, pp 27–62.

10. Shaw, S, Turni, LA, and Katz, KS (eds): Protein reviews on the web. Available on the Internet at http://www.ncbi.nlm.nih.gov/PROW/

11. Melchers, F, and Rolinck, A: B-lymphocyte development and biology. In Paul, WE (ed): Fundamental Immunology, ed. 4. Lippincott Williams & Wilkins, Philadelphia, 1999, pp 183–216.

12. Goldsby, RA, Kindt, TJ, and Osborne, BA: B-cell generation, activation, and differentiation. In Goldsby, RA, et al (eds): Kuby Immunology, ed. 4. WH Freeman, New York, 2000, pp 269–300.

13. Schatz, DG: Developing B-cell theories. Nature 400:614, 1999.

14. Delves, PJ, and Roitt, IM: The immune system. First of two parts. N Engl J Med 343:37, 2000.

15. DeFranco, AL: B-cell development and the humoral immune response. In Stites, DP, Terr, AI, and Parslow, TG (eds): Medical Immunology, ed. 9. Appleton & Lange, Stamford, Conn., 1997, pp 115–129.

16. Glimcher, LH, and Singh, H: Transcription factors in lymphocyte development: T and B cells get together. Cell 96:13, 1999.

17. von Boehmer, H: Positive selection of lymphocytes. Cell 76:219, 1994.

18. Melchers, F: Fit for life in the immune system? Surrogate L chain tests H chains that test L chains. Proc Natl Acad Sci USA 96:2571, 1999.

19. Horejsi, V: Surface antigens of human leukocytes. Adv Immunol 49:75, 1991.

20. Janeway, CA, and Travers, P: Immunobiology: The Immune System in Health and Disease. Garland, New York, 1994.

21. Melamed, D, Benschop RJ, and Cambier, JC, et al: Developmental regulation of B lymphocyte immune tolerance compartmentalizes clonal selection from receptor selection. Cell 92:173, 1998.

22. Cruse, JM, and Lewis, RE (eds): Atlas of Immunology, CRC Press, Boca Raton, Fla., 1998.

23. Rodewald, HR, and Fehling, HJ: Molecular and cellular events in early thymocyte development. In Dixon, FJ (ed): Advances in Immunology. Academic Press, San Diego, 1998.

24. Imboden, JB: T lymphocytes and natural killer cells. In Stites, DP, Terr, AI, and Parslow, TG (eds): Medical Immunology, ed. 9. Appleton & Lange, Stamford, Conn., 1997.

25. Lydyard, P, and Grossi, C: Development of the immune system. In Roitt, IM, Brostoff, J, and Male, DK (eds): Immunology, ed. 5. Mosby, St. Louis, 1996, pp 155–169.

26. Webb, LM, Foxwell, BM, and Feldmann, M: Putative role for interleukin-7 in the maintenance of the recirculating naive CD4+ T-cell pool. Immunology 98:400, 1999.

27. Goldsby, RA, Kindt, TJ, and Osborne, BA: T-cell maturation, activation, and differentiation. In Goldsby, RA, et al (eds): Kuby Immunology, ed. 4. WH Freeman, New York, 2000, pp 239–267.

28. Fink, PJ, and Bevan, MJ: Positive selection of thymocytes. In Dixon, FJ (ed): Advances in Immunology. Academic Press, San Diego, 1995.

29. Hagmann, M: A trigger of natural and other killers. Science 285:645, 1999.

30. van Meerwijk, JP, and Germain, RN: Development of mature CD8+ thymocytes: Selection rather than instruction? Science 261:911, 1993.

31. Barton, GM, and Rudensky, AY: Requirements for diverse, low-abundance peptides in positive selection of T cells. Science 283:67, 1999.

32. Hagmann, M: How the immune system walks memory lane. Science Now July 12:4, 2000.

33. Natural killer cells. In Paul, WE (ed): Fundamental Immunology, ed. 4. Lippincott Williams & Wilkins, Philadelphia, 1999.

34. Lydyard, P, and Grossi, C: Cells involved in the immune response. In Roitt, IM, Brostoff, J, and Male, DK (eds): Immunology, ed. 5. Mosby, St. Louis, 1996, pp 13–30.

35. Moretta, L, Ciccone, E, and Mingari, MC, et al: Human natural killer cells: Origin, clonality, specificity, and receptors. Adv Immunol 55:341, 1994.

36. Goldsby, RA, Kindt, TJ, and Osborne, BA: Cell-mediated effector responses. In Goldsby, RA, et al (eds): Kuby Immunology, ed. 4. WH Freeman, New York, 2000, pp 351–370.

37. Davis, DM, Chiu, I, and Fassett, M, et al: The human natural killer cell immune synapse. Proc Natl Acad Sci USA 96:15062, 1999.

38. Colonna, M: Immunology. Unmasking the killer's accomplice. Nature 391:642, 1998.

39. Wu, J, Song, Y, and Bakker, AB, et al: An activating immunoreceptor complex formed by NKG2D and DAP10. Science 285:730, 1999.

40. Bauer, S, Groh, V, and Wu, J, et al: Activation of NK cells and T cells by NKG2D, a receptor for stress-inducible MICA. Science 285:727, 1999.

41. Rook, G, and Balkwill, F: Cells involved in the immune response. In Roitt, IM, Brostoff, J, and Male, DK (eds): Immunology, ed. 5. Mosby, St. Louis, 1996, pp 121–138.

42. Baseler, MW, et al: Immunologic evaluation of patients with human immunodeficiency virus infection. In Rose, NR, De MacArio, EC, and Folds, JD, et al (eds): Manual of Clinical Laboratory Immunology, ed. 5. American Society for Microbiology, Washington, DC, 1997, pp 764–772.

43. Kidd, PG, and Nicholson, JKA: Immunophenotyping by flow cytometry. In Rose, NR, De MacArio, EC, and Folds, JD, et al (eds): Manual of Clinical Laboratory Immunology, ed. 5. American Society for Microbiology, Washington, DC, 1997, pp 229–244.

44. Flow cytometry. In Stites, DP, Terr, AI, and Parslow, TG (eds): Medical Immunology, ed. 9. Appleton & Lange, Stamford, Conn., 1997.

chapter 4

Nature of Antigens and the Major Histocompatibility Complex

Learning Objectives

After finishing this chapter, the reader will be able to:
1. Define and characterize the nature of immunogens.
2. Differentiate an immunogen from an antigen.
3. Identify the characteristics of a hapten.
4. Describe how an epitope relates to an immunogen.
5. Discuss the role of adjuvants.
6. Differentiate heterophile antigens from alloantigens and autoantigens.
7. Explain what a haplotype is in regard to inheritance of major histocompatibility complex (MHC) antigens.
8. Describe differences in structure of class I and class II proteins.
9. Compare the transport of antigen to cellular surfaces by class I and class II proteins.
10. Describe the role of transporters associated with antigen processing (TAP) in selecting peptides for binding to class I molecules.
11. Discuss the differences in the source and types of antigen processed by class I and class II molecules.
12. Explain the clinical significance of the class I and class II molecules.

Key Terms

Adjuvant	Conformational epitope	Immunogen
Allele	Epitope	Invariant chain (Ii)
Alloantigen	Haplotype	Linear epitope
Antigen	Hapten	Transporters associated
Autoantigen	Heteroantigen	with antigen
Class I MHC (HLA) molecule	Heterophile antigen	processing (TAP)
Class II MHC (HLA)	Major histocompatibility	
molecule	complex (MHC)	

The immune response of lymphocytes is triggered by materials called immunogens. An **immunogen** is a macromolecule capable of eliciting the formation of immunoglobulins (antibodies) or sensitized cells in an immunocompetent host. The immunogen will then specifically react with the antibodies or sensitized cells that have been induced. The term **antigen** is used to refer to a substance that reacts with antibody or sensitized cells but may or may not be able to evoke an immune response in the first place.[1] Thus, all immunogens are antigens, but the converse is not true. However, many times the terms are used synonymously, and the distinction between them is not made. In discussing serologic reactions or particular names of substances such as blood groups, the term antigen is still more commonly used; hence both terms are used in this chapter.

One of the most exciting new areas of research focuses on how and why we respond to particular immunogens. It is now known that this response is caused by a combination of factors: the nature of the immunogen itself, genetic coding of molecules called MHC molecules that must combine with an immunogen before T cells are able to respond, and immunogen processing and presentation. This chapter focuses on all three areas and discusses future clinical implications of some recent findings.

Factors Influencing the Immune Response

Several factors such as age, dose, route of inoculation, overall health, and genetic capacity influence the nature of this response. In general, older individuals are more likely to have a decreased response to antigenic stimulation. At the other end of the age scale, neonates do not fully respond to immunogens because their immune systems are not completely developed. In addition, individuals who are malnourished, fatigued, or stressed are less likely to mount a successful immune response. Generally, the larger the dose of an immungen one is exposed to, the greater the immune response is. However, very large doses can result in T and B cell tolerance, a phenomenon that is not well understood. There also appears to be a genetic predisposition that allows individuals to respond to particular immunogens. This predisposition is linked to the MHC, which is discussed in a later section, and to the receptors generated during T and B lymphocyte development.

Traits of Immunogens

In general, the ability of an immunogen to stimulate a host response depends on the following characteristics: (1) macromolecular size, (2) chemical composition and molecular complexity, (3) foreignness, and (4) the ability to be processed and presented with MHC molecules.[1,2] Usually an immunogen must have a molecular weight of at least 100,000 to be recognized by the immune system.[1,2] There are exceptions, however, because a few substances with a molecular weight of less than 1000 have been known to induce an immune response. For the most part, the rule of thumb is that the greater the molecular weight, the more potent the molecule is as an immunogen.

Immunogenicity is also determined by the chemical composition and molecular complexity of a substance. Proteins and polysaccharides are the best immunogens. Proteins are good immunogens because they are made up of a variety of units known as amino acids. The particular sequential arrangement of amino acids (primary structure) determines the secondary structure (relative orientation of amino acids within the chain) the tertiary structure, which embodies the spatial or three-dimensional orientation of the entire molecule, and the quaternary structure, which is based on the association of two or more chains into a single poly-

meric unit.[2] Because of the variations in subunits, proteins may have an enormous variety of three-dimensional shapes; in contrast, synthetic polymers such as nylon or Teflon are made up of a few simple repeating units with no bending or folding within the molecule, and these materials are nonimmunogenic. For this reason, they are used in making artificial heart valves, elbow replacements, and other medical appliances.

Carbohydrates are somewhat less immunogenic than protein because the units of sugars are more limited than the number of amino acids in protein. As immunogens, carbohydrates most often occur in the form of glycolipids or glycoproteins. Many of the blood group antigens are made up of such carbohydrate complexes. For example, the A, B, and H blood group antigens are glycolipids, and the Rh and Lewis antigens are glycoproteins.[3] Pure nucleic acids and lipids are not immunogenic by themselves, although a response can be generated when they occur in conjunction with other substances.[1] This is the case for autoantibodies to deoxyribonucleic acid (DNA) that are formed in the disease systemic lupus erythematosus. These autoantibodies are actually stimulated by a DNA-protein complex rather than DNA itself.

Another characteristic that all immunogens share is foreignness. The immune system is normally able to distinguish between self and nonself, and those substances recognized as nonself are immunogenic. This ability is acquired as lymphocytes mature in the primary lymphoid organs. Any lymphocyte capable of reacting with self-antigen is normally eliminated. Typically, the more distant taxonomically the source of the immunogen is from the host, the better it is as a stimulus. For example, plant protein is a better immunogen for an animal than is material from a related animal. Occasionally, however, autoantibodies, or antibodies to self-antigens, are known to exist. This is the exception rather than the rule, and this phenomenon is discussed in a later chapter.

Furthermore, for a substance to elicit an immune response, it must be subject to enzymatic digestion to create small peptides or pieces that can be complexed to MHC molecules to present to responsive lymphocytes.[2,3] The particular MHC molecules produced determine genetic responsiveness to individual antigens. T cells are only able to respond to peptides when MHC molecules present them.

Nature of Epitopes

Although an immunogen must have a molecular weight of at least 100,000, only a small part of the immunogen is actually recognized in the immune response. This key portion of the immunogen is known as the determinant site or **epitope.** Epitopes are molecular shapes or configurations that are recognized by antibody or by T cells, and there is evidence that for proteins an epitope may consist of as few as three to six amino acids.[1] Large molecules may have numerous epitopes, and each one may be capable of triggering specific antibody production or a T cell response. These epitopes may be repeating copies, or they may have differing specificities. They may also be sequential or **linear** (i.e., amino acids following one another on a single chain), or they may be conformational. A **conformational epitope** results from the folding of one chain or multiple chains, bringing certain amino acids from different segments of a linear sequence or sequences into close proximity with each other so they can be recognized together (Fig. 4–1).

Epitopes recognized by B cells differ from those recognized by T cells.[1] Surface antibody on B cells may react with both linear and conformational epitopes present on the surface of an immunogen. Anything that is capable of cross-linking surface immunoglobulin molecules is able to trigger B cell activation. The immunogen does not necessarily have to be degraded first. T cells, on the other hand, only recognize an epitope as a part of a complex formed with MHC proteins on the surface of an antigen-presenting cell. The antigen-presenting cell must process an immunogen first and degrade it into small peptides for it to be recognized by T cells (see the section on antigen processing). Thus, T cell epitopes are linear but may be molecules found anywhere in the cell, rather than strictly surface molecules.

Haptens

Some substances are too small to be recognized by themselves, but if they are complexed to larger molecules, they are then able to stimulate a response. **Haptens** are nonimmunogenic materials that, when combined with a carrier, create new antigenic determinants. Once antibody production is initiated, the hapten is capable of reaction with antibody even when the hapten is not complexed to a carrier molecule; however, precipitation or agglutination reactions will not occur. The reason for this is that a hapten has a single determinant site and is not capable of forming the crosslinks with more than one antibody molecule that are necessary for precipitation or agglutination (Fig. 4–2).

Haptens may be complexed artificially with carrier molecules in a laboratory setting, or this may occur naturally within a host and set off an immune response. An example of the latter is an allergic reaction to poison ivy. Poison ivy (*Rhus radicans*) contains chemical substances called catechols, which are haptens. Once in contact with the skin, these are able to couple with tissue proteins to form the immunogens that give rise to contact dermatitis. Drug-protein conjugates can result in a life-threatening allergic response. The best known example of this occurs with penicillin.

The most famous study of haptens was conducted by Karl Landsteiner, a German scientist who was known for his discovery of the ABO blood groups. In his book *The Specificity of Serological Reactions,* published in 1917, he detailed the results of an exhaustive study of haptens that has contributed greatly to our knowledge of antigen–antibody reactions. He discovered that antibodies recognize not just chemical features, such as polarity, hydrophobicity, and ionic charge, but that the overall three-dimensional shape is also important.[1] The spatial orientation and the chemical complementarity are responsible for the lock-and-key relationship that allows for tight binding between antibody and epitope (Fig. 4–3).

Relationship of Antigens to the Host

Antigens can be placed in broad categories according to their relationship to the host. **Autoantigens** are those antigens that belong to the host. These do not evoke an immune response under normal circum-

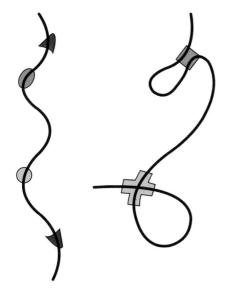

A. Linear epitopes   B. Conformational epitopes

FIG. 4–1. Linear versus conformational epitopes. *(A)* Linear epitopes consist of sequential amino acids on a single polypeptide chain. There may be several different types on one chain. *(B)* Conformational epitopes result from the folding of a polypeptide chain or chains, and nonsequential amino acids are brought into close proximity.

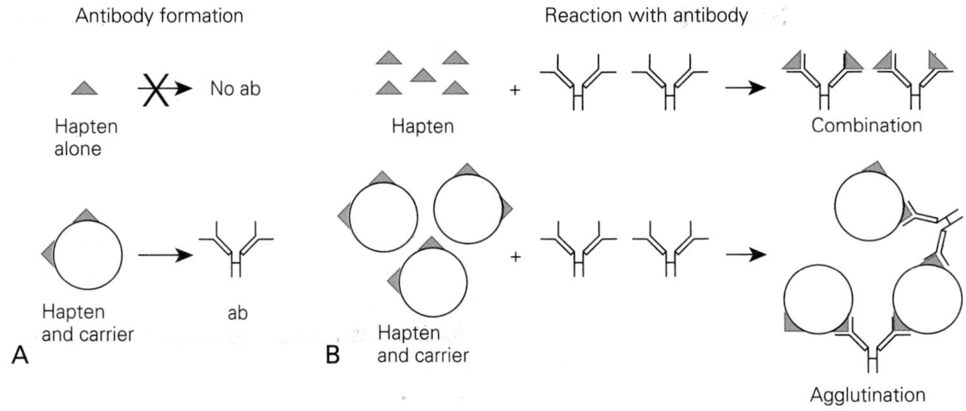

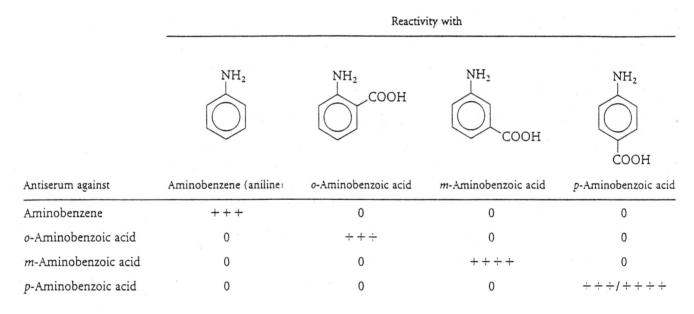

FIG. 4–2. Characteristics of hapten. *(A)* Hapten alone cannot stimulate antibody formation. It can react with antibody, but it is monovalent, so no complexes form. *(B)* When complexed to a carrier, the hapten can stimulate antibody formation. If hapten is complexed to a carrier at multiple sites, then agglutination can take place.

Reactivity with

Antiserum against	Aminobenzene (aniline)	o-Aminobenzoic acid	m-Aminobenzoic acid	p-Aminobenzoic acid
Aminobenzene	+ + +	0	0	0
o-Aminobenzoic acid	0	+ + +	0	0
m-Aminobenzoic acid	0	0	+ + + +	0
p-Aminobenzoic acid	0	0	0	+ + +/+ + + +

FIG. 4–3. Landsteiner's study of the specificity of haptens. Spatial orientation of small groups is recognized because antibodies made against aminobenzene coupled to a carrier will not react with other similar haptens. The same is true for antiserum to o-aminobenzoic acid, m-aminobenzoic acid, and p-aminobenzoic acid. Antibody to a carboxyl group in one location would not react with a hapten, which has the carboxyl group in a different location. (From Landsteiner, K: The Specificity of Serological Reactions, Revised Edition. Dover Press, New York, 1962.)

stances. **Alloantigens** are from other members of the host's species, and these are capable of eliciting an immune response. They are important to consider in tissue transplantation and in blood transfusions. **Heteroantigens** are from other species, such as other animals, plants, or microorganisms.

A **heterophile antigen** is a particular type of heteroantigen. These are antigens that exist in unrelated plants or animals but which are either identical or

closely related in structure so that antibody to one will crossreact with antigen of the other. An example of this is the human blood group A antigen, which is related to pneumococcal polysaccharide type XIV antigen found in pneumococcal bacteria.[4] It is believed that anti-A antibody, which is normally found in individuals with blood types other than A (e.g., type B and type O), is originally formed after exposure to pneumococci or other similar bacteria. Another illustration in nature is the human blood group B antigen, which reacts with antibody to *Escherichia coli*.

Normally in serologic reactions the ideal is to use a reaction that is completely specific, but the fact that crossreactivity exists can be helpful for certain diagnostic purposes. Indeed, the first test for infectious mononucleosis (IM) was based on a heterophile antibody reaction. In IM, during the early states of the disease a heterophile antibody is formed, stimulated by an unknown antigen. This antibody was found to react with sheep red blood cells, and this formed the basis of the Paul-Bunnell screening test for mononucleosis (see Chapter 21). This procedure was a useful screening test when the causative agent of IM had not been identified.

Adjuvants

The power of immunogens to generate an immune response can be increased through the use of adjuvants. An **adjuvant** is a substance administered with an immunogen that increases the immune response. Aluminum salts are the only ones approved for clinical use in the United States, and these are used to complex with the immunogen to increase its size and to prevent a rapid escape from the tissues.[1] Another common adjuvant is Freund's complete adjuvant, which consists of mineral oil, emulsifier, and killed mycobacteria (0.5 mg/mL). Antigen is mixed with adjuvant and then injected. It is released slowly from the injection site. Freund's adjuvant produces granulomas, or large areas of scar tissue, and thus is not used in humans. Adjuvants are thought to enhance the immune response by prolonging the existence of immunogen in the area, increasing the effective size of the immunogen, and increasing the number of macrophages involved in antigen processing.[1,2]

Major Histocompatibility Complex

For years scientists searched to identify postulated immune response genes that would account for differences in how individuals respond to particular immunogens. Recent evidence now indicates that the genetic capability to mount an immune response is linked to a group of molecules originally referred to as human leukocyte antigens (HLA). They were given this name by a French scientist named Dausset because they were first identified on circulating white blood cells.[4] These antigens are also known as MHC molecules because they determine whether transplanted tissue is histocompatible and accepted, or recognized as foreign and rejected. MHC molecules are found not just on white blood cells but on all nucleated cells in the body and play a pivotal role in the development of both humoral and cellular immunity. Their main function is to bring antigen to the cell surface for recognition by T cells because only when antigen is combined with MHC molecules does T cell activation occur. Clinically, they are relevant because they may be involved in transfusion reactions, graft rejection, and autoimmune diseases. Genes controlling expression of these molecules are actually a system of genes known as the **major histocompatibility complex (MHC)**.

Genes Coding for MHC Molecules (HLA Antigens)

The MHC system is the most polymorphic system found in humans.[5,6] Genes coding for the MHC molecules in humans are found on the short arm of chromosome 6 and are divided into three categories or classes. Class I molecules are coded for at three different locations or loci, termed A, B, and C. Class II genes are situated in the D region, and there are several different loci, known as DR, DQ, and DP. For the class II molecules, there is a gene that codes for the alpha chain, and one or more genes that code for the beta chain. Between the class I and class II regions on chromosome 6 is the area of class III genes, which code for complement proteins and cytokines called tumor necrosis factors alpha and beta (Fig. 4–4). Class III proteins are secreted proteins that have an immune function, but they are not expressed on cell surfaces. Class I and II gene products are involved in antigen recognition and influence the repertoire of antigens to which T cells can respond.

At each of these loci, or locations, there is the possibility of multiple alleles. **Alleles** are different forms of a gene that code for slightly different varieties of the same product. The MHC system is described as polymorphic because there are so many possible alleles at each location. For example, at least 266 different alleles of HLA-A, 511 alleles of HLA-B, and 128 alleles of HLA-C have been identified at this time.[7]

The probability that any two individuals will express the same MHC molecules is very low. An individual inherits two copies of chromosome 6, and thus there is a possibility of two different alleles for each gene on the chromosome, unless that individual is homozygous (has the same alleles) at a given location. These genes are described as codominant, meaning that all alleles that an individual inherits code for products that are expressed on cells. For the MHC system, each inherited chromosomal region (called a **haplotype**) consists of a package of genes for A, B, C, DR, DP, and DQ. The full genotype would consist of two of each gene at a particular

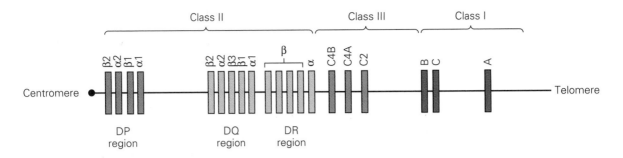

FIG. 4–4. The major histocompatibility complex. Location of the class I, II, and III genes on chromosome 6. Class I consists of loci A, B, and C, while class II has at least three loci, DR, DQ, and DP.

allele. Because there are numerous alleles or varient forms at each locus, an individual's MHC type is about as unique as a fingerprint.

Traditionally, HLA nomenclature has been defined serologically through the use of a battery of antibodies. See Table 4–1 for a listing of current serologically defined HLA groups. Currently, however, advances in DNA analysis have made identification of actual genes possible. The nomenclature has become correspondingly more complex. For instance, the notation HLA DRB1*1301 indicates the actual gene involved in coding for an HLA DR1 antigen, with the B standing for the beta chain, which is a part of the antigen, and the 1301 indicating a specific allele. To simplify matters, serologically defined antigens are used as examples in this chapter.

The uniqueness of the HLA antigens creates a major problem in matching of organ donors because these antigens are highly immunogenic. However, in cases of disputed paternity, polymorphisms can be used as a helpful identification tool. Here HLA testing can show that a man is not a child's father if the child has an HLA allele that is not present in either the mother or the alleged father, or if the child does not possess either of the two alleles that are present in the alleged father at a given locus.[4] If the alleged father does in fact possess all the alleles present in the child that are not from the mother, he is a likely candidate, but paternity cannot be absolutely proven. Consider the following example, which has a simplified list of alleles:

Mother	HLA A2,A3 /B8,B12/ Cw1,Cw3
Child	HLA A3,A9 /B8,B16/ Cw2,Cw1
Father (alleged)	HLA A1,A9 /B7,B14/ Cw2,Cw7

Is it likely that this man is the father of the child? Looking at the child's HLA type, the alleles not found in the mother are A9, B16, and Cw2. The male candidate has A9 and Cw2, but not B16, so this man is excluded as the father of this child.

Structure of Class I Molecules

Each of the MHC genes codes for a protein product that appears on cell surfaces. All of the proteins of a particular class share structural similarities and are found on the same types of cells. **Class I MHC molecules** are expressed on all nucleated cells, although they differ in the level of expression. They are highest on lymphocytes and lowest on liver hepatocytes, neural cells, and muscle cells.[8] This may explain why HLA matching is not done in the case of liver transplants. Additionally, HLA-C antigens are expressed at a lower level than HLA-A and HLA-B antigens, so the latter two are the most important to match for transplantation.[9]

Each class I antigen is a glycoprotein dimer, made up of two noncovalently linked polypeptide chains. The α chain has a molecular weight of 45,000. A lighter chain associated with it, called a β_2-microglobulin, has a molecular weight of 12,000 and is encoded by a single gene on chromosome 15.[9] The α chain is folded into three domains, $\alpha 1$, $\alpha 2$, and $\alpha 3$, and it is inserted into the cell membrane via hydrophobic regions.[8,9] The three external domains consist of about 90 amino acids each, the transmembrane domain has about 25 hydrophobic amino acids along with a short stretch of about 5 hydrophilic amino acids, and an anchor of 30 amino acids (Fig. 4–5). β_2-microglobulin does not penetrate the membrane. X-ray crystallographic studies indicate that the $\alpha 1$ and $\alpha 2$ domains each form an alpha helix, and that these serve as the walls of a deep groove that function as the peptide-binding site in antigen recognition.[8,9] This binding site is able to hold peptides that are between 8 and 10 amino acids long.[8] Most of the polymorphism resides in the $\alpha 1$ and $\alpha 2$

TABLE 4–1. List of Serologically Defined HLA Specificities.

A	B	C	D	DR	DQ	DP
A1	B5	Cw1	Dw1	DR1	DQ1	DPw1
A2	B7	Cw2	Dw2	DR103	DQ2	DPw2
A203	B703	Cw3	Dw3	DR2	DQ3	DPw3
A210	B8	Cw4	Dw4	DR3	DQ4	DPw4
A3	B12	Cw5	Dw5	DR4	DQ5(1)	DPw5
A9	B13	Cw6	Dw6	DR5	DQ6(1)	DPw6
A10	B14	Cw7	Dw7	DR6	DQ7(3)	
A11	B15	Cw8	Dw8	DR7	DQ8(3)	
A19	B16	Cw9(w3)	Dw9	DR8	DQ9(3)	
A23(9)	B17	Cw10(w3)	Dw10	DR9		
A24(9)	B18		Dw11(w7)	DR10		
A2403	B21		Dw12	DR11(5)		
A25(10)	B22		Dw13	DR12(5)		
A26(10)	B27		Dw14	DR13(6)		
A28	B2708		Dw15	DR14(6)		
A29(19)	B35		Dw16	DR1403		
A30(19)	B37		Dw17(w7)	DR1404		
A31(19)	B38(16)		Dw18(w6)	DR15(2)		
A32(19)	B39(16)		Dw19(w6)	DR16(2)		
A33(19)	B3901		Dw20	DR17(3)		
A34(10)	B3902		Dw21	DR18(3)		
A36	B40		Dw22			
A43	B4005		Dw23	DR51		
A66(10)	B41		Dw24	DR52		
A68(28)	B42		Dw25	DR53		
A69(28)	B44(12)		Dw26			
A74(19)	B45(12)					
A80	B46					
	B47					
	B48					
	B49(21)					
	B50(21)					
	B51(5)					
	B5102					
	B5103					
	B52(5)					
	B53					
	B54(22)					
	B55(22)					
	B56(22)					
	B57(17)					
	B58(17)					
	B59					
	B60(40)					
	B61(40)					
	B62(15)					
	B63(15)					
	B64(14)					
	B65(14)					
	B67					
	B70					
	B71(70)					
	B72(70)					
	B73					
	B75(15)					
	B76(15)					
	B77(15)					
	B78					
	B81					
	Bw4					
	Bw6					

From http://www.anthonynolan.com/HIG/lists/specs.html

regions, while the α3 and β2 regions are similar to the constant regions found in immunoglobulin molecules.[10,11] Another group of molecules called the nonclassical class I antigens are designated E, F, and G. This group of molecules, except for G, are not expressed on cell surfaces and do not function in antigen recognition but may play other roles in the immune response. G antigens are expressed on trophoblast cells during the first trimester of pregnancy and are thought to help ensure tolerance for the fetus.[12]

Structure of Class II Molecules

The occurrence of **class II MHC molecules** is much more restricted than that of class I because they are found primarily on antigen-presenting cells which include B lymphocytes, monocytes, macrophages, dendritic cells, and endothelium. The major class II molecules, DP, DQ, and DR, consist of two noncovalently bound polypeptides that are both encoded by genes in the MHC complex. Of the class II molecules, DR is expressed at the highest levels.[7]

Both the α chain, with a molecular weight of 33,000, and the β chain, with a molecular weight of 27,000, are anchored to the cell membrane.[7,8,10,13] Each has two domains, and it is the α1 and the β1 domains that come together to form the peptide-binding site, similar to the one found on class I molecules[7,10] (see Fig. 4–5). However, both ends of the

peptide-binding cleft are open, and this allows for capture of longer peptides than is the case for class I molecules. At least three other class II genes have been described, DM, DN, and DO, the so-called nonclassical class II genes. Products of these genes play a regulatory role in antigen processing.[8]

The main role of the class I and class II antigens is to bind peptides within cells and transport them to the plasma membrane where they can be recognized by T cells. It is thought that the two main classes of these molecules have evolved to deal with two types of infectious agents, those that attack cells from the outside (such as bacteria) and those that attack from the inside (viruses and other intracellular pathogens).[13] Class I molecules present peptides that have been synthesized within the cell to CD8 (cytotoxic) T cells, while class II molecules contribute to antigen recognition by CD4 (helper) T cells. They mainly bind exogenous proteins, those taken into the cell from the outside and degraded.[7,11] Class I molecules are thus the watchdogs of viral, tumor, and certain parasitic antigens within the cell, while the function of the class II molecules is to alert the CD4 T cells to the presence of foreign proteins, such as those produced by bacteria, found outside the cell.[14] In either case, for a T cell response to be triggered, peptides must be available in adequate supply for MHC molecules to bind, they must be able to be bound effectively, and they must be recognized by a T cell receptor.[14,15]

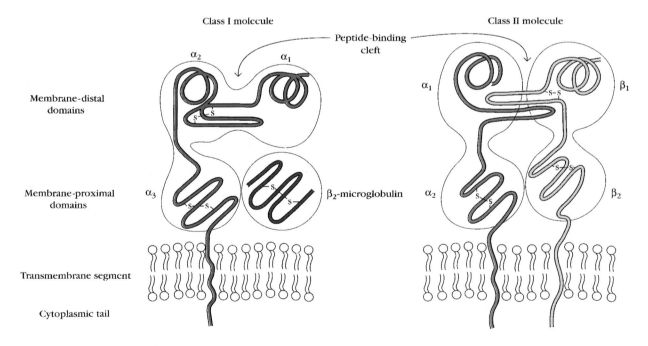

FIG. 4–5. Structure of class I and II MHC products. (From Goldsby, RA, Kindt, TJ, and Osborne, BA: Immunology, ed. 4. WH Freeman, New York, 2000, p 178, with permission.)

The difference in functioning of the two molecules is tied to the mechanisms by which processed antigen is transported to the surface. Both types of molecules, however, must be capable of presenting an enormous array of different antigenic peptides to T cells. The chemistry of the MHC antigens controls what sorts of peptides fit in the binding pockets. These two pathways are discussed in following.

Role of Class I Molecules

Both class I and class II molecules are synthesized in the rough endoplasmic reticulum, and for a time they remain anchored in the endoplasmic reticulum membrane. Class I molecules actually bind peptides while still in the endoplasmic reticulum.[7] In fact, binding helps to stabilize the association of the α chain of class I with the β_2–microglobulin.[16] Before binding with antigen occurs, however, newly synthesized α chains freely bind a molecule called *calnexin*. This 88-kd molecule is membrane-bound in the endoplasmic reticulum, and it keeps the α chain in a partially folded state while it awaits binding to β_2–microglobulin.[8,14] When β_2–microglobulin binds, calnexin is released, and two other chaperone molecules, calreticulin and tapasin, are associated with the complex and help to stabilize it for peptide binding[15] (Fig. 4–6).

Peptides that associate with the class I molecules are approximately nine amino acids in length and derived from partial proteolytic digestion of proteins previously synthesized in the cytoplasm.[8,17] This digestion appears to be carried out by proteases that reside in large cylindrical cytoplasmic complexes called proteosomes.[7,14] Proteosomes consist of approximately 16 to 20 components that degrade proteins in the cytosol.[16] Once cleaved, the peptides are then pumped into the lumen of the endoplasmic reticulum in an ATP-dependent process by specialized transporter proteins.[7] This family of proteins, named **transporters associated with antigen processing (TAP),** are responsible for the adenosine triphosphate-dependent transport, from the cytoplasm to the lumen of the endoplasmic reticulum, of short peptides suitable for binding to class I molecules.[15,16] TAP1 and TAP2 may function as "molecular rulers" to measure the distance between the amino and carboxyl termini of peptides so that only peptides of the correct size are transported. They are most efficient at transporting peptides that are 12 residues or less in length.[14,16,17] Allelic differences in TAP proteins also influence the immune response because they help determine the types of peptides that are best transported. Tapasin may help to bring TAP transporters into close proximity to the newly formed MHC molecules, so that numerous peptides are available to them.[15]

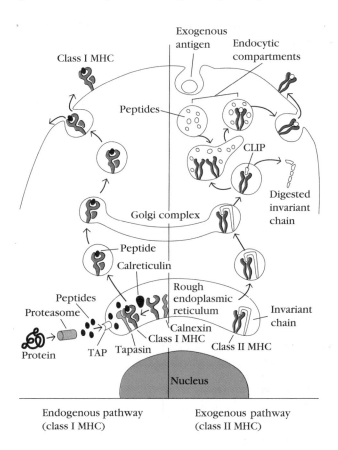

FIG. 4–6. Model of separate antigen-processing pathways for endogenous and exogenous antigens. The mode of antigen entry and the site of processing determines whether peptides associate with class I molecules in the rough endoplasmic reticulum or with class II molecules in endocytic compartments. CLIP = corticotropin-like intermediate lobe peptide; MHC = major histocompatibility complex; TAP = transporters associated with antigen processing. (From Goldsby, RA, Kindt, TJ, and Osborne, BA: Immunology, ed. 4. WH Freeman, New York, 2000, p 209, with permission.)

Tapasin may also help in the loading of peptides into the class I molecules. Once the α chain has bound the peptide, the complex is rapidly transported to the cell surface (see Fig. 4–6).[6]

Of the thousands of peptides that may be processed in this manner, only a small fraction of them (approximately 1 in 2000) actually induce a response in association with class I molecules.[18] These peptides are termed immunodominant. Immunodominant peptides are those that bind with a strong affinity to class I molecules and that produce enough complexes to find CD8+ T cells with a complementary receptor.[18] Binding is based on interaction of only two or three amino acid residues with the class I binding groove. Different class I molecules will have slightly different binding affinities, and it is these small differences that determine to which particular antigens one individual will respond.

It is estimated that a single cell may express about 10^5 copies of each class I molecule, so many different peptides can be captured and expressed in this manner.[19] In healthy cells, these are self-peptides that are ignored by the T cells, while in diseased cells, peptides are derived from viral proteins or proteins associated with cancerous states. Display of hundreds of class I molecules complexed to antigen allows CD8+ T cells to continuously check cell surfaces for the presence of other than self-antigen.[14]

Role of Class II Molecules

Class II molecules, on the other hand, must be transported from the endoplasmic reticulum to an endosomal compartment before they can bind peptides.[7] While still in the endoplasmic reticulum, class II molecules associate with a protein called the **invariant chain (Ii)**, which may cause steric obstruction and prevent interaction of the binding site with any endogenous peptides in the endoplasmic reticulum (ER).[7,13] The invariant chain is a 31-kd protein that is made in excess so that enough is available to bind with all class II molecules shortly after they are synthesized. Ii may be responsible for helping to bring α and β chains together in the ER lumen and then moving them out through the Golgi complex to the endocytic vesicles.[15,20] Because the open structure of class II molecules would permit binding of segments of intact proteins within the ER, Ii may also serve to protect the binding site.[16]

Once bound to the invariant chain, the class II molecule is transported to an endosomal compartment, where it encounters peptides derived from endocytosed, exogenous proteins. Antigen processing may help to unfold molecules and uncover functional sites that are buried deep within the native protein structure.[3] The invariant chain is degraded by a protease, leaving just a small fragment called corticotropin-like intermediate lobe peptide (CLIP) attached to the peptide-binding cleft.[19,21] CLIP is then exchanged for exogenous peptides. Selective binding of peptides may be promoted by the low pH of the endosomal compartment.[16] HLA-DM molecules help to mediate the reaction.[13,19,21] Generally, peptides of approximately 13 to 18 amino acid residues can bind because the groove is open on both ends, unlike class I molecules, which have a closed end.[19,22,23] Conserved amino acids are distributed all along the actual binding site. This allows hydrogen bonding to take place all along the length of the captured peptide, in contrast to class I molecules, which only bond at the amino and carboxy terminal ends.[23,24] There are also several pock-

ets in the class II proteins that easily accommodate amino acid side chains. This gives class II proteins more flexibility in the types of peptides that can be bound.[23,24] Once binding has occurred, the class II protein-peptide complex is transported to the cell surface (see Fig. 4–6). On the cell surface, class II molecules are responsible for formation of a trimolecular complex that occurs between antigen, class II molecule, and an appropriate T cell receptor. If binding occurs with a T cell receptor on a CD4+ T cell, the T helper cell recruits and triggers a B cell response, resulting in antibody formation. The mechanics of this response is discussed in Chapter 6.

Clinical Significance of MHC

Testing for MHC antigens has typically been done because it is known that both class I and class II molecules are capable of inducing a response that leads to graft rejection. Testing methodology has changed from serologic principles to molecular methods, which are much more accurate. The role of the laboratory in transplantation is presented in Chapter 17. MHC antigens also appear to play a role in development of autoimmune diseases. The link between MHC antigens and autoimmune diseases is discussed more fully in Chapter 14.

However, the evidence that both class I and class II molecules play a major role in antigen presentation has more far-reaching consequences. They essentially determine the types of peptides to which an individual can mount an immune response. Although the MHC molecules typically have a broad binding capacity, small differences in these proteins are responsible for differences seen in the ability to react to a specific antigen. It is likely that nonresponders to a particular vaccine, such as hepatitis B, do not have the genetic capacity to respond. Therefore, it will be important to know an individual's MHC type for numerous reasons.

Much of the recent research has focused on the types of peptides that can be bound by particular MHC molecules.[23–25] Future developments may include tailoring vaccines to certain groups of such molecules. As more is learned about antigen processing, vaccines containing certain amino acid sequences that serve as immunodominant epitopes can be specifically developed. This might avoid the risk of using live organisms. Additionally, if an individual suffers from allergies, knowing a person's MHC type might also help predict the types of allergens to which they may be allergic because research in this area is attempting to group allergens according to amino acid structure.[25] It is likely that knowledge of the MHC molecules will affect many areas of patient care in the future.

SUMMARY

To fully comprehend the specificity of antigen–antibody combination, it is essential to understand the principle characteristics of antigens. Antigens are macromolecules that elicit formation of immunoglobulins or sensitized cells in an immunocompetent host. *Immunogen* is a term that is often used synonymously with *antigen*. The term *immunogen* places emphasis on the fact that a host response is triggered, while the term *antigen* is sometimes used to denote a substance that does not elicit a host response but reacts with antibody once it has been formed.

Although immunogenicity is influenced by factors such as age, health, route of inoculation, and genetic capacity, there are certain specific characteristics that are shared by most immunogens: a molecular weight of at least 100,000, molecular complexity, and foreignness to the host. Immunogens themselves are fairly large molecules, but the immune response is keyed to only small portions of these molecules, or epitopes, and very small differences in these epitopes can be detected by the immune system.

Adjuvants are substances that can be mixed with antigen to enhance the immune response. Most adjuvants work by keeping the antigen in the area and by increasing the number of cells involved in the immune response.

The genetic capability to mount an immune response is linked to a group of molecules known as the MHC antigens. The two main classes of these molecules, sometimes referred to as HLA antigens, have evolved to deal with infectious agents that attack cells from the outside (such as bacteria) and those that attack from the inside (viruses and other intracellular pathogens). Class I and class II molecules bind peptides within cells and transport them to the plasma membrane where they can be recognized by T cells. Class I MHC molecules are found on all nucleated cells, and these molecules associate with foreign antigens, such as viral proteins, synthesized within a host cell. Class I molecules are stabilized by the binding of antigen, and the complex is readily transported to the cellular surface. Class II molecules, on the other hand, have a more limited distribution, and these associate with foreign antigens taken into the cell from the outside. Binding of antigen to the class II molecules takes place in endosomal compartments, and then this complex is moved to the outside of the cell. The binding sites on both types of molecules may limit the size and the nature of the antigen bound. Thus, these molecules play a key role in antigen processing and recognition.

Case Study

1. A 25-year-old woman is taking her former boyfriend to court and suing for child support, claiming he is the father of her 3-year-old daughter. The former boyfriend states that the child can't possibly be his. The HLA antigen types of the father, the mother, and the child are submitted as evidence. They are as follows:

Mother   HLA A1A9/B5B12/CW3CW5
Child   HLA A9A11/B5B18/ Cw3Cw8
Father   HLA A9A11/B8B18/Cw5Cw8

Questions:
   a. What are the two likely haplotypes of this child's HLA antigens?
   b. Does one of the haplotypes match that of the alleged father?
   c. Should this man have to pay child support?

Exercise: Specificity of Antigen–Antibody Reactions

PRINCIPLE

Typing serum is an antibody that will react only with the specific red blood cell antigen against which it is directed. Agglutination indicates the presence of that particular antigen.

REAGENTS, MATERIALS, AND EQUIPMENT

- Anti-A typing serum
- Anti-B typing serum
- Group A, group B, and group O reagent red blood cells
- Microscope slides
- Disposable stirrers

PROCEDURE

1. Divide each microscope slide in half, using a wax marking pencil. Label the left side "A" and the right side "B" for the two antisera that will be used.
2. Place one drop of anti-A on the left side of slide and one drop of anti-B to the right side.
3. Add one drop of reagent red blood cell suspension to each side.
4. Mix each side thoroughly with a separate disposable stirrer.
5. Rock slide gently back and forth for 2 minutes.
6. Observe for agglutination.
7. Repeat this procedure for each type of reagent red blood cell.

RESULTS

1. Report any cells that agglutinate with anti-A serum as type A cells and any cells that agglutinate with anti-B serum as type B cells.
2. Agglutination with both types of antisera indicates that both A and B antigens are present, and this is type AB.
3. No agglutination indicates cells have neither antigen, and these belong to group O.

INTERPRETATION OF RESULTS

Red blood cell antigens consist of a lipid–sugar complex that is inserted into the membrane of the cell. The H antigen serves as the building block for both A and B antigens. As can be seen in Figure 4–7, all three antigens differ only by the presence or absence of one sugar. If only H antigen is present, then these cells are typed as O cells. Specific antibody is able to detect the one sugar difference in each of the antigens, and an agglutination reaction will occur only with the antigen against which the antibody is directed.

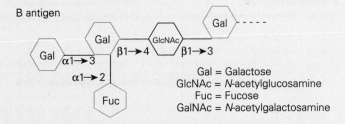

FIG. 4–7. Structure of H, A, and B red cell antigens. (From Walker, R [ed]: Technical Manual of the American Association of Blood Banks, ed. 11. American Association of Blood Banks, Arlington, Vir., 1993, p 207, with permission.)

Review Questions

1. All of the following are characteristic of a good immunogen *except:*
   a. Internal complexity
   b. Large molecular weight
   c. The presence of numerous epitopes
   d. Found on host cells

2. Which of the following best describes a hapten?
   a. Not able to react with antibody
   b. Antigenic only when coupled to a carrier
   c. Has multiple determinant sites
   d. A large chemically complex molecule

3. Which would be the best immunogen?
   a. Protein with a molecular weight of 200,000
   b. Nylon
   c. Polysaccharide with a molecular weight of 250,000
   d. Protein with a molecular weight of 175,000

4. All of the following describe an epitope *except:*
   a. Same as an antigenic determinant site
   b. Area of an immunogen recognized by T cells
   c. Consists of sequential amino acids only
   d. Key portion of the immunogen

5. Adjuvents act by which of the following methods?
   a. Complex to antigen to increase its size
   b. Prevent rapid escape from the tissues
   c. Increase processing of antigen
   d. All of the above

6. A heterophile antigen is one that
   a. Is a self-antigen
   b. Exists in unrelated plants or animals
   c. Has been used previously to stimulate antibody response
   d. Is from the same species but is different from the host

7. Which of the following is true of MHC (HLA) class II antigens:
   a. They are found on all nucleated cells.
   b. They are found on B cells and macrophages.
   c. They all originate at one locus.
   d. They are coded for on chromosome 9.

8. MHC molecules are associated with which of the following:
   a. Graft rejection
   b. Autoimmune diseases
   c. Determining to which antigens an individual responds
   d. All of the above

9. Which of the following best describes the role of TAP?
   a. They bind to class II molecules to help block the antigen-binding site.
   b. They bind to class I proteins in proteosomes.
   c. They transport peptides into the lumen of the endoplasmic reticulum.
   d. They help cleave peptides for transport to endosomes.

10. An individual is recovering from a bacterial infection and tests positive for antibodies to a protein normally found in the cytoplasm of this bacterium. Which of the following statements is true of this situation?
    a. Class I molecules have presented bacterial antigen to CD8+ T cells.
    b. Class I molecules have presented bacterial antigen to CD4+ T cells.
    c. Class II molecules have presented bacterial antigen to CD4+ T cells.
    d. B cells have recognized bacterial antigen without help from T cells.

References

1. Parslow, TG: Immunogens, antigens, and vaccines. In Stites, DP, Terr, AI, and Parslow, TG (eds): Medical Immunology, ed. 9. Appleton & Lange, Stamford, Conn., 1997, pp 74–82.

2. Goldsby, RA, Kindt, TJ, and Osborne, BA: Antigens. In Goldsby, RA, et al (eds): Kuby Immunology, ed. 4. WH Freeman, New York, 2000, pp 63–81.

3. Berzofsky, JA, and Berkower, IJ: Immunogenicity and antigen structure. In Paul, WE (ed): Fundamental Immunology, ed. 4. Lippincott Williams & Wilkins, Philadelphia, 1999, pp 651–698.

4. Bryant, NJ: An Introduction to Immunohematology, ed. 3. WB Saunders, Philadelphia, 1994.

5. Parham, P, and Ohta, T: Population biology of antigen presentation by MHC class I molecules. Science 272:67–74, 1996.

6. Janeway, CA, and Travers, P: Immunobiology: The Immune System in Health and Disease, ed. 2. Garland, New York, 1996.

7. HLA Informatics Group, The Anthony Nolan Trust: The HLA Sequence Database. Accessed January 31, 2003 on the Internet at: http://www.anthonynolan.com/HIG/lists/class1list.html.

8. Brodsky, FM: Antigen presentation and the major histocompatibility complex. In Stites, DP, Terr, AI, and Parslow, TG (eds): Medical Immunology, ed. 9. Appleton & Lange, Stamford, Conn., 1997, pp 83–94.

9. Goldsby, RA, Kindt, TJ, and Osborne, BA: Major histocompatibility complex. In Goldsby, RA, et al (eds): Kuby Immunology, ed. 4. WH Freeman, New York, 2000, pp 173–199.

10. Salter, RD: Structure and function of major histocompatibility complex molecules. In McCluskey, JM (ed): Antigen Processing and Recognition. CRC Press, Boca Raton, Fla., 1991, pp 55–72.

11. Yewdell, JW, and Bennink, JR: Cell biology of antigen processing and presentation to major histocompatibility complex class I molecule-restricted T lymphocytes. Adv Immunol 52:1, 1992.

12. Major histocompatibility complex. In Cruse, JM, and Lewis, RE (eds): Atlas of Immunology, CRC Press, Boca Raton, Fla., 1999, pp 77–89.

13. Pieters, J: MHC class II-restricted antigen processing and presentation. Adv Immunol 75:159–208, 2000.

14. Momburg, F, and Hammerling, GJ: Generation and TAP-mediated

transport of peptides for major histocompatibility complex class I molecules. Adv Immunol 68:191–256, 1998.

15. Germain, RN: Antigen processing and presentation. In Paul, WE (ed): Fundamental Immunology, ed. 4. Lippincott Williams & Wilkins, Philadelphia, 1999, pp 287–336.

16. Germain, RN: MHC-dependent antigen processing and peptide presentation: Providing ligands for T lymphocyte activation. Cell 76:287, 1994.

17. Yewdell, JW, Norbury, CC, and Bennink, JR: Mechanisms of exogenous antigen presentation by MHC class I molecules in vitro and in vivo: implications for generating CD8+ T cell responses to infectious agents, tumors, transplants, and vaccines. Adv Immunol 73:1, 1999.

18. Yewdell, JW, and Bennink, JR: Immunodominance in major histocompatibility complex class I-restricted T lymphocyte responses. Annu Rev Immunol 17:51–88, 1999.

19. Goldsby, RA, Kindt, TJ, and Osborne, BA: Antigen processing and presentation. In Goldsby, RA, et al (eds): Kuby Immunology, ed. 4. WH Freeman, New York, 2000, pp 201–214.

20. Zhong, G, Castellino, F, and Romagnoli, P, et al: Evidence that binding site occupancy is necessary and sufficient for effective major histocompatibility complex (MHC) class II transport through the secretory pathway redefines the primary function of class II-associated invariant chain peptides (CLIP). J Exp Med 184:2061–2066, 1996.

21. Ghosh, P, Amaya, M, and Mellins, E, et al: The structure of an intermediate in class II MHC maturation: CLIP bound to HLA-DR3. Nature 378:457–462, 1995.

22. Brown, JH, Jardetzky, TS, and Gorga, JC, et al: Three-dimensional structure of the human class II histocompatibility antigen HLA-DR1. Nature 364:33, 1993.

23. Jardetzky, TS, Brown, JH, and Gorga, JC, et al: Crystallographic analysis of endogenous peptides associated with HLA-DR1 suggests a common, polyproline II-like conformation for bound peptides. Proc Natl Acad Sci USA 93:734–738, 1996.

24. Stern, LJ, Brown, JH, and Jardetzky, TS, et al: Crystal structure of the human class II MHC protein HLA-DR1 complexed with an influenza virus peptide. Nature 368:215–221, 1994.

25. Aalberse, RC: Structural biology of allergens. J Allergy Clin Immunol 106:228–38, 2000.

Antibody Structure and Function

Learning Objectives

After finishing this chapter, the reader will be able to:
1. Describe the structure of a typical immunoglobulin.
2. Characterize the five immunoglobulin types found in humans.
3. Differentiate between light and heavy chains of immunoglobulins.
4. Describe experimental evidence for the structure of IgG.
5. Relate immunoglobulin structure to function.
6. Compare and contrast the following theories of antibody formation: side-chain theory, template theory, and clonal selection theory.
7. Describe how recent knowledge about immunoglobulin genes supports the clonal selection theory.
8. Discuss the process of monoclonal antibody production.
9. Relate the influence of monoclonal antibodies to current laboratory testing practices.

Key Terms

Allotype	Heavy (H) chain	Kappa (κ) chain
Bence-Jones proteins	Hinge region	Lambda (λ) chain
Class switching	Hybridoma	Light (L) chain
Clonal selection theory	Idiotype	Monoclonal antibody
Constant region	Immunoglobulin	Secretory component (SC)
$F(ab)_2$	Immunoglobulin superfamily	Variable region
Fab fragment	Isotype	
Fc fragment	Joining (J) chain	

When B lymphocytes are stimulated by antigen and undergo differentiation, the end product is antibody or immunoglobulin. **Immunoglobulins** are glycoproteins found in the serum portion of the blood. They are composed of 82- to 96-percent polypeptide and 4- to 18-percent carbohydrate.[1] When subjected to electrophoresis at pH 8.6, the immunoglobulins appear primarily in the gamma (γ) band (Fig. 5–1). Each of the five major classes has slightly different electrophoretic properties. These classes are designated IgG, IgM, IgA, IgD, and IgE. (Ig is an abbreviation for immunoglobulin.)

Immunoglobulins are considered to be the humoral branch of the immune response. They play an essential role in antigen recognition and in biologic activities related to the immune response such as opsonization and the activation of complement. Although each class has unique properties, all immunoglobulin molecules share many common features. In this chapter, the nature of this generalized structure is presented, and then characteristics of each immunoglobulin type are discussed. Specific functions for each of the classes are examined in relation to structural differences.

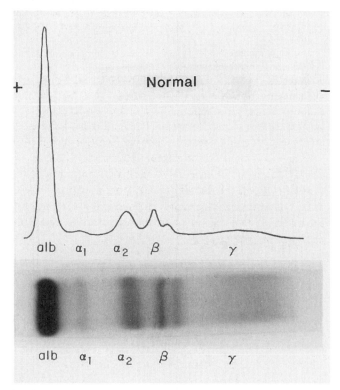

FIG. 5–1. Serum electrophoresis. (From Widmann, FK: An Introduction to Clinical Immunology. FA Davis, Philadelphia, 1989, with permission.)

Tetrapeptide Structure of Immunoglobulins

All immunoglobulin molecules are made up of a basic four-chain polypeptide unit that consists of two large chains, called **heavy** or **H chains,** and two smaller chains, named **light** or **L chains.** These chains are held together by noncovalent forces and disulfide interchain bridges. The basic structure of immunoglobulins was elucidated in the 1950s and 1960s by the efforts of two men, Gerald Edelman working in the United States at the Rockefeller Institute and Rodney Porter at Oxford University in England. For their contributions, these men shared the Nobel Prize in physiology and medicine in 1972. They chose to work with immunoglobulin G.

Edelman's work centered on the use of the analytic ultracentrifuge to separate out immunoglobulins on the basis of molecular weight.[2] He found that intact IgG molecules had a sedimentation coefficient of 7 S. The Svedberg unit (S) is a number that indicates the sedimentation rate in an analytical ultracentrifuge. Larger molecules will travel farther and thus have a larger sedimentation coefficient. On obtaining a purified preparation of IgG, Edelman used 7 M urea to unfold the molecule. Once unfolded, the exposed sulfhydryl bonds could be cleaved by a reducing agent such as mercaptoethanol. After such treatment the material was subjected again to ultracentrifugation, and it was found that two separate fractions, one at 3.5 S and one at 2.2 S, were obtained.

The 3.5 S fraction, with a molecular weight of approximately 50,000, was designated the H chain; the 2.2 S fraction, with a molecular weight of 20,000, was named the L chain. These two pieces occurred in equal amounts, indicating that the formula for IgG had to be H_2L_2. This is the generalized formula for all immunoglobulins.

Cleavage with Papain

Porter's work was based on the use of the proteolytic enzyme papain, which was used to cleave IgG into three pieces of about equal size, each having a sedimentation coefficient of 3.5 S.[1,3] Carboxymethylcellulose ion exchange chromatography separated this material into two types of fragments, one of which spontaneously crystallized at 4°C. This fragment, known as the **Fc fragment** (for fragment crystallizable), had no antigen binding ability and is now known to represent the carboxy-terminal halves of two H chains that are held together by S–S bonding.[4] The Fc fragment is important in effector functions of immunoglobulin molecules, which include opsonization and complement fixation.

The remaining portion was found to have antigen-binding capacity and was named the **Fab fragment** (fragment antigen-binding). Because precipitation would not occur when Fab fragments were allowed to react with antibody, it was guessed that each fragment represented one antigen-binding site and that two such fragments were present in an intact antibody molecule; such a molecule would be able to form a cross-linked complex with antibody, and the complex would precipitate. Each Fab fragment thus consists of one L chain and one half of a H chain, held together by disulfide bonding.[1,3]

Pepsin Digestion

Alfred Nisonoff obtained additional evidence for the structure of immunoglobulins through the use of pepsin.[4] This proteolytic enzyme was found to cleave IgG at the carboxy-terminal side of the interchain disulfide bonds, yielding one piece with all the antigen-binding ability, known as **F(ab)$_2$**, and an additional fragment called Fc', similar to Fc except that it usually disintegrates into several smaller pieces. Thus, a basic picture of the four-chain unit of the immunoglobulin molecule was obtained, which indicated that each L chain was bonded to an H chain by means of an S–S bond, and the H chains were joined to each other by one or more S–S bonds (Fig. 5–2).

The Nature of Light Chains

The difficulty in obtaining a significant amount of a specific immunoglobulin for amino acid analysis was overcome by the discovery that **Bence-Jones proteins,** found in the urine of patients with multiple myeloma, were in fact L chains that were being secreted by the malignant plasma cells.[4] Bence-Jones proteins had been discovered in 1845 by Dr. Henry Bence-Jones, who noted the peculiar behavior of these proteins: When heated to 60°C, they precipitate from urine, but on further heating to 80°C, they redissolve. These characteristics made it possible to isolate the L chains and obtain the amino acid sequence.

Analysis of a number of Bence Jones proteins revealed that there were two main types of L chains, designated **kappa (κ)** and **lambda (λ)**. Each contained between 200 and to 220 amino acids, and from position number 111 on (the amino terminus is

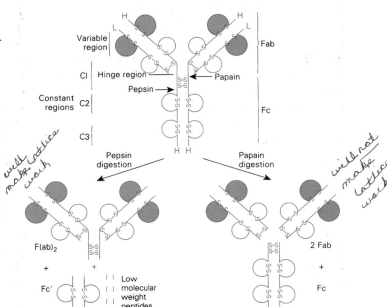

FIG. 5–2. Generalized structure of an immunoglobulin molecule. The basic structure of an immunoglobulin is a tetrapeptide, consisting of two H and two L chains linked by disulfide bonds. Intrachain disulfide bonds create flooded regions or domains. The amino-terminal end of each chain is a variable region, while the carboxy-terminal end is one or more constant regions. Pepsin digestion yields an F(ab)$_2$ fragment, with all the antibody activity, and an Fc$_9$ fragment. Papain digestion yields two F(ab) fragments and an Fc portion.

position number 1), it was discovered that each type had essentially the same sequence. This region was called the constant region, and the amino-terminal end was called the variable region. Thus, all κ L chains have an almost identical carboxy-terminal end, and the same is true of λ chains. The difference between the κ and λ chains lies in the amino acid substitutions at a few locations along the chain. There are no functional differences between the two types. Both κ and λ L chains are found in all five classes of immunoglobulins, but only one type is present in a given molecule.

Heavy Chain Sequencing

H chain sequencing demonstrated the presence of domains similar to those in the L chains; that is, variable and constant regions. The first approximately 110 amino acids at the amino-terminal end constitute the variable domain, and the remaining amino acids can typically be divided up into three or more constant regions with very similar sequences, designated C$_H$1, C$_H$2, and C$_H$3. Constant regions of the H chain are unique to each class and give each immunoglobulin type its name. Hence, IgG has a γ H chain, IgM a μ chain, IgA an α chain, IgD a δ chain, and IgE an ε chain. Each of these represents an **isotype,** a unique amino acid sequence that is common to all immunoglobulin molecules of a given class in a given species. Minor variations of these sequences that are present in some individuals but not others are known as **allotypes** (Fig. 5–3). Allotypes occur for γ, α, ε, and κ chains, but not for μ, δ, or λ chains.[1] These genetic markers are found in the constant region and are inherited in simple Mendelian fashion. Some of the best-known examples of allotypes are variations of the γ chain known as G1m3 and G1m17.

The variable portions of each chain are unique to a specific antibody molecule, and they constitute what is known as the **idiotype** of the molecule. The amino-terminal ends of both L and H chains contain these regions, which are essential to the formation of the antigen-binding site. Together they serve as the antigen recognition unit.

Hinge Region

A segment of the H chain located between the C_H1 and C_H2 regions is known as the **hinge region.** It has a high content of proline and hydrophobic residues; the high proline content allows for flexibility.[5,6] This ability to bend lets the two antigen-binding sites operate independently. The flexibility also assists in effector functions such as initiation of the complement cascade (see Chapter 7 for details).

In addition to the four polypeptide chains, all types of immunoglobulins contain a carbohydrate portion, which is localized between the C_H2 domains of the two H chains. Functions of the carbohydrate include (1) increasing the solubility of immunoglobulin, (2) providing protection against degradation, and (3) enhancing functional activity of the Fc domains. This latter function may be the most important because recognition by Fc receptors has been shown to correlate with the presence of the carbohydrate moiety.[6]

Three Dimensional Structure of Antibodies

The basic four-chain structure of all immunoglobulin molecules does not actually exist as a straight Y shape, but in fact it is folded into compact globular subunits, based on the formation of balloon-shaped loops at each of the domains.[6] Intrachain disulfide bonds stabilize these globular regions. Within each of these regions or domains, the polypeptide chain is folded back and forth on itself to form what is called a β-pleated sheet. The folded domains of the H chains line up with those of the L chains to produce a structure called an immunoglobulin barrel (Fig. 5–4). Antigen is captured within the barrel by binding to a small number of amino acids at strategic locations on each chain known as hypervariable regions.

Three small hypervariable regions consisting of a total of approximately 30 amino acid residues are found within the variable regions of both H and L chains. Each of these regions, called complementarity-determining regions (CDRs), is between 9 and 12 residues long.[4] They occur as loops in the folds of the variable regions of both L and H chains, and the antigen-binding site is actually determined by the apposition of the six hypervariable loops, three from each chain (see Fig. 5–4). Antigen binds in the middle

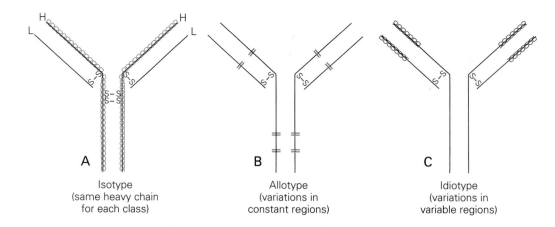

FIG. 5–3. Antibody variations. *(A)* Isotype—the H chain that is unique to each immunoglobulin class. *(B)* Allotype—genetic variations in the constant regions. *(C)* Idiotype—variations in variable regions that give individual antibody molecules specificity.

of the CDRs, with at least four of the CDRs involved in the binding.[7,8] Thus, a small number of amino acids can create an immense diversity of antigen–binding sites.

Not only are all immunoglobulin molecules similar to one another in three-dimensional shape, but they resemble a number of other proteins all involved in molecular recognition or cellular adhesion. These molecules are known as the **immunoglobulin super-family.** Members of this family other than immunoglobulins include the α, β, γ, and ε chains of the T cell receptor, major histocompatibility complex class I and II molecules, CD2, CD4, CD8, and many other cell surface receptors.[4,6] They are all composed of units of globular domains that fold just like immunoglobulin molecules. It has been postulated that there may have been one ancestral gene coding for a polypeptide of 110 amino acids, and this gene reduplicated itself many times, undergoing changes in the process.[1,4] Properties of individual antibody classes are considered in the following.

IgG

IgG is the predominant immunoglobulin in humans, comprising approximately 75 to 80 percent of the total serum immunoglobulins. As seen in Table 5–1, IgG has the longest half-life of any immunoglobulin class, approximately 23 to 25 days, which may help to account for its predominance in serum. There are four major subclasses with a distribution as follows: IgG1, 66 percent; IgG2, 23 percent; IgG3, 7 percent; and IgG4, 4 percent.[9] These subclasses differ mainly in the number and position of the disulfide bridges between the γ chains, as seen in Figure 5–5. Variability in the hinge region affects the ability to reach for antigen and the ability to initiate important biologic functions such as complement activation.[10] IgG3 has the largest hinge region and the largest number of interchain disulfide bonds, and therefore it is the most efficient at binding complement.[1] IgG2 and IgG4 have shorter hinge segments, which tend to make them poor mediators of complement activation.[6,11]

Major functions of IgG include the following: (1) providing immunity for the newborn because IgG can cross the placenta; (2) fixation of complement; (3) opsonization, or coating of antigen for enhanced phagocytosis; (4) neutralization of toxins and viruses; and (5) participation in agglutination and precipitation reactions. All subclasses of IgG appear to be able to cross the placenta, although IgG2 is the least efficient.[1]

Macrophages, monocytes, and neutrophils have receptors on their surfaces that are specific for the Fc

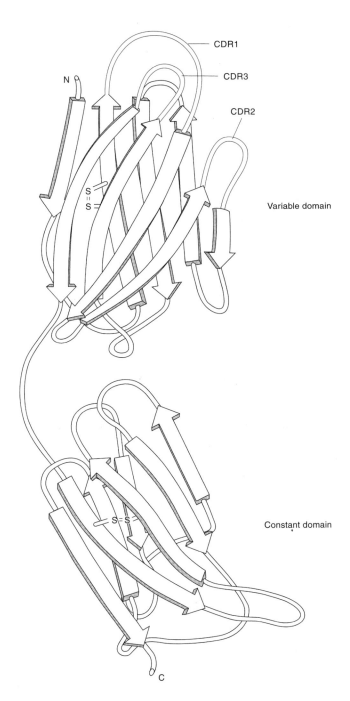

FIG. 5–4. Three-dimensional structure of a L chain. In this ribbon diagram tracing the polypeptide backbone, B strands are shown as wide ribbons, other regions as narrow strings. Each of the two globular domains consists of a barrel-shaped assembly of seven to nine antiparallel B strands. The three hypervariable regions (CDR1, CDR2, and CDR3) are flexible loops that project outward from the amino-terminal end of the V_L domain. (From Parslow, TG, et al: Medical Immunology, ed. 10. McGraw-Hill/Appleton & Lange, 2001, with permission.)

TABLE 5–1. Properties of Immunoglobulins

	IgG	IgM	IgA	IgD	IgE
Molecular weight	150,000	900,000	160,000–	180,000	190,000
Sedimentation coefficient	7 S	19 S	7 S	7 S	8 S
H chain	γ	μ	α	δ	ε
H chain subclasses	γ1,γ2,γ3,γ4	None	α1,α2	None	None
H chain molecular weight	50,000–60,000	70,000	55,000–60,000	62,000	70,000–75,000
Constant domains (H chain)	3	4	3	3	4
Percent of total immunoglobulin	70–75	10	10–15	>1	0.002
Serum concentration (mg/dL)	800–1600	120–150	70–350	1–3	0.005
Serum half-life (days)	23	6	5	1–3	2–3
Carbohydrate content (weight percent)	2–3	12	7–11	9–14	12
Electrophoretic migration	γ2–α1	γ1–β2	γ2–β2	γ1	γ1
Complement fixation	Yes	Yes	No	No	No
Crosses placenta	Yes	No	No	No	No

region of IgG. This enhances contact between antigen and phagocytic cells and generally increases the efficiency of phagocytosis.

IgG has a high diffusion coefficient that allows it to enter extravascular spaces more readily than other immunoglobulin types. Thus, it plays a major role in the neutralization of toxins and viruses.

Agglutination and precipitation reactions take place *in vitro,* although it is not known how significant a role these play *in vivo.* IgG is better at precipitation reactions than agglutination because precipitation involves small soluble particles, which are more easily brought together by the relatively small IgG molecule. Agglutination is the clumping together of larger parti-

cles such as red blood cells, and being a larger molecule, IgM is much more efficient at this than IgG.

IgM

IgM is known as a macroglobulin because it has a sedimentation rate of 19 S, which represents a molecular weight of approximately 900,000. As seen from Table 5–1, the half-life of IgM is about 10 days, much shorter than that of IgG. It accounts for between 5 and 10 percent of all serum immunoglobulins.

If IgM is subjected to treatment with mercaptoethanol, it dissociates into five 7 S units, each having a molecular weight of 180,000 and a four-chain structure that resembles IgG. The molecular weight of the H or μ chain is approximately 70,000. It consists of about 576 amino acids and includes one more constant domain than is found on the γ chain. The pentamer form is found in secretions, while the monomer form occurs on the surface of B cells.[6]

The five monomeric units are held together by a **J** or **joining chain,** which is a glycoprotein with a number of cysteine residues. These serve as linkage points for disulfide bonds between two adjacent monomers. Linkage occurs at the carboxy-terminal end of two of the μ chains, and it appears that the J chain may initiate polymerization by stabilizing Fc sulfhydryl groups so that crosslinking can take place.[9] The molecular weight of the J chain is approximately 15,000. One J chain is present per pentamer.

IgM thus configured assumes a starlike shape (Fig. 5–6) with a total of 10 functional binding sites. In actuality, only about five of these are used unless the antigen is extremely small. When combined with antigen, IgM often assumes a three-dimensional structure that is crablike in appearance.[9] The high valency of IgM anti-

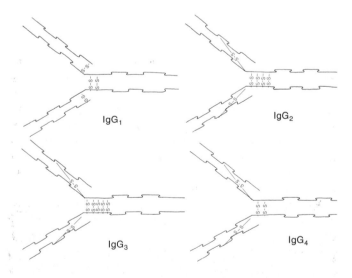

FIG. 5–5. IgG subclasses. There are four subclasses of IgG: IgG1, IgG2, IgG3, and IgG4. These differ in the number and linkages of the disulfide bonds. (From Bryant, NJ: Laboratory Immunology and Serology, ed. 3. WB Saunders, Philadelphia, 1992, p 29, with permission.)

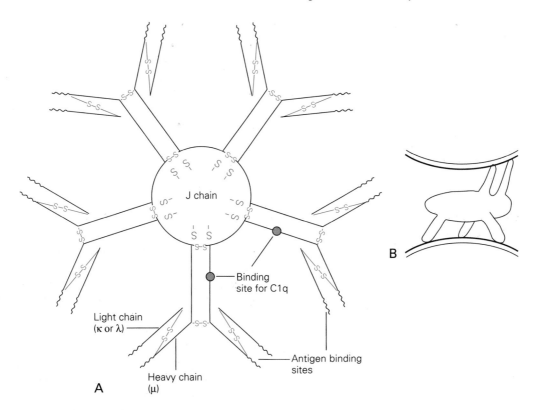

FIG. 5–6. Structure of immunoglobulin M. *(A)* Pentameric structure of IgM, which is linked by a J chain. *(B)* Spacial configuration of IgM. Monomers can extend in different directions. (From Bryant, NJ: Laboratory Immunology and Serology, ed. 3. WB Saunders, Philadelphia, 1992, p 31, with permission.)

bodies contravenes the fact that they tend to have a low affinity for antigen.

Because of its large size, IgM is found mainly in the intravascular pool and not in other body fluids or tissues. It is incapable of crossing the placenta. IgM is known as the primary response antibody because it is the first to appear after antigenic stimulation, and it is also the first to appear in the maturing infant. It is only synthesized as long as antigen remains present because there are no memory cells for IgM. Figure 5–7 depicts the difference between the primary response, which is predominantly IgM, and the secondary response, which is mainly IgG. The primary response is characterized by a long lag phase, while the secondary response has a shortened lag period and a much more rapid increase in antibody titer.

The functions of IgM include: (1) complement fixation, (2) agglutination, (3) opsonization, and (4) neutralization of toxins. IgM is the most efficient of all immunoglobulins at triggering the classical complement pathway (see Chapter 7) because a single molecule can initiate the reaction as a result of its multiple binding sites. This probably represents the most important function of IgM. The larger number of binding

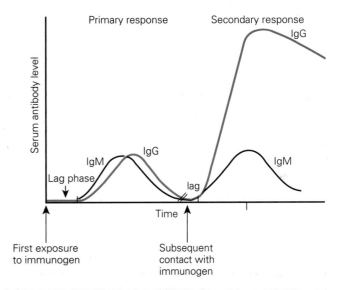

FIG. 5–7. A comparison of the primary and secondary response to immunogen. The primary response is characterized by a long lag phase, slow exponential increase in antibody, and short-lived response. The secondary or anamnestic response has a shortened lag period, antibody rise is much more rapid, and serum levels remain higher for longer periods. This is caused by the large number of antigen-specific memory T and B cells generated during the primary response.

sites also makes IgM more efficient at agglutination reactions, especially with multivalent antigens. Thus, IgM forms a potent defense against many bacterial diseases.

An additional role for IgM is that of a surface receptor for antigen. In the cytoplasm of the pre-B cell μ chains first appear. When they associate with the early surrogate L chains, this sends the signal to exclude rearrangement of the other H chain locus and to begin rearrangement of the genes controlling L chain synthesis.[6] Later, as L chains are synthesized, IgM monomers are formed and become inserted into the plasma membrane. The presence of membrane IgM classifies lymphocytes as mature B cells. (Refer to Chapter 3 for a complete discussion of B cell development.)

IgA

In the serum, IgA appears as a monomer with a molecular weight of approximately 160,000. It has a sedimentation coefficient of 7 S and migrates between the γ and β regions on electrophoresis. The H chain, called the α chain, has a molecular weight of between 55,000 and 60,000 and consists of about 472 amino acids. There are two subclasses, designated IgA1 and IgA2. They differ in content by 22 amino acids, 13 of which are located in the hinge region and are deleted in IgA2.[12] The lack of this region appears to make IgA2 more resistant to some bacterial proteinases that are able to cleave IgA1.[13] Additionally, IgA2 has disulfide bonds that covalently link together the L chains rather than the H chains.[1] The monomer form in serum is primarily IgA1.

IgA, primarily IgA2, is also found as a dimer in body secretions along the respiratory, urogenital, and intestinal mucosa, and in milk, saliva, tears, and sweat. Here it serves to keep antigens from penetrating further into the body. The dimer consists of two monomers held together by a J chain that has a molecular weight of about 15,000. Secretory IgA is synthesized in plasma cells found mainly in mucosal associated lymphoid tissue, and it is released in dimeric form. The J chain regulates the degree of polymerization and may also help in transport to mucosal secretions.[12] IgA is synthesized at a rate that is approximately twice that of IgG, but because it is mainly in secretory form, the serum concentration is much lower.[6]

A **secretory component (SC),** with a molecular weight of about 100,000, is later attached to the Fc region around the hinge portion of the α chains. This protein, consisting of five immunoglobulin-like domains, is derived from epithelial cells found in close

proximity to the plasma cells.[4] As Figure 5–8 indicates, SC precursor, with a molecular weight of 100,000, is actually found on the surface of epithelial cells and serves as a specific receptor for IgA. Plasma cells that secrete IgA actually home to subepithelial tissue, where IgA can bind as soon as it is released from the plasma cells.[4] Once binding takes place, IgA and SC precursor are both taken inside the cell and then released to the opposite surface by a process known as *transcytosis.* The vesicle carrying IgA and the SC receptor fuses with the membrane on the opposite side of the cell, and a small fragment of SC is cleaved to liberate the IgA dimmer with the remaining SC.[14] The SC may thus act to facilitate transport of IgA to mucosal surfaces. It also makes the dimer more resistant to enzymatic digestion.[12]

The main function of secretory IgA is to patrol mucosal surfaces and act as a first line of defense. It plays an important role in neutralization of toxins produced by microorganisms, and it also helps to prevent bacterial adherence to mucosal surfaces. Complexes of IgA and antigen are easily trapped in mucus and then eliminated by the ciliated epithelial cells of the respiratory or intestinal tract.[4]

It appears that IgA is not capable of fixing complement by the classical pathway, although aggregation of immune complexes may trigger the alternate complement pathway.[13] (Refer to Chapter 7 for a complete discussion of the complement pathways.) Lack of complement activation may actually assist in clearing of antigen without triggering an inflammatory response, thus minimizing tissue damage.[12,15]

Additionally, neutrophils, monocytes, and macrophages have been found to possess specific receptors for IgA. Binding to these sites triggers a respiratory burst and degranulation.[16] This occurs for both serum and

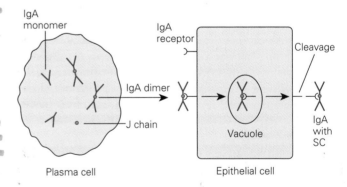

FIG. 5–8. Formation of secretory IgA. IgA is secreted as a dimer from plasma cells and is captured by specific receptors on epithelial cells. The receptor is actually an SC, which binds to IgA and exits the cell along with it.

secretory IgA, indicating that they are capable of acting as opsonins. The success of oral immunizations such the Sabin vaccine, which induces IgA almost exclusively, demonstrates the effectiveness of IgA's protective role on mucosal surfaces.

IgD

IgD was not discovered until 1965 and is extremely scarce in the serum, representing less than 0.2 percent of total immunoglobulins. It is synthesized at a low level and has a half-life of only 2 to 3 days. The molecule has a molecular weight of approximately 184,000, and it migrates as a fast γ protein. The δ H chain has a molecular weight of 62,000 and appears to have an extended hinge region consisting of 58 amino acids.[17]

Most of the IgD present is found on the surface of immunocompetent but unstimulated B lymphocytes. It is the second type of immunoglobulin to appear (IgM being the first), and it may play a role in activation of B cells. The high level of surface expression and its intrinsic flexibility make it an ideal early responder to antigen.[6] It is known that those cells bearing only IgM receptors appear incapable of an IgG response, while those with both IgM and IgD receptors are capable of responding to T cell help and switching to synthesis of IgG, IgA, or IgE.[6]

Because of its unusually long hinge region, IgD is more susceptible to proteolysis than other immunoglobulins. This may be the main reason for its short half-life. Binding of antigen also promotes cleavage, and subsequent changes in the Fc region bound to the B cell may help to trigger proliferation of that cell.[9] In the serum, IgD does not appear to serve a protective function because it does not bind complement, does not bind to

neutrophils or macrophages, and does not cross the placenta.

IgE

IgE is the least abundant immunoglobulin in the serum, accounting for only 0.004 percent of total serum immunoglobulins. It is an 8 S molecule with a molecular weight of approximately 190,000. The ε or H chain is composed of around 550 amino acids that are distributed over one variable and four constant domains. A single disulfide bond joins each ε chain to a L chain, and two disulfide bonds link the H chains to one another.

IgE is the most heat-labile of all immunoglobulins because heating to 56°C for between 30 minutes and 3 hours results in conformational changes and loss of ability to bind to target cells. IgE does not participate in typical immunoglobulin reactions such as complement fixation, agglutination, or opsonization. Additionally, it is incapable of crossing the placenta. Instead, shortly after synthesis, it attaches to basophils and tissue mast cells by means of specific surface proteins, termed high affinity Fcε RI receptors, which are found exclusively on these cells.[6,18] The molecule binds at the C_H4 domain on the Fc region. This leaves the antigen-binding sites free to interact with specific antigen (Fig. 5–9). Plasma cells that produce IgE are located primarily in the lung and the skin.[6]

Mast cells are also found mainly in the skin and in the lining of the respiratory and alimentary tracts. One such cell may have several hundred thousand receptors, each capable of binding an IgE molecule. When two adjacent IgE molecules on a mast cell bind specific antigen, a cascade of cellular events is initiated that

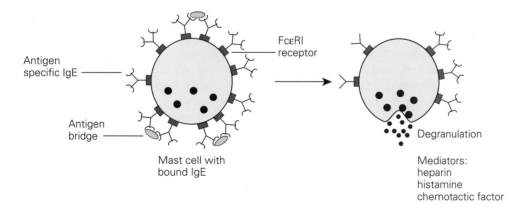

FIG. 5–9. Action of IgE on mast cells. IgE binds to specific ε receptors on mast cells. When antigen bridges two nearby IgE molecules, the membrane is disturbed and degranulation results. Chemical mediators are released.

results in degranulation of the mast cells with release of vasoactive amines such as histamine and heparin. Release of these mediators induces what is known as a type I immediate hypersensitivity or allergic reaction (see Chapter 13). Typical reactions include hay fever, asthma, vomiting and diarrhea, the appearance of hives, and life-threatening anaphylactic shock.

While IgE appears to be a nuisance antibody, it may serve a protective role by triggering an acute inflammatory reaction that recruits neutrophils and eosinophils to the area to help destroy invading antigens that have penetrated IgA defenses.[9] Eosinophils, especially, play a major part in the destruction of large antigens such as parasitic worms that cannot be easily phagocytized (see Chapter 23 for details).

Theories of Antibody Diversity

Attempts to explain the specificity of antibody for a particular antigen began long before the actual structure of immunoglobulins was discovered. The central issue was whether an antigen selected lymphocytes with the inherent capability of producing specific antibody to it or whether the presence of antigen itself added a new specificity to a generalized type of antibody.

Ehrlich's Side-Chain Theory

One of the first theories to be formulated was that of Paul Ehrlich in the early 1900s, termed the *side-chain theory*. Ehrlich postulated that certain cells had specific surface receptors for antigen that were present before contact with antigen occurred.[9] Once antigen was introduced, it would select the cell with the proper receptors, combination would take place, and then receptors would break off and enter the circulation as antibody molecules. New receptors would form in place of those broken off, and this process could be repeated. Although this represented a rather simplistic explanation for antibody synthesis, two key premises emerged. These were (1) the lock and key concept of the fit of antibody for antigen and (2) the idea that an antigen selected cells with the built-in capacity to respond to it. Although this theory did not explain the kinetics of the immune response or the idea of immunologic memory, it laid the foundation for further hypotheses.

The Template Theory

Felix Haurowitz put forth a second major theory, the instructive or template theory, in the early 1930s. According to this theory, antibody-producing cells are capable of synthesizing a generalized type of antibody, and when contact with antigen occurs, the antigen serves as a mold or template and alters protein synthesis so that antibody with a specific fit is made. This now-specific antibody enters the circulation, while the antigen remains behind to direct further synthesis.

The template theory is contradicted by our current knowledge of protein synthesis, which indicates that the three-dimensional structure of a protein is genetically determined and not subject to alteration by factors that bind to it. In addition, the phenomenon of self-tolerance cannot be explained by this theory because there is an abundance of self-antigens that presumably would be capable of serving as templates for antibody production. However, antibody to self-antigens is not detected under normal circumstances.

Clonal Selection

The 1950s saw a return to selective theories when both Niels Jerne and Macfarlane Burnet independently supported the idea of a clonal selection process for antibody formation.[9] The key premise is that individual lymphocytes are genetically preprogrammed to produce one type of immunoglobulin, and that a specific antigen finds or selects those particular cells capable of responding to it, causing these to proliferate. The receptors originally postulated by Ehrlich are the surface immunoglobulins, IgM and IgD, found on unstimulated B lymphocytes. Repeated contact with antigen would continually increase a specific lymphocyte pool. Such a model provides an explanation for the kinetics of the immune response.

The main drawback to the **clonal selection theory** is consideration of the genetic basis for the diversity of antibody molecules. If separate genes were present to code for antibody to every possible antigen, an overwhelming amount of deoxyribonucleic acid (DNA) would be needed. Dryer and Bennett proposed a solution to this dilemma in 1965 by suggesting that the constant and variable portions of immunoglobulin chains are actually coded for by separate genes.[19] There could be a small number coding for the constant region, and a larger number coding for the variable region.[9] This would considerably simplify the task of coding for such variability. This notion implied that although all lymphocytes start out with identical genetic germline DNA, diversity is created by a series of recombination events that take place as the B cell matures. Manipulation of chromosomal DNA with repositioning of fragments was a radical idea then. However, scientific evidence now indicates that this is exactly what happens, as explained in the following discussion.

Genes Coding for Immunoglobulins

Tonegawa made the discovery that chromosomes contain no intact immunoglobulin genes, only building blocks from which genes can be assembled, thus confirming the hypothesis of Dryer and Bennett.[1] He was awarded the Nobel Prize in 1987 for this monumental discovery. Human immunoglobulin genes are found in three unlinked clusters: H chain genes are located on chromosome 14, κ chain genes on chromosome 2, and λ chain genes on chromosome 22. Within each of these clusters, there is a selection process that occurs. The genes cannot be transcribed and translated into functional antibody molecules until this rearrangement takes place.

Rearrangement of Heavy Chain Genes

All H chains are derived from a single region on chromosome 14. The genes that code for the variable region are divided into three groups, V_H, D, and J. There are at least 50 V_H **(variable)** genes, approximately 27 functional D (diversity) genes, and 6 J (joining) genes.[1,9,20,21] In addition, there is a set of genes (C) that codes for the **constant region**. This includes one

gene for each H chain isotype. They are located in the following order: Cμ, Cδ, Cγ3, Cγ1, Cα1, Cα2, Cγ4, Cε, and Cα2. Only one of these constant regions is selected at any one time. For synthesis of the entire H chain, a choice is made from each of the sections so as to include one V_H gene, one D gene, one J gene, and one constant region. During the process of B cell maturation, the pieces are spliced together to commit that B lymphocyte to making antibody of a single specificity.

Joining of these segments probably occurs in two steps: First, at the DNA level one D and one J are joined with deletion of the intervening DNA (Fig. 5–10). Next, a V gene is joined to the DJ complex, resulting in a rearranged V(D)J gene. This rearrangement occurs early in B cell development in pro-B cells.[22] (See Chapter 3 for additional details.) The recombinase enzymes RAG-1 and RAG-2, which are distinctive markers of this stage, are essential for initiating this process.[23] Joining of the V, J, and D segments doesn't always occur at a fixed position, so each sequence can vary by a small number of nucleotides. This contributes additional diversity.[1,22]

The variable and constant regions are joined at the ribonucleic acid (RNA) level, thus conserving the DNA of the constant regions and allowing for a later phenomenon called **class switching,** whereby daughter plasma cells can produce antibody of another type.

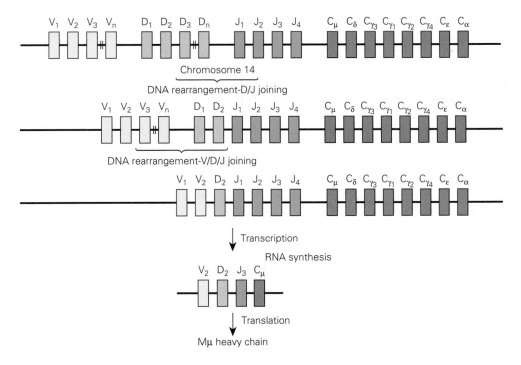

FIG. 5–10. Coding for immunoglobulin H chains. Four separate regions on chromosome 14 code for H chains. DJ regions are spliced first, and then this segment is joined to a variable region. When RNA synthesis occurs, one constant region is attached to the VDJ combination. μ H chains are made first, but the cell retains its capacity to produce immunoglobulin of another class.

During transcription and synthesis of messenger ribonucleic acid (mRNA), a constant region is spliced to the V(D)J complex.[24] In general, the C_H region located immediately next to the V(D)J complex is expressed. Because $C\mu$ is the region closest to J region, μ H chains are the first to be synthesized, and these are the markers of the pre-B lymphocytes.[4] The $C\delta$ region, which lies closest to the $C\mu$ region, is often transcribed along with $C\mu$. The presence of DNA for both the $C\mu$ and $C\delta$ regions allows for RNA for IgD and IgM to be transcribed at the same time. Thus, a B cell could express IgD and IgM with the same variable domain on its surface at the same time. The process of switching to other immunoglobulin classes occurs later, resulting from a looping out and deletion of other constant regions. This produces antibody of a different class (i.e., IgA, IgG, or IgE) but with an identical specificity for antigen. Although the exact mechanism is not clearly defined, contact with T cells and with cytokines provides the signal for switching to take place.[25] Specificity of the antibody is not affected, but the effector functions are.

Light Chain Rearrangement

Because L chain rearrangement occurs only after μ chains appear, μ-chain synthesis represents a pivotal step in the process.[22] L chains exhibit a similar genetic rearrangement, except they lack a D region. Recombination of segments on chromosome 2, coding for κ chains, occurs prior to that on chromosome 22, which codes for λ chains. Chromosome 2 contains approximately 32 functional V_κ regions, 5 J regions, and one C_κ region.[9,21,22] The 5 J regions are in close proximity to the C_κ region, while the V_κ regions are scattered along an area that approximates 1 percent of the length of chromosome 2. The process of VJ joining is accomplished by an excision of intervening DNA. This results in V_κ and J_κ segments becoming permanently joined to one another on the rearranged chromosome. Transcription begins at one end of the V_κ segment and proceeds through the J_κ and C_κ segments. Unrearranged J segments are removed during RNA splicing, which occurs in the translation (Fig. 5-11).

A productive rearrangement of the κ genes with subsequent protein production keeps the other chromosome 2 from rearranging, and in addition, it shuts down any recombination of the λ-chain locus on chromosome 22.[22] This process is known as *allelic exclusion.* Only if a nonfunctioning gene product arises from κ rearrangement does λ-chain synthesis occur.

L chains are then joined with μ chains to form a complete IgM antibody, which first appears in imma-

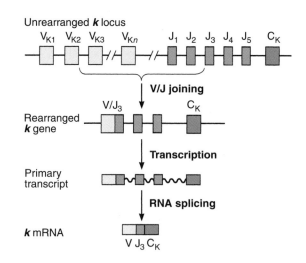

FIG. 5-11. Assembly and expression of the κ L chain locus. A DNA rearrangement fuses one V segment to one J segment. The VJ segment is then transcribed along with a unique C region to form mature κ mRNA. Unarranged J segments are removed during RNA splicing. (From Parslow, TG, et al: Medical Immunology, ed. 10. McGraw-Hill/Appleton & Lange, 2001, with permission.)

ture B cells. Once IgM and IgD are present on the surface membrane, the B lymphocyte is fully mature and capable of responding to antigen (see Chapter 3). The large variety of V, J, D, and C combinations for each type of chain plus the different possibilities for L- and H-chain combination make for more than enough configurations to allow us to respond to any antigen in the environment.

Monoclonal Antibody

The knowledge that B cells are genetically preprogrammed to synthesize very specific antibody has been put to use in the development of antibodies for diagnostic testing known as **monoclonal antibodies.** Normally, the response to an antigen is heterogeneous because even a purified antigen has multiple epitopes that stimulate a variety of B cell clones. In 1975, the discovery of a technique to produce antibody arising from a single B cell has produced a revolution in serologic testing. For their pioneering research, Georges Kohler and Cesar Milstein were awarded the Nobel Prize in 1984.

Kohler and Milstein's technique fuses an activated B cell with a cancerous cell called a myeloma that can be grown indefinitely in the laboratory. Myeloma cells are cancerous plasma cells. Normally plasma cells produce antibody, so a particular cell line that is not capable of producing antibody is chosen. In addition, this cell line has a deficiency of the enzyme hypoxanthine guanine phosphoribosyl transferase (HGPRT) that renders it incapable of synthesizing nucleotides from hypoxanthine and thymidine, which are needed for DNA synthesis.

Hybridoma Production

A mouse is immunized with a certain antigen, and after a time, spleen cells are harvested. Spleen cells are combined with myeloma cells in the presence of polyethylene glycol (PEG), a surfactant. The PEG brings about fusion of plasma cells with myeloma cells, producing a **hybridoma.** Only a small percentage of cells actually fuse, and some of these are like cells—that is, two myeloma cells or two spleen cells. After fusion, cells are placed in culture using a selective medium containing hypoxanthine, aminopterin, and thymidine (HAT). Culture in this medium is used to separate the hybridoma cells by allowing them to grow selectively. Myeloma cells are normally able to grow indefinitely in tissue culture, but in this case they cannot because both pathways for the synthesis of nucleotides are blocked. One pathway is blocked because the myeloma cell line employed is deficient in the required enzymes HGPRT and thymidine kinase.[4] The other pathway is blocked by the presence of aminopterin. Consequently the myeloma cells die out. Normal B cells are not able to be maintained continuously in cell culture, so these too die out. This leaves only the fused hybridoma cells, which have the ability, acquired from the myeloma cell, to reproduce indefinitely in culture and the ability, acquired from the normal B cell, to synthesize nucleotides by the HGPRT and thymidine kinase pathway (Fig. 5–12).

Selection of Specific Antibody-Producing Clones

The remaining hybridoma cells are diluted out and placed in microtiter wells, where they are allowed to grow. Each well, containing one clone, is then screened for presence of the desired antibody by removing the supernatant. Once identified, a hybridoma is capable of being maintained in cell culture indefinitely, and it produces a ready supply of monoclonal antibody that reacts with a single epitope.[4]

Clinical Applications

Monoclonal antibodies were initially used for *in vitro* diagnostic testing. A familiar example is pregnancy testing, which uses antibody specific for the β chain of

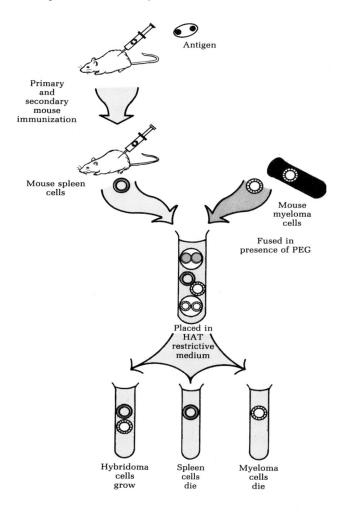

FIG. 5–12. Formation of a hybridoma in monoclonal antibody production. A mouse is immunized, and spleen cells are removed. These cells are fused with nonsecreting myeloma cells and then plated in a restrictive medium. Only the hybridoma cells will grow in this medium, where they synthesize and secrete a monoclonal immunoglobulin specific for a single determinant on an antigen. (From Barrett, JT: Textbook of Immunology, ed. 5. Mosby, St. Louis, 1988, with permission.)

human chorionic gonadotropin, thereby eliminating many false positive reactions. Other examples include detection of tumor antigens and measurement of hormone levels.

Recently, however, there has been an emphasis on the use of monoclonal antibodies as therapeutic agents. One of the biggest success stories is in the treatment of two autoimmune diseases: rheumatoid arthritis and Crohn's disease (a progressive inflammatory colitis). Both of these diseases have been treated with a monoclonal antibody called inflixmab that blocks the action of tumor necrosis factor-alpha.[26–28] Treatment for breast cancer, non-Hodgkin lymphoma, and antiplatelet therapy for coronary syndromes also shows great promise.[29] The fact that monoclonal antibodies can now be humanized by recombinant technology has cut down on reactions to the reagents themselves, which used to be of mouse origin. This area is likely to expand in the future because over one-quarter of the current drugs in development are monoclonal in nature.[29]

SUMMARY

The basic structural unit for all immunoglobulins is a tetrapeptide composed of two L and two H chains joined together by disulfide bonds. While κ and λ L chains are found in all types of immunoglobulins, the H chains differ for each immunoglobulin class. The five classes are IgM, IgG, IgA, IgD, and IgE. IgG, IgD, and IgE exist as monomers, IgA has a dimeric form, and IgM is a pentamer whose subunits are held together by a J chain.

Each immunoglobulin molecule has constant and variable regions. The variable region is at the amino-terminal end, called the *Fab fragment*, and this determines the specificity of that molecule for a particular antigen. The constant region, located at the carboxy-terminal end of the molecule and named the *Fc fragment,* is responsible for binding to effector cells such as neutrophils, basophils, eosinophils, and mast cells to amplify the inflammatory process and speed up antigen removal.

Structural differences determine specific functions for each of the immunoglobulin types. For instance, IgG is relatively small and easily penetrates into tissues, while IgM is much larger and excels at complement fixation. IgA has an SC that protects it from enzymatic digestion while it patrols mucosal surfaces. An extended hinge region gives IgD an advantage as a surface receptor for antigen. IgE binds to mast cells to initiate a local inflammatory reaction.

Theories to explain the diversity seen in immunoglobulin synthesis fall into two main categories: selective and instructive. Ehrlich's side-chain theory is based on selection by the antigen of the correctly programmed B lymphocyte; in contrast, Haurowitz's instructional theory was constructed on the premise that the antigen provides new instructions to lymphocytes secreting a generic type of antibody. The clonal selection theory postulates that lymphocytes are generally pre-endowed to respond to one antigen or a group of antigens, and that IgM and IgD act as surface receptors that interact with specific antigen to trigger proliferation of a clone of identical cells.

Genetic preprogramming of lymphocytes can best be explained by the concept of gene recombination. More than one gene controls synthesis of a particular immunoglobulin, and through a random selection process these individual segments are joined to commit that lymphocyte to making antibody of a single specificity.

A working example of the clonal selection theory is the production of monoclonal antibodies. A cancerous cell or myeloma is fused with an antibody-producing cell to form a hybridoma. Hybridomas formed by fusion of one of each type of cell (e.g., myeloma and B cell) are selected using HAT, a selective medium. Then hybridomas are diluted out and placed in microtiter wells. The clone producing the desired antibody is located by testing the supernatant in each well. Monoclonal antibodies are used both in diagnosis and treatment of disease.

Case Studies

1. A 15-year-old male exhibited symptoms of fever, fatigue, nausea, and sore throat. He went to his primary care physician, and a rapid strep test and a test for infectious mononucleosis were performed in the office. The rapid strep test result was negative, but the test result for infectious mononucleosis was faintly positive. The patient mentioned that he thought he had previously had mononucleosis, but it was never officially diagnosed. His serum was sent to a reference laboratory to test with specific Epstein Barr viral antigens. The results indicated the presence of IgM only. Is this a reactivated case of mononucleosis? Explain your answer.

2. A 10-year-old female experienced one cold after another in the springtime. She had missed a number of days of school, and her mother was greatly concerned. The mother took her daughter to the pediatrician and was concerned that her daughter might be immunocompromised because she couldn't seem to fight off infections. A blood sample was obtained and sent to a reference laboratory for a determination of antibody levels, including an IgE level. The patient's IgM, IgG, and IgA levels were all normal for her age, but the IgE level was greatly increased. What does this indicate about the patient's state of health?

Exercise: Serum Protein Electrophoresis

PRINCIPLE

Electrophoresis is the migration of charged particles in an electrical field through an electrolyte solution toward the electrode of the opposite charge. At a pH of 8.6, all serum proteins are negatively charged, and when placed in an electrical field, they migrate toward the anode at a rate that depends on the net negative charge. Five distinct bands are obtained: albumin, alpha$_1$, alpha$_2$, beta, and gamma. Immunoglobulins are located in the gamma band.

SAMPLE PREPARATION

Obtain serum from whole blood by using a sterile clot tube. Centrifuge and remove the supernatant. Discard any samples that appear to be hemolyzed. Serum is stable for up to 5 days if the specimen is refrigerated. Avoid freezing samples because this tends to denature protein.

REAGENTS, MATERIALS, AND EQUIPMENT

Corning Electrophoresis System (or equivalent), which includes cell base with cover and power supply (90V DC)
Universal agarose film
Universal barbital buffer kit
Amido black stain
Microliter pipette
Stir-stain dishes
5-percent acetic acid
Incubator/oven or drying oven
Optional
Densitometer

PROCEDURE

1. Buffer preparation: Universal barbital buffer consists of 17.7 g sodium barbital, 2.6 g barbital, 1.0 g sodium chloride, and 0.7 g ethylenediaminetetra-acetic acid. Empty the contents of the vial into a clean 2-L volumetric flask about half filled with deionized water. Rinse the vial and empty into the flask. Dilute to volume and mix by stirring with a magnetic stirrer until the powder is completely dissolved. No pH adjustment is required. If stored in the refrigerator, the buffer is stable for up to 4 months. Check for any signs of contamination. The buffer must be at room temperature before using.
2. Five-percent acetic acid: Add 50 mL of glacial acetic acid to 950 mL of deionized water. Stir to mix.
3. Amido black stain: Empty dry powder from one vial into a 1-L flask. Bring volume up to 1 L with 5-percent acetic acid. Cover flask and mix by inversion. If stored in an airtight container at room temperature, the stain is stable for up to 3 months.
4. Fill each side of the electrophoresis chamber with 95 mL of universal PHAB buffer.
5. Connect the filled cell base to the power supply.
6. Gently peel the agarose film from the hard plastic backing.
7. Fill sample wells with 0.8 µL of serum. Use a fresh pipette or tip for each sample. Sample numbers can be recorded on the plastic backing.
8. Insert film into the cassette holder of the cell cover with the agarose side out. Be sure to match the anode (+) side of the film with the anode side of the cell cover.
9. Place the cell cover on the base and electrophorese for approximately 35 minutes. A light on the unit will indicate that current is flowing.
10. Turn on the drying oven, and allow it to warm up for about 30 minutes.
11. Following electrophoresis, remove the cell cover by lifting it straight up from the cassette holder, and drain it without inverting. Grasp the film by the edges, and remove it from the cassette holder.
12. Place the film in amido black stain solution in a stir-stain dish for 15 minutes.
13. Transfer the film to a dish containing 5-percent acetic acid clearing solution. Stir for approximately 30 seconds to remove excess surface stain.
14. Wipe moisture from the back of the film before placing it on a shelf in the drying oven. Let it sit for approximately 15 to 20 minutes or until completely dry.
15. Rinse, with agitation, in the first 5-percent acetic acid cleaning solution for 1 minute.
16. Transfer to a second dish with 5-percent acetic acid, and rinse for 1 minute or until excess dye is removed.
17. Wipe any moisture from the back of the film, and place it back in the drying oven for about 5 to 10 minutes or until completely dry.
18. Interpret visually or quantitatively using a densitometer.

INTERPRETATION OF RESULTS

All serum proteins should migrate toward the anode. The rate of migration is influenced by the net charge on the molecule, size of the molecule, pH of the buffer, ionic strength of the buffer, and gel concentration. Albumin has the greatest negative charge at pH 8.6, and hence it will travel the farthest in a given time. Because it is present in the greatest concentration, a dark compact band should be seen. Next a more faint alpha$_1$ band will be seen, followed by an alpha$_2$ band and the beta band. Immunoglobulins will migrate within the gamma region, but as these are the least charged, they will remain in a diffuse band near the origin.

Protein bands are not visible until after staining with amido black. Once the film is dried and then rinsed in 5-percent acetic acid, the stain will remain localized only on protein bands. If normal controls are run along with patient serum, bands can be visually compared to determine any possible abnormalities in immunoglobulin production. Infection may be indicated by an overall increase in intensity of color within the gamma region. A sharp band within the region would indicate monoclonal gammopathies with specific antibody production. Lack of immunocompetence would be demonstrated by an overall decrease in color in the gamma region.

If a densitometer is available, a more quantitative approach is possible. The following represents a normal distribution for serum proteins: albumin, 58 to 70 percent; $alpha_1$, 2 to 5 percent; $alpha_2$, 6 to 11 percent; beta, 8 to 14 percent; and gamma, 9 to 18 percent. If a total serum protein determination has been made, these percentages can then be turned into actual mg/dL amounts. To determine abnormalities of specific immunoglobulin classes, immunoelectrophoresis must be performed.

Review Questions

1. Which is characteristic of variable domains of immunoglobulins?
   a. They occur on both the H and L chains.
   b. They represent the complement binding site.
   c. They are at the carboxy-terminal ends of the molecules.
   d. All of the above.

2. All of the following are true of IgM *except* that it:
   a. Can cross the placenta
   b. Fixes complement
   c. Has a J chain
   d. Is a primary response antibody

3. How many antigen binding sites does a typical IgM molecule have?
   a. 2
   b. 4
   c. 6
   d. 10

4. Bence-Jones proteins are identical:
   a. H chains
   b. L chains
   c. IgM molecules
   d. IgG molecules

5. An Fab fragment consists of:
   a. Two H chains
   b. Two L chains
   c. One L chain and one-half of a H chain
   d. One L chain and an entire H chain

6. Which of the following pairs represents two different immunoglobulin allotypes?
   a. IgM and IgG
   b. IgM1 and IgM2
   c. Antihuman IgM and antihuman IgG
   d. IgG1m3 and IgG1m17

7. Which of the following are L chains of antibody molecules?
   a. κ
   b. γ
   c. μ
   d. α

8. Members of the immunoglobulin superfamily share which characteristic?
   a. They are all types of antibody.
   b. They are all the same size.
   c. They all have a similar three-dimensional structure.
   d. They are all capable of opsonization.

9. The subclasses of IgG differ mainly in:
   a. The type of L chain
   b. The arrangement of disulfide bonds
   c. The ability to act as opsonins
   d. Molecular weight

10. Which best describes the role of the SC of IgA?
    a. A transport mechanism across endothelial cells
    b. A means of joining two IgA monomers together
    c. An aid to trapping antigen
    d. Enhancement of complement fixation by the classical pathway

11. Which represents the main function of IgD?
    a. Protection of the mucous membranes
    b. Removal of antigens by complement fixation
    c. Enhancing proliferation of B cells
    d. Destruction of parasitic worms

12. Which antibody is best at agglutination and complement fixation?
    a. IgA
    b. IgG
    c. IgD
    d. IgM

13. Which of the following can be attributed to the clonal selection theory of antibody formation?
    a. Plasma cells make generalized antibody.
    b. B cells are preprogrammed for specific antibody synthesis.
    c. Proteins can alter their shape to conform to antigen.
    d. Cell receptors break off and become circulating antibody.

14. All of the following are true of IgE *except* that it:
    a. Fails to fix complement
    b. Is heat stable
    c. Attaches to tissue mast cells
    d. Is found in the serum of allergic persons

15. Which best describes coding for immunoglobulin molecules?
    a. All genes are located on the same chromosome.
    b. L chain rearrangement occurs before H chain rearrangement.
    c. Four different regions are involved in coding of H chains.
    d. λ rearrangement occurs before κ rearrangement.

16. What is the purpose of HAT medium in the preparation of monoclonal antibody?
    a. Fusion of the two cell types
    b. Restricting the growth of unfused myeloma cells
    c. Restricting the growth of unfused spleen cells
    d. Restricting antibody production to the IgM class

References

1. Parslow, TG: Immunoglobulins and immunoglobulin genes. In Stites, DP, Terr, AI, and Parslow, TG (eds): Medical Immunology, ed. 9. Appleton & Lange, Stamford, Conn., 1997, pp 95–114.
2. Edelman, GM: The structure and function of antibodies. Sci Am 223:34, 1970.
3. Porter, RR: The structure of antibodies. Sci Am 217:81, 1967.
4. Goldsby, RA, Kindt, TJ, and Osborne, BA: Immunoglobulins: Structure and function. In Goldsby, RA, et al: Kuby Immunology, ed. 4. WH Freeman, New York, 2000, pp 83–113.
5. Davies, DR, and Metzger, H: Structural basis of antibody function. Annu Rev Immunol 1:87, 1983.
6. Frazer, JK, and Capra, JD: Immunoglobulins: Structure and function. In Paul, WE (ed): Fundamental Immunology, ed. 4. Lippincott Williams & Wilkins, Philadelphia, 1999, pp 37–74.
7. Davies, DR, and Cohen, GH: Interactions of protein antigens with antibodies. Proc Natl Acad Sci USA 93:7–12, 1996.
8. Wedemayer, GJ, Patten, PA, and Wang, LH, et al: Structural insights into the evolution of an antibody combining site. Science 276:1665–1669, 1997.
9. Roitt, I, Brostoff, J, and Male, D: Immunology, ed. 5. Mosby, London, 1998.
10. Harris, LJ, Larson, SB, and McPherson, A: Comparison of intact antibody structures and the implications for effector function. Adv Immunol 72:191–208, 1999.
11. Alzari, PM, Lascombe, MB, and Poljak, RJ: Three-dimensional structure of antibodies. Annu Rev Immunol 6:555, 1988.
12. Burrows, PD, and Cooper, MD: IgA deficiency. Adv Immunol 65:245–276, 1997.
13. Kerr, MA: The structure and function of human IgA. Biochem J 271:285, 1990.
14. Mostov, KE: Transepithelial transport of immunoglobulins. Annu Rev Immunol 12 :63–84, 1994.
15. Mestecky, J, and McGhee, JR: Immunoglobulin A: Molecular and cellular interactions involved in IgA biosynthesis and immune response. Adv Immunol 40:153, 1987.
16. Stewart, WW, and Kerr, MA: The specificity of the human neutrophil IgA receptor determined by measurement of chemiluminescence induced by serum or secretory IgA1 or IgA2. Immunology 71:328, 1990.
17. Cruse, JM, and Lewis, RE (eds): Atlas of Immunology. CRC Press, Boca Raton, Fla., 1999, p 116.
18. Metzger, H: Molecular aspects of receptors and binding factors for IgE. Adv Immunol 43:277, 1988.
19. Dreyer, WJ, and Bennett, JC: The molecular basis of antibody formation: A paradox. Proc Natl Acad Sci USA 54:864, 1965.
20. Delves, PJ, and Roitt, IM: The immune system. First of two parts. N Engl J Med 343:37–49, 2000.
21. Goldsby, RA, Kindt, TJ, and Osborne, BA: Organization and expression of immunoglobulin genes. In Goldsby, RA, et al: Kuby Immunology, ed. 4. WH Freeman, New York, 2000, pp 115–147.
22. Gorman, JR, and Alt, FW: Regulation of immunoglobulin light chain isotype expression. Adv Immunol 69:113–181, 1998.
23. Gellert, M: Recent advances in understanding V(D)J recombination. Adv Immunol 64:39–64, 1997.
24. Lewis, SM: The mechanism of V(D)J joining: Lessons from molecular, immunological, and comparative analyses. Adv Immunol 56: 27–150, 1994.
25. Stavnezer, J: Antibody class switching. Adv Immunol 61:79–146, 1996.
26. Feldmann, M, Elliott, MJ, and Woody, JN, et al: Anti-tumor necrosis factor-alpha therapy in rheumatoid arthritis. Adv Immunol 64:283–350, 1997.
27. Maini, R, St. Clair, EW, and Breedveld, F, et al: Infliximab (chimeric anti-tumour necrosis factor-alpha monoclonal antibody) versus placebo in rheumatoid arthritis patients receiving concomitant methotrexate: A randomised phase III trial. ATTRACT Study Group. Lancet 354:1932–1939, 1999.
28. Present, DH, Rutgeerts, P, and Targan, S, et al: Infliximab for the treatment of fistulas in patients with Crohn's disease. N Engl J Med 340:1398–1405, 1999.
29. Breedveld, FC: Therapeutic monoclonal antibodies. Lancet 355: 735–740, 2000.

Cytokines

Maureane Hoffman, MD, PhD

Learning Objectives

After finishing this chapter, the reader will be able to:

1. Define cytokine.
2. Define pleiotropy and redundancy as they relate to cytokine activities.
3. Distinguish between autocrine, paracrine, and endocrine effects of cytokines.
4. Differentiate innate from specific immune responses.
5. Explain the local and systemic effects of tumor necrosis factor (TNF).
6. Explain the functions of interleukin-1 (IL-1) in mediating the immune response.
7. Compare the cell source and functions of type 1 and type 2 interferons (IFN).
8. Discuss the features and cytokine mediators of the acute phase response.
9. Describe the actions of interleukin-2 (IL-2) on target cells.
10. Discuss the biologic roles of the hematopoietic growth factors.
11. Describe the effects of TNF on virally infected and tumor cells.
12. Describe the biologic role colony stimulating factors.
13. Apply knowledge of interleukins to suggest therapy for certain disease states.

Key Terms

Acute phase response
Adaptive immune response
Autocrine
C-kit ligand
Chemokine
Chemokinesis
Chemotaxis
Colony stimulating factor
  (CSF)
Cytokine
Endocrine
Endogenous pyrogen
Granulocyte-CSF
Granulocyte-macrophage-
  CSF
Innate immune response
Interferons
Interleukin-1 (IL-1)
Interleukin-2 (IL-2)
Interleukin-3 (IL-3)
Ligand
Lipopolysaccharide (LPS)
Macrophage-monocyte-CSF
Paracrine
Pleiotrophy
Redundancy
Tumor necrosis factor (TNF)

Cytokines are chemical messengers that influence the activities of other cells. They play important roles both during the activation and effector phases of the immune response. They act primarily as local mediators. The actions of cytokines often involve **autocrine** stimulation (i.e., affecting the same cell that secreted it) or **paracrine** stimulation (i.e., affecting a target cell in close proximity). Some cytokines also have systemic **(endocrine)** effects, but this is the exception rather than the rule. The local nature of cytokine effects tends to distinguish them from hormones, which generally have effects at a distance from their sites of production and are carried to their sites of action by the blood. Like hormones, the effects of cytokines are mediated by binding to specific protein receptors on their target cells.

Cytokines have a wide variety of actions in the body. Two features that characterize cytokines as a class are pleiotropy and redundancy. **Pleiotropy** means that a single cytokine has many different actions. Not only does a single cytokine usually affect the activities of more than one kind of cell, but it may also have more than one kind of effect on the same cell. **Redundancy** means that different cytokines often have very similar effects. These two features make it quite hard to classify cytokines on the basis of their activities. It is also nearly impossible to classify cytokines based on their cell of origin. In the past some cytokines were referred to as lymphokines (produced by lymphocytes) or monokines (produced by monocytes or macrophages). However, it is now clear that nearly all cytokines are produced by multiple different cell types.

Another characteristic feature of cytokines is that they act in networks. That is, one cytokine may stimulate the release of other cytokines that have similar or overlapping activities. In addition, a cytokine may also produce effects that terminate its activity. For example, cytokines may stimulate release and cleavage of their receptors from target cells. This often counteracts the cytokine's activity by removing the receptor for the cytokine so that the cell can no longer respond. In addition, in some cases the soluble receptors can still bind their target cytokines. Once bound to the soluble receptor, the cytokine is usually inactivated because it cannot also bind to a functional cell-surface receptor. Thus, the effects of a cytokine are not only determined by its local concentration, but also by the local concentration of "antagonists" such as soluble receptors and the level of receptor expression on nearby target cells.

In addition to directly regulating immune responses, many cytokines act as growth factors for hematopoietic cells, regulating both the proliferation and maturation of immature precursors. In this capacity cytokines can modulate the number and composition of cells available to participate in host defense. The various actions of cytokines are summed up in Figure 6–1.

Because of their pleiotropic, redundant, and interactive effects, it can be very difficult to determine the biologically important functions of cytokines. The ability to alter genes in mice has allowed a better understanding of the roles of cytokines *in vivo*. "Knockout" mice, in which a specific cytokine or cytokine receptor gene has been deleted or inactivated, have allowed us to see the biologic consequences of losing a particular cytokine function. In some cases, abolishing a cytokine activity has had surprisingly little effect. In other cases the effects are dramatic, but unexpected. In many cases a cytokine was originally identified as having a particular activity but was later found to play a very different biologic role. Although the use of knockout mouse

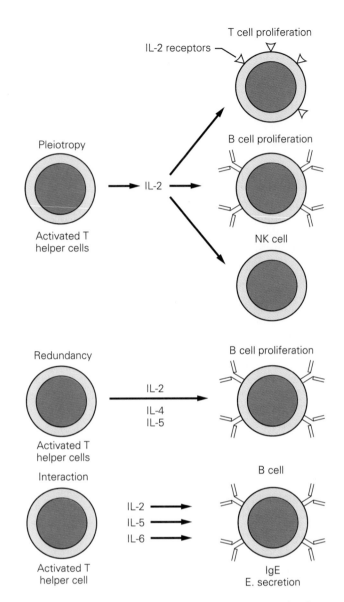

FIG. 6–1. Cytokine characteristics of pleiotropy, redundancy, and interaction. (Adapted from Goldsby, RA, Kindt, TJ, and Osborne, BA: Kuby Immunology, ed. 4. WH Freeman, New York, 2000, with permission.)

models can be a very powerful tool, one must bear in mind that some cytokine systems appear to function differently in mice and humans.

We divide our discussion of cytokines into three segments: (1) cytokines involved in the innate immune response; (2) cytokines involved in the adaptive immune response; and (3) cytokines involved in the growth and differentiation of immature leukocytes. However, because of the pleiotropic effects of cytokines, a single cytokine may have effects in more than one of these areas. In addition, an essential function of cytokines is to regulate the progression from an innate to a specific immune response.

The Role of Cytokines in Innate Immune Responses

Cytokines play a critical role in coordinating the activities of the immune system. The immune system acts to recognize and eliminate foreign organisms. It is composed of innate or "non-specific" immunity and adaptive or "specific" immunity. The innate immune response recognizes a limited repertoire of constituents that are common to a broad range of microorganisms. These constituents are often important to the survival or pathogenicity of the organism. The **innate immune response** is activated within hours of first contact, and its efficacy is not significantly increased on repeated exposure to an organism. The **adaptive immune response,** by contrast, can recognize a nearly unlimited number of different targets but only becomes effective 2 to 4 days after first contact with a given microorganism. Lymphocytes and lymphocyte products specific for that microorganism, however, then persist as immune memory and are rapidly protective on re-exposure to the same infectious agent. Almost all of the effector mechanisms for eliminating infectious organisms are provided by the innate immune system. They may be invoked either directly by innate immune recognition mechanisms or indirectly by cells or products of the adaptive immune systems.

Cytokines produced by mononuclear phagocytes during the innate immune response increase vascular permeability, change the adhesive properties of vascular endothelial lining cells, and recruit additional cells and molecules of the immune system to sites of infection. The actions of cytokines produce the cardinal signs of inflammation: redness, swelling, heat, and pain.

Mononuclear phagocytes and their cytokines also play a critical role in activating the subsequent adaptive immune response. Adaptive immune responses are mediated by lymphocytes. In addition to processing and presenting antigen, macrophages produce cytokines that stimulate both T and B lymphocytes and direct the evolution of specific immunity. T lymphocytes in turn produce cytokines that activate macrophages to kill intracellular pathogens. They also produce cytokines that activate B lymphocytes, thereby enhancing antibody production. Some cytokines also act as direct effector molecules, especially in killing malignant cells. Cytokines involved in the innate immune response are summarized in Table 6–1.

Non-Immune (Type 1) Interferons

Interferons (IFN) were originally named because they "interfere" with viral replication in an infected cell. They also have immunoregulatory effects in addition to antiviral activity. They are grouped into three classes—α, β, and γ—according to their major functions and the cell source. IFN-α and INF-β are considered type 1 or non-immune IFN because they are produced primarily during the initial innate response to viral infection. By contrast, IFN-γ (discussed further later in the chapter) is classified as a type 2 or immune IFN because it is primarily produced as a component of the specific immune response to viral and other pathogens.

IFN-α is a family of about 20 related polypeptides with molecular weights of around 18kD. These molecules are primarily produced by mononuclear phagocytes and therefore are sometimes called leukocyte IFN. IFN-β is produced by fibroblasts *in vitro* and has been called fibroblast interferon. However, both of these molecules can be produced by many different cells in response to viral infection. The presence of viral products that are not normally found in mammalian cells, such as double-stranded ribonucleic acid, stimulate the release of type 1 IFN. The IFN acts primarily in a paracrine fashion to induce the expression of proteins that inhibit viral replication. Thus, IFN induces a viral-resistant state in cells in the vicinity of an infected cell. Type 1 IFN also generally inhibits cell proliferation, perhaps because the mechanisms that interfere with viral replication have a similar effect on host cell replication. This effect is now being therapeutically in the treatment of certain malignancies.

IFN-α and IFN-β are not structurally similar. However, they bind to the same receptor, and they have similar activities. In addition to their antiviral activity, they also increase the ability of natural killer (NK) cells to kill virally infected cells. Type 1 IFN enhances expression of class I major histocompatibility complex (MHC) molecules, which may enhance recognition of virally infected cells by cytotoxic lymphocytes. These IFNs are also produced during specific immune responses to antigens. In this case, antigen-activated T cells stimulate mononuclear phagocytes to produce IFN.

Tumor Necrosis Factor

While type 1 IFN is a major mediator of the defense against viral infection, **tumor necrosis factor (TNF)** is a major mediator of the innate defense against gram-negative bacteria. TNF was named on the basis of the observation that animals treated with bacterial **lipopolysaccharide (LPS)** had a factor in their serum that would cause necrosis of transplanted tumors. This activity is probably primarily the result of an effect of TNF on the tumor vasculature. TNF can also directly trigger apoptotic death of some tumor cells through a receptor-mediated mechanism.[1] However, it is now

TABLE 6–1. Cytokines Involved in Innate Immunity

Name	(Amino Acids)	Primary Source	Primary Action
Type I IFN	166	Mononuclear phagocytes, other cells	Antiviral state, increased MHC class I
TNF	157	Mononuclear phagocytes, T cells	Proinflammatory Fever Acute phase response Catabolism/cachexia
IL-1	159 (α), 153(β)	Mononuclear phagocytes, other cells	Proinflammatory Fever Acute phase response Catabolism/cachexia
IL-6	184	Mononuclear phagocytes, endothelial cells, T cells	Acute phase response
IL-10	160	Mononuclear phagocytes, T cells	Inhibitory
IL-12	750	Mononuclear phagocytes, dendritic cells	Promote IFN-γ synthesis by T cells and cytolytic function of NK cells
IL-15	170	Mononuclear phagocytes, other	Proliferation of NK cells
Chemokines	70–100	Mononuclear phagocytes, endothelial cells, fibroblasts, T cells; platelets	Promote Chemotaxis of:
C-X-C subgroup			
IL-8			Neutrophils
Gro			Neutrophils
Platelet basic protein			Neutrophils
Epithelial-derived neutrophil attractant 78			Neutrophils
Platelet factor 4			?
Interferon-γ protein 10			Lymphocytes
Stromal cell derived factor-1			Neutrophils, monocytes, lymphocytes
C-C subgroup			
Monocyte chemotactic proteins (1,2,3)			Monocyte, T cell, eosinophil
RANTES			
Monocyte inflammatory protein 1			Monocyte, T cell, eosinophil
Eotaxin			Monocyte, T cell, eosinophil
C subgroup			Eosinophil
Lymphotactin			Lymphocyte

IFN = Interferon; MHC = major histocompatibility complex; NK = natural killer; RANTES = regulated on activation, normal T expressed and secreted.

recognized that tumor cell killing is not the primary function of TNF.

TNF is a member of a family of closely related peptides that includes TNF-β (once called lymphotoxin), Fas ligand, CD40 ligand, and others.[2] **Ligand** means the molecule that binds to a specific receptor (e.g., CD40 ligand is the molecule that binds to CD40). These cytokines share structural features, and although they bind to different receptors, they also share the ability to trigger pathways that lead to apoptosis (programmed cell death) in their target cells. Thus, all of these family members could act as effector mechanisms by leading to the death of infected, malignant, or inappropriately responding host cells. The precise physiologic role of the family members other than TNF is not yet clear.

The primary cellular sources of TNF are mononuclear phagocytes, although antigen-activated T cells, activated NK cells, and activated mast cells can also secrete TNF to a limited extent. The major trigger for TNF secretion is LPS from gram-negative bacteria. The terms *LPS* or *bacterial endotoxin* refer to a class of bacterial lipid that is not produced by mammalian cells. LPS is bound by a specific LPS-binding protein (LBP) that is present in plasma. The complex of LPS/LBP binds to a receptor on mononuclear phagocytes, CD14.[3,4] Occupancy of this receptor triggers mononuclear phagocytes to produce TNF and other proinflammatory cytokines, such as IL-1 and interleukin-6 (IL-6). There are almost certainly additional receptors for LPS, but these are less well characterized.

The "secretion" of TNF (and other members of the TNF family) is rather unusual. It is initially produced as a transmembrane protein of about 25 kD. The transmembrane segment of the protein is near the amino-terminus, with only a small portion of the amino-terminal remaining intracellular. The cell-associated TNF molecules assemble into trimers. These TNF trimers are able to engage TNF receptors and transduce a signal to cells in direct contact with the TNF-producing cell. The TNF molecules are cleaved near the transmembrane segment to release soluble, biologically active trimers composed of 17 kD subunits.

When TNF is secreted in low amounts, it acts as an autocrine and paracrine mediator. In this capacity it enhances effector functions of leukocytes and enhances expression of leukocyte adhesion molecules on vascular endothelial cells. It also induces secretion of chemokines by mononuclear phagocytes that recruit additional leukocytes. These activities enhance the number and activity of leukocytes in the local area of an inflammatory reaction.

When secreted in larger amounts, TNF reaches measurable levels in the blood and acts a systemic (endocrine) mediator. In this capacity it acts as an **endogenous pyrogen** (induces fever). It also stimulates secretion of other proinflammatory cytokines, especially IL-1, IL-6, and interleukin-8 (IL-8). Along with IL-1 and IL-6, TNF plays a role in inducing the **acute phase response.** The acute phase response is a rapid alteration in protein synthesis in the liver in response to inflammatory stimuli. The levels of a number of plasma proteins rise during the acute phase response, including C-reactive protein, serum amyloid protein A, and fibrinogen. Levels of albumin and the iron transport protein, transferrin, decline. The acute phase response is reflected in a more rapid sedimentation of red blood cells (RBCs) when the blood is allowed to stand. This can be measured by a technique known as the erythrocyte sedimentation rate (ESR). (See laboratory exercise.)

When secreted at even higher levels, TNF can cause metabolic alterations, depress myocardial contractility, relax vascular smooth muscle and promote intravascular coagulation. These effects can be quite harmful to the host, even being lethal when TNF levels are quite high.

The deleterious effects of TNF are largely responsible for the syndrome of septic shock.[5] Septic shock is caused by the release of huge amounts of TNF in response to gram-negative bacterial infection. Thus, it is the host response that causes the pathologic condition. High levels of TNF have acute and dramatic effects on the host. TNF depression of heart contractility results in a reduction of blood pressure and in the delivery of blood to the tissues. Vascular smooth muscle relaxation further lowers blood pressure. TNF can cause disseminated intravascular coagulation (DIC) by impairing the anticoagulant properties of the blood vessel endothelial lining cells. DIC also reduces tissue perfusion and may lead to uncontrollable bleeding. TNF suppresses the division of hematopoietic stem cells in the bone marrow. While TNF is the most injurious mediator, it also stimulates the production of other inflammatory mediators (especially IL-1) that contribute to the manifestations of sepsis.

In addition to its acute systemic effects in sepsis, chronic TNF release can produce a pattern of systemic metabolic alterations that causes cachexia.[6] This is a catabolic state that results in the wasting of fat and muscle tissue. This syndrome is generally seen in the setting of cancer and chronic infectious or inflammatory diseases.

IFN-α, produced by antigen-activated T cells, increases TNF synthesis by LPS-activated mononuclear phagocytes. Therefore, TNF is linked to both specific and innate immune responses.

Interleukin-1

Many cytokines are called "interleukins." This name was coined when it was thought that cytokines only or primarily served as a means of communication between leukocytes. We now know that most of the interleukins are secreted by multiple cell types. Interleukins are numbered sequentially as they are discovered and studied, but the number is no reflection of a specific cytokine's activities.

Interleukin-1 (IL-1) is produced by macrophages and monocytes in response to bacterial LPS and TNF.[7] IL-1 is the archetypical proinflammatory cytokine. It was initially identified as a product of mononuclear phagocytes that served as a costimulator of T cells. Actions of IL-1 include inducing IL-2 and IL-2 receptors (CD25) in T cells, proliferation and differentiation of B cells, and enhancement of cytotoxicity of NK cells. However, IL-1 has now been extensively studied, and it is generally accepted that the primary role of IL-1 is as a proinflammatory mediator in innate immune responses and a link between innate and adaptive responses.

There are two different forms of IL-1, α and β. Both are synthesized as 31 kD precursors and proteolytically processed to the mature 18 kD forms. The α form possesses activity without further processing, while the β type seems to require cleavage before it is functional. IL-1α primarily remains intracellular.[8] It is released when the cell dies and can be processed to the mature form by extracellular proteases. It can also be cleaved and released from living cells, but it is not clear what the signal is for this *in vivo*. In humans, IL-1α is not found in the circulation except in very severe disease. It has been hypothesized to serve primarily as an autocrine growth factor.

In many respects IL-1β is a very different mediator from IL-1α. Once released from its cell of origin, IL-1β is part of an intricate system of related molecules.[7] Two antagonists are produced: a soluble form of an IL-1 receptor, which binds and inactivates IL-1β, and an IL-1 receptor antagonist, which competes with IL-1β for binding to cell surface receptors. It appears that IL-1β often has systemic, hormone-like effects, while IL-1α acts as a mediator of intracellular events and local inflammation.

Locally, IL-1 acts as a chemotactic agent, attracting neutrophils, lymphocytes, and monocytes to the site of inflammation. It also acts to prime effector and stromal cells so that their responses to inflammatory stimuli are enhanced. For example, exposure to IL-1 results in increased degranulation of neutrophils upon contact with a foreign organism. Additionally, monocytes and fibroblasts show increased prostaglandin release, which enhances capillary permeability.

IL-1 has important systemic effects as well. IL-1 stimulates synthesis of some acute phase reactants. It is also a potent endogenous pyrogen. An increase in temperature enhances T and B cell activity, which may be a reason for the febrile response to infection. Additional effects of IL-1 on the central nervous system include depression of appetite and slow-wave sleep. Many of the effects of IL-1 have been found to be caused by the production of other mediators, especially increased production of inflammatory prostaglandins, leukotrienes, and nitric oxide.

Although most actions of IL-1 enhance the immune response and thus exert a positive effect, there are some negative aspects. Similar to TNF, IL-1 can cause hypoglycemia, hypotension, depressed myocardial contractility, and increased heart rate. Prolonged synthesis of IL-1 contributes to the muscle wasting that occurs in some chronic diseases. IL-1 has a number of activities in common with TNF, and the two cytokines are often produced at the same time *in vivo*. In some cases the two exhibit synergism in producing their proinflammatory effects. However, there are several important differences between IL-1 and TNF. First, IL-1 is produced by a wide range of cell types, not only cells of the immune system. Second, IL-1 by itself does not produce the potentially lethal systemic effects that result from high levels of TNF.

Interleukin-6

Interleukin-6 (IL-6) is a cytokine of about 26 kD that is part of the cascade of cytokines released in response to LPS. It is made by mononuclear phagocytes, vascular endothelial cells, fibroblasts, and some other cells. IL-1 primarily triggers its secretion. It appears later in the course of a gram-negative bacterial infection than TNF and IL-1. Thus, LPS triggers TNF release, which triggers IL-1 release, which in turn triggers IL-6 release. IL-6 is a primary mediator of the acute phase response,[9,10] with TNF and IL-1 also playing roles. IL-6 is the signal for enhanced fibrinogen synthesis by the liver. Fibrinogen levels are the major determinant of the elevated erythrocyte sedimentation rate seen in inflammation.

In addition to its role in the acute phase response, IL-6 is a growth factor for activated B lymphocytes and plasma cells, thereby promoting immunoglobulin secretion. Other effects of IL-6 include the synergistic promotion with interleukin-3 (IL-3) of the growth of hematopoietic progenitor cells, and the activation and generation of cytotoxic T cells.

IL-6 receptors can be released in a soluble form and bind free IL-6. Unlike some ligand–soluble receptor complexes, the IL-6–receptor complex can bind to a signal-transducing subunit on target cells and exert biologic activity.

Chemokines

Chemokines are a large family of homologous cytokines, the archetypical member of which was IL-8.[11] These are **chemo**tactic cyto**kines** that enhance motility **(chemokinesis)** and promote the migration of specific classes of leukocytes toward the source of the chemokine **(chemotaxis)**. Chemokines range in size from 8 to 10 kD and have been classified into two groups by shared structural motifs.[12] Each member of the family has two disulfide bonded loops. If the two amino-terminal cysteine residues involved in disulfide bonding are adjacent to one another, the chemokine is in the "C-C" subfamily. If the two cysteines are separated by another amino acid, the chemokine is in the "C-X-C" subfamily. One chemokine, lymphotaxin, has an unpaired cysteine and is classified as a "C" chemokine. There are several receptors for C-C and C-X-C chemokines that are all structurally related.[13] Some of these receptors are very specific for a single chemokine, while others are more promiscuous and bind several related chemokines. This feature may account for some of the redundancy in chemokine effects.

The C-X-C chemokines are produced primarily by mononuclear phagocytes, endothelial cells, fibroblasts, and megakaryocytes (platelet precursors). Platelets can release several chemokines on activation that act primarily on neutrophils. This is one mechanism linking blood coagulation at a site of injury to the subsequent development of inflammation and an innate immune response.[14]

The C-C chemokines are primarily produced by activated T lymphocytes and act on leukocytes other than neutrophils. Overlapping receptor specificities result in some chemokines having activity for multiple types of leukocytes, while others have a strict specificity for a single cell type. Thus, the pattern of chemokine expression during an inflammatory or immune response is a major determinant of the population of immune cells that will participate in that response. Refer to Table 6–2 for a listing of selected chemokines.

Interleukin-10

In contrast to the cytokines we have discussed so far, interleukin-10 (IL-10) has primarily inhibitory effects on the immune response.[15] It appears to have two major functions. It inhibits production of proinflammatory cytokines by mononuclear phagocytes and inhibits the accessory functions of mononuclear phagocytes for T cell activation. It is interesting that the Epstein-Barr virus contains a gene that encodes a protein homologous to IL-10. This protein appears to play a role in allowing the virus to escape destruction by down-regulating the host immune response.

Interleukin-12

Interleukin-12 (IL-12) was originally characterized as an activator of NK cells produced by mononuclear phagocytes. Active IL-12 is a disulfide-linked dimer of two different subunits, p35 and p40. Many cells synthesize the p35 subunit, but mainly mononuclear phagocytes and dendritic cells produce the p40 subunit. Therefore, it is only the latter cells that produce active IL-12. IL-12 receptors are found on NK cells, T cells, and some B cells.

IL-12 is now recognized to trigger secretion of IFN-γ by T cells and NK cells. It also promotes the differentiation of T helper (Th) cells into Th1 cells that secrete IFN-γ and thus enhances macrophage effector functions. Finally, IL-12 enhances the cytotoxic function of NK cells and CD8+ T cells. Thus, IL-12 fills two roles in the immune response: (1) It links macrophage recognition of microbial products to activation of NK cell functions, and (2) it links innate and adaptive immune responses by promoting a cell-mediated immune response to defend against intracellular pathogens.[16]

Interleukin-15

Interleukin-15 (IL-15) is a 13kD protein that is primarily released by mononuclear phagocytes and some tissue cells.[17] Its release occurs in response to viral infection, LPS, or other products of pathogens that are recognized by the innate immune system. IL-15 was initially identified as a cytokine that could support proliferation of an IL-2–dependent T cell line in the presence of inhibitory IL-2 antibodies. However, its role *in vivo* is not in promoting T cell proliferation. Instead, IL-15 appears to play a unique and important role in supporting the development and proliferation of NK cells.

While IL-15 has little sequence homology to

TABLE 6–2. Cytokines Involved in Adaptive Immunity

Name	(Amino Acids)	Primary Source	Primary Action
IL-2	133	T cell	Proliferation and activation of T, B, and NK cells
IL-4	129	Th cell, mast cell	Isotype switching to IgE; T cell proliferation and differentiation; endothelial cell activation
IL-5	115	T cell	Eosinophil production and activation
TNF-β	240	T cell	Activation of neutrophils and endothelial cells; killing of target cells
Interferon-γ	143	T cell, NK cell	Mononuclear phagocyte activation; enhanced MHC on all cell types

IL = Interleukin; NK = natural killer; Th = T helper; IgE = immunoglobulin E; TNF = tumor necrosis factor; MHC = major histocompatibility complex.

IL-2, computer modeling of its 3-dimensional structure suggested that it was a member of the family (4-helix bindle cytokine family) that includes IL-2, IL-3, IL-6, interleukin-7 (IL-7), granulocyte–colony stimulating factor (G-CSF), granulocyte-macrophage CSF (GM-CSF), and growth hormone. IL-2 and IL-15 receptors consist of three components (α, β, and γ chains).[18] The two types of receptors share the same β and γ chains, but use different α chains. It is the β and γ chains of the receptor complex that are responsible for signaling. Therefore, it is not surprising that IL-2 and IL-15 can mediate similar cellular responses in cell culture. However, the two cytokines appear to fill very different roles *in vivo*. In addition to its role in NK mediated immune responses, IL-15 also seems to play a role in autoimmune processes and the development of adult T cell leukemia.

The Role of Cytokines in Specific Immune Responses

The cytokines that promote and regulate innate immune responses are largely secreted by mononuclear phagocytes. In contrast, the cytokines that regulate acquired immune responses are largely secreted by T cells, especially Th cells. There appear to be several subclasses of Th cells, which have different functions and produce different cytokines. The Th1 subset is thought to be responsible for delayed hypersensitivity reactions and activation of cytotoxic T cells (cell-mediated immunity), while the Th2 subset is the main one responsible for B cell activation (humoral immunity). Th1 cells produce IL-2 and IFN-γ, while Th2 cells produce interleukin-4 (IL-4) and interleukin-5 (IL-5), but not IL-2 or IFN-γ. The delineation between Th1 and Th2 may not be as clear as that, and there may be additional subtypes of Th cells with characteristic patterns of cytokine production. The different populations are thought to induce the appropriate set of regulator functions to eliminate a particular pathogen.[19] For example, killing of a virus requires cell-mediated cytotoxicity that is dominated by Th1 cells, while response to a bacterial cell requires antibodies, facilitated by Th2 cells. Cytokines involved in adaptive immunity are summarized in Table 6–2.

Interleukin-2

Interleukin-2 (IL-2) stimulates activated T cells to proliferate and was originally called T cell growth factor. It is produced by antigen-stimulated Th cells. Contact with an antigen-presenting cell stimulates the Th cell. Costimulatory signaling through the CD28

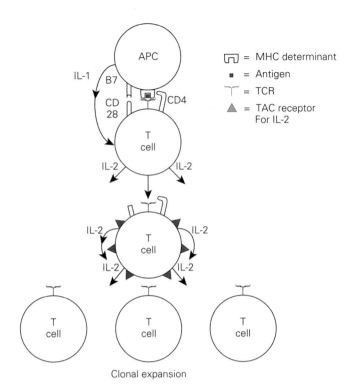

FIG. 6–2. Activation of Th cells by two signals. The T cell receptor (TCR) recognizes antigen with MHC class II on antigen-presenting cells (APCs). CD4 also recognizes MHC class II. The second signal for activation is provided by CD28 on the T cell binding to B7 on the antigen-presenting cell. Activation of the T cell results in IL-2 production and increased IL-2 receptors. IL-2 induces clonal expansion.

molecule and IL-1 released by the antigen presenting cell promote IL-2 secretion and increased IL-2 receptor expression by the Th cell. In essence, the Th cell turns itself on and triggers proliferation. While acting to stimulate the cell that produced it, IL-2 also acts on any other antigen-stimulated T cells in the area, thus amplifying the cellular immune response.[20] IL-2 can be detected 2 to 6 hours after antigen exposure, with maximum production being reached at 12 hours (Fig. 6–2).

In addition to its role as the major growth factor for T cells, IL-2 can promote apoptosis, or destruction, of antigen-stimulated T cells. Although the two effects of IL-2 on T cells may seem antithetical, these effects take place at different stages in T cell development. Thus, IL-2 appears to play a critical role in the elimination of self-reactive T cells. Mice that lack components of the IL-2 receptor develop autoimmunity, presumably because they do not eliminate self-reactive cells through IL-2–dependent activation-induced cell death.

Recall from the section on IL-15 that IL-2 and IL-15 receptors (and a number of other cytokine receptors) consist of α, β, and γ chains.[21] Many cytokine receptors share a common γ chain, but use specific α and β chains. It is the β and -γ chains of the receptor complex that are responsible for signaling. A complex of the IL-2 receptor β- and the common γ chain constitutes a low affinity receptor for IL-2 (and IL-15). Cells that also express the specific IL-2 receptor α chain (also called Tac or T activation antigen) can bind IL-2 with much higher affinity. Resting T cells express the β and γ chains, but not the α chain, of the IL-2 receptor. They only respond to high levels of IL-2. After antigen-mediated stimulation, T cells express the α chain of the receptor and can consequently respond to much lower levels of IL-2.

Two other cell types affected by IL-2 are B cells and NK cells. Proliferation of B cells is enhanced, and B cells are influenced to produce immunoglobulin-G2 (IgG2) antibodies (Fig. 6–3). IL-2 also stimulates proliferation of NK cells and enhances their cytotoxicity, producing lymphokine-activated killer (LAK) cells. LAK cells can destroy cells that are resistant to killing by NK cells, and they do so without regard to MHC restriction.[19] NK cells only express the low–affinity form of the IL-2 receptor. Therefore, high levels of IL-2 are required for generation of LAK cells.

Interleukin-4

Originally called B cell growth factor I, interleukin-4 (IL-4) can trigger activation, proliferation, and differentiation of B cells that have been previously stimulated by antigen.[22] However, the main physiologic functions of IL-4 are to promote growth and differentiation of mast cells and to promote IgE production. IL-4 stimulates isotype switching of B cells to IgE. IL-4 is primarily produced by Th2 cells and also acts as a growth and differentiation factor for Th2 cells. Its production is the main criterion for classifying Th cells as Th2 cells (IFN-γ production is characteristic of Th1 cells).

IL-4 stimulates the expression of adhesion molecules on vascular endothelial cells, thus increasing binding of leukocytes, especially eosinophils. Increased local binding leads to enhanced migration into the adjacent tissue. A less well-characterized cytokine, interleukin-13 (IL-13), shares many of the activities of IL-4,[23] including sharing receptor components similar to the relationship between IL-2 and IL-15.

Interleukin-5

The main physiologic function of interleukin-5 (IL-5) appears to be to promote the growth and differentiation of eosinophils and to activate mature eosinophils to kill parasites more effectively. Studies have demon-

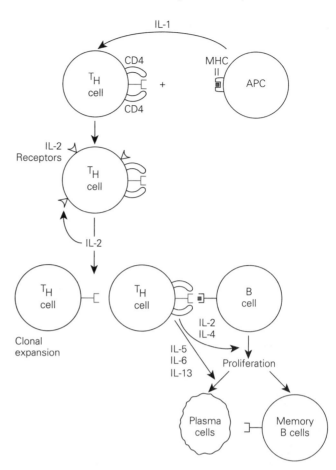

FIG. 6–3. Interaction between Th cells and B cells in the production of antibody. Th cells are stimulated by contact with antigen. The CD4 T cell causes an antigen-activated B cell to proliferate. MHC = Major histocompatibility complex; APC = antigen-presenting cells; IL = interleukin; IFN = interferon.

strated that during helminth infections and allergic encounters, IL-5 is the major cytokine regulating eosinophilia.[24] Thus, IL-4 and IL-5 work together in supporting eosinophil and IgE-mediated immune responses.

IL-5 also has some effects on humoral immunity. It was once known as B cell growth factor II, or B cell differentiating factor, because it can stimulate proliferation of activated B cells. Production and secretion of IgM and class switching to IgA are also enhanced by IL-5, which is secreted by activated Th2 cells and by mast cells.

Immune (Type 2) Interferon

Immune interferon (IFN-γ) is made primarily by activated T cells, and although it also exhibits antiviral activity, its primary importance is as an immune activator. A major role of IFN-γ is to activate macrophages. A number of other cytokines have some macrophage activating effects, including GM-CSF, TNF, and IL-1. However, IFN-γ is the most potent and global macrophage activating factor. In this capacity, it stimulates the phagocytic, cytotoxic, and degradative abilities of these cells, creating "super" macrophages. Such immunologically activated macrophages have an enhanced capability to kill tumor cells, virally infected cells, and intracellular pathogens that are resistant to killing by unactivated macrophages.

IFN-γ also increases expression of class I MHC molecules and causes a variety of cells to express class II MHC antigens. As MHC antigens are recognized along with foreign antigen, increasing the density of these proteins will also increase the likelihood of antigen presentation to lymphocytes. Fragment crystallizable (Fc) receptors on macrophages are also increased because of the influence of IFN-γ. This heightens their ability to combine with immune complexes, thus speeding up the processing and clearing of the antigen from the area.

Additionally, IFN-γ promotes differentiation of T cells into the Th1 subset. Activating mononuclear phagocytes to secrete IL-12 and enhancing expression of IL-12 receptors on T cells probably mediate this effect. IFN-γ also promotes B cell switching from IgM to IgG2a and IgG3 subclasses. Thus, IFN-γ enhances antibody responses that participate in the elimination of microbial organisms by phagocytosis. Neutrophils are also activated by IFN-γ, although less potently than TNF or lymphotoxin.

Tumor Necrosis Factor-β

TNF-β, formerly called lymphotoxin, is produced by both CD4 and CD8 lymphocytes, although it is usually thought of in association with CD8 or cytotoxic lymphocytes.[25,26] It is responsible for the killing of virally infected host cells and tumor cells.

Once recognition of a foreign antigen occurs, cytotoxic T (Tc) cells are induced to proliferate, giving rise to additional Tc cells with the same specificity. In addition, the Tc cells release toxins that kill the target cell. The most important of these toxins is TNF-β, which binds to a specific receptor and triggers apoptosis of the target cell. The activity of TNF-β is short-lived and localized because it has a half-life of only minutes. Once the death of the target cell has been triggered, however, the effector T cell is able to seek other targets because it is not destroyed in the process (Fig. 6–4).

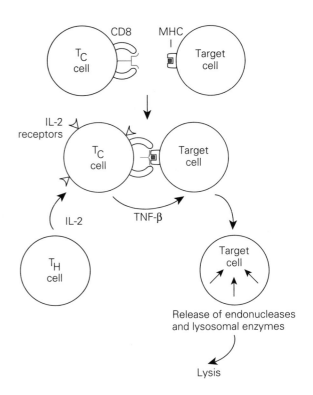

FIG. 6–4. Destruction of target cells by cytotoxic T cells. The cytotoxic Tc recognizes antigen in association with MHC class I protein. With help from a CD4 cell, the cytotoxic Tc produces TNF-β. TNF-α causes the release of enzymes, resulting in killing of the target cell. MHC = Major histocompatibility complex; IL = interleukin; TNF = tumor necrosis factor.

Hematopoietic Growth Factors

A number of cytokines produced during innate and acquired immune responses stimulate the proliferation and differentiation of bone marrow progenitor cells. Thus, the responses that require a supply of leukocytes produce mediators to provide those cells. The primary mediators of hematopoiesis are called **colony stimulating factors (CSFs)** because they stimulate the formation of colonies in cultures of bone marrow cells. The effects of CSFs are also modulated by other inflammatory and immune cytokines, such as IL-1 and TNF. Hematopoietic cells develop from a common precursor in the bone marrow. The proliferation and differentiation of different lineages (i.e., erythrocyte, megakaryocyte, granulocyte, monocyte, and lymphocyte) are controlled by different CSFs. This section primarily covers the growth factors that affect leukocyte lineages. There are many other cytokine growth factors that have their primary effects on non-hematopoietic cells. These are not discussed in this chapter.

C-kit Ligand

The growth factor that affects the growth of the most primitive precursor cells in the bone marrow is called **c-kit ligand** or stem cell factor. This protein was identified originally as the ligand that binds to the cellular oncogene c-kit. It is produced by stromal cells in the bone marrow in cell surface and soluble forms. The cell surface form of c-kit ligand is probably the most important *in vivo*. It appears that c-kit ligand acts to make progenitor cells in the bone marrow responsive to other CSFs. In addition, c-kit ligand has a role in maintaining the viability of T cells in the thymus and of mast cells in mucosal sites.

Interleukin-3

Interleukin-3 (IL-3) is also called multilineage CSF (multi-CSF), and is produced by Th cells of both Th1 and Th2 subtypes.[19] IL-3 stimulates the proliferation of immature marrow cells that are not yet committed to a specific lineage.[27] Most of the studies of IL-3 (and other cytokines) have been done in mice. In the mouse model, IL-3 serves as an important link between the immune system and the hematopoietic system. However, it appears that many of the functions of IL-3 in mice are carried out by GM-CSF in humans. Thus, the specific role of IL-3 in human biology remains unclear.

Lineage-Specific Colony Stimulating Factors

As hematopoietic cells differentiate, they acquire the ability to respond to lineage-specific cytokines such as **granulocyte-macrophage CSF (GM-CSF)**, **macrophage-monocyte CSF (M-CSF)**, and **granulocyte CSF (G-CSF)**. These three CSFs are produced by activated T cells, macrophages, fibroblasts, and endothelial cells. The end result of CSF production is a supply of additional inflammatory leukocytes for the overall immune response. G-CSF and GM-CSF are used clinically to enhance bone marrow recovery after cancer chemotherapy.[28,29] They also promote the movement of progenitor cells from the bone marrow into the peripheral blood. This allows the resulting peripheral blood progenitor cells to be harvested for subsequent transplantation.[30]

While the CSFs are involved in the production of myeloid cells, IL-7 is a product of bone marrow stromal cells that is specifically involved in the production of lymphocytes.[31] A genetically engineered mouse in which the IL-7 gene has been knocked out has a 10- to 20-fold reduction in the total number of B and T cells and impaired maturation of some types of T cells. In addition to its effects on the production of lymphocytes, IL-7 also acts on mature T cells in a similar fashion to IL-2. Thus, it appears that IL-7 is required for normal production and maturation of lymphocytes, especially T cells.

Two other lineage-specific CSFs are erythropoietin and thrombopoietin, which stimulate the production of RBCs and platelets, respectively. These molecules do not have a role in the immune response, so they will not be discussed further. However, they have found clinical utility in stimulating RBC and platelet production in a number of settings.

Clinical Uses of Cytokines

The manipulation of cytokine systems for therapeutic benefit has become well-established during the past 5 years. As mentioned previously, hematopoietic CSFs are routinely used to promote recovery of leukocyte and platelet production by the bone marrow after chemotherapy. Of course, erythropoietin has been used for a relatively long time to promote production of RBCs in a number of clinical settings. Some of the most exciting advances have come in the area of manipulating the immune system to control damaging immune responses and autoimmunity. Strategies to block the activity of TNF appear to be promising in reducing the damaging inflammatory effects of autoimmune responses. Cytokines are also in use to control viral infections that are not controlled by the host, and for which we have no synthetic inhibitors, such as chronic hepatitis C infection. The presence or absence of specific cytokines is best measured by enzyme-linked immunosorbent assay (ELISA) testing. New applications of our evolving understanding of cytokine biology are appearing in clinical trials at a rapid rate.

SUMMARY

Cytokines control the overall immune response by serving as a means of communication between its many components. In this way the responses of different cells are coordinated, and the innate and adaptive immune responses are linked. Cytokines are released on first contact with a foreign antigen to promote an initial inflammatory and innate response. Some cytokines serve as chemotaxins, calling the appropriate cell populations to the sites where they are needed. Many of the cytokines serve as growth factors that enhance proliferation of hematopoietic stem cells or responding lymphocyte subsets. Others act as macrophage-activating factors that enhance effector, antigen processing, and regulatory functions of macrophages. The proinflammatory and immune stimulatory effects of cyto-kines are balanced by immunosupressive cytokines and regulatory systems to terminate cytokine responses. The pleiotrophic and interactive nature of cytokine activities initially made it difficult to alter cytokine responses therapeutically. However, in recent years a number of therapies directed at cytokines have found their way into clinical medicine.

Case Study

1. You are performing complete blood cell counts on an automated analyzer. One of the patient samples is "flagged," indicating a possible instrument error or abnormal cell population in the sample. Previous samples on this patient have been run without problems, although the patient previously had quite low white blood cell (WBC) counts—less than 100 neutrophils and less than 500 total WBC/μL. As per laboratory protocol you review the Wright-stained blood film. On your manual differential count, you find that the monocyte count is slightly increased. You note the presence of immature cells of the granulocyte series, including occasional promyelocytes and myeloblasts. In addition, Dohle bodies, increased granulocyte granulation, and hypersegmented neutrophils are present.

Questions

a. What common clinical conditions can lead to the immature myeloid cells seen in this smear?

b. What should you do to help you interpret this sample?

Exercise: Erythrocyte Sedimentation Rate (Modified Westergren Method)

PRINCIPLE

When well-mixed blood is placed in a vertical tube the erythrocytes (RBCs) settle to the bottom. The distance the top of the column of RBCs has fallen in a given time interval is the ESR. A more rapid ESR results from higher levels of fibrinogen and globulins. These proteins tend to promote rouleaux of the RBCs, which enhances the rate of sedimentation. RBC factors can also affect the ESR. Anemia tends to increase the ESR, while microcytosis tends to decrease the ESR.

SPECIMEN COLLECTION

Collect blood by venipuncture using sterile technique. An ethylenediamine tetraacetate (EDTA)-anticoagulated (purple top) specimen is needed for this procedure. If the test cannot be run immediately, then blood can be stored for up to 24 hours at 4°C.

REAGENTS, MATERIALS, AND EQUIPMENT

The Westergren tube is a straight pipette, 30-cm long, calibrated in millimeters from 0 to 200. It is placed in a Westergren rack.

Sterile saline (0.85 percent sodium chloride) is used as the diluent.

PROCEDURE

1. Two mL of well-mixed EDTA-blood is diluted with 0.5 mL of sterile saline. Undiluted EDTA-blood gives poor precision.
2. A Westergren pipette is filled to the 0 mark (about 1 mL) with diluted blood and placed exactly vertical in the rack. The tube should not be exposed to vibration or direct sunlight. Temperature should be in the range of 20°C to 25°C.
3. After exactly 60 minutes, the distance to the top of the column of RBC is recorded in millimeters as the ESR value. If the demarcation between plasma and RBC is indistinct, the level is taken where the full density of the RBC column is first apparent.

INTERPRETATION OF RESULTS

The ESR gradually increases with age. Normal levels are <15 mm/hour for men under 50 years, <20 mm/hour for women under 50 years, <20 mm/hour for men over 50 years, and <30 mm/hour for women over 50 years. The ESR in elevated in inflammatory disease, hyperfibrinogenemias, multiple myeloma, and macroglobulinemia. False-negative results are rare.

1. When a single cytokine has multiple effects, this is called:
   a. Redundancy
   b. Pleiotropy
   c. Autocrine stimulation
   d. Endocrine effect

2. Which of the following can be attributed to IL-1?
   a. Mediator of the innate immune response
   b. Differentiation of stem cells
   c. Halts growth of virally-infected cells
   d. Stimulation of mast cells

3. Which of the following are target cells for IL-3?
   a. Myeloid precursors
   b. Lymphoid precursors
   c. Erythroid precursors
   d. All of the above

4. A lack of IL-4 might result in which of the following?
   a. Inability to fight off viral infections
   b. Increased risk of tumors
   c. Lack of IgE
   d. Decreased eosinophil count

5. Which of the following represents an autocrine effect of IL-2?
   a. Increased IL-2 receptor expression by the Th cell producing it
   b. Signaling macrophages to the area of antigen stimulation
   c. Proliferation of antigen-stimulated B cells
   d. Increased synthesis of acute phase proteins throughout the body

6. Which of the following might be a reason that IL-2 is being used in cancer therapy?
   a. Increases production of RBCs
   b. Stimulates LAK cells
   c. Mobilizes neutrophils from the marrow
   d. Mediates the acute phase response

7. IFN-α and IFN-β differ in which way from IFN-γ?
   a. IFN-α and IFN-β are so-called immune interferons, and IFN-γ is not.
   b. IFN-α and IFN-β primarily activate macrophages, while IFN-γ halts viral activity.
   c. They are made primarily by activated T cells, while IFN-γ is made by fibroblasts.
   d. IFN-α and IFN-β inhibit cell proliferation, while IFN-γ increases expression of class I MHC molecules.

8. A patient in septic shock caused by a gram-negative bacterial infection exhibits the following symptoms: high fever, very low blood pressure, and disseminated intravascular coagulation. Which cytokine is the most likely contributor to these symptoms?
   a. IL-2
   b. TNF
   c. IL-12
   d. IL-7

9. Selective destruction of Th cells by the human immunodeficiency virus contributes to immuno-suppression by which of the following means?
   a. Decrease in IL-1
   b. Decrease in IL-2
   c. Decrease in IL-8
   d. Decrease in IL-10

10. A cancer patient might be given a colony stimulating factor for which reason?
    a. Stimulating activity of NK cells
    b. Stimulating production of mast cells
    c. Decreasing production of TNF
    d. Increasing the number of leukocytes for the overall immune response

11. Which of the following is a characteristic of cytotoxic T cells?
    a. Recognizes virus apart from the infected cell
    b. Recognizes antigen in association with MHC class II protein
    c. Produces TNF-β, which triggers lysis of the target cell
    d. Destroys itself in the process of killing target cells

12. Which would be the best test to measure a specific IL?
    a. Blast formation
    b. De novo deoxyribonucleic acid synthesis
    c. Measurement of migration inhibition of leukocytes
    d. ELISA testing

References

1. Kuwano, K, and Hara, N: Signal transduction pathways of apoptosis and inflammation induced by the tumor necrosis factor receptor family. Am J Respir Cell Mol Biol 22:147–149, 2000.

2. Gruss, HJ: Molecular, structural, and biological characteristics of the tumor necrosis factor ligand superfamily. Int J Clin Lab Res 26:143–159, 1996.

3. Wright, SD: CD14 and innate recognition of bacteria. J Immunol 155:6–8, 1995.

4. Ingalls, RR, Heine, H, and Lien, E, et al: Lipopolysaccharide recognition, CD14, and lipopolysaccharide receptors. Infect Dis Clin North Am 13:341–353, 1999.

5. van der Poll, T, and Lowry, SF: Tumor necrosis factor in sepsis: Mediator of multiple organ failure or essential part of host defense? Shock 3:1–12, 1995.

6. Tracey, KJ, and Cerami, A: Tumor necrosis factor in the malnutrition (cachexia) of infection and cancer. Am J Trop Med Hyg 47:2–7, 1992.

7. Dinarello, CA: Interleukin-1, interleukin-1 receptors and interleukin-1 receptor antagonist. Int Rev Immunol 16:457–499, 1998.

8. Furutani, Y: Molecular studies on interleukin-1 alpha. Eur Cytokine Netw 5:533–538, 1994.

9. Andus, T, Geiger, T, and Hirano, T, et al: Regulation of synthesis and secretion of major rat acute-phase proteins by recombinant human interleukin-6 (BSF-2/IL-6) in hepatocyte primary cultures. Eur J Biochem 173:287–293, 1988.

10. Castell, JV, Gomez-Lechon, MJ, and David, M, et al: Recombinant human interleukin-6 (IL-6/BSF-2/HSF) regulates the synthesis of acute phase proteins in human hepatocytes. FEBS Lett 232:347–350, 1988.

11. Mukaida, N, Harada, A, and Matsushima, K: Interleukin-8 (IL-8) and monocyte chemotactic and activating factor (MCAF/MCP-1), chemokines essentially involved in inflammatory and immune reactions. Cytokine Growth Factor Rev 9:9–23, 1998.

12. Proudfoot, AE: The chemokine family. Potential therapeutic targets from allergy to HIV infection. Eur J Dermatol 8:147–157, 1998.

13. Rojo, D, Suetomi, K, and Navarro, J: Structural biology of chemokine receptors. Biol Res 32:263–272, 1999.

14. Keane, MP, and Strieter, RM: Chemokine signaling in inflammation. Crit Care Med 28:N13–26, 2000.

15. Pretolani, M: Interleukin-10: An anti-inflammatory cytokine with therapeutic potential. Clin Exp Allergy 29:1164–1171, 1999.

16. Trinchieri, G, and Scott, P: Interleukin-12: Basic principles and clinical applications. Curr Top Microbiol Immunol 238:57–78, 1999.

17. Yoshikai, Y, and Nishimura, H: The role of interleukin 15 in mounting an immune response against microbial infections. Microbes Infect 2:381–389, 2000.

18. Cosman, D, Kumaki, S, and Ahdieh, M, et al: Interleukin 15 and its receptor. Ciba Found Symp 195:221–229, 1995.

19. Vitetta, ES, Fernandez-Botran, R, and Myers, CD, et al: Cellular interactions in the humoral immune response. Adv Immunol 45:1–105, 1989.

20. Semenzato, G, Pizzolo, G, and Zambello, R: The interleukin-2/interleukin-2 receptor system: Structural, immunological, and clinical features. Int J Clin Lab Res 22:133–142, 1992.

21. Sugamura, K, Asao, H, and Kondo, M, et al: The interleukin-2 receptor gamma chain: Its role in the multiple cytokine receptor complexes and T cell development in XSCID. Annu Rev Immunol 14:179–205, 1996.

22. Banchereau, J, Defrance, T, and Galizzi, JP, et al: Human interleukin 4. Bull Cancer 78:299–306, 1991.

23. Defrance, T, Carayon, P, and Billian, G, et al: Interleukin 13 is a B cell stimulating factor. J Exp Med 179:135–143, 1994.

24. Roboz, GJ, and Rafii, S: Interleukin-5 and the regulation of eosinophil production. Curr Opin Hematol 6:164–168, 1999.

25. Aggarwal, BB: Lymphotoxin and tumor necrosis factor: Qualitative and quantitative differences in their receptors and signal transduction in various cell types. Prog Clin Biol Res 349:375–384, 1990.

26. Beutler, B: The tumor necrosis factors: Cachectin and lymphotoxin. Hosp Pract (Off Ed)25:45–56, 1990.

27. Burdach, S, Nishinakamura, R, and Dirksen, U, et al: The physiologic role of interleukin-3, interleukin-5, granulocyte-macrophage colony-stimulating factor, and the beta c receptor system. Curr Opin Hematol 5:177–180, 1998.

28. Tabbara, IA, Ghazal, CD, and Ghazal, HH: The clinical applications of granulocyte colony-stimulating factor in hematopoietic stem cell transplantation: A review. Anticancer Res 16:3901–3905, 1996.

29. Masucci, G: New clinical applications of granulocyte-macrophage colony-stimulating factor. Med Oncol 13:149–154, 1996.

30. Bensinger, WI, Clift, RA, and Anasetti, C, et al: Transplantation of allogeneic peripheral blood stem cells mobilized by recombinant human granulocyte colony stimulating factor. Stem Cells 14:90–105, 1996.

31. Akashi, K, Kondo, M, and Weissman, IL: Role of interleukin-7 in T-cell development from hematopoietic stem cells. Immunol Rev 165:13–28, 1998.

Complement

Learning Objectives

After completing this chapter, the reader will be able to:
1. Describe the nature of the complement components.
2. Differentiate between the classical and the alternative pathways, including proteins and activators involved in each.
3. Discuss formation of the three principal units of the classical pathway: recognition, activation, and membrane attack units.
4. Describe how initiation of the mannose-binding lectin (MBL) pathway occurs.
5. Explain how C3 plays a key role in all pathways.
6. Describe fluid-phase regulators of the complement system.
7. Discuss the role of the following cell membrane receptors: CR1, DAF, MCP, CR2, CR3, CR4, CD59, and C1qR.
8. Relate biologic manifestations of complement activation to generation of specific complement products.
9. Describe the complement deficiency associated with the following conditions: hereditary angioedema and paroxysmal nocturnal hemoglobinuria.
10. Differentiate tests for functional activity of complement from measurement of individual complement components.
11. Analyze laboratory findings and indicate disease implications in relation to complement abnormalities.

Key Terms

Activation unit
Alternative pathway
Anaphylatoxin
Bystander lysis
C1 inhibitor (C1INH)
C4-binding protein
  (C4BP)
Chemotaxin
Classical pathway

Decay-accelerating factor
  (DAF)
Exocytosis
Factor H
Factor I
Hemolytic titration (CH$_{50}$)
  assay
Hereditary angioedema
Immune adherence

Lectin pathway
Mannose-binding lectin
  (MBL)
Membrane attack complex
Paroxysmal nocturnal
  hemoglobinuria (PNH)
Properdin
Recognition unit
S protein

Complement, as described in Chapter 2, is a complex series of more than 30 soluble and cell-bound proteins that interact in a very specific way to mediate and enhance host defense reactions.[1] Originally recognized in the 1890s as a heat-labile substance present in normal nonimmune serum, complement was so named because it augmented specific immune activity by assisting in the destruction of bacteria.[2] Jules Bordet was awarded the Nobel Prize in 1919 for his role in elucidating the nature of complement.

Most plasma complement proteins are synthesized in the liver, with the exception of C1 components, which are mainly produced by intestinal epithelial cells, and factor D, which is made in adipose tissue.[1] Other cells, such as monocytes, macrophages, neutrophils, and T cells also appear to be involved in synthesis of certain individual components, including properdin and C7.[3–5] Most of these proteins are inactive precursors, or zymogens, which are converted to active enzymes in a very precise order. Table 7–1 lists the characteristics of the main complement proteins.

The complement system can be activated in three different ways. One such means of activation, the **classical pathway,** involves nine proteins that are triggered by antigen-antibody combination. Pillemer and colleagues later discovered an antibody-independent pathway in the 1950s, and this plays a major role as a

natural defense system.[2,6] The second pathway, or the **alternative pathway,** was originally called the properdin system because the protein known as properdin was thought to initiate it. Now, however, it is known that the major function of properdin is to stabilize a key enzyme complex formed along the pathway. A third pathway, called the **lectin pathway,** is an additional antibody-independent means of activating complement proteins. Its major constituent, **mannose-** (or **manner-) binding lectin (MBL),** adheres to mannose found mainly in the cell walls or outer coating of bacteria, viruses, yeast, and protozoa.

The complement system plays a major part in the inflammatory response directed against foreign antigens. Although the end product of complement activation is lysis of the invading cell, many other important events take place along the way. Complement fragments acting as opsonins, for which specific receptors are present on phagocytic cells, enhance metabolism and clearance of immune complexes. Recent evidence indicates that uptake of immune complexes in the spleen is, in fact, complement dependent.[7] Complement components are also able to increase vascular permeability, recruit monocytes and neutrophils to the area of antigen concentration, and trigger secretion of immunoregulatory molecules that amplify the immune response.[4] Any deficiencies in the

TABLE 7–1. Proteins of the Complement System

Serum Protein	Molecular Weight, kD	Concentration μg/mL	Function
Classical Pathway			
C1q	410	150	Binds to Fc region of IgM and IgG
C1r	85	50	Activates C1s
C1s	85	50	Cleaves C4 and C2
C4	205	300–600	Part of C3 convertase (C4b)
C2	102	25	Binds to C4b—forms C3 convertase
C3	190	1200	Key intermediate in all pathways
C5	190	80	Initiates membrane attack complex
C6	110	60	Binds to C5b in MAC
C7	100	55	Binds to C5bC6 in MAC
C8	150	55	Starts pore formation on membrane
C9	70	60	Polymerizes to cause cell lysis
Alternative Pathway			
Factor B	93	200	Binds to C3b to form C3 convertase
Factor D	24	1–2	Cleaves factor B
Properdin	53	25	Stabilizes C3bBb–C3 convertase
MBL Pathway			
MBL	200	1 (0.01–20)	Binds to mannose
MASP-1	100	1.5–12	Helps to cleave C4 and C2
MASP-2	76	ND	Cleaves C4 and C2

Fc = Fragment crystallizable; Ig = immunoglobulin; MAC = membrane attack complex; MBL = mannose-binding lectin; MASP = MBL-associated serine protease.

complement system can result in an increased susceptibility to infection or in the accumulation of immune
complexes with possible autoimmune manifestations.
Thus, these proteins play a significant role as a host
defense mechanism.

The Classical Pathway

The classical pathway or cascade is the main antibody-
directed mechanism for triggering complement activation. However, not all immunoglobulins are able to
activate this pathway. Those classes that can do so are
IgM, IgG1, IgG2, and IgG3. IgM is the most efficient
because it has multiple binding sites; thus, it takes only
one molecule attached to two adjacent antigenic determinants to initiate the cascade. Two IgG molecules
must attach to antigen within 30 to 40 nm of each
other before complement can bind, and it may take
hundreds or thousands of attachments before such a
combination is achieved.[4,8] Some epitopes, notably the
Rh group, are too far apart on the cell for this to occur,
and thus they are unable to fix complement. Within the
IgG group, IgG3 is the most effective, followed by
IgG1, and then IgG2.[1,9]

In addition to antibody, there are a few substances
that can bind complement directly to initiate the classical cascade. These include C-reactive protein, certain
viruses such as human immunodeficiency virus,
mycoplasmas, some trypanosomes, *Escherichia coli*, some
schistosomes, and several *Klebsiella* strains.[1] Most infectious agents, however, can directly activate only the
alternative pathway.

Complement activation can be divided into three
main stages, each of which is dependent on the grouping of certain reactants as a unit. The first stage involves
C1, and this is known as the **recognition unit.** Once
C1 is fixed, the next components activated are C4,
C2, and C3, known collectively as the **activation
unit.** C5 through C9 comprise the **membrane attack
complex,** and it is this last unit that completes lysis of
the foreign particle. Each of these is discussed in detail
in the following sections. Figure 7–1 depicts a simplified scheme of the entire pathway.

The Recognition Unit

The first complement component to bind is C1, a
molecular complex of 750,000 d. It consists of three
subunits, C1q, C1r, and C1s, which are stabilized by
calcium.[8] It is made up of one C1q subunit and two
each of the C1r and C1s subunits. Although the C1q unit
is the part that binds to antibody molecules, the C1r and
C1s subunits generate enzyme activity to begin the

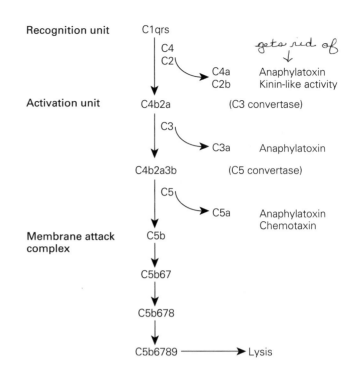

FIG. 7–1. The classical complement cascade. C1qrs is the
recognition unit that binds to the Fc portion of two antibody
molecules. It cleaves C4 and C2 to form C4b2a, which is
known as C3 convertase. C3 convertase cleaves C3 to form
C4b2a3b, known as C5 convertase. The combination of
C4b2b3b is the activation unit. C5 convertase cleaves C5.
C5b attracts C6, C7, C8, and C9, which bind together, forming the membrane attack complex. C9 polymerizes to cause
lysis of the target cell.

cascade. The (C1r, C1s)₂ complex is an S-shaped structure with several domains of unequal size. The
sequence of binding is C1s-C1r-C1r-C1s.[4,10] It is
hypothesized that this structure assumes the shape of a
distorted figure eight, and it wraps itself around the
arms of C1q (Fig. 7–2).

C1q has a molecular weight of 410,000 and is
composed of six strands that form six globular heads
with a collagenlike tail portion.[11] This structure has
been likened to a bouquet with six blossoms extending
outward (see Fig. 7–2). Each of the six heads is
composed of three homologous polypeptide chains, A,
B, and C, which form a triple helix.[4,11] Alanine
residues, which interrupt the triple helix, make a semi-
flexible joint that allows the "stems" to bend. As long as
calcium is present in the serum, C1r and C1s remain
associated with C1q.

C1q "recognizes" the fragment crystallizable (Fc)
region of two adjacent antibody molecules, and at least
two of the globular heads of C1q must be bound to
initiate the classical pathway. This binding occurs at the
C_H2 region for IgG and the C_H3 region for IgM. C1r

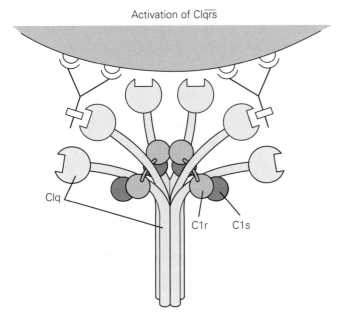

Activation of C1q̄r̄s̄

FIG. 7–2. Structure of C1qrs. When two or more globular heads of C1q attach to bound immunoglobulin molecules, the collagenlike stalks change their configuration. The resulting shape change causes C1r to become a serine protease. This cleaves a small fragment off C1s, uncovering the C1s protease, whose only targets are C4 and C2.

and C1s are both serine protease proenzymes. As binding of C1q occurs, both are converted into active enzymes. Autoactivation of C1r results from a conformational change that takes place as C1q is bound. Formation of the figure eight complex brings together catalytic domains of C1r and C1r, resulting in reciprocal cleavage of each to reveal an active site.[10] Once activated, C1r cleaves a thioester bond on C1s, which activates it. Activated C1r is extremely specific because its only known substrate is C1s. Likewise, C1s has a limited specificity, with its only substrates being C4 and C2. Once C1s is activated, this ends the recognition stage.

The Activation Unit

Phase two, or formation of the activation unit, results in the production of an enzyme known as *C5 convertase*. C4 is the second-most-abundant complement protein, with a serum concentration of approximately 600 μg/mL.[11] It consists of three polypeptide chains and has a molecular weight of approximately 198,000. C1s cleaves C4 to split off a 77-amino acid fragment called C4a. In the process, it opens a thioester-containing active site on the remaining part, C4b.[2] C4b must bind to protein or carbohydrate within a few seconds, or it will react with water molecules to form iC4b, which is rapidly degraded. Thus, C4b binds mainly to antigen in

clusters that are within a 40-nm radius of C1. This represents the first amplification step in the cascade because for every one C1 attached, approximately 30 molecules of C4 are split and attached.[1]

C2 is the next component to be activated. Complement proteins were named as they were isolated, before the sequence of activation was known; hence the irregularity in the numbering system. C2 is a single-chain glycoprotein with a molecular weight of 102,000.[1] The C2 gene is closely associated with the gene for *factor B* (alternative pathway) on chromosome 6 in the major histocompatability complex, and it is believed that the two genes probably arose through gene duplication in the distant past.[12] Each serves a similar purpose in its particular pathway.

When combined with C4b, C2 is cleaved by C1s to form C2a, which has a molecular weight of 70,000, and C2b, with a molecular weight of 34,000. This is the only case for the designation *a* to be given to the cleavage piece with enzyme activity. C2 must be within a 60-nm radius of bound C1s for cleavage to occur. Binding of C2 to C4b can occur in the fluid phase, but C4b attached to antigen is much more efficient in accepting C2. This serves to keep the reaction localized. C1s can cleave free C2, but the product of this cleavage appears to be incapable of binding to C4b, and no convertase activity develops.[12]

The combination of C4b and C2a is known as *C3 convertase* (Fig. 7–3A). This is written as C4b2a to indicate that the complex is an active enzyme. This complex is not very stable. The half-life is estimated to be between 15 seconds and 3 minutes, so C3 must be bound quickly.[12] If binding does occur, C3 is cleaved into two parts, C3a and C3b.

C3 is the major constituent of the complement system, present in the plasma at a concentration of 1200 μg/mL.[11] It serves as the pivotal point for all three pathways, and cleavage of C3 to C3b represents the most significant step in the entire process of complement activation. The molecule has a molecular weight of 190,000, and it consists of two polypeptide chains, one of which contains a highly reactive thioester group. When C3a is removed by cleavage of a single bond in the α chain, the hydrophobic pocket that shelters the thioester is exposed so that it is then capable of reacting with an antigen surface to form an ester or an amide link.[8] In actuality, only a small percentage of the C3 molecules cleaved bind to antigen; most are hydrolyzed by water molecules and decay in the fluid phase. C3b is estimated to have a half-life of 60 microseconds if not bound to antigen.[11,12]

The cleavage of C3 represents a second and major amplification process because about 200 molecules are split for every molecule of C4b2a.[4] In addition to

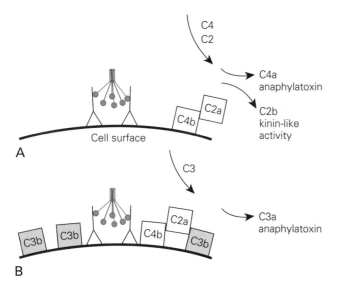

FIG. 7–3. Formation of the activation unit. *(A)* C1qrs is able to cleave C4 and C2. The larger pieces, C4b and C2b, bind to the target cell surface and form the enzyme C3 convertase. This cleaves C3 into C3a and C3b. C3b is a powerful opsonin, and it binds to the target in many places. *(B)* If some remains associated with C4bC2b, the enzyme C5 convertase is formed. The association of C4bC2bC3b is known as the activation unit.

being required for the formation of the membrane attack complex, C3b also serves as a powerful opsonin. Macrophages have specific receptors for it (discussed later in the chapter), and this contributes greatly to the process of phagocytosis. However, a large number of molecules appear to be needed for this to occur; hence the need for amplification.

If C3b is bound within 40 nm of the C4b2a, then this creates a new enzyme known as *C5 convertase*. Figure 7–3*B* depicts this last step in the formation of the activation unit. The cleaving of C5 with deposition of C5b at another site on the cell membrane constitutes the beginning of the membrane attack complex (MAC).

The Membrane Attack Complex

C5 consists of two polypeptide chains, α and β, which are linked by disulfide bonds to form a molecule with a molecular weight of about 190,000. C5 convertase, consisting of C4b2b3b, splits off a 74-amino acid piece known as C5a, and C5b attaches to the cell membrane, forming the beginning of the MAC. The splitting of C5, as well as cleavage of C3, represents the most significant biologic consequences of the complement system, as explained in the section on biologic manifestations of complement activation. C5b is extremely labile, however, because it is inactivated in 2 minutes unless binding to C6 occurs.[4]

Subsequent binding involves C6, C7, C8, and C9. None of these proteins have enzymatic activity, and they are all present in much smaller amounts in serum than the preceding components. C6 and C7 each have molecular weights of approximately 110,000, and both have similar physical and chemical properties. C8 is made up of three dissimilar chains joined by disulfide bonds and has a total molecular weight of about 150,000.[1] C9 is a single polypeptide chain with a molecular weight of 70,000. The carboxy-terminal end is hydrophobic, while the amino-terminal end is hydrophilic. The hydrophobic part probably serves to anchor the MAC within the target membrane.[2] Formation of the membrane attack unit is pictured in Figure 7–4.

Membrane damage appears to be caused by at least two different mechanisms: channel formation and the binding of phospholipids. The latter causes a reordering and reorientation of molecules that results in leaky patches.[13] When complement proteins are bound, membrane phospholipids rearrange themselves into domains surrounding the C5b6789 complex, and the integrity of the membrane is destroyed.

The membrane attack unit begins when C6 binds to C5b, thereby stabilizing it. Then this complex attaches to the cell surface. C7 binds next, forming a trimolec-

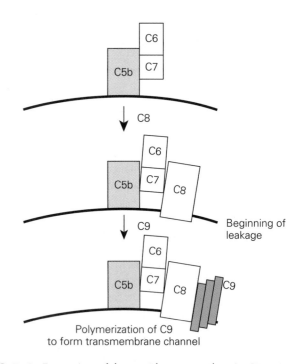

FIG. 7–4. Formation of the membrane attack unit. C5 convertase cleaves C5 into C5a and C5b. C5b binds to the target cell, and C6 and C7 become attached to it. C8 binds to these associated molecules and begins to penetrate the cell membrane. C9 binds to the complex and polymerizes to form the transmembrane channel, which causes lysis of the cell.

ular complex that provides an attachment site for C8. As C7 binds to C5b6, it undergoes a structural transition, exposing hydrophopic regions that can bind to membrane phospholipids. This allows for insertion of the C7 part of the C5b67 complex into the membrane of the target cell.[2,4,11]

Next, C8 interacts with the membrane by means of one of its two chains, and it appears to form a small hole in the membrane as it is inserted. Lysis can be observed at this stage, but the addition of C9 accelerates the process. Binding of C8 causes a loss of potassium from the cell, which is followed by leakage of amino acids and ribonucleotides. The pore formed by the binding of C5b678 is a small one, capable of lysing erythrocytes but not nucleated cells.[2] For lysis of nucleated cells to be achieved, C9 must bind to the complex.

When C9 binds to the C5–C8 complex, it unfolds, becomes inserted into the lipid bilayer, and polymerizes. Anywhere from 1 to 12 molecules of C9 can bind to one C8 molecule. C9 only polymerizes when bound, and it is believed that the C5–C8 complex acts as a catalyst to enhance the rate of reaction.[1] Polymerized C9 forms a hollow thin-walled cylinder, which can be seen on electron microscopy and constitutes the transmembrane channel.[13] The completed MAC unit has a functional pore size of 70 to 100Å.[4] One such unit is able to lyse erythrocytes, but lysis of nucleated cells is a multihit phenomenon. Originally, it was believed that lysis of all cells was a single-hit phenomenon. Destruction of target cells actually occurs through an influx of water and a corresponding loss of electrolytes.

The Alternative Pathway

Pathogens can be destroyed in the absence of antibody by means of the alternative pathway, which acts as natural defense against infection. Phylogenetically, this represents the oldest of the C3 activating pathways. First described by Pillemer and his associates in the early 1950s, the pathway was originally named for the protein **properdin,** a constituent of normal serum with a concentration of approximately 5 to 15 μg/mL.[5] Now it is known that properdin does not initiate this pathway, but rather stabilizes the C3 convertase formed from activation of other factors. In addition to properdin, the serum proteins that are unique to this pathway include factor B and factor D. C1, C2, and C4, found in the classical pathway, are not used at all in this system. C3, however, is a key component of both pathways. The alternative pathway is summarized in Figure 7–5.

Triggering substances for the alternative pathway include bacterial cell walls, especially those containing

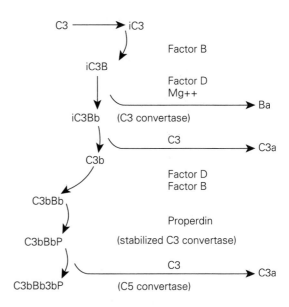

FIG. 7–5. The alternative pathway. C3 is hydrolyzed by water to produce iC3. This molecule can bind factor B. When factor B is bound to iC3, B is cleaved to form iC3Bb, an enzyme with C3 convertase activity. More C3 is cleaved to form more C3bBb. This enzyme is stabilized by properdin, and it continues to cleave additional C3. If a molecule of C3 remains attached to the C3bBbP enzyme, the convertase now has the capability to cleave C5. The C5 convertase thus consists of C3bBb3bP. After C5 is cleaved, the pathway is exactly the same as the classical pathway.

lipopolysaccharide, fungal cell walls, yeast, viruses, virally infected cells, tumor cell lines, and some parasites, especially trypanosomes.[4] All of these are able to serve as sites for binding the complex C3bBb, one of the end products of this pathway. The conversion of C3 is the first step in this pathway.

In plasma, native C3 is not stable. Water is able to hydrolyze a thioester bond and, thus, spontaneously activates a small number of these molecules.[2,8] This ability of C3 to activate spontaneously is known as *tickover,* and it results in a molecule called iC3, which has the ability to bind factor B just as C3b does.[14] However, this reaction takes place in a soluble phase because iC3 cannot bind covalently to cell surfaces as does C3b.[15] Factor B has a molecular weight of 93,000 and is fairly abundant in the serum at a level of 200 μg/mL.[11] iC3 is able to bind factor B in a magnesium-dependent reaction. Only bound factor B can be cleaved by factor D. The role of factor B is thus analogous to that of C2 in the classical pathway because it forms an integral part of a C3 convertase.

Factor D is a plasma protein that circulates in active enzyme form. It is a serine protease with a molecular weight of 24,000, and its only substrate is bound factor

B. The concentration of factor D in the plasma is the lowest of all the complement proteins, approximately 1 μg/mL.[11] It cleaves factor B into two pieces, Ba, with a molecular weight of 33,000, and Bb, whose molecular weight is approximately 60,000. Bb remains attached to iC3, forming the initial C3 convertase of the alternative pathway. Bb is rapidly inactivated unless it becomes bound to a site on one of the triggering cellular antigens.

As the alternative pathway convertase, *iC3Bb* is then capable of cleaving additional C3 into C3a and C3b. Some C3b attaches to cellular surfaces and acts as a binding site for more factor B. This results in an amplification loop that feeds C3b into the classical pathway and the alternative one. All C3 present in plasma would be rapidly converted by this method were it not for the fact that the enzyme C3bBb is extremely unstable unless properdin binds to the complex.[2] Binding of properdin increases the half-life of C3bBb from 5 to 30 minutes.[4] In this manner, optimal rates of alternative pathway activation are achieved.[5] If some of the C3b produced remains bound to the C3 convertase, the enzyme is altered to form *C3bBb3bP*, which exhibits C5 convertase activity.[15] C5 is cleaved in the same manner as in the classical pathway. From this point on, both pathways are identical.

The Lectin Pathway

The lectin pathway represents a second means of activating complement without antibody being present. Lectins are proteins that bind to carbohydrates. This pathway provides another important link between the innate and acquired immune response because it involves nonspecific recognition of carbohydrates that are common constituents of microbial cell walls and are distinct from those found on human cell surfaces.[16] One key lectin, called MBL, binds to mannose or related sugars such as *N*-acetylglucosamine to initiate this pathway. These sugars are found in glycoproteins or carbohydrates of various microorganisms such as bacteria, yeasts, viruses, and some parasites. MBL is considered an acute phase protein because it is normally present in the serum but increases during an initial inflammatory response. It resembles C1q in both structure and function because its structure consists of six subunits, each of which is composed of three chains twisted around each other with a globular domain at the carboxy-terminal end. This creates the appearance of a bouquet of tulips, similar to C1q.[1,17,18] Several of the globular domains must attach to neighboring sugar residues to activate the cascade.

After MBL is bound to the surface of a cell, two MBL-associated serine proteases (MASPs), MASP-1 and MASP-2, become activated. Although some MBL forms a complex with MASP-1 and MASP-2 in serum, it appears that over 95 percent of total MASP found in serum is unbound. Binding of the serine proteases mainly takes place after MBL attaches to a cell surface.[17,19] MASP-1 and MASP-2 are homologous to C1r and C1s in that a conformational change takes place after binding to a cell, and this leads to activation of both serine proteases.[2,20,21] Although the exact nature of the reaction that takes place is not known, current research indicates that both MASP-1 and MASP-2 are able to cleave C4 and C2.[22] This leads to formation of the same C3 convertase found in the classical complement pathway. The rest of the pathway is exactly the same as that of the classical pathway. Figure 7–6 shows the convergence of all three pathways.

System Controls

Activation of complement could cause tissue damage and have devastating systemic effects if it were allowed to proceed uncontrolled. To ensure that infectious agents and not self-antigens are destroyed and that the reaction remains localized, a number of plasma proteins act as regulators of the system. In addition, there are specific receptors on certain cells that also exert a controlling influence on the activation process. In fact, approximately one-half of the complement components serve as controls for critical steps in the activation process.[23] Because activation of C3 is the pivotal step in all pathways, the majority of the control proteins are aimed at halting accumulation of C3b. Spontaneous inactivation of many labile components as they diffuse away from target cells is an additional means of regulation. Plasma regulators are discussed first. A brief summary of these is found in Table 7–2.

Fluid Phase Regulators

C1 inhibitor, or **C1INH,** is a glycoprotein with a molecular weight of 105,000. Like most of the other complement proteins, it is mainly synthesized in the liver, but monocytes also may be involved to some extent in its manufacture. Its main role is to inactivate C1 by binding to the active sites of C1r and C1s. C1r and C1s become instantly and irreversibly dissociated from C1q.[1,11] C1q remains bound to antibody, but all enzymatic activity ceases.

C1INH also inhibits plasmin, kallikrein, and activated factor XII (Hageman factor), all essential in clot formation.[11] Thus, the normal activities of coagulation

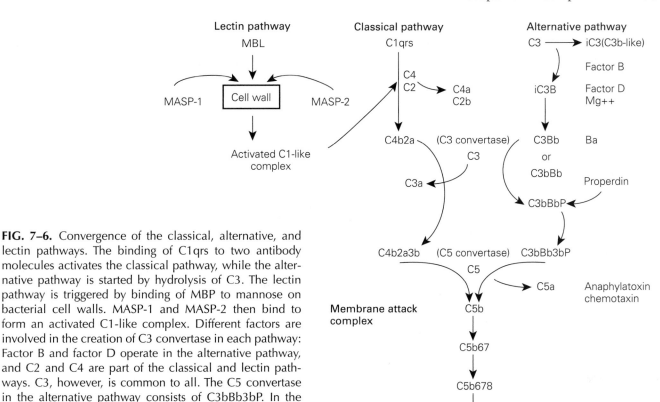

FIG. 7–6. Convergence of the classical, alternative, and lectin pathways. The binding of C1qrs to two antibody molecules activates the classical pathway, while the alternative pathway is started by hydrolysis of C3. The lectin pathway is triggered by binding of MBP to mannose on bacterial cell walls. MASP-1 and MASP-2 then bind to form an activated C1-like complex. Different factors are involved in the creation of C3 convertase in each pathway: Factor B and factor D operate in the alternative pathway, and C2 and C4 are part of the classical and lectin pathways. C3, however, is common to all. The C5 convertase in the alternative pathway consists of C3bBb3bP. In the classical pathway, C5 convertase is made up of C4b2b3b. After C5 is cleaved, the pathway is common to all.

and inflammation depend on maintaining a delicate balance between activators and inhibitors.

A second control protein, **factor H,** which has a molecular weight of 160,000, inhibits convertase activity in the fluid or plasma phase. It does so by binding to C3b, thus preventing the binding of factor B. C3b in the fluid phase has a 100-fold greater affinity for factor H than for factor B, but on cell surfaces, C3b preferentially binds factor B. However, factor H also accelerates the dissociation of the C3bBb complex on cell surfaces.[24] When factor H binds to C3bBb, Bb becomes displaced.[23] In this manner, C3 convertase activity is curtailed in plasma and on cell surfaces as well.

Additionally, factor H acts as a cofactor that allows factor I to break down C3b. **Factor I** (molecular weight, 88,000) is a serine protease that inactivates C3b and C4b only when they are associated with factor H. It appears that only those molecules with tightly bound factor H acquire high-affinity binding sites for factor I.[24] When factor I binds, a conformational change takes place and allows it to cleave C3b.[24] On cellular surfaces, C3b is cleaved to C3f, a small piece that is released into the plasma, and iC3b, which remains attached but is no longer an active enzyme. iC3b is further broken down to C3c and C3dg by factor I in conjunction with another cofactor, the CR1 receptor (Fig. 7–7).[1]

C4-binding protein, or **C4BP,** also serves as a cofactor for factor I in the inactivation of C4b. C4BP is abundant in the plasma and has a molecular weight

Serum Protein	Molecular Weight	Concentration mg/mL	Function
C1 inhibitor (C1INH)	105	240	Dissociates C1r and C1s from C1q
Factor I	88	35	Cleaves C3b and C4b
Factor H	150	300–450	Cofactor with I to inactivate C3b; prevents binding of B to C3b
C4-binding protein	550	250	Acts as a cofactor with I to inactivate C4b (C4bp)
S protein (vitronectin)	84	500	Prevents attachment of the C5b67 complex to cell membranes

TABLE 7–2. Plasma Complement Regulators

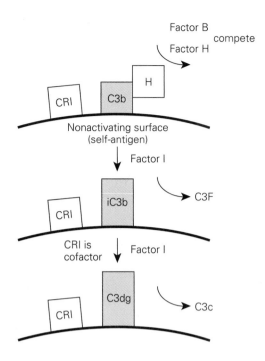

FIG. 7–7. Complement controls. CR1 receptor acts as cofactor in the inactivation of C3b. Factor I cleaves C3b to form C3dg and C3c. C3dg is not an effective opsonin, and it is not capable of further participation in the complement cascade.

of about 520,000. It is capable of combining with either fluid-phase or bound C4b, so that C4b cannot bind C2 and is made available for degradation by factor I.[11,23] If C4BP attaches to cell-bound C4b, it can dissociate it from C4b2a complexes, thus causing the cessation of the classical pathway. C4BP can also interact with C3b in a way similar to that of factor H. This inhibits convertase activity in the plasma phase.

S protein is a control protein that acts at a further level of complement activation. Also known as vitronectin, S protein interacts with the C5b67 complex as it forms in the fluid phase and prevents its binding to cell membranes.[2,11] Binding of C8 and C9 still proceeds, but polymerization of C9 does not occur, and the complex is unable to insert itself into the cell membrane or to produce lysis.[11,23]

Cell-Bound Regulators

Specific proteins found on cell surfaces act both as cofactors to control the proliferation of complement products and as mediators that assist in the destruction of foreign particles that originally triggered complement activation. These glycoproteins, called regulators

of complement activation, have many structural similarities, suggesting the possibility of a common genetic ancestry.[14,23] They are found on host-cell membranes, where their main function is to protect host cells from the phenomenon known as **bystander lysis.** This occurs when C3b fragments generated due to the presence of an infectious agent become deposited on host cells. Control of the production of C3b occurs in two ways—inactivation of C3 convertase and inactivation of C3b itself. A few other receptors act on a later stage of the complement pathway, blocking formation of the membrane attack complex. Table 7–3 lists the receptors and indicates the type of cell on which they are found.

CR1, also known as CD35, is a large polymorphic glycoprotein with a molecular weight of between 190,000 and 250,000. It is found mainly on peripheral blood cells, including neutrophils, monocytes, macrophages, erythrocytes, eosinophils, B lymphocytes, some T lymphocytes, and follicular dendritic cells.[1,11] It binds C3b, iC3b, and C4b, but has the greatest affinity for C3b.[1] Once bound, these molecules can then be degraded by factor I. Thus, it functions as a cofactor similar to factor H in the fluid phase. In addition, recent evidence indicates that CR1 on neutrophils participates in mediating a signal that induces particle uptake to aid in phagocytosis.[25]

Perhaps one of the main functions of CR1, however, is to act as a receptor on platelets and red blood cells and to mediate transport of C3b-coated immune complexes to the liver and spleen.[2,14,23] It is there that fixed tissue macrophages strip the immune complexes from the red blood cells, process the complexes, and return the red blood cells intact to circulation. The ability of cells to bind complement-coated particles is referred to as **immune adherence.** In addition, CR1 on follicular dendritic cells in lymph nodes and the spleen helps to stimulate immunological memory by trapping complement-coated immune complexes so that antigen persists longer in germinal centers.[1,26]

Decay-accelerating factor (DAF), or CD55, a 70,000 d membrane glycoprotein, is another receptor with a wide tissue distribution. It is not only found on peripheral blood cells, but also on endothelial cells and fibroblasts, as well as on numerous epithelial cell surfaces such as that of the cornea, the gastrointestinal mucosa, renal tubules, and pleural cavity.[23,27] DAF is capable of dissociating both classical and alternative pathway C3 convertases. It does not prevent initial binding of either C2 or factor B to the cell, but is able to rapidly dissociate both from their binding sites and so prevent the assembly of an active C3 convertase.

The carboxy-terminal portion of DAF is covalently

TABLE 7–3. Receptors on Cell Membranes for Complement Components

Receptor	Ligand	Cell Type	Function
CR1	C3b, iC3b, C4b	RBCs, neutrophils, monocytes, macrophages, eosinophils, B and T cells, follicular dendritic cells	Cofactor for factor I; mediates transport of immune complexes
CR2	C3dg, C3d	B cells, follicular dendritic cells, epithelial cells	Not clear; may stimulate immune response
CR3	iC3b	Monocytes, macrophages, neutrophils, NK cells	Adhesion and aggregation of phagocytic cells
CR4	iC3b	Monocytes, macrophages, neutrophils, NK cells	Mediate clearance of opsonized particles
DAF	C3b, C4b	Erythrocytes, neutrophils, platelets, monocytes, endothelial cells, fibroblasts, T cells, B cells	Dissociates C2b or Bb from binding sites, thus preventing formation of C3 convertase
Factor H	Factor H	B cells, monocytes, neutrophils	Not clear; may stimulate lymphocyte blastogenesis
Clq	Clq	Neutrophils, monocytes, macrophages, B cells, platelets, endothelial cells	Enhance binding of Clq to Fc receptors on immunoglobulins

Adapted from Widmann, FK: An Introduction to Clinical Immunology. FA Davis, Philadelphia, 1989.
RBC = Red blood cell; NK = natural killer.

attached to a glycophospholipid anchor that is inserted into the outer layer of the membrane lipid bilayer. This arrangement allows DAF mobility within the membrane, so it is able to reach C3 convertase sites that are not immediately adjacent to it[27] (Fig. 7–8). The presence of DAF on host cells protects them from bystander lysis and is one of the main mechanisms used in discrimination of self from nonself because foreign cells do not possess this substance.[14] It does not, however, permanently modify C3b or C4b; thus, they are capable of reforming elsewhere as active convertases.

An additional complement receptor that assists in the inactivation of C3b and C4b has been characterized. Named *membrane cofactor protein (MCP)*, or *CD46*, it has a molecular weight of between 60,000 and 70,000 and is located on endothelial cells, fibroblasts, and certain peripheral blood cells.[23] Although not found on erythrocytes, it is carried by platelets, monocytes, and B and T lymphocytes. MCP is the most efficient cofactor for factor I-mediated cleavage of C3b. It also serves as a cofactor for cleavage of C4b, but it is not as effective as C4BP.[2] In addition, binding of C2 to C4b and of factor B to C3b is inhibited, thus limiting the formation

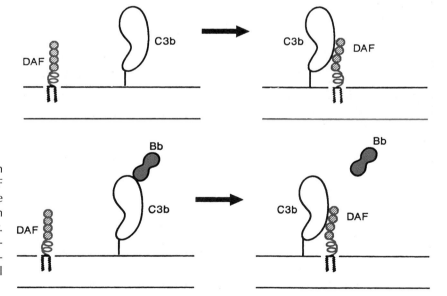

FIG. 7–8. Inhibitory effects of DAF. When C3b binds to cell surfaces that have DAF present, the DAF is actually able to migrate to the C3b and help dissociate Bb from binding to C3b in the alternative pathway. (From Lublin, DM, and Atkinson, J: Decay-accelerating factor: Biochemistry, molecular biology, and function. Adv Immunol 7:35, 1989, with permission.)

of the enzyme C3 convertase on autologous cell membranes.[15]

A receptor known by various terms, including membrane inhibitor of reactive lysis (MIRL), or CD59, may play an important role further along the complement pathway by blocking formation of the membrane attack complex.[23] MIRL is widely distributed on cell membranes of all circulating blood cells including red blood cells, and on endothelial, epithelial, and many other types of cells.[1,23] Its main function is to bind to C8 and prevent insertion of C9 into the cell membrane.

Receptors that Amplify the Immune Response

A second major category of complement receptors found on host cells amplifies and enhances the immune response by augmenting phagocytosis and stimulating accessory cells, rather than acting as regulators. Table 7–3 summarizes the main characteristics of each and describes the cell types on which they are found. The first of these proteins, *CR2, or CD21,* is found mainly on B lymphocytes, follicular dendritic cells, some T cells, and certain epithelial cells.[1] Ligands for CR2 include degradation products of C3b, such as C3dg, C3d, and iC3b.[23] In addition, the Epstein-Barr virus gains entry to B cells by binding to this receptor. CR2 is present only on mature B cells, and it is lost when conversion to plasma cells occurs. CR2 has been found to play an important role as part of the B cell coreceptor for antigen. Acting in concert with several other cell-bound receptors, it binds complement-coated antigen and cross-links it to membrane immunoglobulin to activate B cells. In this manner, immune complexes are more effective at enhancing B cell differentiation and production of memory cells than is antigen by itself.[26,28,29]

Monocytes, macrophages, neutrophils, and natural killer cells have a receptor that combines specifically with particles opsonized with iC3b, a C3b degradation product.[2] The *CR3 (CD11b/CD18)* receptor plays a key role in mediating phagocytosis of particles coated with these complement fragments. CR3 consists of an α and a β chain with respective molecular weights of 165,000 and 95,000.[30] These proteins may trigger surface adhesion and aggregation of phagocytic cells.[26] They are also responsible for producing an oxidative burst and increased activity in phagocytic cells.[1]

Patients whose white blood cells lack these receptors fail to exhibit functions such as chemotaxis, surface adherence, and aggregation. Deficiencies in phagocytosis are also noted. These individuals have an impaired capacity to bind iC3b-coated particles and are subject to recurrent infections.

The *CR4 (CD11c/CD18)* receptor is very similar to CR3 in that it binds iC3b fragments but in a calcium-dependent fashion. CR4 proteins are found on neutrophils, monocytes, tissue macrophages, T cells, mast cells, and activated B cells.[2,30] Neutrophils and monocytes, however, possess smaller amounts of CR4 than of CR3. Their function appears to be similar to that of CR3.

Receptors specific for C1q are found on neutrophils, monocytes, macrophages, B cells, platelets, and endothelial cells.[30,32] These receptors, known as collectin receptors, bind the collagen portion of C1q and generally enhance the binding of C1q to Fc receptors. Interacting only with bound C1q, the receptors appear to increase the uptake by phagocytic cells of immune complexes opsonized with C1q. Additionally, on neutrophils, they may act to enhance the respiratory burst triggered by IgG binding to Fc receptors.

Biologic Manifestations of Complement Activation

Activation of complement is a very effective means of amplifying the inflammatory response to destroy and clear foreign antigens. The cycle does not always have to proceed to lysis for this to be accomplished; hence, some of the initiating proteins are much more plentiful than proteins that take part in formation of the membrane attack complex. The complement proteins also serve as a means of linking innate and natural immunity. They not only act as opsonins to facilitate destruction by phagocytic cells, but they also play a major role in uptake and presentation of antigens so a specific immune response can occur. They also facilitate B cell activation and may, in fact, be necessary for maintaining immunological memory. Effector molecules generated earlier in the cascade play a major role in all these areas. Such molecules can be classified into three main categories: anaphylatoxins, chemotaxins, and opsonins.

An **anaphylatoxin** is a small peptide that causes increased vascular permeability, contraction of smooth muscle, and release of histamine from basophils and mast cells. Proteins that play such a part are C3a, C4a, and C5a. All of these have a molecular weight of between 9,000 and 11,000, and they are formed as cleavage products from larger complement components. Of these molecules, C5a is the most potent, at least 100 times more powerful than C3a, while C4a is the least effective.[2]

C3a, C4a, and C5a attach to specific receptors on neutrophils, basophils, mast cells, eosinophils, smooth muscle cells, and vascular endothelium.[4,30] C3a and C4a attach to the C3a receptor (C3aR), and C5a attaches to the C5a receptor (C5aR).[30] Histamine is released from basophils and mast cells, thereby increasing vascular permeability and causing contraction of smooth muscles. In addition, C5a causes neutrophils to release hydrolytic enzymes, oxygen radicals, and prostaglandins, aiding in destruction of foreign antigens.[4,30]

C5a also serves as a **chemotaxin** for neutrophils, basophils, eosinophils, mast cells, and monocytes.[2,11] In this manner, these cells are directed to the source of antigen concentration. Because of increased vascular permeability, neutrophils migrate from blood vessels to the tissues and tend to aggregate.

Binding of C5a to monocytes causes them to undergo an oxidative burst that includes increased production of hydrolytic enzymes, neutrophil chemotactic factor, platelet activating factors, and interleukin-1.[2] Interleukin-1 is a protein that enhances T cell activation. This may produce fever and an increase in acute phase reactants, both of which are characteristic of an inflammatory response.

As a means of localizing and controlling the effects of C3a, C4a, and C5a, these substances are rapidly inactivated by an enzyme in the plasma called *carboxypeptidase N*. C3a and C4a are cleaved in seconds, while conversion of C5a takes place more slowly.

The last major effect of complement-derived peptides is opsonization. C4b, C3b, and iC3b, which accumulate on cell membranes as complement activation proceeds, bind to specific receptors on erythrocytes, neutrophils, monocytes, and macrophages, as discussed earlier. This facilitates phagocytosis and clearance of foreign substances and is one of the key functions of the complement system. In addition, attachment of C3 products to an antigen has been found to enhance the B cell response, as mentioned earlier.

Complement and Disease States

Although complement acts as a powerful weapon to combat infection by amplifying phagocytosis, in some cases it can actually contribute to tissue damage or death. Complement can be harmful: (1) if activated systemically on a large scale as in gram-negative septicemia, (2) if it is activated by tissue necrosis such as

myocardial infarction, or (3) if there is a buildup of immune complexes.[2] In the case of septicemia due to a gram-negative organism, large quantities of C3a and C5a are generated, leading to neutrophil aggregation and clotting. Damage to the tiny pulmonary capillaries and interstitial pulmonary edema may result.[31]

Tissue injury following obstruction of the blood supply, such as occurs in myocardial infarction or heart attack, can cause complement activation and deposition of membrane attack complexes on cell surfaces.[2] This has been demonstrated in experimental models of myocardial infarction and in patients with congestive heart failure. Soluble CR1 receptors have been used on an experimental basis to block the activity of complement.[30]

In autoimmune diseases, such as Goodpasture's syndrome, myasthenia gravis, and systemic lupus erythematosus (SLE), immune complexes trigger activation and degranulation of neutrophils, basophils, and mast cells. Complement also plays a harmful role in demyelinating diseases such as multiple sclerosis and Guillain-Barré syndrome.[32] If immune complexes adhere to tissue surfaces, a process called **exocytosis** produces tissue damage due to the release of hydrolytic and lysosomal enzymes from phagocytes.[2] Glomerulonephritis, which results in destruction of endothelial cells in the kidney, may be caused by deposition of immune complexes on the basement membrane of the glomerulus with a subsequent accumulation of the C5b-9 membrane attack complex.[33,34]

Lysis may be another end result of complement activation. Hemolytic diseases such as cold autoimmune hemolytic anemia are characterized by the presence of an autoantibody that binds at low temperatures. When these cells warm up, complement fixation results in lysis (see Chapter 14 for a more complete discussion of complement-mediated autoimmune diseases).

Complement Deficiencies

Major Pathway Components

Although excess activation of the complement system can result in disease states, lack of individual components also has a deleterious effect. Hereditary deficiency of any complement protein, with the exception of C9, usually manifests itself in increased susceptibility to infection and delayed clearance of immune complexes. Most of these conditions are inherited on an autosomal recessive gene, and they are quite rare. The deficiency that occurs most often is that of C2, which is found in 1 in 10,000 individuals.[4] The factor B locus is nearby, and often C2-deficient patients are reported to have decreases in factor B.[35] Other types of complement deficiencies are less common.

The most serious deficiency is that of C3 because it is the key mediator in all pathways. Patients with a C3 deficiency are prone to developing severe recurrent life-threatening infections with encapsulated bacteria and may also be subject to immune complex diseases.[36] It appears that a deficiency of any of the terminal components of the complement cascade (C5–C8) causes increased susceptibility to systemic *Neisseria* infections, including meningococcal meningitis and disseminated gonorrheal disease.[4] Table 7–4 lists the complement components and the disease states associated with the absence of each individual factor.

Regulatory Factor Components

A prime example of a disease due to a missing or defective regulatory component is **paroxysmal nocturnal hemoglobinuria (PNH).** Patients with this disease have red blood cells that are deficient in DAF; hence, the cells are subject to lysis by means of the bystander effect once the complement system has been triggered.[14] These individuals appear to have a deficiency in the glycophosphopholipid anchor of the DAF molecule that prevents its insertion into the cell membrane.[27] When C3b is deposited on erythrocytes because of activation of either pathway, the result is complement-mediated intravascular and extravascular hemolysis resulting in a chronic hemolytic anemia.

Some studies indicate that a deficiency of DAF alone may not be enough to cause enhanced hemolysis, and that a lack of CD59 (MIRL/HRF20) may also be implicated in PNH.[23,37] As mentioned previously, CD59 prevents insertion of C9 into the cell membrane, thus inhibiting formation of transmembrane channels. Presence of both DAF and CD59 appears to be important in protection of red blood cells against bystander lysis.

Recurrent attacks of angioedema that affect the extremities, the skin, the gastrointestinal tract, and other mucosal surfaces are characteristic of the disease called **hereditary angioedema.** This is caused by a deficiency or lack of C1INH, which results in excess cleavage of C4 and C2. This allows perpetuation of the classical pathway and produces kinin-related proteins that increase vascular permeability.[11] Thus, the response to a localized antigen is continued swelling or edema. If this occurs in the area of the oropharynx, life-threatening upper airway obstruction may develop.

The condition may be either hereditary or acquired. It is inherited as an autosomal dominant gene that codes for either a dysfunctional protein or an inactive one. One normal gene does not produce enough inhibitor to keep up with the demand, and the condition is apparent in the heterozygous state. If the condition is hereditary, laboratory results indicate normal levels of C1q and C3 but reduced levels of C4 and C2.[2]

Patients with an acquired C1INH deficiency, in contrast, show reduced levels of C1q because of excess activation of the classical cascade by antibody. This may result from a B cell malignancy, presence of an autoimmune disease, or in some rare instances, appearance of an autoantibody that binds to the active site of C1 inhibitor.[16] In each instance, C1INH is present but quickly becomes depleted.

Other inhibitors for which there are genetic deficiencies include factors H and I. Lack of either component produces a constant turnover of C3 to the point of depletion.[2] Recurrent bacterial infections may ensue.

Laboratory Detection of Complement Abnormalities

Determination of the levels of complement components can be a useful adjunct in the diagnosis of disease. Not only can hereditary deficiencies be identified, but also much can be learned about inflammatory or autoimmune states by following the consumption of complement proteins. Techniques to determine complement abnormalities generally fall into two categories: (1) measurement of components as antigens in serum, and (2) measurement of functional activity.[8] There are both advantages and disadvantages to each.

TABLE 7–4. Deficiencies of Complement Components	
Deficient Component	**Associated Disease**
C1 (q, r, or s)	Lupus erythematosus-like syndrome
C2	Lupus erythematosus-like syndrome, recurrent infections
C3	Severe recurrent infections
C4	Lupuslike syndrome
C5	*Neisseria* infections
C6	*Neisseria* infections
C7	*Neisseria* infections
C8	*Neisseria* infections
C9	No known disease association
C1INH	Hereditary angioedema
DAF	Paroxysmal nocturnal hemoglobinuria
HFR	Paroxysmal nocturnal hemoglobinuria
Factor H or factor I	Recurrent bacterial infections
C1INH = C1 inhibitor; DAF = decay accelerating factor.	

Immunologic Assays of Individual Components

The methods most frequently used to assay individual components include radial immunodiffusion (RID) and nephelometry.[8,38] Components that are usually measured and for which there are standardized reagents include Clq, C4, C3, C5, factor B, factor H, factor I, and C1 inhibitor.[8] Radial immunodiffusion uses agarose gel into which specific antibody is incorporated. Serum serves as the antigen and is placed in wells that are cut in the gel. Diffusion of the antigen from the well occurs in a circular pattern. The radius of the resulting circle can be related to antigen concentration (see Chapter 9 for further details on RID). This is a sensitive technique when performed correctly, but it takes at least 24 hours before test results are available.

Nephelometry measures concentration according to the amount of light scattered by a solution containing a reagent antibody and a measured patient sample (refer to Chapter 9 for more details on nephelometry). Generally, the more antigen-antibody complexes that are present, the more a beam of light will be scattered as it passes through the solution. Such systems have a high degree of accuracy, results are available quickly, and processing is easy because of the use of automation. The purchase of expensive equipment is necessary, however. Nephelometry and RID achieve approximately the same precision.[38]

None of the assays for individual components are able to distinguish whether or not the molecules are functionally active. Thus, although the preceding techniques give quantitative results and are relatively easy to perform, test results must be interpreted carefully.

Assays for the Classical Pathway

Assays that measure lysis, the endpoint of complement activation, are functional assays that are frequently run in conjunction with testing of individual components. The **hemolytic titration (CH$_{50}$) assay** is the one most often used for this purpose.[38] This measures the amount of patient serum required to lyse 50 percent of a standardized concentration of antibody-sensitized sheep erythrocytes. Because all proteins from C1 to C9 are necessary for this to occur, absence of any one component will result in an abnormal CH$_{50}$, essentially reducing this number to zero.

The titer is expressed in CH$_{50}$ units, which is the reciprocal of the dilution that is able to lyse 50 percent of the sensitized cells.[8] The 50 percent point is used because this is the point at which the change in lytic activity per unit change in complement is a maximum. When absorbance is plotted against the complement concentration, an S-shaped curve results (Fig. 7–9A). This can be converted to a linear curve by using semi-log paper (Fig. 7–9B). The reciprocal of the dilution is plotted on the y-axis or log axis, and the percent of lysis is plotted on the x-axis. The percent of lysis is obtained by dividing the corrected optical density of the sample by the optical density of the tube with 100-percent lysis. A best-fit line is drawn, and the *y* value obtained where the line crosses the 50-percent lysis point is the CH$_{50}$ value.[38] This technique primarily determines functional activity of the classical cascade.

A microtiter lytic assay can also be performed using 96-well microtiter plates. Doubling dilutions are made, and the results are read from an enzyme-linked immunosorbent assay (ELISA) reader set at a wavelength of 405 to 410 nm. The results are not quite as reproducible as those obtained from the tube assay, but it may be a useful screening test.[38]

Lytic assays in general are complicated to perform and lack sensitivity. Individual labs must establish their own normal values. When the results are abnormal, the reasons cannot be determined. Such procedures, however, are useful in establishing functional activity or lack thereof. Additional testing for individual components should be performed to follow up on any abnormality.

ELISAs have also been designed to measure activation of the classical pathway.[39,40] Solid-phase IgM attached to the walls of microtiter plates is used to initiate complement activation. Antihuman antibody to C9 conjugated to alkaline phosphatase is the indicator of complement activation. When a substrate is added, if any C9 is present and the antibody conjugate has attached, a color change will be evident. (Refer to Chapter 11 for a complete discussion of the principle of ELISA techniques.) This type of testing, which is very sensitive, shows promise for the future because of its simplicity and capability for achieving standardization.

Alternative Pathway Assays

Alternative pathway activation can be measured by several different means. An AH$_{50}$ can be performed in the same manner as the CH$_{50}$, except magnesium chloride and ethylene glycol tetra-acetic acid are added to the buffer, and calcium is left out.[38] This buffer chelates calcium, which blocks classical pathway activation. Another test system uses radial hemolysis in agarose plates. Rabbit red blood cells that have been sensitized with antibody are implanted in agarose, and patient serum is added to wells punched in the gel. Lysis appears as a clear zone around each well, and if complement standards are run, the size of the zone can be related to complement concentration.

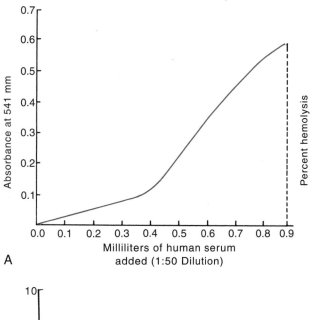

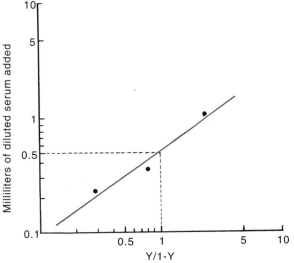

B   Y=Corrected O.D. (Correct with O.D. of tube with 100% lysis)

FIG. 7–9. CH_{50} absorbance curve. *(A)* Curve that relates the percent of hemolysis to various concentrations of a 1:50 serum dilution read at 541 nm. *(B)* Semilog plot of CH_{50} curve, because CH_{50} cannot be calculated from the absorbance curve.

A third means of testing for alternative pathway function is through the use of ELISA. One such test is able to detect C3bBbP or C3bP complexes in very small quantities.[8] Microtiter wells are typically coated with bacterial polysaccharide to trigger activation of the alternative pathway.

Interpretation of Laboratory Findings

Decreased levels of complement components or activity may be due to any of the following: (1) decreased production, (2) consumption, or (3) in vitro consump-

tion.[39] The third condition must be ruled out before either of the other two is considered. Specimen handling is extremely important. Once the blood has been collected in a clot tube, it should be spun down, and the serum should be frozen or placed on dry ice if it is not tested within 1 to 2 hours.[38] If a specimen has been inadequately refrigerated, subjected to multiple freeze-thaws, or been in prolonged storage, the results may be invalid, and the test needs to be repeated with a fresh specimen. Control serum should also be included with each batch of test sera.

A phenomenon called coagulation-associated complement consumption must also be taken into consideration. In certain disease states, notably chronic liver disease, consumption of C1, C2, and C3 occurs when the blood clots.[38] Thus, if test results suggest a complement deficiency, plasma should also be run. Although the ethylenediaminetra-acetic acid present in tubes used to collect plasma chelates calcium, buffers used for testing replace magnesium and calcium so that activation of either pathway should not be affected. If both plasma and serum are tested and the concentrations of C1, C2, and C3 are decreased in the serum sample only, this is an indicator that coagulation-associated complement consumption is taking place.

A typical screening test for complement abnormalities usually includes determination of the following: C3, C4, and factor B levels as well as hemolytic content.[39] Testing for products of complement activation such as C3a, C4a, C5a, and Ba as well as breakdown products including C3dg, iC3b, and C4d can also be performed as a means of monitoring inflammatory processes. This is especially helpful for patients with rheumatoid arthritis, systemic lupus, angioedema, gram-negative sepsis, and chronic hepatitis because these conditions may not show a decrease in individual complement components.[39] Table 7–5 presents some of the possible screening results and correlates these with disease states. An understanding of these patterns may be helpful in differentiating hereditary deficiencies from activational states that consume available complement components. Additional testing would be necessary, however, to actually pinpoint hereditary deficiencies.

Complement Fixation Testing

Complement itself can actually be used as a reagent in the test known as complement fixation. Because complement fixation occurs after the binding of antigen and antibody, uptake of complement can be used as an indicator of the presence of either specific antigen or antibody. This technique has been used in the detection of viral, fungal, and rickettsial antibodies. The test involves a two-stage process: (1) a test system with antigen and antibody, one of which is unknown, and (2) an

CH$_{50}$	Alternate Pathway	C3	C4	Indications
↓	N or ↓	↓	↓	Immune complexes triggering classical pathway—SLE, RA, serum sickness, chronic hepatitis endocarditis, malaria
N or ↓	↓	↓	N	Alternative pathway activation–poststrep GN, MPGN, deficiency of C3, factor I, or factor H
↓	N	N	↓	Mild classical activation C1INH deficiency, C4 deficiency
↓	↓	N	N	Improperly handled sera, coagulation-associated abnormality, hereditary component

TABLE 7–5. Diagnosis of Complement Abnormalities

Adapted from Luskin, AT and Tobin, MC: Alterations of complement components in disease. America Journal of Medical Technology 48:749, 1982.

↓ = Decrease or lack of functioning; N = normal; GN = glomerulonephritis; RA = rheumatoid arthritis; SLE = systemic lupus erythematosus; MPGN = membranoproliferative glomerulonephritis.

indicator system consisting of sheep red blood cells coated with hemolysin, which will lyse in the presence of complement.

To destroy any complement present, patient serum must be heated to 56°C for 30 minutes prior to testing. Then dilutions of the serum are combined with known antigen and a measured amount of guinea pig complement. Guinea pig complement can be used for testing because complement is not species-specific. If patient antibody is present, it will combine with the reagent antigen, and complement will be bound. The test can also be performed with reagent antibody to detect the presence of antigen in the sample.

The second step involves addition of sheep red blood cells that are coated with hemolysin. After an additional incubation, the tubes are centrifuged and then read for hemolysis. If hemolysis is present, this means that no patient antibody was present, and this is a negative test. Lack of hemolysis is a positive test (Fig. 7–10). Results are expressed as the highest dilution showing no hemolysis.

The use of controls is extremely important to ensure the accuracy of test results. These include running known positive and negative sera, an antigen control, a patient serum control, a cell control, and a complement control. The antigen and patient serum controls test for the ability of complement to bind in the absence of antibody. These controls should show lysis with the sheep red blood cells. The cell control is a check on spontaneous lysis. Lysis should be absent or extremely low. The complement control tube should show lysis to indicate that the complement is working correctly. Due to the amount of manipulation required and the need for standardization and numerous controls, the use of complement fixation in the clinical laboratory is limited.

SUMMARY

The complement system is a series of more than 30 proteins normally found in serum that play a major role

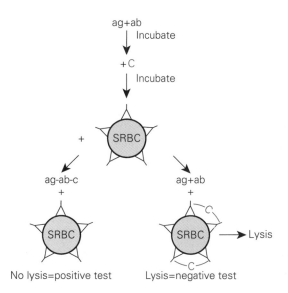

FIG. 7–10. Patient serum and antigen are incubated, and then a measured amount of complement is added. After a second incubation, sheep red blood cells, which are coated with antibody, are added to the reaction tube. If patient antibody to the specific antigen is present, no hemolysis occurs. Lack of patient antibody allows the complement to combine with coated sheep red blood cells, and lysis occurs.

in phagocytosis and clearance of foreign antigens from the body. While the end product of complement activation is lysis, other important events, such as opsonization, increase in vascular permeability, and chemotaxis of monocytes and neutrophils take place along the way and enhance host defense mechanisms. Most of the proteins of the complement system are inactive enzyme precursors, or zymogens, that are converted to active enzymes in a very precise order. One such means of activation is the classical pathway, which is triggered by antigen–antibody combination and involves nine of the proteins.

The alternative pathway acts as a natural means of defense against infection; it is triggered not by antigen-antibody combination but by the presence of microorganisms themselves. The lectin pathway also involves nonspecific recognition microorganisms by means of sugars such as mannose that are common constituents of microbial cell walls but distinct from those found on human cell surfaces. Although initial activation of these pathways involves proteins that are unique to each, C3 serves a major role in linking all three pathways. Cleavage of C3 to C3a and C3b represents one of the most significant steps in all pathways because C3b is a powerful opsonin that greatly enhances phagocytosis. C3a is an anaphylatoxin that causes release of reactants from mast cells that amplify the inflammatory response. The end result is lysis of cells due to production of a membrane attack complex that drills holes in the cell membrane.

If activation of the complement system were to proceed uncontrolled, tissue damage and life-threatening systemic effects might result. Therefore, several proteins act as regulators to keep the reaction localized and ensure that infectious agents and not self-antigens are destroyed. Some of these are free floating in the plasma, while others are found on cell surfaces as specific receptors.

One class of membrane receptors on host cells acts in conjunction with complement components to amplify the immune response. These receptors bind antigen-antibody complexes and facilitate phagocytosis. Other functions may include enhancing activity of phagocytes and production of increased memory cells.

Complement plays a major role in a number of disease states. Decreased complement levels or decline in lytic activity can indicate either hereditary deficiencies or extreme activation of the system. Paroxysmal nocturnal hemoglobinuria and hereditary angioedema are two conditions that result from missing or very low production of certain components. Autoimmune diseases such as SLE are characterized by the presence of numerous antigen-antibody complexes that tie up available components.

Several laboratory assays have been devised to detect abnormal complement levels. One of these, the CH_{50} hemolytic assay, uses 50 percent lysis of a standard concentration of antibody-sensitized sheep erythrocytes as an endpoint. This measures the presence of all proteins involved in the classical pathway. A similar assay, the AH50 assay, measures the functioning of the alternative pathway. Other assays using RID or ELISA techniques measure levels of individual components.

Proper handling of specimens is essential to ensure correct interpretation of laboratory testing.

Complement fixation tests use complement as a reagent to detect the presence of antigen or antibody. Antigen and antibody are allowed to combine with a measured amount of complement. Then indicator sheep red blood cells are added. These are coated with hemolysin (anti-sheep cell antibody) and, if complement has not been tied up in the first reaction, then lysis of the cells occurs. Thus, lysis is a negative test, indicating that either antigen or antibody was not present. As in all complement testing, the use of standards and control is necessary for accurate results.

Case Studies

1. A 3-year-old child has a history of serious infections and is currently hospitalized with meningitis. The doctor suspects that he may have a complement deficiency and orders testing. The following results are obtained: decreased CH_{50}, normal C4 and C3 levels, and decreased radial hemolysis in agarose plates using a buffer that chelates calcium.

Questions

   a. What do the results indicate about possible pathway(s) affected?
   b. Which component(s) are likely to be lacking?
   c. What sort of additional follow-up would be recommended?

2. A 25-year-old female patient appeared at the emergency room with symptoms that included abdominal pain with severe vomiting and swelling of the legs and hands. She stated that she has had these symptoms on several previous occasions. After ruling out appendicitis, a battery of tests, including some for abnormalities of complement components, were performed. The following results were obtained: red and white blood cell count normal, total serum protein normal, CH_{50} decreased, alternative pathway function normal, C3 level normal, C4 and C2 levels decreased.

Questions

   a. What symptoms led physicians to consider a possible complement abnormality?
   b. What are possible reasons for a decrease in both C4 and C2?
   c. What other testing would confirm your suspicions?

Exercise: Ez Complement CH$_{50}$ Assay

PRINCIPLE

Total hemolytic complement activity is measured by calculating the dilution of patient serum that is needed to lyse 50 percent of a standard concentration of optimally sensitized sheep red blood cells. Sheep erythrocytes have been previously sensitized with specific antibody. The value obtained is compared with those reported for a normal control. The degree of hemolysis is directly proportional to the total complement activity.

SAMPLE PREPARATION

Collect at least 2 mL of blood by venipuncture using sterile technique. Do not use any anticoagulants. Allow the blood to clot at room temperature. Separate the serum from the clot. If not used within a few hours, the serum can be aliquoted in 0.5-mL portions and quick-frozen at −70°C. Do not use plasma.

REAGENTS, MATERIALS, AND EQUIPMENT

Sheep erythrocytes sensitized with anti-sheep antibody and preserved with sodium azide (Diamedix Corp., Miami, FL). These should be stored upright at 2°C to 8°C.
Complement reference serum (Diamedix or in-house controls)
High and low controls (Diamedix)
Pipette and disposable tips to dispense 5 μL
Centrifuge
Photometer that will read absorbance at 415 nm

CAUTION

The sensitized cells contain sodium azide. Azides are reported to react with lead and copper in plumbing to form compounds that may detonate on percussion. When disposing of solutions containing sodium azide, flush with large volumes of water to minimize the buildup of metal azide compounds.

PROCEDURE*

1. Reconstitute the standard with cold (2°C to 8°C) distilled water for immediate use. Discard any unused portion.
2. Reconstitute high and low controls with cold distilled water for immediate use. Discard the unused portion.
3. Place test tubes with sensitized cells in a rack and allow them to warm to room temperature. Set up one tube for each specimen, one for the reference serum, one each for the high and low controls, and one for the spontaneous lysis control. It is recommended that no more than 12 tubes be run at once.
4. Vortex tubes or shake vigorously for 10 seconds to resuspend cells.
5. Remove the stopper and transfer 5 μL of sample or standard into a tube. Replace the stopper and mix immediately by inverting tube three to four times. The spontaneous lysis tube receives no sample, but should also be mixed.
6. Allow tubes to stand at room temperature for 60 minutes.
7. Mix contents of all tubes again by inverting three to four times, or vortexing.
8. Centrifuge the tubes at approximately 1000 rpm for at least 5 minutes.
9. Read the absorbance of the supernatants at 415 nm within 15 minutes. If possible, read directly through the original tube, or use a photometer with a sipping device that can withdraw the supernatant without disturbing the sedimented cells.
   a. To read the absorbance, zero the photometer with a water blank.
   b. Read and record the absorbance of the spontaneous lysis control. If the absorbance value is greater than 0.1, the results of the assay will not be valid, and the test must be repeated with a new lot of sensitized cells.
   c. Zero the photometer again with the spontaneous lysis control. This will correct for any spontaneous lysis in test specimens.
   d. Read and record the absorbance value of the reference serum.
   e. Read and record the absorbance value of each test sample.
   Note: The volume of individual tubes is at the lowest limit of detection on Spectrometer 20 instruments used in many clinical laboratory science programs. An EZ Reader photometer designed specifically to read these tubes is available from Diamedix.
10. Calculate test results as follows: Divide the absorbance value of the supernate by the absorbance value of the reference serum and multiply by 100 to give the percent of reference.

RESULTS

Percent of Reference	Standard Complement Level
0–50	Absent or low
51–150	Normal
≥150	High

* From the package insert for the EZ Complement CH$_{50}$ Assay by Diamedix Corporation, Miami, FL.

INTERPRETATION OF RESULTS

This test will provide a quantitative value for the functional activity of total complement. It cannot identify the individual component or components that are abnormal. Abnormal specimens should be assayed for levels of each of the individual components of complement (C1–C9).

Depressed complement levels may be due to any of the following: genetic deficiencies, decreased complement synthesis accompanying liver disease, or fixation of complement due to chronic glomerulonephritis, rheumatoid arthritis, hemolytic anemias, graft rejection, SLE, or other autoimmune phenomena. Elevated levels are found in acute inflammatory conditions, leukemia, Hodgkin's disease, sarcoma, and Behçet's disease.

1. The classical complement pathway is activated by:
   a. Most viruses
   b. Antigen-antibody complexes
   c. Fungal cells walls
   d. All of the above

2. All of the following are characteristic of complement components *except*:
   a. Normally present in serum
   b. Mainly synthesized in the liver
   c. Present as active enzymes
   d. Heat-labile

3. All of the following are true of the recognition unit *except*:
   a. It consists of Clq, Clr, and Cls.
   b. The subunits require calcium for binding together.
   c. Binding occurs at the Fc region of antibody molecules.
   d. Clq becomes an active esterase.

4. Which is referred to as C3 convertase?
   a. C4b2a
   b. C3bBb
   c. iC3Bb
   d. All of the above

5. Mannose-binding protein in the lectin pathway is most similar to which classical pathway component?
   a. C3
   b. C1rs
   c. C1q
   d. C4

6. Which of the following describes the role of properdin in the alternative pathway?
   a. Stabilization of C3/C5 convertase
   b. Conversion of B to Bb
   c. Inhibition of C3 convertase formation
   d. Binding to the initiating antigen

7. All but which one of the following are true of the MAC?
   a. The same components are used in both pathways.
   b. C9 must be attached for lysis to occur.
   c. C8 becomes inserted into the membrane.
   d. C9 polymerizes to form the transmembrane channel.

8. All of the following represent functions of the complement system *except*:
   a. Decreased clearance of antigen-antibody complexes
   b. Lysis of foreign cells
   c. Increase in vascular permeability
   d. Migration of neutrophils to the tissues

9. Which of the following is true of the amplification loop in complement activation?
   a. It is found in the alternative pathway.
   b. iC3 binds factor B to generate amplification.
   c. C3b is the product that is increased.
   d. All of the above.

10. Factor H acts by competing with which of the following for the same binding site?
    a. Factor B
    b. Factor D
    c. C3B
    d. Factor I

11. A lack of CR1 receptors on red blood cells would result in which of the following?
    a. Decreased binding of C3b to red blood cells
    b. Lack of clearance of immune complexes by the spleen
    c. Increased breakdown of C3b to C3d and C3dg
    d. All of the above

12. A lack of CR2 on cell membranes would result in which of the following?
    a. Decrease in hemolysis
    b. Increased susceptibility to infection
    c. Decreased antibody production
    d. Increase in antibody of the IgG class

13. Why is complement not activated with anti-Rh (D) antibodies?
    a. Rh antigens stimulate little antibody production.
    b. Rh antigens are too far apart on red blood cells.
    c. Rh antibodies are not capable of fixing complement.
    d. DAF protects red blood cells from buildup of antibody.

14. The CH_{50} test measures which of the following?
    a. The dilution of patient serum required to lyse 50 percent of a standard concentration of sensitized sheep red blood cells
    b. Functioning of both the classical and the alternative pathway
    c. Genetic deficiencies of any of the complement components
    d. All of the above

15. Which of the following would be most effective in preventing bystander lysis of red blood cells?
    a. C1INH
    b. Factor B
    c. DAF
    d. Factor H

16. Decreased CH_{50} levels may be caused by:
    a. Inadequate refrigeration of specimen
    b. Coagulation-associated complement consumption
    c. Autoimmune disease process
    d. All of the above

References

1. Prodinger, WM, et al: Complement. In Paul, WE (ed): Fundamental Immunology, ed. 4. Lippincott-Raven, Philadelphia, 1999, pp 967–995.
2. Walport, M: Complement. In Roitt, I, Brostoff, J, and Male, D (eds): Immunology. Mosby, London, 1998, pp 43–60.
3. Cole, FS, and Colten, HR: Complement biosynthesis: Factors of the classical pathway. In Rother, K, and Till, GO (eds): The Complement System. Springer-Verlag, Berlin, 1988, pp 44–70.
4. Goldsby, RA, Kindt, TJ, and Osborne, BA: Immunology, ed. 4. WH Freeman and Co., New York, 2000, pp 329–350.
5. Schwaeble, WJ, and Reid, KBM: Does properdin crosslink the cellular and the humoral response? Immunology Today 20:17–21, 1999.
6. Pillemer, L, et al: The properdin system and immunity: Demonstration and isolation of a new serum protein, properdin, and its role in immune phenomena. Science 120:279, 1954.
7. Davies, KA, et al: Splenic uptake of immune complexes in man is complement-dependent. J Immunol 151:3866, 1993.
8. Khan, WA, Wigfall, DR, and Frank, MM: Complement and kinins: Mediators of infection. In Henry, JB (ed): Clinical Diagnosis and Management by Laboratory Methods, ed. 19. WB Saunders, Philadelphia, 1996, pp 928–946.
9. Loos, M: Reactivity in immune hemolysis: Classical pathway of activation. In Rother, K, and Till, GO (eds): The Complement System. Springer-Verlag, Berlin, 1988, pp 136–141.
10. Arlaud, G, Colomb, MG, and Gagnon, J: A functional model of the human C1 complex. Immunol Today 8:106, 1987.
11. Frank, MM: Complement and kinin. In Stites, DP, Terr, AI, and Parslow, TG (eds): Medical Immunology, ed. 9. Appleton & Lange, Stamford, Conn., 1997, pp 169–181.
12. Vogt, W: Formation of the C3/C5 convertase. In Rother, K, and Till, GO (eds): The Complement System. Springer-Verlag, Berlin, 1988, pp 141–154.
13. Hansch, GM: The complement attack phase. In Rother, K, and Till, GO (eds): The Complement System. Springer-Verlag, Berlin, 1988, pp 202–230.
14. Atkinson, JP, and Farries, T: Separation of self from non-self in the complement system. Immunol Today 8:212, 1987.
15. Sim, RB, et al: Complement factor I and cofactors in control of complement system convertase enzymes. In Lorand, L, and Mann, KG (eds): Methods Enzymol 223:13, 1993.
16. Medzhitov, R, and Janeway, C: Innate immunity. New Engl J Med 343:338–343, 2000.
17. Matsushita, M, Endo, Y, Nonaka, M, and Fujita, T: Complement-related serine proteases in tunicates and vertebrates. Current Opinion in Immunology 10:29–35, 1998.
18. Epstein, J, et al: The collectins in innate immunity. Current Opinion in Immunology 8:29–35, 1996.
19. Thiel, S, et al: Interaction of C1q and mannan-binding lectin (MBL) with C1r, C1s, MBL-associated serine proteases 1 and 2, and the MBL-associated protein Map19. J Immunol 165:878–887, 2000.
20. Reid, KBM, Colomb, MG, and Loos, M. Complement components C1 and the collectins: Parallels between routes of acquired and innate immunity. Immunol Today 19:56–59, 1998.
21. Thiel, S, et al: A second serine protease associated with mannan-binding lectin that activates complement. Nature 386:506–510, 1997.
22. Matsushita, M, et al: Proteolytic activities of two types of mannose-binding lectin-associated serine protease. J Immunol 165:2637–2642, 2000.
23. Liszewski, MK, et al: Control of the complement system. In Dixon, FJ (ed): Advances in Immunology 61:201–283, 1996.
24. DiScipio, RG: Ultrastructures and interactions of complement factors H and I. J Immunol 149:2592, 1993.
25. Fallman, M, Andersson, R, and Andersson, T: Signaling properties of CR3 and CR1 in relation to phagocytosis of complement-opsonized particles. J Immunol 151:330, 1993.
26. Lubin, DM, and Atkinson, J: Decay-accelerating factor: Biochemistry, molecular biology, and function. Adv Immunol 7:35, 1989.
27. Carroll, MC, and Fischer, MB: Complement and the immune response. Curr Opin Immunol 9:64–69, 1997.
28. Morgan, BP: Complement regulatory molecules: Application to therapy and transplantation. Immunol Today 16:257–259, 1995.
29. Kozono, Y, et al: Cross-linking CD21/CD35 or CD19 increases both B7-1 and B7-2 expression on murine splenic B cells. J Immunol 160:1565–1572, 1998.
30. Sun, X, et al: Role of decay-accelerating factor in regulating complement activation on the erythrocyte surface as revealed by gene targeting. Proc Natl Acad Sci, USA 96:628–633, 1999.
31. Lukacs, NW, and Ward, PA: Inflammatory mediators, cytokines, and adhesion molecules in pulmonary inflammation and injury. In Dixon, FJ (ed): Adv Immunol 62:257–304, 1996.
32. Asghar, SS, and Pasch, MC: Complement as a promiscuous signal transduction device. Lab Invest 78:1203–1225, 1998.
33. Wurzner, R, and Dierich, MP: Complement in human disease. Immunol Today 18:460–463, 1997.
34. Pascual, M, and French, LE: Complement in human diseases: Looking towards the 21st century. Immunol Today 16:58–61, 1995.
35. Hughes, J, et al: C5-9 membrane attack complex mediates endothelial cell apoptosis in experimental glomerulonephritis. Am J Physiol Renal Physiol 278:F747–F757, 2000.
36. Walport, MJ, et al: Complement deficiency and autoimmunity. Ann NY Acad Sci 815:267–281, 1997.
37. Frank, MM: Complement deficiencies. In Stites, DP, Terr, AI, and Parslow, TG (eds): Medical Immunology, ed. 9. Appleton & Lange, Stamford, Conn., 1997, pp 371–375.
38. Giclas, PC: Complement tests. In Rose, NR, et al (eds): Manual of Clinical Laboratory Immunology, ed. 5. ASM Press, Washington, D.C., 1997, pp 181–186.
39. Rabson, AR: Complement Activation. In Rose, NR, et al (eds): Manual of Clinical Laboratory Immunology, ed. 5. ASM Press, Washington, D.C., 1997, pp 187–191.
40. Fredrikson, GN, Truedsson, L, and Sjoholm, AG: New procedure for the detection of complement deficiency by ELISA. J Immunol Methods 166:263, 1993.

Part II

Basic Immunologic Procedures

chapter 8

Safety and Specimen Preparation

By Susan K. Strasinger, DA, MT(ASCP) and Christine Stevens

Learning Objectives

On completion of this chapter, the reader will be able to:

1. List the components of the chain of infection and the safety precautions that will break the chain.
2. Correctly perform routine handwashing.
3. Describe the types of the personal protective equipment used by laboratory personnel.
4. Differentiate among Universal Precautions (UP), body substance isolation (BSI), and Standard Precautions.
5. Describe the acceptable methods for disposal of biological waste in the laboratory.
6. Safely dispose of sharp objects.
7. Describe the components of the Occupational Exposure to Bloodborne Pathogens Standard.
8. Describe safety precautions used when handling chemicals.
9. Discuss the components of chemical hygiene plans.
10. Identify the symbol for radiation.
11. Describe the following: serial dilution, solute, diluent, and compound dilution.
12. Explain how an antibody titer is determined.
13. Calculate the amount of diluent needed to prepare a specific dilution of a serum specimen.

Key Terms

Biohazardous
Body substance isolation
  (BSI)
Centers for Disease Control
  and Prevention (CDC)
Chain of infection
Chemical Hygiene Plan
Diluent

Material Safety Data Sheet
  (MSDS)
Occupational Safety and
  Health Administration
  (OSHA)
Personal protective
  equipment (PPE)
Postexposure prophylaxis

Serial dilution
Solute
Standard Precautions
Titer
Universal Precautions (UP)

The clinical laboratory contains a wide variety of safety hazards, many capable of producing serious injury or life-threatening disease. To work safely in this environment, the clinical laboratorian must learn what hazards exist, the basic safety precautions associated with them, and finally how to apply the basic rules of common sense required for everyday safety. Some hazards are unique to the health-care environment, and others are encountered routinely throughout life (Table 8–1).

Biologic Hazards

In the immunology laboratory, the most significant hazard exists in obtaining and testing of patient specimens. An understanding of the transmission (**chain of infection**) of microorganisms is necessary to prevent infection. The chain of infection requires a continuous link between three elements—a source, a method of transmission, and a susceptible host. The most likely source of infection in serologic testing is through contact with patient specimens, and the main concern is exposure to viruses such as the hepatitis viruses and human immunodeficiency virus (HIV). Therefore, safety precautions are designed to protect health-care workers from exposure to potentially harmful infectious agents. The ultimate goal of biologic safety is to prevent completion of the chain by preventing transmission. Figure 8–1 uses the universal symbol for **biohazardous** material to illustrate the chain of infection and demonstrates how it can be broken by following safety practices.

Preventing the transmission of microorganisms from infected sources to susceptible hosts is critical in controlling the spread of infection. Procedures used to prevent microorganism transmission include: handwashing, the wearing of **personal protective equipment (PPE)**, isolation of highly infective or highly susceptible patients, and proper disposal of contaminated materials. Strict adherence to guidelines published by the **Centers for Disease Control and Prevention (CDC)** and the **Occupational Safety and Health Administration (OSHA)** is essential.

Handwashing

Hand contact represents the number one method of infection transmission. Hands should always be washed at the following times: before patient contact, when gloves are removed, prior to leaving the work area, at any time when they have been knowingly contaminated, before going to designated break areas, and before and after using bathroom facilities.

Correct routine handwashing technique includes:

- Wetting hands with warm water
- Applying soap, preferably antimicrobial
- Rubbing to form a lather, creating friction, and loosening debris
- Thoroughly cleaning between fingers and under fingernails and rings for at least 15 seconds and cleaning up to the wrist
- Rinsing hands in a downward position
- Drying with a paper towel
- Turning off faucets with the paper towel to prevent recontamination

Personal Protective Equipment

PPE encountered by the laboratorian includes gloves, gowns, laboratory coats, masks, goggles, face shields, and plexiglass countertop shields. Gloves are worn to protect the health-care worker's hands from contamination by patient body substances and to protect the patient from possible microorganisms on the health-

TABLE 8–1. Types of Safety Hazards		
Type	**Source**	**Possible Injury**
Biologic	Infectious agents	Bacterial, fungal, viral, or parasitic infections
Sharp	Needles, lancets, and broken glass	Cuts, punctures, or bloodborne pathogen exposure
Chemical	Preservatives and reagents	Exposure to toxic, carcinogenic, or caustic agents
Radioactive	Equipment and radioisotopes	Radiation exposure
Electrical	Ungrounded or wet equipment and frayed cords	Burns or shock
Fire/explosive	Bunsen burners and organic chemicals	Burns or dismemberment
Physical	Wet floors, heavy boxes, and patients	Falls, sprains, or strains

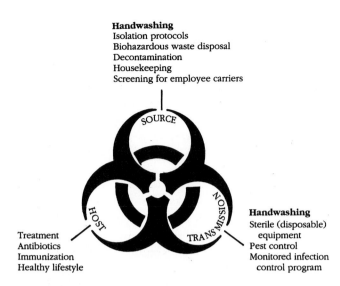

Handwashing
Isolation protocols
Biohazardous waste disposal
Decontamination
Housekeeping
Screening for employee carriers

SOURCE

HOST

TRANSMISSION

Treatment
Antibiotics
Immunization
Healthy lifestyle

Handwashing
Sterile (disposable)
    equipment
Pest control
Monitored infection
    control program

FIG. 8–1. Chain of infection and safety practices related to the biohazard symbol. (From Strasinger, SK, and DiLorenzo, MA: Phlebotomy Workbook for the Multiskilled Healthcare Professional, ed. 2. FA Davis, Philadelphia, 2003, with permission.)

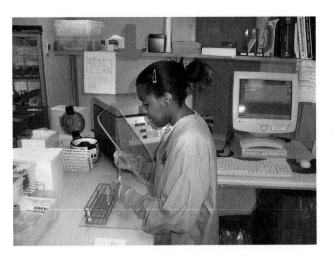

FIG. 8–2. Personal protective equipment. (From Strasinger, SK, and DiLorenzo, MA: Phlebotomy Workbook for the Multiskilled Healthcare Professional ed. 2. FA Davis, Philadelphia, 2003, with permission.)

care worker's hands. Wearing gloves is not a substitute for handwashing. Hands must always be washed when gloves are removed. A variety of gloves are available, including sterile and nonsterile, powdered and unpowdered, and latex and nonlatex.

Allergy to latex is increasing among health-care workers, and laboratorians should be alert for symptoms of reactions associated with latex contact. Reactions to latex include irritant contact dermatitis that produces patches of dry, itchy irritation on the hands; delayed hypersensitivity reactions resembling poison ivy that appear 24 to 48 hours following exposure; and true immediate hypersensitivity reactions often characterized by respiratory difficulty (see Chapter 13). Handwashing immediately after removal of gloves and avoiding powdered gloves may aid in preventing the development of latex allergy. Replacing latex gloves with nitrile gloves provides an acceptable alternative. Any signs of a latex reaction should be reported to a supervisor because true latex allergy can be life threatening.[1]

Gowns or laboratory coats are worn to protect the clothing and skin of health-care workers from contamination by patient body substances. Fluid-resistant gowns or laboratory coats should be worn when the possibility of encountering splashes or large amounts of body fluids is anticipated. Gowns usually tie in the back at the neck and the waist and have tight-fitting cuffs. Laboratory coats should be completely buttoned, with gloves pulled over the cuffs. Coats and gowns should be changed when they become visibly soiled.

Masks are worn to protect against inhalation of droplets containing microorganisms from infective patients. Masks and goggles are worn to protect the mucous membranes of the mouth, nose, and eyes from splashing of body substances (Fig. 8–2). Face shields and countertop plexiglass shields also protect the mucous membranes from splashes. They are most commonly worn when processing blood and body fluids in the laboratory.

Procedure Precautions

Universal Precautions (UP) were instituted by the CDC in 1985 to protect health-care workers from exposure to bloodborne pathogens; primarily hepatitis B virus (HBV) and HIV. Under UP, all patients are assumed to be possible carriers of bloodborne pathogens. Transmission may occur by skin puncture from a contaminated sharp object or by passive contact through open skin lesions or mucous membranes. The guideline recommends wearing gloves when collecting or handling blood and body fluids contaminated with blood, wearing face shields when there is danger of blood splashing on mucous membranes, and disposing of all needles and sharp objects in puncture-resistant containers without recapping.

A modification of UP, **body substance isolation (BSI)** is not limited to bloodborne pathogens and considers all body fluids and moist body substances to be potentially infectious. Personnel should wear gloves at all times when encountering moist body substances. A disadvantage of the BSI guideline is that it does not recommend handwashing following removal of gloves unless visual contamination is present.

The major features of UP and BSI have now been combined and are called **Standard Precautions**. Standard Precautions should be used for the care of all patients and include the following[2]:

- Handwashing
  Wash hands after touching blood, body fluids, secretions, excretions, and contaminated items, whether or not gloves are worn. Wash hands immediately after gloves are removed, between patient contacts, and when otherwise indicated to avoid transfer of microorganisms to other patients or environments. It may be necessary to wash hands between tasks and procedures on the same patient to prevent crosscontamination of different body sites.
- Gloves
  Wear gloves (clean, nonsterile gloves are adequate) when touching blood, body fluids, secretions, excretions, and contaminated items. Change gloves between tasks and procedures on the same patient after contact with material that may contain a high concentration of microorganisms. Remove gloves promptly after use, before touching noncontaminated items and environmental surfaces, and before going to another patient. Wash hands immediately to avoid transfer of microorganisms to other patients or environments.
- Mask, Eye Protection, and Face Shield
  Wear a mask and eye protection or a face shield to protect mucous membranes of the eyes, nose, and mouth during procedures and patient-care activities that are likely to generate splashes or sprays of blood, body fluids, secretions, and excretions.
- Gown
  Wear a gown (a clean, nonsterile gown is adequate) to protect skin and to prevent soiling of clothing during procedures and patient-care activities that are likely to generate splashes of blood, body fluids, secretions, or excretions. Select a gown that is appropriate for the activity and amount of fluid likely to be encountered. Remove a soiled gown as promptly as possible, and wash hands to avoid transfer of microorganisms to other patients or environments.
- Patient-Care Equipment
  Handle used patient-care equipment soiled with blood, body fluids, secretions, and excretions in a manner that prevents skin and mucous membrane exposures, contamination of clothing, and transfer of microorganisms to other patients and environments. Ensure that reusable equipment is not used for the care of another patient until it has been cleaned and reprocessed appropriately. Ensure that single-use items are discarded properly.
- Environmental Control
  Ensure that the hospital has adequate procedures for the routine care, cleaning, and disinfection of environmental surfaces, beds, bed rails, bedside equipment, and other frequently touched surfaces, and ensure that these procedures are being followed.
- Linen
  Handle, transport, and process used linen soiled with blood, body fluids, secretions, and excretions in a manner that prevents skin and mucous membrane exposures and contamination of clothing, and that avoids transfer of microorganisms to other patients and environments.
- Occupational Health and Bloodborne Pathogens
  Take care to prevent injuries when using needles, scalpels, and other sharp instruments or when handling sharp instruments after procedures; when cleaning used instruments; and when disposing of used needles. Never recap used needles or otherwise manipulate them using both hands, and never use any other technique that involves directing the point of a needle toward any part of the body; rather, use either a one-handed "scoop" technique or a mechanical device designed for holding the needle sheath. Do not remove used needles from disposable syringes by hand, and do not bend, break, or otherwise manipulate used needles by hand. Place used disposable syringes and needles, scalpel blades, and other sharp items in appropriate puncture-resistant containers, which are located as close as practical to the area in which the items were used, and place reusable syringes and needles in a puncture-resistant container for transport to the reprocessing area.
- Patient Placement
  Place a patient who contaminates the environment or who does not (or cannot be expected to) assist in maintaining appropriate hygiene or environmental control in a private room. If a private room is not available, consult with infection control professionals regarding patient placement or other alternatives.

Biologic Waste Disposal

All biologic waste, except urine, must be placed in appropriate containers labeled with the biohazard symbol. This includes not only specimens, but also the materials with which the specimens come in contact. Any supplies contaminated with blood and body fluids must also be disposed of in containers clearly marked with the biohazard symbol or red or yellow color-coding. This includes alcohol pads, gauze, bandages, disposable tourniquets, gloves, masks, gowns, and plastic tubes and pipettes. Disposal of needles and other sharp objects is discussed in the next section.

Contaminated nondisposable equipment, blood spills, and blood and body fluid processing areas must be disinfected. The most commonly used disinfectant is a 1:10 dilution of sodium hypochlorite (household bleach) prepared weekly and stored in a plastic, not glass, bottle. The bleach should be allowed to air dry on the contaminated area prior to removal. National Committee for Clinical Laboratory Standards (NCCLS) states that a 1:100 dilution can be used for routine cleaning.[3]

Sharps Hazards

Sharp objects in the laboratory, including needles, lancets, and broken glassware, present a serious biologic hazard for possible exposure to bloodborne pathogens caused by accidental puncture. Although bloodborne pathogens also are transmitted through contact with mucous membranes and nonintact skin, a needle or lancet used to collect blood has the capability to produce a very significant exposure to bloodborne pathogens. It is essential that safety precautions be followed at all times when sharps hazards are present.

The number one personal safety rule when using needles is to *never* manually recap a needle. Many safety devices are available for needle disposal, and they provide a variety of safe guards. These include needle holders that become a sheathe, needles that automatically resheath or become blunt, and needles with attached sheathes. All sharps must be disposed of in puncture-resistant, leak-proof containers labeled with the biohazard symbol (Fig. 8–3). Containers should be located in close proximity to the work area. Containers must always be replaced when the safe capacity mark is reached.

Government Regulations

The federal government has enacted regulations to protect health-care workers from exposure to bloodborne pathogens. These regulations are monitored and enforced by OSHA. The Occupational Exposure to Bloodborne Pathogens Standard became law in 1991.[4] It requires all employers to have a written Bloodborne Pathogen Exposure Control Plan and to provide necessary protection free of charge for employees. Specifics of the OSHA standard include:

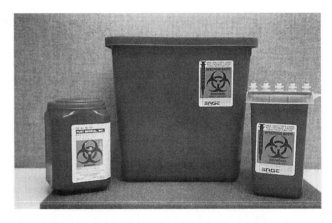

FIG. 8–3. Examples of puncture-resistant containers. (From Strasinger, SK, and DiLorenzo, MA: Phlebotomy Workbook for the Multiskilled Healthcare Professional, ed. 2. FA Davis, Philadelphia, 1996, with permission.)

- Requiring all employees to practice UP (Standard Precautions).
- Providing lab coats, gowns, face shields, and gloves to employees, and laundry facilities for nondisposable protective clothing.
- Providing sharps disposal containers and prohibiting recapping of needles.
- Prohibiting eating, drinking, smoking, and applying cosmetics in the work area.
- Labeling all biohazardous materials and containers.
- Providing immunization for HBV free of charge.
- Establishing a daily work surface disinfection protocol. The disinfectant of choice for bloodborne pathogens is sodium hypochlorite (household bleach, freshly diluted 1:10).
- Providing medical follow-up to employees who have been accidentally exposed to bloodborne pathogens.
- Documenting regular training of employees in safety standards.

The exposure control plan must be available to employees. It must be updated annually and identify procedures and individuals at risk of exposure to bloodborne pathogens. The plan must identify the engineering controls (e.g., sharps containers) and the procedures in place to prevent exposure incidents.

In 1999, OSHA issued a new compliance directive, Enforcement Procedures for the Occupational Exposure to Bloodborne Pathogens Standard.[5] The new directive placed more emphasis on the use of engineering controls to prevent accidental exposure to bloodborne pathogens. Additional changes to the directive were mandated by passage of the Needlestick Safety and Prevention Act, signed into law in 2001.[6] Under the new law employees must:

- Document their evaluations and implementation of safer needle devices.
- Involve employees in the selection and evaluation of new devices.
- Maintain a log of all injuries from contaminated sharps.

In June 2002, OSHA issued a revision to the Bloodborne Pathogens Standard compliance directive.[7] In the revised directive, the agency requires that all blood holders (adapters) with needles attached be immediately discarded into a sharps container after the device's safety feature is activated. Rationale for the new directive is based on the exposure of workers to the unprotected stopper-puncturing end of evacuated tube needles, the increased needle manipulation required to remove it from the holder, and the possible worker exposure from the use of contaminated holders.

Occupational Exposure to Bloodborne Pathogens

Any accidental exposure to blood through needlestick, mucous membranes, or nonintact skin must be reported to a supervisor and a confidential medical examination immediately be started. Evaluation of the incident must begin right away to insure appropriate **postexposure prophylaxis.** Needlesticks are the most frequently encountered exposure and place the laboratorian in danger of contracting HIV, HBV, and hepatitis C virus (HCV). Each health-care institution is responsible for designing and implementing its own Exposure Control Plan.[8]

Chemical Hazards

General Precautions

Serologic testing may involve use of chemical reagents that must be handled in a safe manner to avoid injury. General rules for safe handling of chemicals include: taking precautions to avoid getting chemicals on your body, clothes, and work area; wearing PPE, such as safety goggles, when pouring chemicals; observing strict labeling practices; and carefully following instructions. Preparing reagents under a fume hood is a recommended safety precaution. Chemicals should never be mixed together unless specific instructions are followed, and they must be added in the order specified. This is particularly important when combining acid and water because acid should always be added to water to avoid the possibility of sudden splashing.

When skin or eye contact occurs, the best first aid is to immediately flush the area with water for at least 15 minutes and then seek medical attention. Laboratorians must know the location of the emergency shower and eyewash station in the laboratory. Do not try to neutralize chemicals spilled on the skin.

Material Safety Data Sheets

All chemicals and reagents containing hazardous ingredients in a concentration greater than 1 percent are required to have a **Material Safety Data Sheet (MSDS)** on file in the work area. By law, vendors must provide these sheets to purchasers; however, it is the responsibility of the facility to obtain and keep them available to employees. An MSDS contains information on physical and chemical characteristics, fire, explosion reactivity, health hazards, primary routes of entry, exposure limits and carcinogenic potential, precautions for safe handling, spill clean-up, and emergency first aid information. Containers of chemicals that pose a high risk must be labeled with a chemical hazard symbol representing the possible hazard, such as flammable, poison, or corrosive. State and federal regulations should be consulted for the disposal of chemicals.

Chemical Hygiene Plan

OSHA requires that all facilities that use hazardous chemicals have a written **Chemical Hygiene Plan** available to employees.[9] The purpose of the plan is to detail the following:

- Appropriate work practices
- Standard operating procedures
- PPE
- Engineering controls, such as fume hoods and flammables safety cabinets
- Employee training requirements
- Medical consultation guidelines

Each facility must appoint a chemical hygiene officer, who is responsible for implementing and documenting compliance with the plan. Examples of chemical safety equipment and information are shown in Figure 8–4.

Chemical Waste Disposal

Hazardous chemical waste should be disposed of by following current Environmental Protection Agency (EPA) regulations. Local regulations and the Department of Transportation also track disposal of hazardous chemical waste. Many kits used in testing

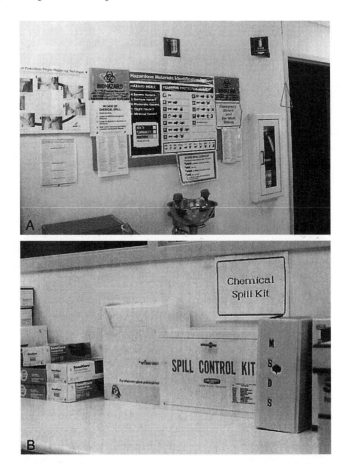

FIG. 8–4. Examples of chemical safety equipment and information. (From Strasinger, SK, and DiLorenzo, MA: Urinalysis and Body Fluids, ed. 4. FA Davis, Philadelphia, 2001, with permission.)

contain sodium azide, which can be disposed of by flushing down the drain with plenty of water to avoid buildup in plumbing.

Radioactive Hazards

General Precautions

Radioactivity is encountered in the clinical laboratory when procedures using radioisotopes, such as radioimmunoassay, are performed. The amount of radioactivity present in most medical situations is very small and represents little danger. However, the effects of radiation are related to the length of exposure and are cumulative. Exposure to radiation is dependent on the combination of time, distance, and shielding. Persons working in a radioactive environment are required to wear measuring devices to determine the amount of radiation they are accumulating.

Laboratorians should be familiar with the radioactive symbol. This symbol must be displayed on the doors of all areas where radioactive material is present. Exposure

to radiation during pregnancy presents a danger to the fetus and personnel who are pregnant or think they may be should avoid areas with this symbol.

Radioactive Waste Disposal

Disposal of radioactive waste is regulated by the Nuclear Regulatory Commission (NRC). Such waste must be separated from other waste materials in the laboratory and may be disposed of by storage in a locked, labeled room until the background count is reduced by a specified number of half-lives. Typically, ^{125}I is the most frequently encountered radiolabel, and this can be disposed of in this manner.

Serologic Testing

Specimen Preparation and Processing

The most frequently encountered specimen in immunologic testing is serum. Blood is collected aseptically by venipuncture into a clean, dry, sterile tube.

Care must be taken to avoid hemolysis because hemolysis may produce false-positive results. The blood specimen is allowed to clot at room temperature or at 4°C and then centrifuged. Serum should be promptly separated into another tube without transferring any cellular elements. Fresh non–heat inactivated serum is usually recommended for testing. However, if testing cannot be performed immediately, serum may be stored between 2°C and 8°C for up to 72 hours. If there is any additional delay in testing, the serum should be frozen at −20°C or below.

Simple Dilutions

For many tests, a measured amount of a serum sample is used directly for detection of antibodies. However, for a visible endpoint to occur in a serologic reaction, the relative proportions of antigen and antibody present are important. Sometimes in a serologic test too much antibody may be present, and an endpoint may not be reached. In this case, serum that contains antibody must be made less concentrated by means of dilution. Therefore, knowledge of serial dilutions is essential to the understanding of all serologic testing in the clinical laboratory.

A dilution involves two entities: the **solute,** which is the material being diluted, and the **diluent,** the medium making up the rest of the solution. The relationship between these two is expressed as a fraction. For example, if a 1:20 dilution is called for, this implies 1 part of solute and 19 parts of diluent. The number on the bottom of the fraction is the total volume, reached by adding the volumes of the solute and diluent together.

$$1/\text{dilution} = \text{Amount of solute/total volume}$$

To create a certain volume of a specified dilution, it is helpful to know how to manipulate this relationship. An algebraic equation can be set up to find the total volume, the amount of solute, or the amount of diluent needed to make a dilution. Consider the following example:

2 mL of a 1:20 dilution is needed to run a specific serologic test. How much serum and how much diluent are needed to make this dilution?

The equation is set up using the fraction for the dilution, indicating the relationship between the total volume and the solute, or amount of serum needed:

$$1/20 = x/2 \text{ mL}$$

Note that the 20 represents the total number of parts in the solution, and that 2 mL is the total volume desired.

Solving this equation for x gives 0.1 mL for the amount of serum needed to make this dilution. The amount of diluent is obtained by subtracting 0.1 mL from 2.0 mL to give 1.9 mL of diluent. To check the answer, simply set up a proportion between the amount of solute over the total volume. This should equal the dilution desired.

Thus the correct answer has been obtained.

If, on the other hand, the amount of serum that is to be used is known, a problem can be set up in the following manner:

A 1:5 dilution of patient serum is necessary to run a serologic test. There is 0.1 mL of serum that can be used. What amount of diluent is necessary to make this dilution using all of the serum?

A slightly different formula can be used to solve this problem.

$$1/\text{dilution} - 1 = \text{Amount of solute/amount of diluent}$$
$$1/4 = 0.1 \text{ mL}/x$$
$$x = 0.4 \text{ mL of diluent}$$

Note that the final volume is obtained by adding 0.1 mL of solute to the 0.4 mL of diluent. Dividing the volume of the solute by the total volume of 0.5 mL yields the desired 1:5 ratio.

Depending on the unknown being solved for, either of these formulas can be used. To calculate the total volume, the total dilution factor must be used. If, however, the amount of diluent is to be calculated, the formula using dilution −1 can be used. Further problems are given at the end of the chapter to allow practice with calculation of dilutions.

Compound Dilutions

The previous examples represent simple dilutions. Occasionally in the laboratory it is necessary to make a very large dilution, and it is more accurate and less costly to do this in several steps rather than all at once. Such a process is known as a compound dilution. The same approach is used, but the dilution occurs in several stages. For example, if a 1:500 dilution is necessary, it would take 49.9 mL of diluent to accomplish this in one step with 0.1 mL of serum. If only a small amount of solution is needed to run the test, this is wasteful; furthermore, inaccuracy may occur if the solution is not properly mixed. Therefore, it is helpful to make several smaller dilutions.

To calculate a compound dilution problem, the first step is to plan the number and sizes of simple dilutions necessary to reach the desired endpoint. To use the example above, a 1:500 dilution can be achieved by making a 1:5 dilution of the original serum, a 1:10

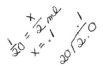

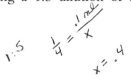

dilution from the first dilution, and another 1:10 dilution. This can be shown as follows:

Serum:

1:5 dilution:	1:10 dilution:	1:10 dilution
0.1 mL serum	0.1 mL of 1:5 dilution	0.1 mL of 1:10 dilution
0.4 mL diluent	0.9 mL diluent	0.9 mL diluent

Multiplying $5 \times 10 \times 10$ equals 500, or the total dilution. Each of the simple dilutions is calculated individually by doing mental arithmetic or by using the formula given for simple dilutions. In this example, the 1:500 dilution was made using very little diluent in a series of test tubes, rather than having to use a larger volume in a flask. The volumes were kept small enough so that mixing could take place easily, and the final volume of 1.0 mL is all that is necessary to perform a test.

If, in each step of the dilution, the dilution factor is exactly the same, this is known as a **serial dilution.** Serial dilutions are often used to obtain a **titer,** or indicator of the strength of an antibody. A series of test tubes is set up with exactly the same amount of diluent in each (Fig. 8–5). The most common serial dilution is a doubling dilution, in which the amount of serum is cut in half with each dilution. For example, six test tubes can be set up with 0.2 mL of diluent in each. If 0.2 mL of serum is added to the first tube, this becomes a 1:2 dilution

0.2 mL serum/0.2 mL serum plus 0.2 mL diluent = 0.2mL/0.4mL = 1/2

Then when 0.2 mL of the 1:2 dilution is added to 0.2 mL of diluent, a 1:4 dilution is obtained. The final dilution is obtained by counting the number of tubes and setting up a multiplication series in which the original dilution factor is raised to a power equal to the number of tubes. In this example, if the first tube contains a 1:2 dilution, the dilution in tube number six is:

$$\frac{1}{2} \times \frac{1}{2} \times \frac{1}{2} \times \frac{1}{2} \times \frac{1}{2} \times \frac{1}{2} = \frac{1}{64}$$

If, in this instance, an endpoint was reached at tube number five, the actual titer would be 1:32. To avoid confusion this is customarily written as the reciprocal of the dilution, that is 32.

Serial dilutions do not always have to be doubling dilutions. Consider the following set of test tube dilutions:

$$1:5 \rightarrow 1:25 \rightarrow 1:125 \rightarrow 1:625 \rightarrow 1:3125$$

For each successive tube, the dilution is increased by a factor of 5, so this would indeed be considered a serial dilution. Having the ability to work with simple and compound dilutions and interpret serial dilutions is a necessary skill for laboratory work. The laboratory exercise at the end of this chapter illustrates the principle of serial dilutions.

SUMMARY

Laboratory personnel are most frequently exposed to biologic, sharp, chemical, and radiation hazards. Transmission of biologic hazards that are encountered when testing patient specimens requires a chain of infection consisting of a source, a method of transmission, and a host. Handwashing and the wearing of PPE are essential to prevent transmission of infectious organisms. Standard Precautions should be followed at all times. Specimens, except urine, and contaminated supplies must be disposed of in a biohazard container. Sodium hypochlorite is the recommended disinfectant for blood and body fluid contamination of counter tops and nondisposables. All sharps including needles and adaptors must be disposed of in puncture proof containers. Recapping of needles is prohibited.

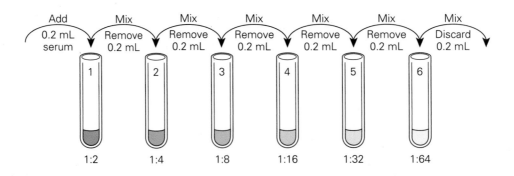

FIG. 8–5. Serial dilution. Each tube contains 0.2 mL of diluent. Patient serum (0.2 mL) is added to tube one. This is carefully mixed, and then 0.2 mL is withdrawn and added to tube two. The process is continued until the last tube is reached. The sample is mixed, and 0.2 mL is discarded. Note that in this dilution, the amount of antibody is cut in half in each successive tube.

Accidental exposure to blood and body fluids must be reported immediately to a supervisor.

Follow specific directions when mixing chemicals and always add acid to water. When chemical contact with skin or eyes occurs, immediately flush the area with water. An MSDS and a Chemical Hygiene Plan must be available to employees. Dispose of chemicals following EPA guidelines. Laboratorians who are pregnant should avoid areas with a radioactive symbol. Dispose of radioactive material following NRC guidelines.

Serum is typically the specimen used in serologic testing to look for the presence or absence of antibody. For a visible endpoint to occur in antigen–antibody reactions, often a dilution needs to be made. Patient serum, the solute, is made weaker by adding diluent so that the antibody present is not as concentrated. The relationship between the serum and the total volume is expressed as a fraction, 1:20 for example. When several dilutions are made in which the dilution factor is the same in each case, this is called a serial dilution. Serial dilutions are used to determine the titer, or strength, of an antibody. The last tube in which a visible reaction is seen is considered the endpoint.

Case Study

The serology supervisor is reviewing safety precautions with the department staff. Briefly state what the supervisor should cover in the following topics:
A. Centrifuging of specimens
B. Use of paper towel during handwashing
C. Discarding of needles used for specimen collection
D. Cleaning up a blood spill
E. UP versus Standard Precautions

Exercise: Serial Dilutions

PRINCIPLE

Serial dilutions are a set of dilutions in which the dilution factor is exactly the same at each step. These are used to make high dilutions with a small number of test tubes and a minimal amount of diluent. This is commonly done to determine the strength or titer of a particular antibody in patient serum as a part of the diagnosis of a disease state. Traditionally, serologic pipettes have been used in this process, but now it is more common to employ micropipettes for this purpose. In this experiment, a series of doubling dilutions will be made with both serologic pipettes and micropipettes, and the results will be compared.

SAMPLE PREPARATION

None.

REAGENTS, MATERIALS, AND EQUIPMENT

Anti-A antiserum
Serologic pipettes, 1 mL
Micropipettes
Disposable plastic microtiter plates
Disposable glass test tubes, 12×75 mm
Saline solution (0.85 percent)
Type A red blood cells (3 percent to 4 percent solution)
Centrifuge

PROCEDURE*

Macrotiter

1. Make a 1:10 dilution of reagent anti-A antiserum by adding 1 mL of anti-A to 9 mL of saline for every 10 mL of reagent desired. Allow approximately 1.5 mL of antiserum per student. This will be enough to run the dilutions with a little extra for repeat testing.
2. If type A red blood cells are not purchased, a 4 percent solution of red blood cells can be made using type A blood collected in ethylenediaminetetraacetic acid (EDTA). Spin the collection tube in a centrifuge for approximately 10 minutes at 1500 revolutions per minute (rpm). Remove the serum and add saline to the remaining red blood cells. Transfer the solution to a disposable conical centrifuge tube that has graduations marked on it. Spin again for 10 minutes, and note the color of the saline wash on top. Remove saline wash and

resuspend in additional saline. Make sure all cells are uniformly resuspended. Repeat this procedure for three washes or until the saline supernatant is clear. Note the final volume of the packed red blood cells. Make a 4-percent solution by suspending 4 mL of packed red cells in 96 mL of saline. Each student needs approximately 4 mL of the final solution.

3. Label eight 12- × 75-mm test tubes as follows: 10, 20, 40, 80, 160, 320, 640, 1280.
4. Using a 1-mL serologic pipette, add 0.25 mL of saline to tubes two through eight.
5. Add 0.25 mL of anti-A antiserum to tubes one and two, using a clean serologic pipette.
6. With a new serologic pipette, mix tube two by drawing fluid up and down 5 to 10 times.
7. Transfer 0.25 mL from tube two to tube three and mix.
8. Repeat the transfer and mixing process with tubes three and four, and so on through tube eight. After tube eight is mixed, discard the last 0.25 mL of the dilution.
9. Using a 1-mL serologic pipette, add 0.25 mL of 4-percent type A red blood cells to each tube.
10. Centrifuge for 30 to 45 seconds.
11. Observe for agglutination by gently shaking the red blood cell button loose from the side of each test tube. A positive reaction is indicated by cells that remain clumped together after shaking. Note that the size of the clumps decreases with further dilution, but any visible clumping is considered positive.
12. Record the titer. This is the last tube in which visible agglutination can be discerned. The titer is written as the reciprocal of the dilution; that is, if the 1:160 tube is the last positive one, the titer is written as 160.

Microtiter

1. Label one row of a microtiter plate as follows: 10, 20, 40, 80, 160, 320, 640, 1280.
2. Add one drop of saline to wells two through eight on the microtiter plate.
3. Add one drop of anti-A antiserum to wells one and two.
4. Using a 20-μl micropipette, mix well number two by drawing up and down in the pipette several times. Wipe the outside of the pipette tip, and transfer 20 μL to well number three.
5. Repeat this process with successive wells through well number eight.
6. After well eight is mixed, discard 20 μL from it.
7. Add one drop of 4-percent type A red blood cells to all wells.
8. Rotate plate on the lab bench for 1 minute, making a concentric circular pattern. Let the plate sit for 30 minutes at room temperature.
9. Observe for agglutination with a microtiter plate reader, or carefully hold up to the light. A smooth button on the

* Acknowledgment: This experiment was originally designed by Dan Southern of the Clinical Laboratory Sciences Program, Western Carolina University, Cullowhee, N.C.

bottom of a well indicates that the red blood cells have settled out with no agglutination. If agglutination has occurred, an irregular or crenulated pattern is seen at the bottom of the well (Fig. 8–6).

10. Report the titer as the last well in which agglutination can be seen. Compare the results with those from the macrotiter. The titers obtained should be within (plus or minus) one dilution of each other.

INTERPRETATION OF RESULTS

This experiment introduces the student to the concept and techniques involved in making serial dilutions. This is a procedure often used to determine the titer of an antibody. The titer is defined as the reciprocal of the last tube in which a positive reaction is seen. The titer is an indicator of the concentration of an antibody, and this is important in diagnostic testing. In some diseases, the mere presence of the antibody is enough to confirm the diagnosis. For other diseases, however, it is necessary to find a titer that is significantly elevated beyond what

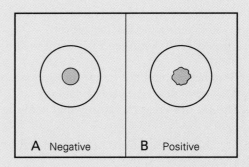

FIG. 8–6. Microtiter agglutination patterns. *(A)* A negative result is indicated by a smooth button. *(B)* Agglutination is a positive result and is indicated by a ragged edge as the cells settle out.

might be found in the normal population to link the antibody to an active disease state. Whenever a titer is reported, the accuracy is assumed to be plus or minus one tube.

 Exercise: Laboratory Safety

INSTRUCTIONS

Explore the student laboratory or the area designated by the instructor, and provide the following information.

1. Location of the fire extinguishers
2. Instructions for operation of the fire extinguisher
3. Location of the fire blanket
4. Location of the eye wash station
5. Location of the emergency shower
6. Location of the first aid kit
7. Location of the master electric panel
8. Location of the fire alarm
9. The emergency exit route
10. Location of the MSDS pertaining to serology
11. Location of the emergency spill kit
12. Location of the Bloodborne Pathogen Exposure Control Plan
13. Disinfectants available for cleaning work areas
14. Location of PPE

1. A technologist who observes a red rash on the hands after removing his/her gloves:
   a. Should apply antimicrobial lotion to the hands
   b. May be washing the hands too frequently
   c. May have developed a latex allergy
   d. Should not create friction when washing the hands

2. In the chain of infection, a contaminated work area would serve as the:
   a. Source
   b. Method of transmission
   c. Host
   d. All of the above

3. Which of the following is not a criterion for lab coats?
   a. They must be made of cotton.
   b. They must have long sleeves.
   c. They must be completely buttoned.
   d. They must have tight fitting cuffs.

4. The only biologic waste that does not have to be discarded in a container with a biohazard symbol is:
   a. Urine
   b. Serum
   c. Feces
   d. None of the above

5. The Occupational Exposure to Bloodborne Pathogens Standard developed by OSHA requires employers to provide all of the following except:
   a. HBV immunization
   b. Safety training
   c. HCV immunization
   d. Laundry facilities for nondisposable lab coats

6. An employee who receives an accidental needlestick should immediately:
   a. Apply sodium hypochlorite to the area.
   b. Notify a supervisor.
   c. Receive HIV prophylaxis.
   d. Receive an HBV booster shot.

7. The first thing to do when acid is spilled on the skin is to:
   a. Notify a supervisor.
   b. Neutralize the area with a base.
   c. Apply burn ointment.
   d. Flush the area with water.

8. When combining acid and water:
   a. Acid is added to water.
   b. Water is added to acid.
   c. Water is slowly added to acid.
   d. Both solutions are added simultaneously.

9. To determine the chemical characteristics of a particular chemical, an employee would consult the:
   a. Chemical hygiene plan
   b. Merck manual
   c. MSDS
   d. NRC guidelines

10. A technician who is pregnant should avoid working with:
    a. Organic chemicals
    b. Radioisotopes
    c. HIV-positive serum
    d. Needles and lancets

11. How much diluent needs to be added to 0.2 mL of serum to make a 1:20 dilution?
    a. 19.8 mL
    b. 4.0 mL
    c. 3.8 mL $\quad \frac{1}{19} = \frac{.2}{x} \quad = 3.8$
    d. 10.0 mL

12. A 1:750 dilution of serum is needed to perform a serologic test. Which of the following series of dilutions would be correct to use in this situation?
    a. 1:5, 1:15, 1:10
    b. 1:5, 1:10, 1:5
    c. 1:15, 1:10, 1:3
    d. 1:15, 1:3, 1:5

13. A tube containing a 1:80 dilution of serum is accidentally dropped. A 1:4 dilution of the specimen is still available. A volume of 4 mL is needed to run the test. How much of the 1:4 dilution is needed to make 4 mL of a 1:80 dilution?
    a. 5.0 mL
    b. 0.2 mL
    c. 0.05 mL
    d. 2.0 mL

14. A 4-percent solution of red blood cells is needed for diagnostic testing in the laboratory. What dilution of packed red cells does this represent?
    a. 1:25
    b. 1:4
    c. 1:96
    d. 4:1

References

1. National Institute for Occupational Safety and Health (NIOSH) Alert: Preventing Allergic Reactions to Natural Rubber Latex in the Workplace. DHHS (NIOSH) Publication 97–135. National Institute for Occupational Safety and Health, Cincinnati, Ohio, 1997.

2. Guidelines for Isolation Precautions in Hospitals. Parts I and II. Atlanta, 1996. http://www.cdc.gov.

3. National Committee for Clinical Laboratory Standards: Protection of Laboratory Workers from Instrument Biohazards and Infectious Disease Transmitted by Blood, Body Fluids, and Tissue: Approved Guideline M29-A, NCCLS, Wayne, Penn., 1997.

4. Occupational Exposure to Bloodborne Pathogens, Final Rule. Federal Register 56(235), 1991.

5. OSHA: Enforcement Procedures for the Occupational Exposure to Bloodborne Pathogens Standard. Directive 2-2.44D. Washington, D.C., 1999. http://www.osha.gov/oshdoc/Directive data/cpl_2-2_69.html.

6. OSHA: Needlestick Requirements Take Effect April 18. OSHA, Washington, D.C., 2001. http://www.osha.gov/media/oshnews/apr01/national-20010412.html.

7. OSHA: OSHA Clarifies Position on the Removal of Contaminated Needles. OSHA, Washington, D.C., 2002. http://www.osha.gov/media/oshnews/june02/trade-20020612A.html.

8. CDC: Updated U.S. Public Health Service Guidelines for the Management of Occupational Exposures to HBV, HCV, and HIV and Recommendations for Postexposure Prophylaxis. MMWR 2001:50 (RR11); 1–42. http:// www.cdc.gov.

9. Occupational Exposure to Hazardous Chemicals in Laboratories, Final Rule. Federal Register 55(Jan 31), 1990.

chapter 9

Precipitation Reactions

Learning Objectives

After completion of this chapter, the reader will be able to:

1. Describe and differentiate primary, secondary, and tertiary immune phenomena.
2. Distinguish precipitation and agglutination.
3. Discuss affinity and avidity and their influence on antigen–antibody reactions.
4. Explain how the zone of equivalence is related to the lattice hypothesis.
5. Differentiate between turbidity and nephelometry and discuss the role of each in measurement of precipitation reactions.
6. Explain the difference between single diffusion and double diffusion.
7. Give the principle of the endpoint method of radial immunodiffusion.
8. Determine the relationship between two antigens by looking at the pattern of precipitation resulting from Ouchterlony immunodiffusion.
9. Describe how rocket immunoelectrophoresis differs from radial immunodiffusion.
10. Compare immunoelectrophoresis and immunofixation electrophoresis regarding placement of reagents, time to obtain results, and limitations of each method.

Key Terms

Affinity	Immunoelectrophoresis	Precipitation
Agglutination	Immunofixation electrophoresis	Prozone phenomenon
Avidity	Law of Mass Action	Radial immunodiffusion
Complement fixation	Nephelometry	Rocket immunoelectrophoresis
Cross-reactivity	Ouchterlony double diffusion	Single diffusion
Electrophoresis	Passive immunodiffusion	Turbidimetry
Endosmosis	Postzone phenomenon	Zone of equivalence

The combination of antigen with specific antibody can be thought of as occurring in three distinct phases: primary, secondary, and tertiary. The primary phenomenon involves the combination of an individual binding site on an antibody molecule with a single epitope or determinant site on an antigen.[1] These reactions are reversible and can occur in milliseconds.[2] They are usually not easily detectable, although they can be measured indirectly by techniques such as immunofluorescence, radioimmunoassay, and enzyme immunoassay. Secondary phenomena, however, can be measured more readily, and these include precipitation, agglutination, and complement fixation. Inflammation, phagocytosis, deposition of immune complexes, immune adherence, and chemotaxis are all in vivo reactions that are classified as tertiary phenomena.

Although early immunologists often used tertiary reactions, especially skin testing, as endpoints for measurement of immune activity, the secondary phenomena form the basis for many of the serologic tests that are performed in the clinical laboratory today. **Precipitation** involves combination of soluble antigen with soluble antibody to produce insoluble complexes that are visible. **Agglutination** is the process by which particulate antigens such as cells aggregate to form larger complexes when a specific antibody is present. **Complement fixation** is the triggering of the classical complement pathway due to combination of antigen with specific antibody, as discussed in Chapter 7. This chapter focuses on precipitation, and the following chapter presents agglutination.

Precipitation was first noted in 1897 by Kraus, who found that culture filtrates of enteric bacteria would precipitate when they were mixed with specific antibody. For such reactions to occur, both antigen and antibody must have multiple binding sties for one another, and the relative concentration of each must be equal. Binding characteristics of antibodies, that is, affinity and avidity, also play a major role, and these are discussed, along with theoretical considerations of binding, including the Law of Mass Action and the principle of lattice formation. Such considerations are related to conditions for testing in the clinical laboratory.

Antigen–Antibody Binding

Affinity

The primary union of binding sites on antibody with specific epitopes on an antigen depends on two characteristics of antibody known as affinity and avidity. **Affinity** is the initial force of attraction that exists between a single Fab site on an antibody molecule and a single epitope or determinant site on the corresponding antigen.[1] As epitope and binding site come into close proximity to one another, several types of noncovalent bonds hold them together. These include ionic bonds, hydrogen bonds, hydrophobic bonds, and Van der Waals forces.[1,2] Ionic bonds occur between oppositely charged particles. Hydrogen bonds involve an attraction between polar molecules that have a slight charge separation and in which the positive charge resides on a hydrogen atom. Hydrophobic bonds occur between nonpolar molecules that associate with one another and exclude molecules of water as they do so. Van der Waals forces occur because of the interaction between the electron clouds of oscillating dipoles. All of these are rather weak bonds, and dissociation can easily occur.[3]

The strength of attraction depends on the specificity of antibody for a particular antigen. One antibody molecule may initially attract a number of different antigens, but it is the shape of the epitope and the way it fits together with the binding sites on an antibody molecule that determines whether the bonding will be stable. Antibodies are capable of reacting with antigens that are structurally similar to the original antigen that induced antibody production. This is known as **cross-reactivity.** The more the cross-reacting antigen resembles the original antigen, the stronger the bond will be between the antigen and the binding site. However, if the epitope and the binding site have a perfect lock-and-key relationship, as is the case with the original antigen, the affinity will be maximal. This is because of the fact that all types of attractions only operate over very small distances, approximately 1 Å or less[1] (Fig. 9–1).

Avidity

Avidity represents the sum of all the attractive forces between an antigen and an antibody. This involves the strength with which a multivalent antibody binds a multivalent antigen, and it is a measure of the overall stability of an antigen–antibody complex.[1,3,4] In other words, once binding has occurred, it is the force that keeps the molecules together. A high avidity can actually compensate for a low affinity. Stability of the antigen–antibody complex is essential to detection of the presence of an unknown, whether it is antigen or antibody.

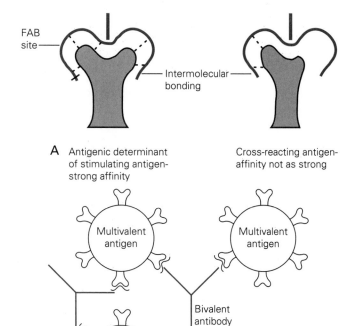

FIG. 9–1. Affinity and avidity. *(A)* Affinity is the fit of one antigenic determinant with one antibody binding site. The original stimulating antigen is a better fit than cross-reacting antigen. *(B)* Avidity is the sum of the forces binding multivalent antigens to multivalent antibodies.

Law of Mass Action

All antigen–antibody binding is reversible and is governed by the **Law of Mass Action.** This law states that free reactants are in equilibrium with bound reactants.[2] The equilibrium constant represents the difference in the rates of the forward and reverse reactions according to the following equation.

$$Ag + Ab \underset{K_2}{\overset{K_1}{\rightleftharpoons}} AgAb$$

where
Ag = antigen
Ab = antibody
K_1 = rate constant for the forward reaction
K_2 = rate constant for the reverse reaction

The equilibrium constant is thus

$$K = K_1/K_2 = [AgAb]/[Ab][Ag]$$

where [AgAb] = concentration of the antigen–antibody complex (mol/L)

[Ab] = concentration of antibody (mol/L)
[Ag] = concentration of antigen (mol/L)

This constant can be seen as a measure of the goodness of fit.[3] Its value depends on the strength of binding between antibody and antigen. As the strength of binding, or avidity, increases, the tendency of the antigen–antibody complexes to dissociate decreases, and the value of K_2 decreases. This increases the value of K_1. The higher the value of K, the larger the amount of antigen–antibody complex and the more visible or easily detectable the reaction is. The ideal conditions in the clinical laboratory would be to have an antibody with a high affinity, or initial force of attraction, as well as a high avidity, or strength of binding. The higher the values are for both of these and the more antigen–antibody complexes that are formed, the more sensitive the test will be.

Precipitation Curve

Zone of Equivalence

In addition to the affinity and avidity of the antibody involved, precipitation depends on the relative proportions of antigen and antibody present. The zone in which optimum precipitation occurs is called the **zone of equivalence,** in which the number of multivalent sites of antigen and antibody are approximately equal. In this zone, precipitation is the result of random, reversible reactions whereby each antibody binds to more than one antigen and vice versa, forming a stable network or lattice.[5] The so-called lattice hypothesis, as formulated by Marrack, is based on the assumptions that each antibody molecule must have at least two binding sites, and antigen must be multivalent. As they combine, this results in a multimolecular lattice that increases in size until it precipitates out of solution.[4]

Prozone and Postzone

Heidelberger and Kendall performed the classic quantitative precipitation reactions that established proof for this theory.[4] On either side of the equivalence zone, precipitation is actually prevented because of an excess of either antigen or antibody. In the case of antibody excess, the **prozone phenomenon** occurs, in which antigen combines with only one or two antibody molecules, and no cross-linkages are formed (Fig. 9–2). At the other side of the zone, where there is antigen excess, the **postzone phenomenon** occurs, in which

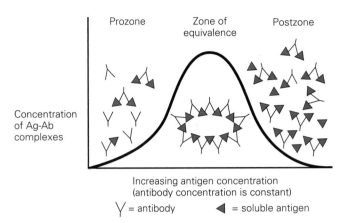

Prozone   Zone of equivalence   Postzone

Concentration of Ag-Ab complexes

Increasing antigen concentration
(antibody concentration is constant)

Y = antibody   ◄ = soluble antigen

FIG. 9–2. Precipitin curve. The precipitin curve shows how the amount of precipitation varies with varying antigen concentration when the antibody concentration is kept constant. Excess antibody is the prozone, and excess antigen concentration is called the postzone.

small aggregates are surrounded by excess antigen, and again no lattice network is formed.[1] Thus, for precipitation reactions to be detectable, they must be run in the zone of equivalence.

The prozone and postzone phenomena must be taken into consideration in the clinical setting, because negative reactions occur in both. A false-negative reaction may take place in the prozone due to the presence of a high concentration of antibody. If it is suspected that the reaction is a false-negative, diluting out antibody and performing the test again may produce a positive result. In the postzone, excess antigen may obscure the presence of a small amount of antibody. Typically, such a test is repeated with an additional patient specimen taken about a week later. This would give time for the further production of antibody. If the test is negative on this occasion, it is unlikely that the patient has that particular antibody.

Measurement of Precipitation by Light Scattering

Turbidimetry

Precipitation is one of the simplest methods of detecting antigen–antibody reactions because most antigens are multivalent and thus capable of forming aggregates in the presence of the corresponding antibody. When antigen and antibody solutions are mixed, the initial turbidity is followed by precipitation. Precipitates in fluids can be measured by means of turbidimetry or

nephelometry. **Turbidimetry** is a measure of the turbidity or cloudiness of a solution. A detection device is placed in direct line with the incident light, collecting light after it has passed through the solution. It thus measures the reduction in light intensity due to reflection, absorption, or scatter.[6] Scattering of light occurs in proportion to the size, shape, and concentration of molecules present in solution. It is recorded in absorbance units, a measure of the ratio of incident light to that of transmitted light. Measurements are made using a spectrophotometer or an automated clinical chemistry analyzer.

Nephelometry

Nephelometry measures the light that is scattered at a particular angle from the incident beam as it passes through a suspension[6] (Fig. 9–3). The amount of light scattered is an index of the concentration of the solution. Beginning with a constant amount of antibody, increasing amounts of antigen result in an increase in antigen–antibody complexes.[6,7] Thus, the relationship between antigen concentrations, as indicated by antigen–antibody complex formation, and light scattering approaches linearity.[6] Light scatter may be recorded in arbitrary units of "relative light scatter," or it may be directly extrapolated by a computer to give actual concentrations in milligrams per deciliter (mg/dL) or international units per milliliter (IU/mL), based on established values of standards. Nephelometers measure light scatter at angles ranging from 10 degrees to about 90 degrees. If a laser beam is used, light deflected only a few degrees from the original path can be measured. Although the sensitivity of turbidity has increased, nephelometry is still the preferred method for measurement of low-level antigen–antibody reactions.[8]

Uses of nephelometry include quantification of serum proteins such as IgG, IgA, IgM, and IgE, complement components C3, C4, and C1 inhibitor, haptoglobin, C-reactive protein, transferrin, albumin, alpha$_1$-antitrypsin, alpha$_2$-macroglobulin, fibrinogen, ceruloplasmin, and rheumatoid factor.[6] This method can be used to detect either antigen or antibody, but it is usually run with antibody as the reagent and the patient antigen as the unknown. In *endpoint nephelometry*, the reaction is allowed to run essentially to completion, but large particles tend to fall out of solution and decrease the amount of scatter. Thus, another method called kinetic or rate nephelometry was devised, in which the rate of increase of scattering is measured immediately after the reagent is added. This rate change is directly related to antigen concentration if the concentration of antibody is kept constant.[6] Several automated instruments utilize this principle for the

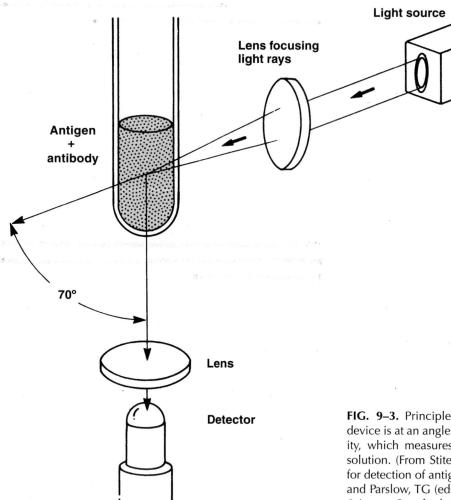

FIG. 9–3. Principles of nephelometry. The light detection device is at an angle to the incident light, in contrast to turbidity, which measures light rays passing directly through the solution. (From Stites, DP, et al: Clinical laboratory methods for detection of antigens and antibodies. In Stites, DP, Terr, AI, and Parslow, TG (eds): Medical Immunology, ed. 9. Appleton & Lange, Stamford, Conn., 1997, p 230, with permission.)

measurement of immunoglobulins, complement components, C-reactive protein, and other serum proteins, including several clotting factors. It provides accurate and precise quantitation of serum proteins.[7] The sensitivity, however, is limited to the range between 0.1 and 0.5 mg/dL.[4]

Passive Immunodiffusion Techniques

The precipitation of antigen–antibody complexes can also be determined in a support medium such as a gel. Agar, a high-molecular-weight complex polysaccharide derived from seaweed, and agarose, a purified agar, are used for this purpose. Agar and agarose help stabilize the diffusion process and allow visualization of the precipitin bands.[2]

Reactants are added to the gel, and antigen–antibody combination occurs by means of diffusion. When no electrical current is used to speed up this process, it is

known as **passive immunodiffusion.** The rate of diffusion is affected by size of the particles, temperature, gel viscosity, amount of hydration, and interactions between the matrix and reactants.[2,7] An agar concentration of from 0.3 percent to 1.5 percent allows for diffusion of most reactants. Agarose is often preferred to agar because agar has a strong negative charge, while agarose has almost none, so that interactions between the gel and the reagents are minimized. Immunodiffusion reactions can be classified according to the number of reactants diffusing and the direction of diffusion.

Radial Immunodiffusion

Oudin was the first to use gels for precipitation reactions, and he pioneered the technique known as **single diffusion.**[7] A modification of the single-diffusion technique, **radial immunodiffusion,** has been commonly used in the clinical laboratory. Antibody is uniformly distributed in the support gel, and antigen is

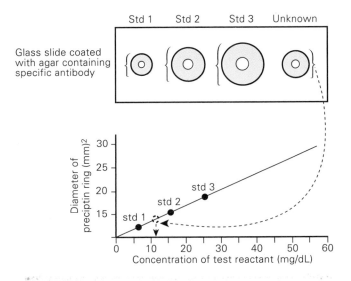

Std 1   Std 2   Std 3   Unknown

Glass slide coated
with agar containing
specific antibody

FIG. 9–4. Radial immunodiffusion. The amount of precipitate formed is in proportion to the antigen present in the sample. In the Mancini endpoint method, concentration is in proportion to the diameter squared. (From Nakamura, RM, Tucker, ES III, and Carlson, IH: Immunoassays in the clinical laboratory. In Henry, JB: Clinical Diagnosis and Management by Laboratory Methods, ed. 18. WB Saunders, Philadelphia, 1991, p 858, with permission.)

taken at about 18 hours, and this is known as the kinetic method.

It is essential, for either method, that monospecific antiserum with a fairly high affinity be used. This increases the clarity of the precipitation reaction. In addition, the precision of the assay is directly related to accurate measurement of samples and standards. Sources of error include overfilling or underfilling the wells, nicking the side of the wells when filling, spilling sample outside the wells, improper incubation time and temperature, and incorrect measurement.[11] Radial immunodiffusion has been used to measure IgG, IgM, IgA, and complement components. It is simple to perform and requires no instrumentation. However, immunodiffusion has largely been replaced by more sensitive and automated methods such as nephelometry and enzyme-linked immunosorbent assays except for low-volume analytes such as IgD or IgG subclasses.[11]

Ouchterlony Double Diffusion

One of the older immunochemical techniques but also one of the most useful is the classic **Ouchterlony double diffusion** technique.[7] Both antigen and antibody diffuse independently through a semisolid medium in two dimensions, horizontally and vertically. Agar gel is the usual support medium, and the reaction can be run on a glass slide or in a Petri dish.[4,7] Wells are cut in the gel, and reactants are added to the wells. After an incubation period of between 12 and 48 hours in a moist chamber, precipitin lines form where the moving front of antigen meets that of antibody. The density of the lines reflects the amount of immune complex formed.[7]

Most Ouchterlony plates are set up with a central well surrounded by four to six equidistant outer wells. Antibody that is multispecific is placed in the central well, and different antigens are placed in the surrounding wells. This is essentially a qualitative technique because the position of the precipitin bands between wells allows for the antigens to be compared with one another. Several patterns are possible: (1) Fusion of the lines at their junction to form an arc represents serologic identity or the presence of a common epitope, (2) a pattern of crossed lines demonstrates two separate reactions and indicates that the compared antigens share no common epitopes, and (3) fusion of two lines with a spur indicates partial identity. In this last case, the two antigens share a common epitope, but some antibody molecules are not captured by antigen and travel through the initial precipitin line to combine with additional epitopes found in the more complex antigen. Therefore, the spur always points to the simpler antigen[1] (Fig. 9–5). Uses for this technique include the

applied to a well cut into the gel. As the antigen diffuses out from the well, antigen–antibody combination occurs in changing proportions until the zone of equivalence is reached and a stable lattice network is formed in the gel. The area of the ring obtained is a measure of antigen concentration, and this can be compared to a standard curve obtained by using antigens of known concentration.[2,4] Figure 9–4 depicts some typical results.

There are two techniques for the measurement of radial immunodiffusion. The first was developed by Mancini and is known as the *endpoint method.* In this technique, antigen is allowed to diffuse to completion, and when equivalence is reached, there is no further change in the ring diameter.[9] This occurs between 24 and 72 hours.[7] The square of the diameter is then directly proportional to the concentration of the antigen. A graph is obtained by plotting concentrations of standards on the x-axis versus the diameter squared on the y-axis, and a smooth curve is fit to the points.[7] The major drawback to this method is the time it takes to obtain results.

The Fahey and McKelvey method uses measurements taken before the point of equivalence is reached. In this case, the diameter is proportional to the log of the concentration.[10,11] A graph is drawn on semilog paper by plotting antigen concentration on the log axis and diameter on the arithmetic axis. Readings are

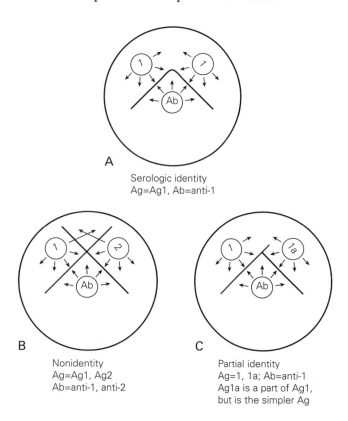

A
Serologic identity
Ag=Ag1, Ab=anti-1

B
Nonidentity
Ag=Ag1, Ag2
Ab=anti-1, anti-2

C
Partial identity
Ag=1, 1a; Ab=anti-1
Ag1a is a part of Ag1,
but is the simpler Ag

FIG. 9–5. Ouchterlony diffusion patterns. Antibody that is a mixture of anti-1 and anti-2 is placed in the central well. Unknown antigens are placed in the outside wells. (A) Serologic identity. The arc indicates that the two antigens are identical. (B) Nonidentity. Two crossed lines represent two different precipitation reactions. The antigens share no identical determinants. (C) Partial identity. Antigen 1a shares a determinant that is part of antigen 1, but it is not as complex. The spur formed always points to the simpler antigen.

identification of fungal antigens and detection of antibodies to extractable nuclear antigens.[7]

It is important to perform this technique with care because several problems may arise. Irregular patterns of precipitation may be due to overfilling the wells, irregular hole punching, or nonlevel incubation.[7] Other factors affecting the accuracy of results include drying out of the gels; inadequate time for diffusion, resulting in weakness of band intensity; and fungal or bacterial contamination of the gel.

Electrophoretic Techniques

Diffusion can be combined with electrophoresis to speed up or sharpen the results. **Electrophoresis** separates molecules according to differences in their elec-

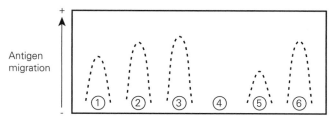

FIG. 9–6. Rocket immunoelectrophoresis. Standards are in wells 1 to 3. Patient samples are in wells 4 to 6. Note that well 4 contains no antigen because no ring is formed. Well 5 has a low concentration of antigen, and well 6 has a high concentration of antigen.

tric charge when they are placed in an electric field. A direct current is forced through the gel, causing antigen, antibody, or both to migrate. As diffusion takes place, distinct precipitin bands are formed. This technique can be applied to both single and double diffusion.

Rocket Immunoelectrophoresis

One-dimension electroimmunodiffusion, an adaptation of radial immunodiffusion (RID), was developed by Laurell in the early 1960s.[4] Antibody is distributed in the gel, and antigen is placed in wells cut in the gel, just as in RID. However, instead of allowing diffusion to take place at its own rate, electrophoresis is used to facilitate migration of the antigen into the agar. When the antigen diffuses out of the well, precipitation begins. As the concentration of antigen changes, there is dissolution and reformation of the precipitate at ever-increasing distances from the well. The end result is a precipitin line that is conical in shape, resembling a rocket, hence the name **rocket immunoelectrophoresis.** The height of the rocket, measured from the well to the apex, is directly in proportion to the amount of antigen in the sample. If standards are run, a curve can be constructed to determine concentrations of unknown specimens[4] (Fig. 9–6).

Rocket immunoelectrophoresis is much more rapid than RID because results can be obtained in a few hours. It is essential, however, to determine the net charge of the molecules at the pH used for the test because this determines the direction of migration within the gel. This technique is most often used to quantitate immunoglobulins, using a buffer of pH 8.6. At this pH, immunoglobulins are electrically neutral, but they are carried toward the anode by the movement of the buffer particles, a phenomenon known as **endosmosis.**

Other applications include assay of proteins whose concentration is too low to be detected by nephelometry and too high for RID. Examples include alphafetoprotein in amniotic fluid, immunoglobulins in urine and spinal fluid, and complement components in body fluids.

Immunoelectrophoresis

Immunoelectrophoresis is a double-diffusion technique that utilizes an electric current to enhance results. Introduced by Grabar and Williams in 1953,[7] this is performed as a two-step process and can be used for semiquantitation of a wide range of antigens.[4] Typically, the source of the antigens is serum, which is electrophoresed to separate out the main protein fractions; then a trough is cut in the gel parallel to the line of separation. Antiserum is placed in the trough, and the gel is incubated for 18 to 24 hours. Double diffusion occurs at right angles to the electrophoretic separation, and precipitin lines develop where specific antigen–antibody combination takes place. These lines or arcs can be compared in shape, intensity, and location to that of a normal serum control to detect abnormalities.[5]

This procedure has been used as a screening tool for the differentiation of more than 30 serum proteins, including the major classes of immunoglobulins. It is both a qualitative and a semiquantitative technique and has been used in clinical laboratories for the detection of myelomas, Waldenström's macroglobulinemia, malignant lymphomas, and other lymphoproliferative disorders.[4] (See Chapter 15 for further details on lymphoproliferative diseases.) In addition, immunodeficiencies can be detected in this manner, if no precipitin band is formed for a particular immunoglobulin. Deficiencies of complement components can also be identified. Figure 9–7 (Color Plate 8) shows an example of an abnormal pattern. This technique is gradually being replaced, however, by immunofixation electrophoresis, which gives quicker results and is easier to interpret.[12]

Immunofixation Electrophoresis

Immunofixation electrophoresis, as first described by Alper and Johnson,[13] is similar to immunoelectrophoresis except that after electrophoresis has taken place, antiserum is applied directly to the surface of the gel, rather than being placed in a trough. Agarose or cellulose acetate can be used for this purpose. Immunodiffusion takes place in a shorter time and results in a higher resolution than when antibody diffuses from a trough.[12] Because diffusion is only

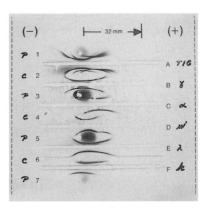

FIG. 9–7. Immunoelectrophoresis film showing normal controls (odd-numbered wells) and patient serum (even-numbered wells). Trough A contains antitotal immunoglobulin, and troughs B through F contain the following monospecific antisera: B, anti-γ; C, anti-α; D, anti-μ; E, anti-λ; and F, anti-κ. The restricted electrophoretic mobility seen in well 1 with antitotal immunoglobulin and in well 5 with anti-μ and anti-λ immunoglobulins indicate that the patient has an IgM monoclonal gammopathy with λ light chains. (From Harr, R: Clinical Laboratory Science Review, ed. 2, FA Davis, Philadelphia, 2000, Color Plate 4, with permission.) See Color Plate 8.

across the thickness of the gel, approximately 1 mm, the reaction usually takes place in less than 1 hour.[12]

Most often, an antibody of known specificity is used to determine whether or not patient antigen is present. The unknown antigen is placed on the gel, electrophoretic separation takes place, and then the reagent antibody is applied. Immunoprecipitates form only where specific antigen–antibody combination has taken place and the complexes have become trapped in the gel. The gel is washed to remove any nonprecipitating proteins and can then be stained for easier visibility. This method is especially useful in demonstrating those antigens present in serum or spinal fluid in low concentrations (Fig. 9–8 and Color Plate 9). Although it is more sensitive than immunoelectrophoresis, dilutions may need to be made to avoid the zones of antigen or antibody excess.[12]

Perhaps one of the best-known adaptations of this technique is the so-called Western blot, used as a confirmatory test to detect antibodies to human immunodeficiency virus 1 (HIV-1). A mixture of HIV antigens is placed on a gel and electrophoresed to separate the individual components. The components are then transferred to nitrocellulose paper by means of blotting or laying the nitrocellulose over the gel so that the electrophoresis pattern is preserved. Patient serum is applied to the nitrocellulose and allowed to react. The strip is then washed and stained to detect precipitin

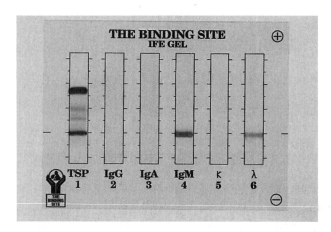

FIG. 9–8. Immunofixation electrophoresis. A complex antigen mixture such as serum proteins is separated by electrophoresis. An antiserum template is aligned over the gel. Then protein fixative and monospecific antisera, IgG, IgA, IgM, κ, and λ are applied to the gel. After incubating for 30 minutes, the gel is stained and examined for the presence of paraproteins. Precipitates form where specific antigen–antibody combination has taken place. In this case, the patient has an IgM monoclonal antibody with λ chains. (Courtesy of The Binding Site Ltd., Birmingham, UK.) See Color Plate 9.

bands. It is simpler to visualize the reaction on the nitrocellulose, and in this manner, antibodies to several antigens can be detected. Refer to Figure 22–1 for a specific example of a Western blot used to determine the presence of antibody to HIV-1. This technique is characteristically used to determine the presence of antibodies to organisms of complex antigenic composition. If antibodies to more than one disease-associated antigen are identified in patient serum, this usually confirms presence of the suspected disease.

Other important uses for immunofixation include detecting the presence of a monoclonal antibody component in diseases such as multiple myeloma, Waldenstrom's macroglobulinemia, and other benign lymphoproliferative processes.[7,14] Additionally, cerebrospinal fluid is the specimen of choice for diagnosis of multiple sclerosis, and urine is used to detect the presence of Bence-Jones proteins.[14]

Sources of Error in Electrophoresis

Many of the sources of error are similar for all the electrophoretic techniques, so they are discussed together. One problem that can arise is the application of the current in the wrong direction. If this occurs, samples may either run off the gel or not be separated. Incorrect pH of the buffer and incorrect electrophoresis time also hinder proper separation. Concentrations

of antigen and antibody must be carefully chosen so that lattice formation and precipitation is possible. If either is too concentrated, no visible reaction will result. The amount of current applied also influences the efficiency of the separation. If the current is not strong enough, separation may be incomplete. On the other hand, if the current is too strong, heat will be generated and may denature proteins. As in diffusion techniques, wells must be carefully filled.

Comparison of Precipitation Techniques

Each type of precipitation technique has its own distinct advantages and disadvantages. Some techniques are technically more demanding, and others are more automated. Each type of precipitation testing has particular applications for which it is best suited. Table 9–1 presents a comparison of the techniques discussed in this chapter.

SUMMARY

Antigen–antibody combination can be separated into three distinct phases: primary, secondary, and tertiary. The primary phenomenon represents the initial antigen–antibody binding, while the secondary phase includes aggregation of complexes to produce precipitation, agglutination, and complement fixation. The tertiary phase is the reaction of the body to immune complexes and includes inflammation, phagocytosis, chemotaxis, and complex deposition.

Union of antigen and antibody depends on affinity, or the force of attraction that exists between one antibody-binding site and a single epitope on an antigen. Avidity is the sum of all attractive forces occurring between multiple binding sites on antigen and antibody. For testing purposes, it is important to have an antibody with high affinity and high avidity for the antigen in question.

Maximum binding of antigen and antibody occurs when the aggregate number of multivalent sites of antigen and antibody are approximately equal. The concentrations of antigen and antibody that yield maximum binding represent the zone of equivalence. When antibody is in excess (the prozone) or antigen is in excess (the postzone), manifestations of antigen–antibody combination such as precipitation and agglutination are present to a much lesser degree. All testing should take place in the zone of equivalence, where a reaction is most visible.

Precipitation can be detected in the laboratory by several different means. Light scatter produced by

TABLE 9–1. Comparison of Precipitation Techniques

Technique	Application	Comment
Nephelometry	Immunoglobulins, complement, C-reactive protein, other serum proteins	Automated, sensitive, expensive equipment needed
Radial immunodiffusion	Immunoglobulins, complement	Quantitative, slow, not as sensitive as nephelometry
Ouchterlony double	Complex antigens such as fungal antigens diffusion	Semiquantitative, slow, may be difficult to interpret
Rocket electrophoresis	Immunoglobulins, complement, alpha-fetoprotein	Fast, quantitative, technically demanding
Immunoelectrophoresis	Differentiation of serum proteins	Slow, semiquantitative, difficult to interpret
Immunofixation electrophoresis	HIV, Lyme disease, syphilis	Fairly rapid, semiquantitative sensitive

HIV = Human immunodeficiency virus.

immune complexes in solution can be measured as a reduction in light intensity (turbidimetry) or as the amount of light scattered at a particular angle (nephelometry). Several automated instruments are based on these principles.

Other precipitation techniques utilize a support medium such as a gel, and antigen–antibody combination takes place by means of passive diffusion. In single diffusion, only one of the reactants travels, while the other is incorporated in the gel. An example is radial immunodiffusion, in which antibody is incorporated in a gel in a plate or Petri dish. The amount of precipitate formed is directly related to the amount of antigen present.

Ouchterlony diffusion is a double-diffusion technique in which both antigen and antibody diffuse from wells and travel toward each other. Precipitin lines may indicate identity, nonidentity, or partial identity, depending on the pattern formed.

Electrophoresis can be combined with diffusion to speed up the process and enhance the reaction patterns. Rocket immunoelectrophoresis applies an electric charge to single diffusion, with resultant precipitation patterns that look like rockets that project upward from the sample wells. In immunoelectrophoresis, the antigen is first electrophoresed by itself to separate out different components, and then antibody is placed in a trough to allow diffusion to take place. Specific reaction patterns indicate presence or absence of certain antigens. A related technique, immunofixation electrophoresis, differs in that antibody is applied directly to the gel after electrophoresis has taken place. Compared to immunoelectrophoresis, precipitation occurs in a shorter time, and bands with higher resolution are obtained.

Precipitation is adaptable to both automated technologies as well as individually processed testing. Thus, it is a versatile and practical method for use in the clinical laboratory.

Case Study

1. A 4-year-old female was hospitalized for pneumonia. She has a history of upper respiratory tract infections and several bouts of diarrhea since infancy. Due to her recurring infections, the physician decided to measure her immunoglobulin levels. The following results were obtained by nephelometry:

Immunoglobulin	Normal level (3–5 yrs) (mg/dL)	Patient level (mg/dL)
IgG	550–1700	800
IgA	50–280	20
IgM	25–120	75

Questions

a. What do these results indicate?

b. How do they explain the symptoms?

c. How do nephelometry measurements compare with the use of RID?

Exercise: Radial Immunodiffusion

PRINCIPLE

Radial immunodiffusion is a single-immunodiffusion technique based on incorporation of antibody into an agarose gel. Antigen, usually human serum, is placed in wells that are punched in the gel. As diffusion of the antigen occurs, a ring of precipitate forms. This continues to move out from the well until the point of equivalence, representing maximum antigen–antibody combination, is reached. According to the endpoint or Mancini method, the area of the precipitin zone, as measured by the diameter squared, is directly in proportion to antigen concentration. If a standard curve is plotted using antigens of known concentration, concentration of the unknown specimen can be determined from the graph.

SAMPLE PREPARATION

Collect blood by venipuncture using sterile technique. Care should be taken to avoid dilution or gross contamination as the serum is removed from the specimen. The sample may be kept in the refrigerator for 2 days before testing. If it needs to be held longer, it should be frozen at −70°C. Repeated freezing and thawing will cause variable results. Cerebrospinal fluid or urine can also be used for testing.

REAGENTS, MATERIALS, AND EQUIPMENT

Immunodiffusion plates for IgG, IgA, and IgM (available in kits from Helena Laboratories, Beaumont, TX; The Binding Site, San Diego, CA; Behring Diagnostics, Inc., Westwood, MA; and others)
High and low serum controls
Reference sera for plotting standard curve
Microcapillaries or micropipetter capable of delivering a volume of 5 μL
Plastic boxes with lids for incubation chambers
Ocular viewer or magnifying system for reading ring diameters
Measuring device (ruler or calibrated magnifier)
Graph paper for plotting standard curve

Precautions

Serum used for the reference standards and controls have been found to be negative when tested for hepatitis B surface antigen and HIV by Food and Drug Administration–required tests. However, the standards and controls should be handled with the same precautions as those used in handling human sera. The standards should be stored at 2°C to 6°C and are stable until the expiration date indicated. Failure to obtain a linear reference curve may indicate product deterioration.

PROCEDURE

1. Remove plates from the refrigerator and allow the plates to stand at room temperature for about 20 to 30 minutes to equilibrate to room temperature.
2. Remove each plate from the plastic storage bag and take off the lid. Inspect the wells for moisture. If moisture is present, it can be carefully removed by placing a capillary tube into each individual well and allowing the liquid to flow into the tube by capillary action.
3. With a micropipetter or microcapillary tube, withdraw 5 μL from each control or serum sample, using a new microcapillary for each specimen. Wipe off the outside of each capillary tube.
4. Deliver the sample into a well by touching the tip of the capillary to the bottom of the well and pushing the plunger past the capillary tip. Hold the pipetter perpendicular to the surface of the gel.
5. Replace the cover tightly on the plate, and place the plate in a moist incubation chamber. A plastic box with a tightly fitting lid and a moist paper towel in the bottom will serve the purpose.
6. Incubate at room temperature for 48 hours.
7. After incubation, measure the precipitin ring diameters to the nearest 0.1 mm, using a ruler and magnifier or other suitable measuring device.
8. Using regular arithmetic graph paper, plot the square of the ring diameter on the y-axis versus concentration on the x-axis. Draw a straight line to connect the points.
9. Values for patient samples are determined by interpolation from this reference curve.

RESULTS

Normal immunoglobulins are as follows.

Immunoglobulins	mg/dL	IU/mL
IgG	700–1700	80–195
IgA	70–350	40–200
IgM	45–210	82–246

Decreased levels of immunoglobulins may indicate an immunodeficiency. Most of these have a hereditary basis and are more pronounced in childhood. The most common immunodeficiency seen is selective IgA deficiency. Other deficiencies may be acquired, and these are seen in monoclonal gammopathies, chronic lymphocytic leukemia, or during immunosuppressive therapy.

Increased levels may be due to immunoproliferative conditions such as multiple myeloma or Waldenström's macroglobulinemia. In these cases, a monoclonal increase in one immunoglobulin type is noted. A polyclonal increase may be caused by chronic infections, liver disease, or autoimmune diseases such as multiple sclerosis, lupus erythematosus, or rheumatoid arthritis.

INTERPRETATION OF RESULTS

An early readout method, based on the kinetic method, can be used to obtain qualitative results as early as 6 hours after incubation. In this case, all ring diameters are measured to the nearest 0.1 mm, and the results are compared to the high and low controls. If a ring diameter is below the low-level control, concentration of the specimen is below normal. Conversely, if the diameter is above the high-level control, the concentration is above normal. These readings are approximate.

Most kits also contain a table of reference values relating ring diameters to concentration for each of the three immunoglobulin types; therefore, it is not necessary to plot a reference curve. However, it may be useful for students to do so and then compare the results with the table.

Results are dependent on accurate pipetting. If wells are nicked as the sample is added, the diameter reading will be affected. If the high- and low-level control values are not within those specified on the label of each vial, then the test is invalidated. High- and low-level controls should be run on each plate to ensure the accuracy of the test system.

This technique must be performed with care because irregular precipitation patterns may result from overfilling the wells, irregularly punched holes, or drying out of the gels.

1. In a precipitation reaction, how can the ideal antibody be characterized?
   a. Low affinity and low avidity
   b. High affinity and low avidity
   c. High affinity and high avidity
   d. Low affinity and high avidity

2. Precipitation differs from agglutination in which way?
   a. Precipitation is a primary phenomenon, while agglutination is a secondary phenomenon.
   b. Precipitation occurs with univalent antigen, while agglutination requires multivalent antigen.
   c. Precipitation does not readily occur because few antibodies can form aggregates with antigen.
   d. Precipitation involves a soluble antigen, while agglutination involves a particulate antigen.

3. When soluble antigens diffuse in a gel that contains antibody, in which zone does optimum precipitation occur?
   a. Prozone
   b. Zone of equivalence
   c. Postzone
   d. Prezone

4. Which of the following statements apply to rate nephelometry?
   a. Readings are taken before equivalence is reached.
   b. It is more sensitive than turbidity.
   c. Measurements are time dependent.
   d. All of the above

5. Which of the following is characteristic of the endpoint method of RID?
   a. Readings are taken before equivalence.
   b. Concentration is directly in proportion to the square of the diameter.
   c. The diameter is plotted against the log of the concentration.
   d. It is primarily a qualitative rather than a quantitative method.

6. Which statement is true of measurements of turbidity?
   a. It indicates the ratio of incident light to transmitted light.
   b. Light that is scattered at an angle is detected.
   c. It is recorded in units of relative light scatter.
   d. It is not affected by large particles falling out of solution.

7. Which of the following refers to the force of attraction between an antibody and a single antigenic determinant?
   a. Affinity
   b. Avidity
   c. Van der Waals attraction
   d. Covalence

8. Which technique is typified by radial immunodiffusion combined with electrophoresis?
   a. Countercurrent electrophoresis
   b. Rocket electrophoresis
   c. Immunoelectrophoresis
   d. Southern blotting

9. Immunofixation electrophoresis differs from immunoelectrophoresis in which way?
   a. Electrophoresis takes place after diffusion has occurred.
   b. Better separation of proteins with the same electrophoretic mobilities is obtained.
   c. Antibody is directly applied to the gel instead of being placed in a trough.
   d. It is mainly used for antigen detection.

10. In which zone might an antibody screening test be falsely negative?
    a. Prozone
    b. Zone of equivalence
    c. Postzone
    d. None of the above

11. In an Ouchterlony immunodiffusion reaction with antigens 1 and 2, if crossed lines result, what does this indicate?
    a. Antigens 1 and 2 are identical.
    b. Antigen 2 is simpler than antigen 1.
    c. Antigen 2 is more complex than antigen 1.
    d. The two antigens are unrelated.

12. Which might affect the outcome of immunodiffusion procedures?
    a. Improper dilution of antigen in the wells
    b. Overfilling the wells
    c. Nonlevel incubation of plates
    d. All of the above

13. Which technique represents a single-diffusion reaction?
    a. Radial immunodiffusion
    b. Ouchterlony diffusion
    c. Immunoelectrophoresis
    d. All of the above

14. Which best describes the Law of Mass Action?
   a. Once antigen–antibody binding takes place, it is irreversible.
   b. The equilibrium constant only depends on the forward reaction.
   c. The equilibrium constant is related to strength of antigen–antibody binding.
   d. If an antibody has a high avidity, it will dissociate from antigen easily.

References

1. Goldsby, RA, Kindt, TJ, and Osborne, BA: Kuby Immunology, ed. 4. WH Freeman and Co., New York, 2000, pp 149–156.
2. Kricka, LJ: Principles of Immunochemical Techniques. In Burtis, CA, and Ashwood, ER (eds): Tietz Fundamentals of Clinical Chemistry, ed. 5. WB Saunders, Philadelphia, 2001, pp 177–194.
3. Roitt, IM, Brostoff, J, and Male, DK: Immunology, ed. 5. Mosby, St. Louis, 1998.
4. Kasahara, Y, and Nakamura, RM: Immunoassays and immunochemistry. In Henry, JB (ed): Clinical Diagnosis and Management by Laboratory Methods, ed. 19. WB Saunders, Philadelphia, 1996, pp 851–876.
5. Miller, LE, et al: Manual of Laboratory Immunology, ed. 2. Lea & Febiger, Philadelphia, 1991.
6. Van Lente, F: Light-scattering immunoassays. In Rose, NR, et al (eds): Manual of Clinical Laboratory Immunology, ed. 5. American Society for Microbiology Press, Washington, D.C., 1997, pp 13–19.
7. Stites, DP, et al: Clinical laboratory methods for detection of antigens and antibodies. In Stites, DP, Terr, AI, and Parslow, TG (eds): Medical Immunology, ed. 9. Appleton & Lange, Stamford, Conn., 1997, pp 211–253.
8. Tiffany, TO: Light emission and scattering techniques. In Burtis, CA, and Ashwood, ER (eds): Tietz Fundamentals of Clinical Chemistry, ed. 5. WB Saunders, Philadelphia, 2001, pp 74–90.
9. Mancini, G, Carbonara, AO, and Heremans, JF: Immunochemical quantitation of antigens by single radial immunodiffusion. Immunochem 2:235, 1965.
10. Fahey, JL, and McKelvey, EM: Quantitative determination of serum immunoglobulins in antibody-agar plates. J Immunol 94:84, 1965.
11. Check, IJ, and Papadea, C: Immunoglobulin quantitation. In Rose, NR, et al (eds): Manual of Clinical Laboratory Immunology, ed. 5. American Society for Microbiology Press, Washington, D.C., 1997, pp 134–146.
12. Ledue, TB, and Garfin, DE: Immunofixation and immunoblotting. In Rose, NR, et al (eds): Manual of Clinical Laboratory Immunology, ed. 5. American Society for Microbiology Press, Washington, D.C., 1997, pp 54–64.
13. Alper, CA, and Johnson, AM: Immunofixation electrophoresis: A technique for the study of protein polymorphism. Vox Sanguinis 17:445, 1969.
14. Keren, DF: Clinical indications for electrophoresis and immunofixation in serum. In Rose, NR, et al (eds): Manual of Clinical Laboratory Immunology, ed. 5. American Society for Microbiology Press, Washington, D.C., 1997, pp 65–74.

Agglutination

Learning Objectives

After completion of this chapter, the reader will be able to:
1. Differentiate between agglutination and precipitation.
2. Discuss how IgM and IgG differ in ability to participate in agglutination reactions.
3. Describe physiologic conditions that can be altered to enhance agglutination.
4. Describe and give an example of each of the following:
   a. Direct agglutination
   b. Passive agglutination
   c. Reverse passive agglutination
   d. Agglutination inhibition
   e. Hemagglutination inhibition
   f. Coagglutination
5. Explain and give an application for the direct Coombs' test.
6. Discuss reasons for the use of the indirect Coombs' test.
7. Describe the principle of measurement used in particle-counting immunoassay (PACIA).
8. Discuss conditions that must be met for optimal results in agglutination testing.

Key Terms

Agglutination inhibition
  reactions
Agglutinin
Coagglutination
Direct agglutination
Direct antiglobulin test

Hemagglutination
Hemagglutination inhibition
  reactions
Indirect antiglobulin test
Lattice formation
Low ionic strength saline

Particle-counting
  immunoassay (PACIA)
Passive agglutination
Reverse passive agglutination
Sensitization

Whereas precipitation reactions involve soluble antigens, agglutination is the aggregation of particulate matter caused by combination with specific antibody. Antibodies that produce such reactions are often called **agglutinins.** Because this reaction takes place on the surface of the particle, antigen must be exposed and able to bind with antibody. Agglutination is actually a two-step process, involving sensitization or initial binding followed by lattice formation, or formation of large aggregates. Types of particles participating in such reactions include erythrocytes, bacterial cells, and inert carriers such as latex particles. Each particle must have multiple antigenic or determinant sites, which are crosslinked to sites on other particles through the formation of antibody bridges.[1]

The first published report about the ability of antibody to clump cells was made by Gruber and Durham in 1896, based on observations of agglutination of bacterial cells by serum.[2] This finding gave rise to the use of serology as a tool in the diagnosis of disease, and it also led to the discovery of the ABO blood groups. Widal and Sicard developed one of the earliest diagnostic tests in 1896 for the detection of antibodies occurring in typhoid fever, brucellosis, and tularemia.[2] Agglutination reactions now have a wide variety of applications in the detection of both antigens and antibodies. Such testing has a high degree of sensitivity, and the endpoints can easily be read visually.[3]

Agglutination reactions can be classified into several distinct categories: direct, passive, reverse passive, agglutination inhibition, and coagglutination. Principles of each of these types of reactions are discussed, including their current use in today's clinical laboratory.

Steps in Agglutination

Sensitization

Agglutination, like precipitation, is a two-step process that results in the formation of a stable lattice network. The first reaction involves antigen–antibody combination through single antigenic determinants on the particle surface and is often called the **sensitization** step.[4] This initial reaction is rapid and reversible.[5] The second step is the formation of crosslinks that form the visible aggregates. This represents the stabilization of antigen–antibody complexes with the binding together of multiple antigenic determinants.[5] Each stage of the process is affected by different factors, and it is important to understand these to be able to manipulate and enhance endpoints for such reactions.

Sensitization is affected by the nature of the antibody molecules themselves. The affinity and avidity (discussed in Chapter 9) of an individual antibody determine how much antibody remains attached. The class of immunoglobulin is also important; IgM with a potential valence of 10 is over 750 times more efficient in agglutination than is IgG with a valence of 2.[2]

The nature of the antigen-bearing surface is also a key factor in the initial sensitization process. If epitopes are sparse or if they are obscured by other surface molecules, they are less likely to interact with antibody.

Lattice Formation

The second stage, representing the sum of interactions between antibody and multiple antigenic determinants on a particle, is dependent on environmental conditions and the relative concentrations of antigen and antibody.[4] Bordet hypothesized that **lattice formation** is governed by physicochemical factors such as ionic strength of the milieu, pH, and temperature.[2] Antibody must be able to bridge the gap between cells in such a way that one molecule can bind to a site on each of two different cells. The above factors can be manipulated to facilitate such attachment. Figure 10–1 depicts the two-stage process.

Erythrocytes and bacterial cells have a slight negative surface charge, and because like charges tend to repel one another, it is difficult to bring such cells together into lattice formation. This ability to link cells together depends in part on the nature of the antibody. Originally, a distinction was made between complete antibody, which is capable of both primary and secondary interactions that result in visible aggregation of cells, and nonagglutinating antibody, or incomplete antibody, which produces no visible agglutination.

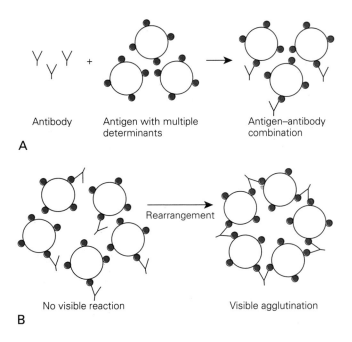

FIG. 10–1. Phases of agglutination. *(A)* Sensitization. Antigen and antibody unite through antigenic determinant sites. *(B)* Lattice formation. Rearrangement of antigen and antibody bonds to form stable lattice.

Incomplete antibody was thought to have only one active site for combining with antigen, and this was why it was incapable of agglutination. Now it is known that incomplete antibody has two active sites with the potential to bind two cells together, but it cannot bridge the distance between particles, so there is no lattice formation. This occurs most often with antibodies of the IgG class because their small size and restricted flexibility at the hinge region often prohibits multivalent binding.[6] However, a number of enhancement techniques, which vary physicochemical conditions, usually allow such a reaction to take place. Therefore, the term is not really applicable in the modern serology laboratory.

Enhancement of Lattice Formation

The surface charge must be controlled for lattice formation, or a visible agglutination reaction, to take place. One means of accomplishing this is by decreasing the ionic strength of the buffer through the use of **low ionic strength saline**.[4] The addition of albumin in concentrations of 5 to 30 percent is also thought to neutralize surface charges and facilitate agglutination.

Other techniques that enhance agglutination, especially that of red blood cells, include increasing the viscosity, use of enzymes, and agitation or centrifugation. Viscosity can be increased by adding agents such as dextran, polyvinyl pyrrolidone, or serum albumin.[7] Bromelin, papain, and ficin are the enzymes most often used, and these are thought to enhance agglutination by reducing the surface charge on red blood cells through cleaving of chemical groups and decreasing hydration.[4] Ficin cleaves sialoglycoproteins from the red blood cell surface, and in addition to reducing the charge, this may change the external configuration of the membrane to reveal more antigenic determinant sites.[2] Agitation and centrifugation provide a physical means to increase cell–cell contact and thus heighten agglutination.[5] All of these techniques plus the use of antiglobulin reagents (discussed in a separate section) are used in the blood bank to better detect antigen–antibody reactions, especially in selecting blood for transfusion.

The temperature at which the antigen–antibody reaction takes place must also be considered because it has an influence on the secondary or aggregation phase. Antibodies belonging to the IgG class agglutinate best at 30°C to 37°C, while IgM antibodies react best at temperatures between 4°C and 27°C. Because naturally occurring antibodies against the ABO blood groups belong to the IgM class, these reactions are best run at room temperature. Antibodies to other human blood groups usually belong to the IgG class, and reactions involving these must be run at 37°C. These latter reactions are the most important to consider in selecting compatible blood for a transfusion because these are the ones that will actually occur in the body.

An additional physicochemical factor that can be manipulated when performing agglutination reactions is pH. Most reactions produce optimal antigen–antibody combination when the pH is between 6.7 and 7.2, but there are some exceptions, such as human anti-M, which reacts best at a lower pH.[4]

Types of Agglutination Reactions

Agglutination reactions are easy to carry out, require no complicated equipment, and can be performed as needed in the laboratory without the necessity of batching specimens. Batching specimens is done if a test is expensive or complicated; then a large number are run at one time, which may result in a time delay. Many kits are available for standard testing, so reagent preparation is minimal, and agglutination reactions are an often used serologic test. They can be used to identify either antigen or antibody. Typically, most agglutination tests are qualitative, simply indicating absence or presence of antigen or antibody, but dilutions can be made to obtain semiquantitative results. Many variations exist, and these can be categorized according to the type of particle used in the reaction and whether antigen or antibody is attached to it.

Direct Agglutination

So-called **direct agglutination** occurs when antigens are found naturally on a particle. Identification of bacterial types represents a classic example of a direct agglutination reaction that is still used today. A suspension of bacteria is prepared and combined with standardized antiserum. Cloudiness that forms in the test tube is indicative of a positive reaction. Sometimes tubes are left to incubate overnight in the refrigerator to facilitate reading the reaction. The Kauffmann and White scheme for serotyping of Salmonella species is an example of such a reaction. Serotyping is done on the basis of two main types of antigen, O and H. *H antigens* are flagellar antigens that form a loosely woven network of clumped cells, called snowflake agglutination. *O antigens* are somatic antigens that are an integral part of the cell wall, and this type of agglutination is compact and granular.

Direct agglutination testing can also be set up with known bacterial antigens used to test for the presence of unknown antibodies in the patient. Typically, patient serum is diluted into a series of tubes and reacted with bacterial antigens specific for the suspected disease. Detection of antibodies is primarily used in diagnosis of diseases for which the bacterial agents are extremely difficult to cultivate. A prime example is the febrile agglutinin test, a rapid screening test to help determine the cause of a fever of unknown origin. The antigens used in this procedure include Salmonella O (somatic) and H (flagellar) antigens, Brucella abortus antigen, and Proteus OX19 antigen.[8] The Salmonella antigens test for typhoid fever, and Brucella antigens screen for brucellosis and tularemia. Proteus OX 19 is used to detect antibodies formed during rickettsial diseases such as Rocky Mountain Spotted Fever because these antibodies crossreact with Proteus antigens. A significant finding is a fourfold increase in antibody titer over time when paired dilutions of serum samples are tested with any of these antigens.[8] The febrile agglutinin series is no longer routinely used because there are more specific tests on the market now.

If an agglutination reaction involves red blood cells, then it is called **hemagglutination.** The best example of this occurs in ABO blood group typing of human red blood cells. Antisera of the IgM type can be used to determine the presence or absence of the A and B antigens, and this reaction is usually performed at room temperature without the need for any enhancement techniques.[5] This type of agglutination reaction is simple to perform, relatively sensitive, and easy to read.[5] A titer that yields semiquantitative results can be performed in test tubes or microtiter plates by making serial dilutions of the antibody. The reciprocal of the last dilution still exhibiting a visible reaction is the titer, indicating strength of the antibody.

Interpretation of the test is done on the basis of the cell sedimentation pattern. If there is a dark red, smooth button at the bottom of the well, the result is negative. A positive result, on the other hand, will have cells that are spread across the bottom of the well, usually in a jagged pattern with an irregular edge. Test tubes also can be centrifuged and then shaken to see if the cell button can be evenly resuspended. If it is resuspended with no visible clumping, then the result is negative. Positive reactions can be graded to indicate the strength of the reaction (Fig. 10–2). Hemagglutination kits are now available for detection of antibodies to hepatitis B virus (HBV), hepatitis C virus (HCV), and human immunodeficiency virus (HIV) I and II, to cite just a few examples.[1]

Passive Agglutination

Passive agglutination employs particles that are coated with antigens not normally found on their surfaces. Until the 1970s, erythrocytes were the major particle carrier used.[2] Now, however, a variety of particles, including polystyrene latex, bentonite, and charcoal are used for this purpose.[5] The use of synthetic

beads or particles provides the advantage of consistency, uniformity, and stability.[3] Reactions are also easy to read visually. Particle sizes vary from 7 microns for red blood cells all the way down to 0.05 microns for very fine latex particles.[1]

Many antigens, especially polysaccharides, adsorb to red blood cells spontaneously, so they are relatively easy to manipulate. However, stability of red cells has been a problem, and to overcome the possibility of spontaneous lysis, most red blood cells are treated with formalin or glutaraldehyde.[2] To coat red blood cells with antigens other than polysaccharides, pretreatment is often necessary. Proteins are more easily attached after processing of the cells with tannic acid. Tannic acid treatment, however, makes cells more susceptible to spontaneous lysis or nonspecific agglutination, so reactions must be carefully controlled.[5]

For some antigenic groups, chemical coupling is required. Bisdiazobenzidine (BDB) links protein through a diazo reaction. Other chemicals used include carbodiimide (CDI), glutaraldehyde, and 1,3 difluoro-4-6-dinitrobenzene.[2,3,5] Problems encountered with the use of erythrocytes as carrier particles include the possibility of crossreactivity, especially with heterophile antibody (see Chapter 4) if the cells used are nonhuman.

In 1955, Singer and Plotz found by happenstance that IgG was naturally adsorbed to the surface of polystyrene latex particles. While other substances such as polysaccharides and highly charged proteins are not

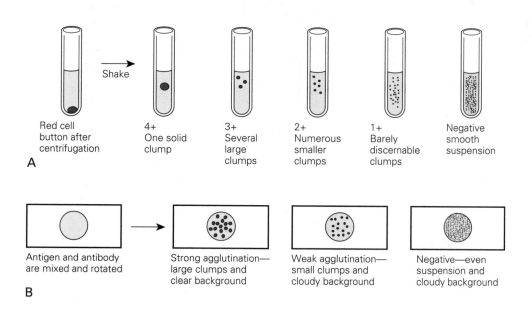

FIG. 10–2. Grading of agglutination reactions. *(A)* Tube method. If tubes are centrifuged and shaken to resuspend the button, reactions can be graded from negative to 41 depending on the size of clumps observed. *(B)* Slide method. Reactions can be graded from negative to strongly reactive depending on the size of the clumps in the suspension.

naturally adsorbed by these particles, manipulation with the same types of chemicals used in red blood cell processing are usually successful in coating latex particles with these substances. Latex particles are inexpensive, relatively stable, and are not subject to crossreactivity with other antibodies.[2] A large number of antibody molecules can be bound to the surface of latex particles, so the number of antigen-binding sites is large.[1] Additionally, the large particle size facilitates reading of the test.[5]

Passive agglutination tests have been used to detect rheumatoid factor, antinuclear antibody occurring in the disease lupus erythematosus, antibodies to group A streptococcus antigens, antibodies to *Trichinella spiralis,* and antibodies to viruses such as cytomegalovirus, rubella, and varicella-zoster.[9–12] Because many of these kits are designed to detect IgM antibody, and there is always the risk of nonspecific agglutination caused by the presence of other IgM antibodies, reactions must be carefully controlled and interpreted. Commercial tests are usually performed on cardboard cards or glass slides, and reactions can be graded on a scale of 1+ to 4+. Often control latex particles are tested alongside antigen-coated beads, and if the patient specimen reacts with both types of particles, the test is not valid.[1] Such tests are typically used as screening tools to be followed by more extensive testing if the results are positive.

Reverse Passive Agglutination

In **reverse passive agglutination,** antibody rather than antigen is attached to a carrier particle. The antibody must still be reactive and is joined in such a manner that the active sites are facing outward. Adsorption may be spontaneous, or it may require some of the same manipulation as is used for antigen attachment. This type of testing is often used for the detection of microbial antigens. Figure 10–3 shows the differences between passive and reverse passive agglutination.

Numerous kits are available today for the rapid identification of antigens from such infectious agents as group B streptococcus, *Staphylococcus aureus, Neisseria meningitidis,* group A streptococcus, *Haemophilus influenzae,* rotavirus, *Cryptococcus neoformans, Mycoplasma pneumoniae,* and *Candida albicans.*[2,9,13,14] Rapid agglutination tests have found the widest application in detecting soluble antigens in urine, spinal fluid, and serum.[14] The principle is the same for all these tests: Latex particles coated with antibody are reacted with a patient sample containing the suspected antigen. In some cases, an extraction step is necessary to isolate antigen before the reagent latex particles are added. Organisms can be identified in a few minutes with

fairly high sensitivity and specificity. For example, the sensitivity of latex agglutination kits for the detection of Cryptococcal antigen has been reported to be as high as 99 percent.[15] Use of monoclonal antibodies has greatly cut down on cross-reactivity, but there is still the possibility of interference or nonspecific agglutination. Such tests are most often used for organisms that are difficult to grow in the laboratory, or for instances when rapid identification will allow treatment to be initiated more promptly. However, direct testing of specimens for the presence of viral antigens has still not reached the sensitivity of enzyme immunoassays.[14]

Reverse passive agglutination testing has also been used to measure levels of certain therapeutic drugs, hormones, and plasma proteins such as haptoglobin and C-reactive protein. In all of these reactions, rheumatoid

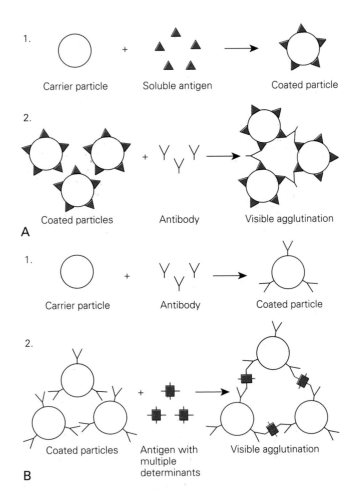

FIG. 10–3. Passive and reverse passive agglutination. *(A)* Passive agglutination. Antigen is attached to the carrier particle, and agglutination occurs if patient antibody is present. *(B)* Reverse passive agglutination. Antibody is attached to the carrier particle, and agglutination occurs if patient antigen is present.

factor will cause a false positive as it reacts with any IgG antibody, so this must be taken into account.

Agglutination Inhibition

Agglutination inhibition reactions are based on competition between particulate and soluble antigens for limited antibody combining sites, and a lack of agglutination is an indicator of a positive reaction. Typically, this type of reaction involves haptens that are complexed to proteins; the hapten–protein conjugate then is attached to a carrier particle. The patient sample is first reacted with a limited amount of reagent antibody that is specific for the hapten being tested. Indicator particles that contain the same hapten one wishes to measure in the patient are then added. If the patient sample has no free hapten, the reagent antibody is able to combine with the carrier particles and produce a visible agglutination. In this case, however, agglutination is a negative reaction, indicating that the patient did not have sufficient hapten to inhibit the secondary reaction (Fig. 10–4). Either antigen or antibody can be attached to the particles. The sensitivity of the reaction is governed by the avidity of the antibody itself. It can be a highly sensitive assay capable of detecting small quantities of antigen.[6]

The classic example of agglutination inhibition is pregnancy testing. Human chorionic gonadotropin (hCG), a hormone that appears in serum and urine early in pregnancy, is attached to carrier latex particles. A urine specimen from the patient is mixed with antibody to hCG. Reagent latex particles are then added. If hCG is present, no agglutination will occur, indicating that the patient is pregnant. Use of monoclonal antibody directed against the β subunit of hCG has lessened the crossreactivity with other hormones, such as luteinizing hormone and follicle-stimulating hormone. Latex agglutination tests for pregnancy have largely been replaced by enzyme immunoassays, however, because enzyme tests are much more sensitive.

Hemagglutination inhibition reactions use the same principle, except red blood cells are the indicator particles. This type of testing has been used for detection of antibodies to certain viruses, such as rubella, mumps, measles, influenza, parainfluenzae, HBV, herpesvirus, respiratory syncytial virus, and adenovirus.[3,6,9,14] Red blood cells have naturally occurring viral receptors. When virus is present, spontaneous agglutination occurs because the virus particles link the red blood cells together. Presence of patient antibody inhibits the agglutination reaction.

To perform a hemagglutination inhibition test, patient serum is first incubated with a viral preparation.

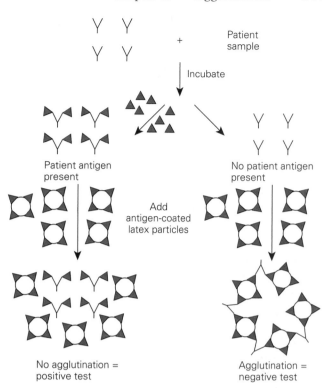

FIG. 10–4. Agglutination inhibition. Reagent antibody is added to the patient sample. If patient antigen is present, antigen–antibody combination results. When antigen-coated latex particles are added, no agglutination occurs, which is a positive test. If no patient antigen is there, the reagent antibody combines with latex particles, and agglutination results, which is a negative test.

Then red blood cells that the virus is known to agglutinate are added to the mixture. If antibody is present, this will combine with viral particles and prevent agglutination, so a lack of or reduction in agglutination indicates presence of patient antibody. Controls are necessary because there may be a factor in the serum that causes agglutination, or the virus may have lost its ability to agglutinate.

Coagglutination

Coagglutination is the name given to systems using bacteria as the inert particles to which antibody is attached.[2] *Staphylococcus aureus* is most frequently used because it has a protein on its outer surface, called protein A, which naturally adsorbs the fragment crystallizable (Fc) portion of antibody molecules. The active sites face outward and are capable of reacting with specific antigen (Fig. 10–5). These particles exhibit greater stability than latex particles and are more refractory to changes in ionic strength.[2] However, because

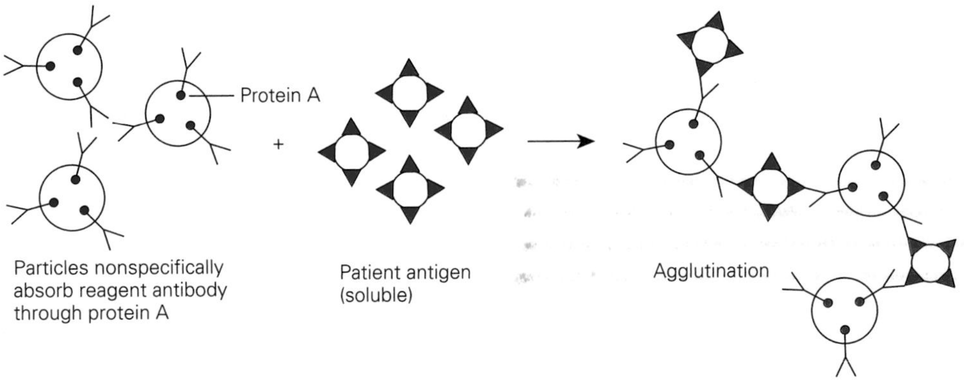

FIG. 10–5. Coagglutination with *Staphylococcus aureus*. *Staphylococcus aureus* particles nonspecifically bind the Fc portion of immunoglobulin molecules. When reagent antibody is used, combination with patient antigen produces a visible agglutination reaction.

bacteria are not colored, reactions are often difficult to read. Such testing is highly specific, but it may not be as sensitive for detecting small quantities of antigen, as is latex agglutination.[9] Coagglutination reagents have been used in identification of streptococci, *Neisseria meningitidis, Neisseria gonorrhoeae,* and *Haemophilus influenzae.*[9,14,16]

Antiglobulin-Mediated Agglutination

Antibody-mediated agglutination, also known as the *Coombs' test,* is a technique that detects nonagglutinating antibody by means of coupling with a second antibody. It remains one of the most widely used procedures today in blood banking.[3] The key component of the test is antibody to human globulin that is made in animals. Such antibody will react with the Fc portion of the human antibody attached to red blood cells. Agglutination takes place because the antihuman globulin is able to bridge the distance between cells that IgG alone cannot do. The strength of the reaction is proportional to the amount of antibody coating the red blood cells.[4] The Coombs' test can be divided into two different types, direct and indirect, each of which has a different purpose.

Direct Antiglobulin Test

The **direct antiglobulin test** is used to demonstrate *in vivo* attachment of antibody or complement to an individual's red blood cells.[3] This test serves as an indicator of autoimmune hemolytic anemia, hemolytic disease of the newborn, sensitization of red blood cells caused by the presence of drugs, or a transfusion reac-

tion. The test is called *direct* because red blood cells are tested directly as they come from the body. A blood sample is obtained from the patient, the red blood cells are washed to remove any antibody that is not specifically attached, and then cells are tested directly with antibody to IgG or complement components. If IgG or complement is present on the red blood cells, the antihuman globulin (Coombs' reagent) is able to bridge the gap between red blood cells and cause a visible agglutination (Fig. 10–6).

Polyspecific antiserum will react with IgG and with complement components C3d, C3b, C4b, or C4d.[4] If such a reaction is positive, then monospecific antibody, which will react with only one component, is used. This will differentiate between IgG and individual complement components on the patient's red blood cells. A positive test indicates that an immune reaction is taking place in that individual.

Indirect Antiglobulin Test

The **indirect antiglobulin test,** or Coombs' test, is used to determine the presence of a particular antibody in a patient, or it can be used to type patient red blood cells for specific blood group antigens. This is a two-step process, in which red blood cells and antibody are allowed to combine at 37°C and the cells then are carefully washed to remove any unbound antibody. When antihuman globulin is added, a visible reaction occurs where antibody has been specifically bound.

This test is most often used to check for the presence of unexpected antibody in patient serum when performing compatibility testing for a blood transfusion.[5] In this case, patient serum is used to combine with reagent red blood cells of known antigenicity. All reactions are run at 37°C to detect clinically significant

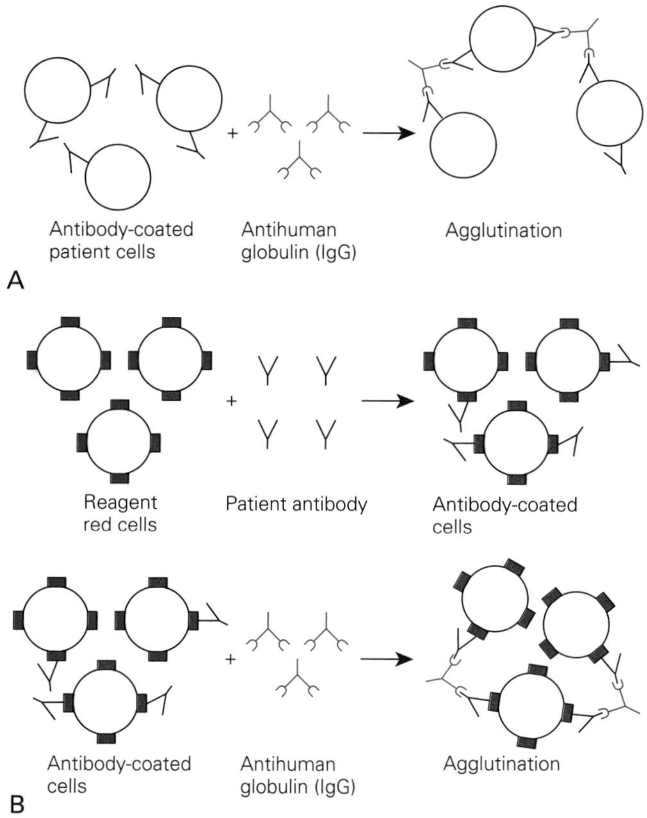

A

B

FIG. 10–6. Direct and indirect antiglobulin tests. *(A)* Direct antiglobulin test (DAT). Antihuman globulin is combined with patient cells that have become coated with antibody *in vivo*. *(B)* Indirect antiglobulin test (IAT). Reagent cells are reacted with patient antibody. These are washed, and then antihuman globulin is added to enhance agglutination.

antibodies. Cells are then washed, and antihuman globulin is added. Tubes are centrifuged and read for agglutination (see Fig. 10–6).

Possible sources of error in performing the Coombs' test include failure to wash cells, improper centrifugation, and use of reagents that are expired or not properly stored.[4] Thus, it is important to use quality controls and to interpret results carefully.

Instrumentation

While agglutination reactions require no complicated instrumentation to read, several systems have been developed using automation to increase sensitivity. Many of these use turbidimetry, which is based on the principle that as particles combine, light scatter increases, and the absorbance of the solution increases proportionally.[2] Refer to Chapter 9 for further discussion of the principles of turbidimetry. Nephelometry

has also been applied to the reading of agglutination reactions, and the term *particle-enhanced immunoassay* is used to describe such reactions. Nephelometry without the use of particles is capable of detecting soluble antigen–antibody complexes at a sensitivity of between 1 and 10 μg/mL.[7] If particles are used, the sensitivity can be increased to subnanograms/mL.[7] For this type of reaction, small latex particles with a diameter of less than 1 μm are used. One such type of instrumentation system is called a PACIA.

Particle-counting immunoassay (PACIA) involves measurement of the number of residual nonagglutinating particles in a specimen. These are counted by means of a laser beam in an optical particle counter similar to one that is designed to count blood cells. Nephelometric methods are used to measure forward light scatter. Very large and very small particles are excluded by setting certain thresholds on the instrument. Latex particles of less than 1 μm are usually used in this assay.[1]

Latex particles are coated with whole antibody molecules or with F(ab)$_2$ fragments. Use of the latter reduces interference and nonspecific agglutination. If antigen is present, complexes will form and will be screened out by the counter because of their large size. An inverse relationship exists between the number of unagglutinated particles counted and the amount of unknown in the patient specimen. Measurements can be made by looking at the rate at which the number of unagglutinated particles decrease, called a rate assay, or the total number of unagglutinated particles left at the end, known as an endpoint assay.[1] PACIAs have been used to measure several serum proteins, therapeutic drugs, tumor markers, and viral antigens, such as those associated with measles and herpes simplex.[7] Although PACIA is extremely sensitive, a disadvantage is the need to invest in expensive equipment.

Quality Control and Quality Assurance

Although agglutination reactions are simple to perform, interpretation must be carefully done. Techniques must be standardized as to concentration of antigen, incubation time, temperature, diluent, and the method of reading. The possibility of cross-reactivity and interfering antibody should always be considered. Cross-reactivity is caused by the presence of antigenic determinants that resemble one another so closely that antibody formed against one will react with the other. Most cross-reactivity can be avoided through the use of monoclonal antibody directed against an antigenic determinant that is unique to a particular antigen. In pregnancy testing, the use of monoclonal antibody directed against the β subunit of human chorionic gonadotropin is a good example of increased specificity using this technique. Refer to the exercise on pregnancy testing at the end of this chapter for more details.

Heterophile antibody and rheumatoid factor are two interfering antibodies that may produce a false-positive result. Heterophile antibodies (Chapter 4) are most often a consideration when red blood cells are used as the carrier particle. Patients may have an antibody that is capable of reacting with an antigen on the red blood cell other than the antigen that is being tested for. Such cross-reactions can be controlled by preadsorption of test serum on red blood cells without the test antigen or by treating red blood cells to remove possible interfering antigens. Rheumatoid factor, as mentioned previously, will react with any IgG present and is especially a problem in reverse passive agglutination tests. Thus, the use of positive and negative control sera is essential in agglutination testing, but it cannot rule out all false-positive reactions.

Other considerations include proper storage of reagents and close attention to expiration dates. Reagents should never be used beyond the expiration date. Each new lot should be evaluated before use, and the manufacturer's instructions for each kit should always be followed. The sensitivity and specificity of different kits may vary, and thus must be taken into account.

Advantages of agglutination reactions include rapidity, relative sensitivity, and the fact that if the sample contains a microorganism, it does not need to be viable.[2] In addition, most tests are simple to perform and require no expensive equipment. A wide variety of antigens and antibodies can be tested for in this manner. It must be kept in mind, however, that agglutination tests are screening tests only, and that a negative result does not rule out presence of the disease or the antigen. The quantity of antigen or antibody may be below the sensitivity of the test system. Refer to Table 10–1 for a list of false-positive and false-negative reactions.

SUMMARY

Agglutination, first observed in 1896 when antibody was found to react with bacterial cells, is a versatile technique that is simple to perform. The process of agglutination can be divided into two steps: (1) sensitization or initial binding, which depends on the nature of the antibody and the antigen-bearing surface, and (2) lattice formation, which is governed by such factors as pH, ionic strength, and temperature. Decreasing the

ionic strength of the milieu, running the reaction at a pH between 6.7 and 7.2, and choosing the correct temperature for the particular immunoglobulin type can all enhance lattice formation. Many of these manipulations are necessary to overcome the fact that many particles in solution are charged, and like charges tend to repel one another. Incomplete antibody is capable of complexing with antigenic determinants on particles but is unable to bridge the gap and bring two such charged particles together. Often IgG acts as an incomplete antibody, while IgM, because of its larger size, is usually able to effect lattice formation without additional enhancement.

Agglutination reactions can be divided into several distinct categories: (1) direct, (2) passive, (3) reverse passive, (4) agglutination inhibition, and (5) coagglutination. In direct agglutination, antigens are found naturally on the indicator particle, but in passive agglutination, antigens are artificially attached to such a particle. Reverse passive agglutination is so called because antibody is attached to the indicator particle. Agglutination inhibition is based on competition between antigen-coated particles and soluble patient antigen for a limited number of antibody sites. This is the only instance in which agglutination represents a negative test. Coagglutination uses bacteria as the carrier particle to which antibody is attached.

Coombs' tests involve the use of antihuman globulin to enhance agglutination. Two distinct techniques, direct and indirect testing, are frequently used in the blood bank, and each has a specific purpose. The direct Coombs' test is used to detect *in vivo* coating of patient cells with antigen. The indirect Coombs' test, on the other hand, amplifies *in vitro* antigen–antibody combination. Typically, it is employed to detect unexpected patient antibody to red blood cells intended for a transfusion.

Several automated agglutination techniques have been employed in the clinical laboratory to increase the sensitivity of agglutination reactions. PACIA looks at residual nonagglutinating particles by means of nephelometry. As agglutination occurs, clumps of antigens increase in size, and these large clumps are not counted. The amount of unknown in a patient specimen is therefore indirectly proportional to the number of unagglutinated particles because an increase in unknown results in a decrease in particles that do not agglutinate.

Quality control is an important aspect of the performance of agglutination reactions. Concentration of antigen, incubation time, temperature, diluent used, and the method of reading should be standardized for each particular test done. This helps to cut down on the occurrence of false-positive and false-negative results.

TABLE 10–1. Causes of False-Positive and False-Negative Reactions in Agglutination Testing

Cause	Correction
FALSE-POSITIVE REACTIONS	
Overcentrifugation: Button is packed too tight and is difficult to resuspend.	Regulate centrifuge to proper speed and time.
Contaminated glassware, slides, or reagents: Contaminants (dust, dirt, or fingerprints) may cause cells to clump.	Keep supplies covered in storage and handle with care.
Autoagglutination: Test cells clump without specific antibody present; mainly a problem with red cells.	Use a control with saline and no antibody present. If the control is positive, test is invalidated.
Saline stored in glass bottles: Colloidal silica may leach out and cause agglutination.	Store saline in plastic containers.
Presence of cross-reactivity.	Use purified antigen preparations and specific monoclonal antibody whenever possible.
Presence of rheumatoid factor.	Test specifically for rheumatoid factor to rule out its presence. If rheumatoid factor is present, agglutination results must be interpreted carefully.
Presence of heterophile antibody: This occurs mainly when red blood cells are used as the carrier particle.	Preabsorb serum with red blood cells without specific antigen; or pretreat red blood cells to remove other antigens.
Delay in reading a slide test: Dried out antigen may look like agglutination.	Follow directions and read reactions immediately after incubation.
FALSE-NEGATIVE REACTIONS	
Under centrifugation: If sample is undercentrifuged, cells may not be close enough to interact.	Regulate centrifuge to proper speed and time.
Inadequate washing of cells, especially in antiglobulin testing: Unbound immunoglobulins may neutralize the antihuman globulin.	Wash cells thoroughly, according to the procedure being followed. Use control cells on negative reactions.
Reagents not active: This may be caused by improper storage.	Refrigerate antisera, but do not freeze because loss of activity may occur.
Delays in testing procedures: This especially pertains to antiglobulin testing. Antibody may be eluted from red blood cells.	Once a procedure is begun, follow through to the end without delay.
Incorrect incubation temperature: Too low a temperature, may result in the lack of association of antigen and antibody.	Check temperature at which test is carried out.
Insufficient incubation time: Antigen and antibody may not have time for association.	Follow instructions carefully.
Prozone phenomenon: Too much patient antibody for amount of test.	If this is suspected, dilute antibody and repeat the test.
Failure to add antiglobulin reagent: This occurs mainly in direct and indirect antiglobulin testing.	Add check cells that are antibody-coated to see if agglutination occurs after a negative test. If there is still no agglutination, disregard the results and repeat.

Agglutination reactions are typically used as screening tests; they are fast and sensitive and can yield valuable information when interpreted correctly.

Case Study

1. A 25-year-old female who was 2 months pregnant went to her physician for a prenatal workup. She had been vaccinated against rubella, but her titer was never established. She was concerned because a friend of hers who had never been vaccinated for rubella thought she might have the disease. The patient had previously been on an all-day shopping trip with her friend. The physician ordered a rubella test as a part of the prenatal workup. The results on an undiluted serum specimen were positive.

Questions

a. What does the positive rubella test indicate?
b. How should this be interpreted in the light of the patient's condition?
c. Is a semiquantitative test indicated?

Exercise: Color Slide Test for Rubella

PRINCIPLE

Rubella virus is the etiologic agent of German measles. It generally causes a mild viral infection with a slight rash. However, it is recommended that all women of childbearing age be tested for the presence of rubella antibodies to determine their immune status because viral infection during the first trimester of pregnancy can result in birth defects or stillbirth. Colored latex particles that are coated with disrupted rubella virus are used to allow a visible observation of the antigen–antibody reaction. When patient serum is mixed with the latex reagent, if specific antibody is present, a visible agglutination reaction will result.

SPECIMEN COLLECTION

Collect blood aseptically by venipuncture into a clean, dry, sterile tube and allow it to clot. Separate the serum without transferring any cellular elements. Do not use grossly hemolyzed, excessively lipemic, or bacterially contaminated specimens. Fresh non–heat inactivated serum is recommended for the test. However, if the test cannot be performed immediately, serum may be stored between 2°C and 8°C for up to 48 hours. If there is any additional delay, freeze the serum at −20°C.

For diagnosis of current or recent rubella infection, paired sera (acute and convalescent) should be obtained. The acute sera should be collected as soon after rash onset as possible or at the time of exposure. Convalescent sera should be obtained 10 to 21 days after the onset of the rash or at least 30 days after exposure if no clinical symptoms appear. Test acute and convalescent sera simultaneously using the semiquantitative procedure.

REAGENTS, MATERIALS, AND EQUIPMENT

Kit containing the following:

  Color slide rubella reagent A—protein stabilizer
  Color slide rubella reagent B—latex suspension
  Color slide rubella diluent
  Color slide rubella control—strongly positive
  Color slide rubella control—positive
  Color slide rubella control—negative
  Plastic stirrers
  Disposable slides

Materials required but not provided:

A pipette or pipettes capable of providing 10-, 20-, 35-, and 50-μL volumes.
Timer

PRECAUTIONS

Latex reagent controls and buffer contain 0.1-percent sodium azide as a preservative. Sodium azide may react with lead and copper plumbing to form highly explosive metal azides. On disposal, flush with a large volume of water to prevent azide buildup.

The virus strain used in the preparation of the latex reagent has been previously inactivated. However, it is recommended that users follow the same safety precautions in effect for the handling of other types of potentially infectious material.

Each donor unit used in the preparation of control material was tested by a Food and Drug Administration–approved method for the presence of antibodies to HIV, HBV surface antigen, and HCV and found to be negative. However, the controls should be handled as recommended for any potentially infectious human serum or blood specimen.

PROCEDURE★

Qualitative Slide Test:

1. Allow reagents, controls, and specimens to reach room temperature.
2. Label test slide for each sample and control to be tested. Avoid touching surface inside the circles.
3. Place one drop of reagent A onto each control or test circle needed.
4. Pipette 10 μL of sample or control into the reagent A drop.
5. Resuspend the latex reagent by gently mixing the vial until the suspension is homogeneous. Using the dropper provided, hold the dropper perpendicular to the slide, and place one drop of latex reagent beside but not touching reagent A containing specimen or control.
6. Using a new plastic stirrer for each circle, mix each specimen and control until the entire area of each oval is filled.
7. Rotate the slide back and forth in a figure eight pattern, slowly and evenly, for 2 minutes. Place the slide on a flat surface and observe for agglutination using a direct light source.

Semiquantitative Slide Test

If a positive reaction is obtained, the specimen may be serially diluted with diluent to obtain a semiquantitative estimate of the rubella antibody level.

★ From Seradyn Color Slide Rubella, Package insert, Remel, 12076 Santa Fe Drive, Lenexa, KS 66215.

1. Label the test slide from 1:1 to 1:128, using twofold serial dilutions (e.g., 1:2, 1:4, 1:8) for the high positive control and for each positive serum sample to be tested. The low positive control and negative control are not subject to serial twofold dilutions.

2. Place one drop of reagent A onto one of the circles of the disposable slide. Pipette 10 μL of negative control (or low positive control) into the reagent A drop.

3. Pipette 50 μL of diluent onto the circle marked 1:1 and 35 μL to each circle marked 1:2 through 1:128. Pipette 20 μL of positive serum (or high positive control) onto the diluent drop in each circle marked 1:1.

4. Using a pipette set at 35 μL, mix contents in 1:1 circle by drawing up and down in the pipette tip four times. Transfer 35 μL directly into diluent in circle marked 1:2. Mix four times, and repeat the procedure through the circle marked 1:128.

5. Discard 35 μL from the circle marked 1:128.

6. Resuspend the latex reagent by gently mixing the vial until the suspension is homogeneous. Using the dropper provided, hold the dropper perpendicular to the slide and place one drop of reagent B beside but not touching the drop of reagent A containing specimen or control.

7. Using a separate plastic stirrer for each set of samples or controls, mix each specimen and control until the entire area of each oval is filled. Start at the highest dilution of each sample or control, and proceed to the next lower dilution with the same stirrer until all circles are spread. Stir gently to minimize bubbles.

8. Rotate the slide back and forth in a figure eight pattern, slowly and evenly, for 2 minutes. Place the slide on a flat surface and observe for agglutination using a direct light source.

RESULTS

The presence of any visible agglutination significantly different from the negative control indicates the presence of antibodies against rubella virus in the serum sample. Both the low and high positive controls should show agglutination different from the uniform appearance of the negative control. The negative control should show no agglutination. In the semiquantitative test, the rubella titer will correspond to the highest serum dilution that produces visible agglutination. The high positive control should give a titer within one doubling dilution of that indicated on the label.

INTERPRETATION OF RESULTS

Undiluted serum will give a positive reaction if at least 10 ± 1 IU/mL of antibody is present. This indicates that the individual has immunity to rubella. When a semiquantitative test is performed with acute and convalescent sera from the same patient, a fourfold increase in titer is considered to be significant. This typically indicates infection. Some individuals previously exposed to rubella may demonstrate a rise in antibody titer. Seroconversion can also be seen after a vaccination procedure. All test results must be evaluated by a physician in light of the clinical symptoms shown by the patient.

Review Questions

1. Which of the following best describes agglutination?
   a. A combination of soluble antigen with soluble antibody
   b. A combination of particulate antigen with soluble antibody
   c. A reaction that produces no visible endpoint
   d. A reaction that requires instrumentation to read

2. All of the following could be used to enhance an agglutination reaction *except:*
   a. Increasing the viscosity of the medium
   b. Use of albumin
   c. Increasing the ionic strength of the medium
   d. Centrifugation

3. Agglutination of dyed bacterial cells represents which type of reaction?
   a. Direct agglutination
   b. Passive agglutination
   c. Reverse passive agglutination
   d. Agglutination inhibition

4. In which of the following circumstances would the indirect Coombs' test by employed?
   a. Identification of the ABO blood groups
   b. Identification of cold-reacting antibody
   c. Identification of an unexpected IgG antibody
   d. Identification of hemolytic disease of the newborn

5. In an agglutination reaction, if cells are not centrifuged long enough, which of the following might occur?
   a. False-negative result
   b. False-positive result
   c. No effect
   d. Slight effect but can be ignored

6. Agglutination inhibition could best be used for which of the following types of antigens?
   a. Large cellular antigens such as erythrocytes
   b. Soluble haptens
   c. Bacterial cells
   d. Antigen attached to latex particles

7. Which of the following correctly describes reverse passive agglutination?
   a. It is a negative test.
   b. It can be used to detect autoantibodies.
   c. It is used for identification of bacterial antigens.
   d. All of the above.

8. In which of the following tests is patient antigen determined by measuring the number of nonagglutinating particles left after the reaction has taken place?
   a. Direct agglutination
   b. Coagglutination
   c. PACIA
   d. Coombs' testing

9. IgG is sometimes referred to as incomplete antibody because:
   a. It is only active at 25°C.
   b. It may be too small to produce lattice formation.
   c. It only has one antigen-binding site.
   d. It is not able to produce visible *in vitro* agglutination.

10. For which of the following tests is a lack of agglutination a positive reaction?
    a. Hemagglutination
    b. Passive agglutination
    c. Reverse passive agglutination
    d. Agglutination inhibition

11. All of the following would be considered good quality control procedures *except:*
    a. Proper storage of reagents
    b. Standardizing temperature of reactions
    c. Allowing the reaction to go as long as possible
    d. Use of monoclonal antibody to avoid cross-reactivity

12. A positive direct Coombs' test could occur under which circumstances?
    a. Hemolytic disease of the newborn
    b. Autoimmune hemolytic anemia
    c. Antibodies to drugs that bind to red cells
    d. Any of the above

References

1. Kasahara, Y: Agglutination immunoassays. In Rose, NR, De MacArio, EC, and Folds, JD, et al (eds): Manual of Clinical Laboratory Immunology, ed. 5. American Society for Microbiology, Washington, D.C., 1997, pp 7–12.

2. Tinghitella, TJ, and Edberg, SC: Agglutination tests and limulus assay for the diagnosis of infectious diseases. In Balows, A, Hausler, WJ, and Hermann, KL, et al (eds): Manual of Clinical Microbiology, ed. 5. American Society for Microbiology, Washington, D.C., 1991, pp 61–72.

3. Stites, DP, et al: Clinical laboratory methods for detection of antigens and antibodies. In Stites, DP, Terr, AI, and Parslow, TG (eds): Medical Immunology, ed. 9. Appleton & Lange, Stamford, Conn., 1997, pp 211–253.

4. Vengelen-Tyler, V (ed): The Technical Manual of the American Association of Blood Banks, ed. 12. American Association of Blood Banks, Bethesda, 1996, pp 213–227.

5. Miller, LE, et al: Manual of Laboratory Immunology, ed. 2. Lea & Febiger, Philadelphia, 1991, pp 48–57.

6. Goldsby, RA, Kindt, TJ, and Osborne, BA: Kuby Immunology, ed. 4. WH Freeman, New York, 2000, pp 157–159.

7. Kasahara, Y, and Nakamura, RM: Immunoassays and Immunochemistry. In Henry, JB (ed): Clinical Diagnosis and Management by Laboratory Methods, ed. 19. WB Saunders, Philadelphia, 1996, pp 851–876.

8. Difco Manual: Bacto Febrile Antigen Set, ed. 11. Difco Laboratories, Detroit, 1999, pp 637–642.

9. Forbes, BA, Sahm, DF, and Weissfeld, AS: Bailey and Scott's Diagnostic Microbiology, ed. 10. Mosby, St. Louis, 1998, pp 211–214.

10. Hodinka, RL: Human cytomegalovirus. In Murray, PR, Baron, EJ, and Pfaller, MA, et al (eds): Manual of Clinical Microbiology, ed. 7. American Society for Microbiology, Washington, D.C., 1999, pp 888–899.

11. Chernesky, MA, and Mahoney, JB: Rubella virus. In Murray, PR, Baron, EJ, and Pfaller, MA, et al (eds): Manual of Clinical Microbiology, ed. 7. American Society for Microbiology, Washington, D.C., 1999, pp 964–969.

12. Gershon, AA, LaRussa, P, and Steinberg, SP: Varicella-Zoster virus. In Murray, PR, Baron, EJ, and Pfaller, MA, et al (eds): Manual of Clinical Microbiology, ed. 7. American Society for Microbiology, Washington, D.C., 1999, pp 900–911.

13. Park, CH et al: Detection of Group B streptococcal colonization in pregnant women using direct latex agglutination testing of selective broth. J Clin Micro 39:408–409, 2001.

14. Mahoney, JB, and Chernesky, MA: Immunoassays for the diagnosis of infectious diseases. In Murray, PR, Baron, EJ, and Pfaller, MA, et al (eds): Manual of Clinical Microbiology, ed. 7. American Society for Microbiology, Washington, D.C., 1999, pp 202–214.

15. Merz, WG, and Roberts, GD: Algorithms for detection and identification of fungi. In Murray, PR, Baron, EJ, and Pfaller, MA, et al (eds): Manual of Clinical Microbiology, ed. 7. American Society for Microbiology, Washington, D.C., 1999, pp 1167–1183.

16. Campos, JM: Haemophilus. In Murray, PR, Baron, EJ, and Pfaller, MA, et al (eds): Manual of Clinical Microbiology, ed. 7. American Society for Microbiology, Washington, D.C., 1999, pp 604–613.

Labeled Immunoassays

Learning Objectives

After finishing this chapter, the reader will be able to:
1. Describe the typical constituents of a labeled assay.
2. Identify characteristics that an antibody must have to be used for immunoassay.
3. Discuss different separation methods used in heterogeneous assays.
4. Explain the principle of competitive binding in radioimmunoassays.
5. Distinguish between heterogeneous and homogeneous enzyme immunoassay.
6. Explain the principle of sandwich or capture immunoassays.
7. Describe uses for membrane-bound cassette assays.
8. Describe applications for homogeneous enzyme immunoassay.
9. Compare and contrast enzyme immunoassay and radioimmunoassay regarding ease of performance, shelf life, sensitivity, and clinical application.
10. Discuss how cloned enzyme donor immunoassay (CEDIA) differs from other types of enzyme immunoassays.
11. Describe the difference between direct and indirect immunofluorescence techniques.
12. Relate the principle of fluorescence polarization immunoassay.
13. Discuss advantages and disadvantages of each type of immunoassay.
14. Choose an appropriate immunoassay for a particular analyte.

Key Terms

Analyte
Capture assay
Chemiluminescence
Cloned enzyme donor
immunoassay
Direct immunofluorescent assay
Enzyme-linked immuno-
sorbent assay (ELISA)

Fluorescence
Fluorescence polarization
immunoassay (FPIA)
Homogeneous enzyme
immunoassay
Immunofluorescent assay (IFA)
Immunoradiometric assay
(IRMA)

Indirect immuno-
fluorescent assay
Radioimmunoassay
(RIA)
Sandwich
immunoassays

The need to develop rapid, specific, and sensitive assays to determine the presence of important biologically active molecules ushered in a new era of testing in the clinical laboratory. Labeled immunoassays are designed for antigens and antibodies that may be small in size or present in very low concentrations. The presence of such antigens or antibodies is determined indirectly by using a labeled reactant to detect whether or not specific binding has taken place.

The substance to be measured is known as the **analyte.** Examples include bacteria antigens, hormones, drugs, tumor markers, specific immuno-globulins, and many other substances. Analytes are bound by molecules that react specifically with them. Typically, this is antibody. One reactant, either the antigen or antibody, is labeled with a marker so that the amount of binding can be monitored. Labeled immunoassays have made possible rapid quantitative measurement of many important entities such as virus antigens in patients infected with human immunodeficiency virus (HIV). The ability to detect antigen or antibody very early during the course of an illness has revolutionized diagnosis, monitoring, and determining treatment options for numerous diseases.

Constituents of Labeled Assays

Current techniques include the use of fluorescent, radioactive, chemiluminescent, and enzyme labels. The underlying principles of all these techniques are essentially the same. For detection of an analyte, the following are usually a part of the assay: (1) labeled and nonlabeled analytes, (2) specific antibody, (3) standards or calibrators, (4) a means of separation of the bound from free components, and (5) a means of detection of the label. The role of each of these is discussed.

Labeled Analyte

In a competitive assay in which labeled and unlabeled analytes typically compete with each other for a limited number of binding sites on antibody molecules, the analytes should be indistinguishable from one another serologically. In other words, the label must not alter the reactivity of the molecule, and it should remain stable for the shelf life of the reagent. Radioactivity, enzymes, fluorescent, and chemiluminescent tags have all been used as labels. Each of these is discussed in a later section.

Antibodies

In any assay, it is essential for the antibody used to have a high affinity for the antigen in question. As discussed in Chapter 9, affinity is the strength of the primary interaction between a single antibody-combining site and an antigenic determinant or epitope. In competitive binding assays, there is random interaction between individual antigen and antibody molecules. Therefore, the higher the affinity of antibody for antigen, the larger the amount of antigen bound to antibody, and the more accurately specific binding can be measured. The ultimate sensitivity of the immunoassay, in fact, depends largely on the magnitude of affinity.[1,2]

The antibody used should also be very specific for the antigen involved in the reaction. If a polyspecific antiserum is used, it often has to be purified to cut down on crossreactivity with other substances in the patient specimen.[3] The era of monoclonal antibodies, however, has made available a constant source of highly specific antibody and has decreased the need for pretreatment.

Standards or Calibrators

Standards, also known as *calibrators,* a third constituent of most assays, are unlabeled analytes that are made up in known concentrations of the substance to be measured. They are used to establish a relationship between the labeled analyte measured and any unlabeled analyte that might be present in patient specimens.[4] Differing amounts of standards are added to antibody–antigen mixtures to ascertain their effect on binding of the labeled reagent. Most instruments then extrapolate this information and do a best-fit curve (one that is not absolutely linear) to determine the concentration of the unknown analyte.

Separation Methods

In most assays, once the reaction between antigen and antibody has taken place, there must be a partitioning step, or a way of separating reacted from unreacted analyte. This can be accomplished by several different means. Unreacted analyte can be removed by adsorption on particles such as dextran-coated charcoal, talc, silica, or cellulose.[2,4] These adsorb out the smaller unbound molecules, which are then physically separated from bound molecules by centrifugation or filtration. The amount of label remaining in the supernatant provides an indirect measure of analyte present in the patient's sample.

Another means of separation involves precipitation of antigen–antibody complexes. If the antigen is small, usually less than 30,000 d, complexes can be precipitated out by adding concentrated solutions of ammonium sulfate, ethanol, or polyethylene glycol.[2,4] Antigen–antibody complexes can also be removed from a solution by the use of a second or precipitating antibody. For this method, sometimes called the sandwich technique, antibody to human immunoglobulins is made in another species, usually goats. This second antibody combines with all immunoglobulins present, thereby precipitating out labeled antigen–antibody complexes and leaving unbound labeled analyte in solution (Fig. 11–1).

Currently most immunoassays use a *solid-phase* vehicle for separation. Numerous substances, such as polystyrene test tubes, microtiter plates, glass or polystyrene beads, magnetic beads, or cellulose membranes, have been used for this purpose.[2,3] Antigen or antibody is attached by physical adsorption, and when specific binding takes place, complexes remain attached to the solid phase. This provides a simple way to separate bound and free reactants. It has been found that the size and shape of the solid phase not only affects the kinetics of the reaction, but it also influences the capturing capacity of the attached antigen or antibody. Small spherical particles usually work best because they actually provide a larger surface area than most microtiter wells.[5]

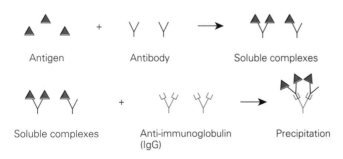

FIG. 11–1. Anti-immunoglobulin as precipitating antibody. Small soluble antigens combine with antibody to produce soluble complexes. To remove these complexes from solution, an antihuman immunoglobulin is added. This combines with the fragment crystallizable (Fc) portion of antibody molecules to produce larger, insoluble complexes.

In all assays in which a separation step is necessary, the efficiency with which this is accomplished may be a limiting factor in the assay. Either the bound or free analyte may be measured. Regardless of which means is chosen, the procedure must be precise and reproducible and must clearly distinguish bound and free fractions. The fractions are usually separated by physical means, including decanting, centrifugation, or filtration.[4] This is followed by a washing step to remove any remaining unbound analyte. Great care must be taken to perform this correctly because incomplete washing leads to incomplete removal of the labeled analyte and inaccurate results.

Detection of the Label

The last step common to all immunoassays is detection of the labeled analyte. For radioimmunoassays, this involves a system for counting radioactivity, while for other labels such as enzymes, fluorescence, or chemiluminescence, typically a change in absorbance in a substrate is measured by spectrophotometry. All systems must use stringent quality controls.

Quality Control

When measuring analytes that are present in very limited quantities, it is essential that quality control procedures be established. Because the goal of testing is to establish whether patient levels are increased or decreased over normal values, test performance must be monitored to limit random errors. Such errors may include temperature fluctuations, minor changes in the concentration of reagents, and changes in detector efficiency.[4] One means of doing this is to run a blank tube, usually phosphate-buffered saline, with every test. This is not expected to have any detectable label but serves as a check for nonspecific adsorption and for inadequate washing between steps. Any readings indicative of label in the blank are known as *background*. If the background is too high, wash steps need to be made more efficient. The purity of the labeled reagent also needs to be considered.[3]

A negative control and a high and a low positive control should be run in addition.[3] This serves as a check on the quality of the reagents to make sure that the label is readily detectable under current testing conditions.[4] All controls as well as the patient sample are usually run in duplicate. If any controls are out of range, test values should not be reported. Automated procedures have cut down on many performance variables. Individual testing procedures are now considered in the following sections.

Radioimmunoassay

Competitive Binding Assays

Radioimmunoassay (RIA), first developed by Yalow and Berson in the late 1950s,[6] uses a radioactive substance as a label. Radioactive elements have nuclei that decay spontaneously, emitting matter and energy. Several radioactive labels, including ^{131}I, ^{125}I, and tritiated hydrogen, or ^{3}H, have been used, but ^{125}I is the most popular.[5] It has a half-life of 60 days, and because it has a higher counting rate than that of ^{3}H, the total counting time is less. It is easily incorporated into protein molecules, and it emits gamma radiation, which is detected by a gamma counter.

RIA was originally based on the principle of competitive binding. This means that the analyte being detected competes with a radiolabeled analyte for a limited number of binding sites on a high-affinity antibody.[2,5] The concentration of the radioactive analyte is in excess, so that all binding sites on antibody will be occupied. If patient antigen is present, some of the binding sites will be filled with unlabeled analyte, thus decreasing the amount of bound radioactive label (Fig. 11–2). When bound and free radiolabeled antigens are separated and a washing step has occurred, the amount of label in the bound phase is indirectly proportional to the amount of patient antigen present. This can be illustrated by the following equation:

$$6Ag\star + 2Ag + 4Ab \rightarrow 3Ag\star Ab + 1AgAb + 3Ag\star + 1Ag$$

In this example, labeled and unlabeled antigens occur in a 3:1 ratio. Binding to a limited number of antibody sites will take place in the same ratio. Thus, on the right side of the equation, three of the four binding sites are occupied by labeled antigen, while one site is filled by unlabeled antigen. As the amount of patient antigen increases, fewer binding sites will be occupied by labeled antigen, as demonstrated by the next equation:

$$6Ag\star + 18Ag + 4Ab \rightarrow 1Ag\star Ab + 3AgAb + 5Ag\star + 15Ag$$

In this case, the ratio of labeled to unlabeled antigen is 1:3. Binding to antibody sites takes place in the same ratio, and the amount of bound label is greatly decreased in comparison to the first equation. In this type of RIA, use of a constant amount of radiolabeled antigen with standards of known concentration will result in a graph that can be used to extrapolate the concentration of the unknown patient antigen. The detection limits of competitive assays are largely determined by the affinity of the antibody.[7] These limits have been calculated to be as low as 10 fmol/L, or 600,000 molecules in a sample volume of 100 μL.[2]

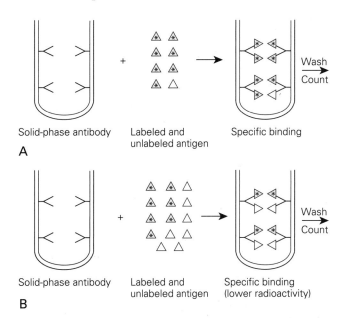

FIG. 11–2. Principle of RIA. Labeled antigen competes with patient antigen for a limited number of binding sites on solid-phase antibody. *(A)* Very little patient antigen is present, making radioactivity of the solid phase high. *(B)* More patient antigen is present, and the radioactivity of the solid phase is reduced in proportion to the amount of patient antigen bound.

Noncompetitive Immunoradiometric Assay

A second type of radioassay, **immunoradiometric assay (IRMA),** uses labeled antibody that is present in excess, thus representing a noncompetitive immunoassay. Miles and Hales pioneered this technique in the late 1960s.[8] In this system, unreacted antibody is removed by the addition of excess analyte coupled to a solid phase (Fig. 11–3). The supernatant, containing the bound complexes, is counted, and the amount of bound labeled antibody is in direct proportion to the amount of patient analyte. Advantages of IRMA include a faster reaction rate and an increased sensitivity because the antibody excess allows all of the unknown analyte to be involved in the reaction.[5] There may, however, be a loss of specificity because the increase in antibody concentration can result in cross-reactivity with other antigens.[7]

Advantages and Disadvantages of Radioimmunoassay

Substances that are measured by RIA include the following: human chorionic gonadotropin (hCG), follicle-stimulating hormone, gastrin, insulin, carci-

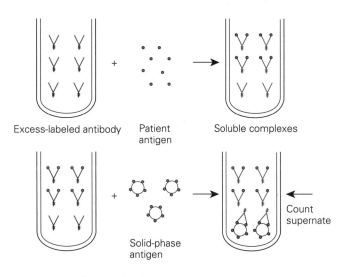

FIG. 11–3. IRMA with excess labeled antibody. Patient antigen is added to a tube with excess labeled antibody. After incubation, solid-phase antigen is added. This will combine with any labeled antibody that has not bound patient antigen. The tube is centrifuged, and the solid-phase antigen goes to the bottom. Radioactivity remaining in the supernate is determined. The count obtained is directly proportional to the amount of patient antigen present in the specimen.

noembryonic antigen, thyroxine, thyroid-stimulating hormone, estrogens, androgens, and IgE.[2,5,9] RIA is an extremely sensitive and precise technique for determining trace amounts of analytes that are small in size.

Chief among the disadvantages of all RIA techniques, however, is the health hazard involved in working with radioactive substances. Laboratories have found it more and more difficult and expensive to maintain a license and to be in compliance with federal regulations.[9] In addition, disposal problems, short shelf life, and the need for expensive equipment has caused laboratorians to explore other techniques for identification of analytes in low concentration.[9] Enzyme immunoassays have largely taken the place of RIA because of its comparable sensitivity and recent developments in automated instrumentation that allow for processing of a large number of samples in less time.[2,10]

Enzyme Immunoassay

Enzymes are naturally occurring molecules that catalyze certain biochemical reactions. They react with suitable substrates to produce breakdown products that may be chromogenic, fluorogenic, or luminescent. Some type of spectroscopy can then be used to measure the changes involved. As labels for immunoassay,

they are cheap and readily available, have a long shelf life, are easily adapted to automation, and cause changes that can be measured using inexpensive equipment.[5] Sensitivity can be achieved without disposal problems or the health hazards of radiation, as mentioned previously.[10] Because one molecule of enzyme can generate many molecules of product, little reagent is necessary to produce high sensitivity.[5] Enzyme labels can either be used qualitatively to determine the presence of an antigen or antibody or quantitatively to determine the actual concentration of an analyte in an unknown specimen.

Enzymes used as labels for immunoassay are chosen according to the following criteria: (1) number of substrate molecules converted per molecule of enzyme, (2) purity, (3) sensitivity, (4) ease and speed of detection, (5) stability, and (6) absence of interfering factors in patient samples.[3,5] In addition, availability and cost of enzyme and substrate play a role in the choice of a particular enzyme as reagent. Typical enzymes that have been used as labels include horseradish peroxidase, glucose oxidase, glucose-6-phosphate dehydrogenase, alkaline phosphatase, urease, and β-D-galactosidase.[2,10] End products of glucose-6-phosphate dehydrogenase activity need to be determined by fluorometric means. Alkaline phosphatase and horseradish peroxidase have the highest turnover (conversion of substrate) rates, high sensitivity, and are easy to detect, so they are most often used in such assays.[3] Alkaline phosphatase, however, is expensive, while horseradish peroxidase is readily available and cheap, is easily coupled to proteins, and reacts with a number of available chromogens (substrates that produce a colored end product).

The enzyme label is linked to antibody or analyte by several means. Glutaraldehyde is often used as a crosslinker to join amino groups of the enzyme and the molecule to be labeled. Maleimide derivatives are also used to attach the enzyme label.[5]

Enzyme assays are classified as either heterogeneous or homogeneous on the basis of whether or not a separation step is necessary. Heterogeneous enzyme immunoassays require a step to physically separate free from bound analyte. In homogeneous assays, on the other hand, no separation step is necessary because enzyme activity diminishes when binding of antibody and antigen occurs. The principles underlying each of these types of assays are discussed next.

Heterogeneous Enzyme Immunoassay

Competitive ELISA

The first **ELISAs,** or **enzyme-linked immunosorbent assays,** were competitive assays based on the principles of RIA. Enzyme-labeled antigen competes with unlabeled patient antigen for a limited number of binding sites on antibody molecules that are attached to a solid phase. After carefully washing to remove any nonspecifically bound antigen, enzyme activity is determined. Enzyme activity is inversely proportional to the concentration of the test substance, meaning that the more patient antigen is bound, the less enzyme-labeled antigen can attach. In this manner, a sensitivity of nanograms (10^{-9} g)/mL can be achieved.[3] This method is used for measurement of small molecules that are relatively pure, such as insulin and estrogen.[10]

Noncompetitive ELISA

Although competitive tests have a high specificity, the tendency in the laboratory today is toward the use of noncompetitive assays because they have a higher sensitivity.[10] Many such assays are capable of detecting concentrations of less than 1 pg/mL, achieving a sensitivity actually higher than most RIAs.[3] Noncompetitive assays are often referred to as indirect ELISA tests because the enzyme-labeled reagent does not participate in the initial antigen–antibody-binding reaction. This type of assay is one of the most frequently used immunoassays in the clinical laboratory.[10] Either antigen or antibody may be bound to solid phase. When antigen is used for coating, patient antibody is added and given time to react. After a wash step, an enzyme-labeled antiglobulin is added. This second antibody reacts with any patient antibody that is bound to solid phase. If no patient antibody is bound to the solid phase, the second labeled antibody will not be bound. After a second wash step, the enzyme substrate is added. The amount of enzyme label detected is directly proportional to the amount of antibody in the specimen (Fig. 11–4). This type of assay has been used to measure the status of immunity to infectious agents and for autoantibody testing.[10] Virus infections especially are often more easily diagnosed by this method than by other more traditional testing. This technique remains the method of choice for detection of antibody to the HIV. Additionally, Epstein-Barr–specific antibody detection is more sensitive than conventional immunofluorescent assay (IFA),[11] and hepatitis C antibody detection has been reported to be as sensitive as polymerase chain reaction.[12] (See Chapter 12 for a description of the polymerase chain reaction.)

Capture Assays

If antibody is bound to the solid phase, these assays are often called **sandwich immunoassays,** or **capture assays.** Antigens captured in these assays must have multiple epitopes. Excess antibody attached to solid

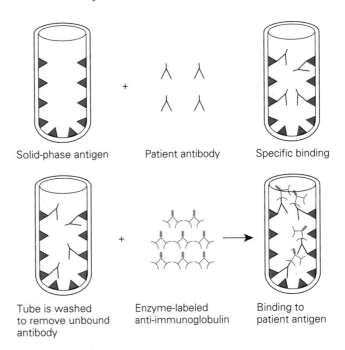

FIG. 11–4. Noncompetitive ELISA. Patient antibody is incubated with solid-phase antigen. After a wash step, enzyme-labeled anti-immunoglobulin is added. This will bind to the patient antibody on solid phase. A second wash step is performed to remove any unbound anti-immunoglobulin, and substrate for the enzyme is added. Color development is directly proportional to the amount of patient antibody present.

phase is allowed to combine with the test sample. After an appropriate incubation period, enzyme-labeled antibody is added. This second antibody may recognize the same or a different epitope than the solid-phase antibody.[10,13] Enzymatic activity is directly proportional to the amount of antigen in the test sample (Fig. 11–5).

Capture assays are best suited to antigens that have multiple determinants, such as antibodies, polypeptide hormones, proteins, tumor markers, and microorganisms, especially viruses.[5] When used with microorganisms, the epitope must be unique to the organism being tested, and it must be present in all strains of that organism. Use of monoclonal antibodies has made this a very sensitive test system. Rotavirus in stool and respiratory syncytial virus in respiratory tract secretions are two examples of capture assays.[14] In addition, recently developed ELISAs have made detection of parasites in the stool, such as *Giardia lamblia* and *Cryptosporidium,* much easier.[14]

Another major use of capture assays is in the measurement of immunoglobulins, especially those of certain classes. For instance, the presence of IgM can be specifically determined, thus indicating an acute

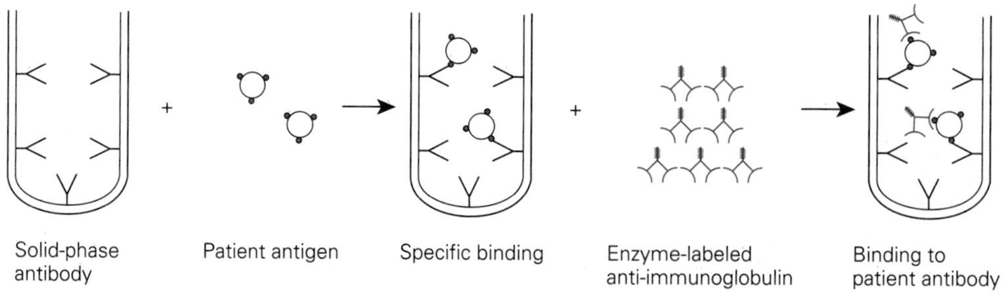

Solid-phase antibody + Patient antigen → Specific binding + Enzyme-labeled anti-immunoglobulin → Binding to patient antibody

FIG. 11–5. Noncompetitive ELISA: sandwich technique with solid-phase antibody. Patient antigen is incubated with solid-phase antibody. After washing, enzyme-labeled immunoglobulin is added, which combines with additional determinant sites on the bound patient antigen. After a second wash step, substrate for the enzyme is added. Color development is directly proportional to the amount of patient antigen present.

infection. Measurement of IgE, including allergen-specific IgE, which appears in minute quantities in serum, can also be accomplished with this system.[15] Chapter 13 provides a more detailed discussion on detection of IgE. When capture assays are used to measure immunoglobulins, the specific immunoglobulin class being detected is actually acting as antigen, and the antibody is antihuman immunoglobulin.

Indirect ELISA tests are more sensitive than their direct counterparts because all patient antigen has a chance to participate in the reaction. However, there is more manipulation than in direct tests because there are two incubations and two wash steps.

Heterogeneous enzyme assays, in general, achieve a sensitivity similar to that of RIA[1,3,13]; however, there may be problems with nonspecific protein binding and cross-reactivity. In addition, test conditions must be carefully controlled because temperature variations may have an effect on the results.[4] In sandwich assays, capture antibody on solid phase must have both a high affinity and a high specificity for this test system to be effective. It may be necessary to preabsorb serum with antirheumatoid factor to eliminate interference from IgM rheumatoid factor.[3] Sandwich assays are also subject to the hook effect, an unexpected fall in the amount of measured analyte when an extremely high concentration is present.[7] If this condition is suspected, serum dilutions must be made and then retested.

Membrane-Based Cassette Assays

Membrane-based cassette assays are a relatively new type of enzyme immunoassay. They are rapid, are easy to perform, and give reproducible results.[5] Although designed primarily for point-of-care or home testing, many of these have been modified for increased sensitivity and can be made semiquantitative for use in a clinical laboratory by reading the color reaction with a densitometer.[10] Typically these are designed as single-use, disposable assays in a plastic cartridge. The membrane is usually nitrocellulose, which is able to easily immobilize proteins and nucleic acids.[16] The rapid flow through and large surface area of the membrane enhance the speed and sensitivity of ELISA reactions.[16]

Either antigen or antibody can be coupled to the membrane, and the reaction is read by looking for the presence of a colored reaction product. Some test devices require the separate addition of patient sample, wash reagent, labeled antigen or antibody, and finally, the substrate. Another type of rapid assay, called immunochromatography, combines all the previously mentioned steps into one. The analyte is applied at one end of the strip and migrates toward the distal end, where there is an absorbent pad to maintain a constant capillary flow rate.[5] The labeling and detection zones are set between the two ends. As the sample is loaded, it reconstitutes the labeled antigen or antibody, and the two form a complex that migrates toward the detection zone. An antigen or antibody in the detection zone captures the immune complex and forms a colored line for a positive test (Fig. 11-6). This may be in the form of a plus sign. Excess labeled immunoreactant migrates to the absorbent pad. This type of test device has been used for identification of microorganisms such as *Streptococcus pyogenes* and *Streptococcus agalactiae,* for pregnancy testing, testing for troponin in a heart attack, and testing for hepatitis B surface antigen, to name just a few examples. Test results are most often qualitative rather than quantitative.

Homogeneous Enzyme Immunoassay

A **homogeneous enzyme immunoassay** is any antigen–antibody system in which no separation step is necessary. Homogeneous assays are generally less sensitive than heterogeneous assays, but they are rapid, are

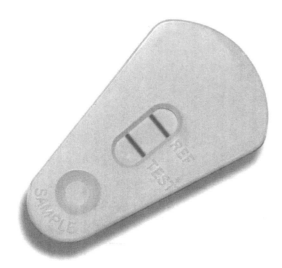

FIG. 11–6. Example of a membrane cassette assay. (Courtesy of Wampole Laboratories, Div. of Carter-Wallace, Inc., Cranbury, NJ, 08512.)

simple to perform, and adapt easily to automation.[5] No washing steps are necessary. Their chief use has been in the determination of low-molecular-weight analytes such as hormones, therapeutic drugs, and drugs of abuse in both serum and urine.[4,5,10] An example of a homogeneous immunoassay is the enzyme-multiplied immunoassay developed by the Syva Corporation.

Homogeneous assays are based on the principle of change in enzyme activity as specific antigen–antibody combination occurs.[5] Reagent antigen is labeled with an enzyme tag. When antibody binds to specific determinant sites on the antigen, the active site on the enzyme is blocked, resulting in a measurable loss of activity. Free analyte (antigen) competes with enzyme-labeled analyte for a limited number of antibody-binding sites, so this is a competitive assay. Enzyme activity is directly in proportion to the concentration of patient antigen or hapten present in the test solution. A physical separation of bound and free analyte is thus not necessary.

The sensitivity of homogeneous assays is determined by the following: (1) detectability of enzymatic activity, (2) change in that activity when antibody binds to antigen, (3) the strength of binding of the antibody, and (4) susceptibility of the assay to interference from endogenous enzyme activity, crossreacting antigens, or enzyme inhibitors. Typically, a sensitivity of micrograms per milliliter is reached, far less than that achievable by heterogeneous enzyme assays because the amplification properties of enzymes are not utilized.[5,10] They are, however, quick and easy to perform, and they are easily automated.[17] This technique is usually applied only to detection of small molecules that could not be easily measured by other means.

Other considerations include the fact that only certain enzymes are inhibited in this manner. Enzymatic activity may be altered by steric exclusion of the substrate, or there may also be changes in the conformation structure of the enzyme, especially in the region of the active site. Enzymes that are subject to this type of alteration include lysozyme, amylase, hexokinase, trypsin, papain, bromelain, glucose-6-phosphate dehydrogenase (G-6-PD), and β-D-galactosidase.[5,18]

Cloned Enzyme Donor Immunoassay

A completely different type of homogeneous immunoassay is the **cloned enzyme donor immunoassay,** the first enzyme immun-oassay developed through genetic engineering technology. It is based on the enzyme β-galactosidase, which has been reengineered into two subunits. The large polypeptide is called the enzyme acceptor, and the smaller subunit is the enzyme donor.[5] When the two pieces bind together, enzyme activity is restored. The small piece is attached as a label to antigen, which competes with patient antigen for antibody-binding sites. When antibody binds to labeled antigen, the enzyme cannot be reconstituted, and enzyme activity will be reduced. If, however, the patient specimen contains the analyte being tested for, the less the labeled analyte will be bound to antibody, and hence the greater the enzyme activity (Fig. 11-7). This type of system has been used for digoxin testing,[5] and it is adaptable to many clinical chemistry analyzers.[18]

Advantages and Disadvantages of Enzyme Immunoassay

Enzyme immunoassays have achieved a sensitivity similar to that of RIA without creating a health hazard or causing disposal problems. The use of nonisotopic enzyme labels with high specific activity in noncompetitive assays not only increases sensitivity but does so using shorter incubation times than the original RIAs.[7] There is no need for expensive instrumentation because most assays can be read by spectrophotometry or by simply noting the presence or absence of color. Reagents are inexpensive and have a long shelf life. Although homogeneous assays are not as sensitive as heterogeneous assays, they are simple and require no separation step.

Disadvantages include the fact that some specimens may contain natural inhibitors. Additionally, the size of the enzyme label may be a limiting factor in the design of some assays. Nonspecific protein binding and the sensitivity of enzymes to temperature are other

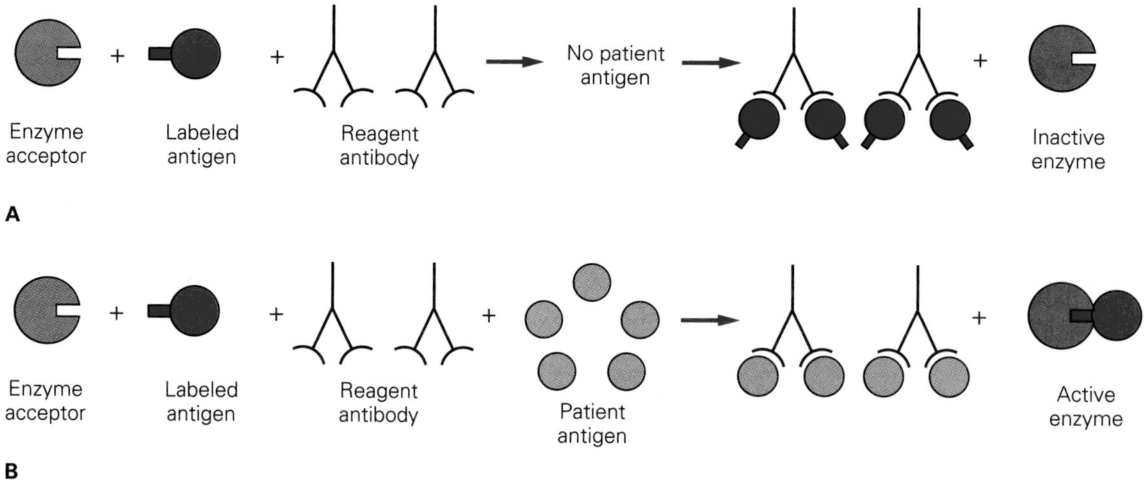

A

B

FIG. 11–7. Cloned donor enzyme immunoassay. Enzyme subunit, called the enzyme donor, is used as a label on antigen. If no patient antigen is present *(A)*, all the labeled antigen will bind and the enzyme cannot be reconstituted. If patient antigen is present, however, it will bind to antibody, allowing the enzyme to recombine.

difficulties encountered with the use of enzyme labels.[10] However, this technique has been successfully applied to a wide range of assays, and its use will continue to increase.

Fluorescent Immunoassay

In 1944 Albert Coons demonstrated that antibodies could be labeled with molecules that fluoresce.[13] These fluorescent compounds are called *fluorophores* or *fluorochromes*. They have the ability to absorb energy from an incident light source and convert that energy into light of a longer wavelength and lower energy as the excited electrons return to the ground state.[19] Fluorophores are typically organic molecules with a ring structure, and each has a characteristic optimum absorption range. The time interval between absorption of energy and emission of fluorescence is very short and can be measured in nanoseconds.[19]

Ideally, a fluorescent probe should exhibit high intensity, which can be distinguished easily from background fluorescence.[2] It should also be stable and have a high molar extinction coefficient.[5] The two compounds most often used are fluorescein and rhodamine, usually in the form of isothiocyanates because these can be readily coupled with antigen or antibody. Fluorescein absorbs maximally at 490 to 495 nm and emits a green color at 517 nm. It has a high intensity, good photostability, and a high quantum yield. Tetramethylrhodamine absorbs at 550 nm and emits red light at 580 to 585 nm. Because their absorbance and emission patterns differ, fluorescein and

rhodamine can be used together. Newer compounds that are beginning to be used are phycobiliproteins derived from algae, porphyrins, and chlorophylls, all of which exhibit red fluorescence at over 600 nm.[13]

Fluorescent tags or labels were first used for histochemical localization of antigen in tissues. This technique is called **immunofluorescent assay (IFA),** a term restricted to qualitative observations involving the use of a fluorescence microscope. In this manner, many types of antigens can be detected either in fixed tissue sections or live cell suspensions with a high degree of sensitivity and specificity. A short discussion of fluorescence microscopy is followed by coverage of newer developments using fluorescence in quantitative techniques.

Fluorescence Microscopy

A **fluorescence** microscope uses a light source that emits light in the appropriate wavelength necessary to excite the fluorochrome used. A high-intensity light source such as that of a tungsten halogen or mercury vapor arc lamp is usually used. Two filters are placed in the system. The first filter, located between the light source and the specimen, is used to remove wavelengths of light other than the one necessary to excite the fluorochrome. When this light strikes the specimen, the fluorochrome is excited and emits light at a new, longer wavelength. The second, or barrier, filter, placed between the specimen and the ocular lens, screens out light other than that produced by the fluorochrome. A typical fluorescence microscope is shown in Figure 11–8.

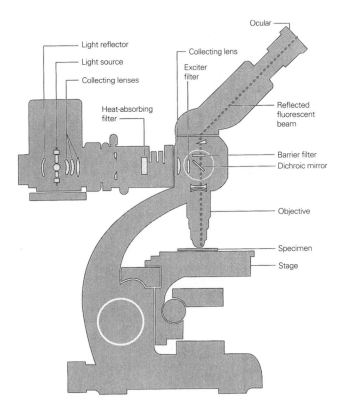

FIG. 11–8. Fluorescent microscope with epi-illumination. The light beam is directed through the exciter filter and down onto the specimen. A dichroic mirror allows passage of selected wavelengths in one direction but not another. After reaching the specimen, the light is reflected through the dichroic mirror, and emitted fluorescent light is visualized at the ocular. (From Stites, DP, Terr, AI, Parslow, TG et al: Medical Immunology, ed. 9. Appleton & Lange, Stamford, Conn., 1997, with permission.)

The presence of a specific antigen is determined by the appearance of localized color against a dark background. This method is used for rapid identification of microorganisms in cell culture or infected tissue, identification of tumor-specific antigens on neoplastic tissue, identification of transplantation antigens, and identification of CD antigens on T and B cells through the use of cell flow cytometry.[16] (See Chapter 3 for a more complete discussion of the principles of cell flow cytometry.)

Fluorescent staining can be categorized as direct or indirect, depending on whether or not the original antibody has a fluorescent tag attached. In a **direct immunofluorescent assay,** antibody that is conjugated with a fluorescent tag is added directly to unknown antigen that is fixed to a microscope slide. After incubation and a wash step, the slide is read using a fluorescence microscope. Antigens are typically visu-

alized as bright apple green or orange-yellow objects against a dark background. Direct immunofluorescent assay is best suited to antigen detection, while indirect assays can be used for both antigen and antibody identification.[14] Examples of antigens detected by this method include *Legionella pneumophila, Pneumocystis carinii, Chlamydia trachomatis,* and respiratory syncytial virus (RSV).[20]

Indirect immunofluorescent assays involve reaction of patient serum with a known antigen attached to a solid phase. The slide is washed, and an antihuman immunoglobulin containing a fluorescent tag is added. This combines with the first antibody in an adaptation of the antiglobulin technique of Coombs.[4] In this manner, one antibody conjugate can be used for many different types of reactions, eliminating the need for numerous purified, labeled reagent antibodies. Indirect assays result in increased staining because multiple molecules can bind to each primary molecule, thus making this a more sensitive technique.[13] Such assays are especially useful in antibody identification and have been used to detect treponema, antinuclear, chlamydial, and toxoplasma antibodies, as well as antibodies to viruses such as herpes simplex, Epstein-Barr, and cytomegalovirus, to cite some examples.[3,14,20] Figure 11–9 depicts the difference between the two techniques.

Both techniques allow for a visual assessment of the adequacy of the specimen. This is especially helpful in testing for chlamydia and RSV antigens.[20] Immunofluorescent assays in general, however, face the issue of subjectivity in the reading of slides. Only experienced clinical laboratorians should be responsible for reporting out slide results.

Heterogeneous Fluorescent Immunoassays

Quantitative fluorescent immunoassays (FIAs) can be classified as heterogeneous or homogeneous, corresponding to similar types of enzyme immunoassays. Heterogeneous assays, which require a separation step, include the following: indirect, competitive, and sandwich or capture assays.[19] These are based on the same principles as those of enzyme immunoassay (EIA), but in this case the label is fluorescent. Such a label can be applied to either antigen or antibody.

Use of solid phase is the typical means of separation in heterogeneous assays. Microbeads made of polysaccharides, polyacrylamides, or magnetizable cellulose particles have been used by a number of manufacturers. Either antigen or antibody can be attached to the beads and reacted with analyte and a fluorescent

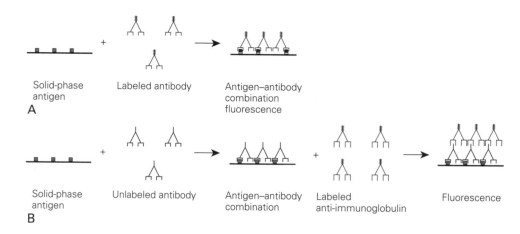

FIG. 11–9. Direct versus indirect immunofluorescent assays. *(A)* Direct fluorescent assay. Solid-phase antigen fixed to a microscope slide is incubated directly with a fluorescent-labeled antibody. The slide is washed to remove unbound antibody. If specific antigen is present in the patient sample, fluorescence will be observed. *(B)* Indirect fluorescence. Patient antibody is reacted with specific antigen fixed to a microscope slide. A wash step is performed, and a labeled antihuman immunoglobulin is added. After a second wash step to remove any uncombined anti-immunoglobulin, fluorescence of the sample is determined. The amount of fluorescence is directly in proportion to the amount of patient antibody present.

labeled analyte in a competitive or noncompetitive manner. Then the reaction mixture is centrifuged, the supernatant is discarded, and the beads are analyzed for fluorescence. In the case of magnetizable beads, rather than being centrifuged, the reaction tube is placed on a magnetic surface that attracts all the beads to the bottom of the tube.

Another type of solid phase used in fluorescent assays is the dipstick. This is coated with antigen or antibody and reacted with patient sample. A labeled antibody is then added. One side of the dipstick is not coated, and this can be used as a control to measure any nonspecific binding.

Solid-phase fluorescent assays have been developed for the identification of antibodies to nuclear antigen, toxoplasma antigen, rubella virus, and numerous other virus antigens.[19] In addition, heterogeneous fluorescent assays are used in detection of such important biologic compounds as cortisol, progesterone, and serum thyroxine (T4).[5]

Homogeneous Assays

Many of the newer developments in fluorescent immunoassay, however, have been related to homogeneous immunoassays. Homogeneous FIA, just like the corresponding EIAs, requires no separation procedure, so it is rapid and simple to perform. There is only one incubation step and no wash step, and usually competitive binding is involved. This basis for this technique is the change that occurs in the fluorescent label on antigen when it binds to specific antibody. Such changes may be related to wavelength emission, rotation freedom,

polarity, or dielectric strength. There is a direct relationship between the amount of fluorescence measured and the amount of antigen in the patient sample. As binding of patient antigen increases, binding of the fluorescent analyte decreases, and hence more fluorescence is observed.

Typically homogeneous assays, including enzyme assays, have suffered from a lack of sensitivity. Hence, most research has aimed at increasing sensitivity, and newer procedures have been developed that include fluorescence polarization immunoassay (FPIA), fluorescence excitation transfer immunoassay, and time-resolved fluorescence immunoassay. All of these require specific instrumentation. The principles of FPIA are discussed as a representative example of recently developed techniques.

Fluorescence Polarization Immunoassay

Fluorescence polarization immunoassay (FPIA) is based on the change in polarization of fluorescent light emitted from a labeled molecule when it is bound by antibody.[5] Incident light directed at the specimen is polarized with a lens or prism so the waves are aligned in one plane. If a molecule is small and rotates quickly enough, when it is excited by polarized light, the emitted light is unpolarized.[2,5] If, however, the labeled molecule is bound to antibody, the molecule is unable to tumble as rapidly, and it emits an increased amount of polarized light. Thus, the degree of polarized light reflects the amount of labeled analyte that is bound.

In FPIA, labeled antigens compete with unlabeled

antigen in the patient sample for a limited number of antibody binding sites. The more antigen that is present in the patient sample, the less the fluorescence-labeled antigen is bound and the less the polarization that will be detected. Hence, the degree of fluorescence polarization is inversly proportional to concentration of the analyte (Fig. 11–10).

This technique is limited to small molecules that tumble freely in solution, usually those analytes with a molecular weight under 20,000 d.[4,5,16] An additional consideration is nonspecific binding of the labeled conjugate to other proteins in serum. Binding to these molecules would increase polarization, thus falsely decreasing values.

This method has been used to determine concentrations of therapeutic drugs and hormones. It requires sophisticated instrumentation and is the basis for several automated analyzers on the market today.

Advantages and Disadvantages of Fluorescent Immunoassay

In principle, the use of fluorescence has the potential for increased sensitivity over radiolabels and enzyme reactions.[18] The methodology is fairly simple, and there is no need to deal with and dispose of hazardous substances. The main problem, however, has been separation of the signal on the label from background fluorescence because of different organic substances normally present in serum. Another difficulty encountered is the fact that nonspecific binding to substances in serum can cause quenching or diminishing of the signal and change the amount of fluorescence generated.[19] Any bilirubin or hemoglobin present can absorb either the excitation or emission energy. Fluorescence polarization has been developed to overcome some of these problems, and this technique has seen more widespread use.[2] It does, however, require expensive dedicated instrumentation, which may limit its use in smaller laboratories.

Chemiluminescent Immunoassays

Several recently developed immunoassays use the principle of chemiluminescence to follow antigen–antibody combination. **Chemiluminescence** is the emission of light caused by a chemical reaction producing an excited molecule that decays back to its original ground state.[18,21] A large number of molecules are capable of chemiluminescence, but some of the most common substances used are luminol, acridium esters, peroxyoxalates, ruthenium derivatives, and dioxetanes.[18,22] When these substances are oxidized, typically

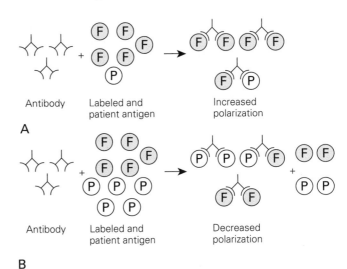

FIG. 11–10. Fluorescence polarization immunoassay. Reagent antibody is combined with patient antigen and fluorescent-labeled antigen. *(A)* If little or no patient antigen is present, antibody will bind to the labeled antigen. Binding causes these molecules to rotate more slowly in solution, increasing the amount of polarized light that they return. *(B)* When patient antigen is present, more labeled antigen will be unbound. These molecules will rotate more quickly in solution, giving off light in many directions, and polarization will be decreased.

using hydrogen peroxide and an enzyme for a catalyst, intermediates are produced that are of a higher energy state. These intermediates spontaneously return to their original state, giving off energy in the form of light.[21] Light emissions range from a rapid flash of light to a more continuous glow that can last for hours. Acridinium esters, for example, emit a quick burst or flash of light, while with luminol and dioxetane, the light remains for a longer time.[21] Different types of instrumentation are necessary for each kind of emission.

This type of labeling can be used for heterogeneous as well as homogeneous assays because labels can be attached to either antigen or antibody. In heterogeneous assays, competitive and sandwich formats are the ones most often used.[22] Smaller analytes such as therapeutic drugs and steroid hormones are measured using competitive assays, while the sandwich format is used for larger analytes such as protein hormones.

Advantages and Disadvantages of Chemiluminescent Assays

Chemiluminescent assays have an excellent sensitivity, comparable to EIA and RIA, and the reagents are stable and relatively nontoxic.[5,21,22] The sensitivity of some assays has been reported to be in the range of attamoles (10^{-18} mol) to zeptomoles (10^{-21} mol). Because very little reagent is used, they are also quite inexpensive to perform. The relatively high speed of detection also means a faster turnaround time. Detection systems basically consist of photomultiplier tubes, which are simple and relatively inexpensive.[22]

False results may be obtained, however, if there is lack of precision in injection of the hydrogen peroxide or if some biologic materials such as urine or plasma cause quenching of the light emission. This method has begun to be more widely applied to immunologic testing and has great potential for the future.

SUMMARY

Labeled immunoassays were developed to measure antigens and antibodies that may be small in size or present in very low concentrations. Labeling techniques include the use of radioactivity, enzymes, fluorescence, and chemiluminescence. The following constituents are a necessary part of most assays: labeled and unlabeled analytes, specific antibody, standards, a means of separation of bound and unbound label, and a means of detection of the bound label.

Antibodies used in immunoassays must be very specific and have a high affinity for the antigen in question. Specificity helps to cut down on cross-reactivity, and the affinity determines how stable the binding is between antigen and antibody. These two factors help to determine the sensitivity of such assays.

Bound and unbound label can be separated by several means. These include the use of absorbing particles such as charcoal, silica, or cellulose; a second antibody to precipitate out antigen–antibody complexes; and a solid phase, which uses a rigid medium, such as glass beads, cellulose membranes, polystyrene test tubes, or microtiter plates, to attach either antigen or antibody. The use of solid phase is the most popular method.

Radioimmunoassay was the first type of immunoassay to be applied to quantitative measurements of analytes in the clinical laboratory. The original technique was based on competition between labeled and unlabeled antigen for a limited number of antibody-binding sites. The more analyte that is present in the patient sample, the lower the amount of radioactivity that is detected.

A second type of radioimmunoassay called IRMA was developed using labeled antibody present in excess. After antigen–antibody combination takes place, the excess label is removed by solid-phase antigen, usually bound to glass beads. This noncompetitive method allows the entire unknown antigen to participate in the reaction, thus increasing the sensitivity of the assay.

Enzymes can be used as labels in much the same manner as radioactivity. Competitive assays involve the use of labeled analyte and a limited number of antibody-binding sites. Once separation of bound and unbound analyte has been achieved, substrate for the enzyme is added to the reaction mix, and the presence of the enzyme is detected by a color change in the substrate.

Most enzyme assays used in the laboratory today are noncompetitive assays. Often, it is antigen that is bound to solid phase and patient antibody that is being detected. After allowing sufficient time for binding to occur, a second enzyme-labeled antibody is added. The sensitivity of noncompetitive assays is greater than that of competitive assays.

Homogeneous enzyme assays require no separation step. They are based on the principle that enzyme activity changes as specific antigen–antibody binding occurs. When antibody binds to enzyme-labeled antigen, steric hindrance results in a loss in enzyme activity.

Fluorochromes are fluorescent compounds that are used as markers in immunologic reactions. Direct immunofluorescent assays involve antigen detection through a specific antibody that is labeled with a fluorescent tag. In indirect immunofluorescent assays, the original antibody is unlabeled. Incubation with antigen is followed by addition of a second labeled anti-immunoglobulin that detects antigen–antibody complexes.

Heterogeneous fluorescent immunoassays are similar to those described for other labels. Recent research has been directed toward improvement of homogeneous fluorescent immunoassays to reduce the background fluorescence normally found in serum. FPIA takes advantage of the fact that when an antigen is bound to antibody, polarization of light increases.

Chemiluminescence is the production of light energy by certain compounds when they are oxidized. Substances that do this can be used as markers in reactions that are similar to RIA and EIA.

Each type of system has advantages and disadvantages related to the particular nature of the label. Some are better for large multivalent antigens, while others are capable of detecting only small haptens. These limitations must be kept in mind in choosing the technique that is most sensitive and best suited for a particular analyte.

Case Study

1. A 2-year-old male child has symptoms that include fatigue, nausea, vomiting, and diarrhea. These symptoms have persisted for several days. Stool cultures for bacteria pathogens such as Salmonella and Shigella were negative. The stool was also checked for ova and parasites, and the results were negative. The day-care center that the child attends has had a previous problem with contaminated water, and the physician is suspicious that this infection might be caused by *Cryptosporidium,* a waterborne pathogen. However, because no parasites were found, he is not certain how to proceed.

Questions

   a. Does a negative finding rule out the presence of a parasite?

   b. What other type of testing could be done?

   c. How does the sensitivity of testing such as enzyme immunoassay compare with visual inspection of stained slides?

   d. What are other advantages of enzyme immunoassay tests?

Exercise: Enzyme Immunoassay Determination of Human Chorionic Gonadotropin

PRINCIPLE

Membrane cassette tests for pregnancy determination are one-step solid-phase enzyme immunoassays designed to detect the presence of hCG in urine or serum. hCG is a hormone, secreted by the trophoblast of the developing embryo, which rapidly increases in the urine or serum during the early stages of pregnancy. In a normal pregnancy, hCG can be detected in serum as early as 7 days following conception, and the concentration doubles every 1.3 to 2 days. It is subsequently excreted into the urine. Levels of hCG reach a peak of approximately 200,000 mIU/mL at the end of the first trimester.

Because the test cassette contains all necessary reagents, this is called immunochromatography. The test band region is precoated with antialpha hCG antibody to trap hCG as it moves through the membrane caused by capillary action. When the patient specimen is added, it reconstitutes an antibeta hCG antibody, which is complexed to colloidal gold particles. This complex is trapped by the antialpha hCG and forms a colored complex in the test region. This may be in the form of a straight line or a plus sign. A positive test results if a minimum concentration of approximately 25 mIU/mL is present. The control region contains a second antibody directed against the antibeta hCG antibody. This second antibody reacts with the excess antibeta hCG antibody gold particles to indicate that the test is working correctly.

SAMPLE PREPARATION

Serum, plasma, or urine may be used for testing. Any urine specimen may be used, but the first morning specimen is preferable because it is the most highly concentrated. Plasma collected with ethylenediaminetetra-acetic acid, heparin, or citrate may be used. Specimens may be stored for up to 72 hours at 2°C to 8°C. If specimens need to be held longer, freezing at 220°C is recommended. Freezing and thawing is not recommended.

REAGENTS, MATERIALS, AND EQUIPMENT

Test kit containing test cassettes
Marked pipettes or sample dispensers
Urine control
Serum control
Timer
NOTE: There are numerous kits on the market.

Examples are SureStep, QuickView, Concise, and Clearview.

PROCEDURE

1. Remove the test device from its protective pouch.
2. Allow the test device to equilibrate to room temperature.
3. Draw sample up to the mark on the pipette.
4. Dispense a certain number of drops or the entire contents of the pipette, depending on kit instructions.
5. Wait for the sample to completely run through the membrane.
6. Colored bands will usually appear in 1 to 3 minutes.
7. A colored band should also appear in the control region. If it does not, the test is invalidated.

RESULTS

A sample is positive if a line forms in the test region. A negative specimen will produce a line in the control region only. If no color develops in the control region, either the reagents are not active or the test procedure was incorrect.

INTERPRETATION OF RESULTS

The hCG hormone consists of two subunits, called alpha and beta. The beta subunit is unique to hCG, while the alpha subunit can be found in other hormones. In this test system, as soon as a patient sample containing hCG is added, it binds to monoclonal antibeta hCG antibody, which is complexed to an indicator such as colloid gold particles. The monoclonal antibody to the alpha portion of hCG on the cassette membrane binds the hCG complex as the patient sample travels along the membrane. A second antibody directed against the antibeta hCG antibody is bound in the control region.

False negatives caused by crossreactivity with other hormones such as luteinizing hormone and follicle-stimulating hormone are avoided through the use of monoclonal antibody that is directed against the β chain of hCG. Note that the actual procedure and reagents present will vary slightly with individual kits. This type of testing is a visual qualitative test only.

NOTE: There are numerous other kits on the market that can be used to demonstrate EIA reactions readily. Some of these are available for infectious agents such as *Streptococcus pyogenes* and *Streptococcus agalactiae*. Another alternative is an EIA kit that simulates HIV testing, available from Edvotek, Inc. (see Chapter 22 for the procedure).

1. Which of the following statements accurately describes competitive binding assays?
   a. Excess binding sites for the analyte are provided.
   b. Labeled and unlabeled analyte are present in equal amounts.
   c. The concentration of patient analyte is inversely proportional to bound radioactive label.
   d. All the patient analyte is bound in the reaction.

2. Which statement best describes how heterogeneous assays differ from homogeneous assays?
   a. Heterogeneous assays require a separation step.
   b. Heterogeneous assays are easier to perform than homogeneous assays.
   c. The concentration of patient analyte is directly proportional to bound label in homogeneous assays.
   d. Homogeneous assays are more sensitive than heterogeneous ones.

3. All of the following would be present in a labeled assay *except:*
   a. Specific antibody
   b. Standard that differs from the analyte
   c. Labeled analyte
   d. Means of detection of the label

4. In the following equation, what is the ratio of bound radioactive antigen (Ag★) to bound patient antigen (Ag)?

   12Ag ★ 1 4Ag 1 4Ab 9:___Ag ★ Ab 1___AgAb 1 Ag★ 1___Ag

   a. 1:4
   b. 1:3
   c. 3:1
   d. 8:4

5. Which of the following characterizes a capture enzyme assay?
   a. More sensitive than heterogeneous enzyme assays
   b. Requires two wash steps
   c. Best for high-molecular-weight substances
   d. Requires no separation step

6. How does cloned donor enzyme immunoassay differ from other types of enzyme immunoassays?
   a. It only detects large multivalent antigens.
   b. A wash step is necessary.
   c. Two enzyme subunits reassociate.
   d. It is a type of heterogeneous assay.

7. All of the following statements apply to sandwich assays *except:*
   a. Antigens with multiple epitopes are used.
   b. There are a limited number of antibody sites on the solid phase.
   c. Enzyme activity is directly proportional to the amount of antigen in the test sample.
   d. This technique can be used to measure immunoglobulins of a certain class.

8. Advantages of EIA over RIA include all *except* which one of the following?
   a. Decrease in hazardous waste
   b. Shorter shelf life of kit
   c. No need for expensive equipment
   d. Ease of adaptation to automated techniques

9. Which of the following is characteristic of direct fluorescent assays?
   a. The anti-immunoglobulin has the fluorescent tag.
   b. Antibody is attached to a solid phase.
   c. Microbial antigens can be rapidly identified by this method.
   d. The amount of color is in inverse proportion to the amount of antigen present.

10. Which of the following is true of fluorescence polarization immunoassay?
    a. Both antigen and antibody are labeled.
    b. Large molecules polarize more light than smaller molecules.
    c. When binding occurs, there is quenching of the fluorescent tag.
    d. The amount of fluorescence is directly proportional to concentration of the analyte.

11. All of the following are desirable characteristics of antibodies used in immunoassays *except:*
    a. High affinity
    b. High specificity
    c. High cross-reactivity
    d. Not found in the patient sample

12. All of the following are solid phase separation methods *except:*
    a. Precipitating antibody
    b. Glass beads
    c. Cellulose membranes
    d. Microtiter plates

References

1. Law, B, Malone, MD, and Biddlecomb, RA: Enzyme-linked immunosorbent assay (ELISA) development and optimization. In Law, B (ed): Immunoassay: A Practical Guide. Taylor and Francis, Bristol, Penn., 1996, pp 127–149.

2. Kricka, LJ: Principles of immunochemical techniques. In Burtis, CA, and Ashwood, ER (eds): Tietz Fundamentals of Clinical Chemistry, ed. 5, WB Saunders, Philadelphia, 2001, pp 177–194.

3. Mahoney, JB, and Chernesky, MA: Immunoassays for the diagnosis of infectious diseases. In Murray, PR, et al. (eds): Manual of Clinical Microbiology, ed. 7, American Society for Microbiology, Washington, D.C., 1999, pp 202–214.

4. Stites, DP, et al: Clinical laboratory methods for detection of antigens and antibodies. In Stites, DP, Terr, AI, and Parslow, TG (eds): Medical Immunology. Appleton & Lange, Stamford, Conn., 1997, pp 211–253.

5. Ashihara, Y, Kasahara, Y, and Nakamura, RM: Immunoassays and immunochemistry. In Henry, JB (ed): Clinical Diagnosis and Management by Laboratory Methods, ed. 20. WB Saunders, Philadelphia, 2001, pp 821–849.

6. Yalow, RS, and Berson, SA: Immunoassay of endogenous plasma insulin in man. J Clin Invest 39:1157, 1960.

7. Ekins, RP: Immunoassay, DNA analysis, and other ligand binding assay techniques: From electropherograms to multiplexed, ultrasensitive microarrays on a chip. J Chem Ed. 76:769–780, 1999.

8. Miles, CEM, and Hales, CN: Labelled antibodies and immunological assay systems. Nature 219:186, 1968.

9. Becker, S, and Border, BG. Clinical laboratory radioimmunoassay usage. CLS 11:9–12, 1998.

10. Carpenter, AB: Enzyme-linked immunoassays. In Rose, NR, et al (eds): Manual of Clinical Laboratory Immunology, ed. 5. American Society for Microbiology, Washington, D.C., 1997, pp 20–29.

11. Tang, YM, et al: Detection of Epstein-Barr virus-specific antibodies by an automated enzyme immunoassay: Performance evaluation and cost analysis. Diagn Microbiol Infect Dis 31:549–554, 1998.

12. Huber, KR, et al: Detection of HCV subtypes with a third-generation enzyme immunoassay. Hepatology 24:471–474, 1996.

13. Goldsby, RA, Kindt, TJ, and Osborne, BA: Kuby Immunology, ed. 4, WH Freeman and Co., New York, 2000, pp 159–163.

14. Koneman, EW, et al: Color Atlas and Textbook of Diagnostic Microbiology, ed. 5, Lippincott, Philadelphia, 1997, pp 33–43.

15. Peace-Brewer, AL, Craft, DW, and Schmitz, JL: Immunologic techniques in the clinical microbiology laboratory. Lab Med 31:24–29, 2000.

16. Henderson, CW: Reverse ELISA measures specific immunoglobulin E to major allergens. Vaccine Weekly, 06/14/2000–6/21/2000, p 16, 2000.

17. Slagle, KM, and Ghosn, SJ: Immunoassays: Tools for sensitive, specific, and accurate test results. Lab Med 27:177–183, 1996.

18. Persoon, T: Immunochemical assays in the clinical laboratory. Clinical Laboratory Science 5:31, 1992.

19. Nakamura, RM, and Bylund, DJ: Fluorescence immunoassays. In Rose, NR, et al (eds): Manual of Clinical Laboratory Immunology, ed. 5. American Society for Microbiology, Washington, D.C., 1997, pp 39–48.

20. Forbes, BA, Sahm, DF, and Weissfeld, AS: Bailey and Scott's Diagnostic Microbiology, ed. 10, Mosby, St. Louis, 1998, pp 214–216.

21. Kricka, LJ: Chemiluminescence immunoassays. In Rose, NR, et al (eds): Manual of Clinical Laboratory Immunology, ed. 5. American Society for Microbiology, Washington, D.C., 1997, pp 49–53.

22. Jandreski, MA: Chemiluminescence technology in immunoassays. Lab Med 29:555–560, 1998.

Molecular Biology Techniques

Learning Objectives

After finishing this chapter, the reader will be able to:
1. Describe the structure of deoxyribonucleic acid (DNA) and ribonucleic acid (RNA).
2. Discuss the primary function of each in the cell.
3. Explain what a nucleic acid probe is and how it is used.
4. Define hybridization and discuss the conditions that influence its specificity.
5. Differentiate dot-blot from a Southern blot.
6. Describe the role of restriction endonucleases in DNA analysis.
7. Explain the basis of DNA chip technology.
8. Discuss the principles of the polymerase chain reaction (PCR).
9. Differentiate target amplification from probe amplification and give examples of each.
10. Compare the relative advantages and disadvantages of amplification systems in general.
11. Correlate individual nucleic acid techniques with actual use in clinical settings.
12. Determine when nucleic acid technology is appropriate for clinical testing.

Key Terms

Branched chain signal
    amplification
Deoxyribonucleic acid
    (DNA)
Dot-blot
Gel electrophoresis
Hybridization
In situ hybridization
Ligase chain reaction (LCR)

Northern blot
Nucleic acid probe
Polymerase chain reaction
    (PCR)
Primer
Purine
Pyrimidine
Qβ replicase reaction
Restriction endonuclease

Restriction fragment length
    polymorphisms (RFLPs)
Ribonucleic acid (RNA)
Sandwich hybridization
Southern blot
Stringency
Transcription-mediated
    amplification (TMA)

Characteristics of Nucleic Acids

Molecular biology assays are powerful new tools used to gain information to aid in diagnosis and monitoring of disease. These techniques are based on the detection of specific nucleic acid sequences in microorganisms or particular cells. Tools used in biotechnology to identify unique nucleic acid sequences include enzymatic cleavage of nucleic acids, gel electrophoresis, enzymatic amplification of target sequences, and nucleic acid probes. All of these will be discussed in this chapter along with an overview of the structure and functions of deoxyribonucleic acid (DNA) and ribonucleic acid (RNA). Advantages and disadvantages of each type of detection method will be presented along with examples of use in actual clinical settings.

Composition of DNA and RNA

The two main types of nucleic acids are **deoxyribonucleic acid (DNA)** and **ribonucleic acid (RNA).** DNA carries the primary genetic information within chromosomes found in each cell. The entire sequence of the human genome is more than 3 billion DNA bases long.[1] It represents more than 100,000 genes, each of which is present in duplicate. DNA is what makes each individual unique.

RNA, on the other hand, is an intermediate that helps convert the genetic information into proteins that are the primary cellular structure. DNA acts as the template for synthesis of RNA. Both nucleic acids are polymers made up of repeating nucleotides, or bases, that are linked together to form long molecules. Each nucleotide consists of a cyclic, 5-carbon sugar, with a phosphate group at the 5' C, and one of four nitrogenous bases at the 1' C. The sugar deoxyribose is present in DNA, while ribose is the primary sugar found in RNA.

DNA and RNA have the same two **purine** bases, adenine and guanine, but the **pyrimidine** bases differ. DNA uses cytosine and thymine, while in RNA, uracil takes the place of thymine. DNA exists primarily as a double-stranded molecule with very specific base pair linkages: adenine pairs with thymine, and cytosine pairs with guanine. Any other combinations of base pairs are either too large or too small and do not fit together. The bases are found on the inside of the molecule, and the sugars are linked together via alternating phosphate groups to form the outside backbone. Nucleotides are joined together by phosphodiester bonds that link the

5' phosphate group of one sugar to the 3' hydroxyl group of an adjacent sugar.[2] The two strands are twisted into a so-called alpha helix (Fig. 12–1). Hydrogen bonding between adjacent bases holds the two chains together.

Replication of DNA

DNA is a very stable molecule, which makes it ideal for a clinical specimen. It loses its conformational structure only under extremes of heat, pH, or the presence of destabilizing agents.[2] Replication of the DNA molecule is very straightforward. It is characterized as a *semiconservative* process because one strand of the molecule acts as a template for creation of a complementary strand. Two daughter molecules result, each of which is an exact copy of the original molecule. This process can be artificially initiated in the laboratory because the hydrogen bonds that hold the two strands together are relatively weak.[3] The double helix can easily be separated or *denatured* by using heat or an alkaline solution. When heat is used to separate the strands, the process is known as *melting*. As the DNA strands are returned to normal physiological conditions, complementary strands spontaneously rejoin or *anneal*. It is these characteristics that are exploited in molecular testing.

Types of RNA

A single strand of DNA can also serve as a template for the production of messenger RNA. All forms of RNA are single stranded polymers with an irregular three-dimensional structure, and they are in much shorter lengths than DNA. Messenger RNA is used to translate the DNA code into making functional proteins. The two other types of RNA are transfer RNA, which transports different amino acids to make proteins, and ribosomal RNA, which acts as the site for protein synthesis directed by the messenger RNA. Generally, RNA is less stable than DNA because it is more susceptible to alkaline hydrolysis and is rapidly degraded by RNase enzymes found in abundance in the environment.[2] However, RNA can easily be replicated and is also used in molecular diagnostic techniques.

Nucleic Acid Probes

Spontaneous pairing of complementary DNA strands forms the basis for techniques that are used to detect

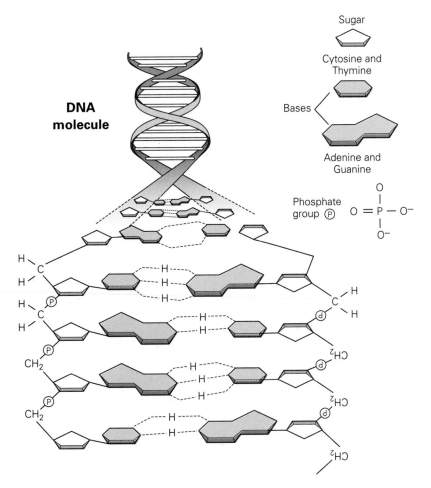

FIG. 12–1. DNA molecule. The double helix of the DNA is shown along with details of how the bases, sugars, and phospates connect to form the structure of the molecule. DNA is a double-stranded molecule twisted into a helix (think of a spiral staircase). Each spiraling strand, composed of a sugar-phosphate backbone and attached bases, is connected to a complementary strand by noncovalent hydrogen bonding between paired bases. The bases are adenine (A), thymine (T), cytosine (C), and guanine (G). A and T are connected by two hydrogen bonds. G and C are connected by three hydrogen bonds.

and characterize genes. Probe technology is typically the basis for identification of individual genes or DNA sequences. A **nucleic acid probe** is a short strand of DNA or RNA of a known sequence that is used to identify the presence of a complementary single strand of DNA in a patient specimen. Binding of two such complementary strands is known as **hybridization** and is very specific. Two DNA strands must share at least 16 to 20 consecutive bases of perfect complementarity to form a stable hybrid.[1] The probability of such a match occurring as a result of chance is less than 1 in 1 billion, so there is an extraordinary degree of specificity to this process.[1] Probes are labeled with a marker such as a radioisotope, a fluorochrome, an enzyme, or a chemiluminescent substrate to make detection of hybridization possible. Hybridization can take place either in a solid support medium or in solution.

Hybridization Techniques

Solid Support Hybridization

Dot-blot and **sandwich hybridizations** are the simplest types of solid support hybridization assays.[1] In the dot-blot assay, clinical samples are applied directly to a membrane surface. The membrane is heated to denature or separate DNA strands, and then labeled probes are added. After careful washing to remove any unhybridized probe, presence of remaining probe is detected by autoradiography or enzyme assays (Fig. 12–2). A positive result indicates presence of a specific gene sequence. This permits qualitative testing of a clinical specimen because it only indicates presence or absence of a particular genetic sequence. It is much easier to handle multiple samples in this manner.[4]

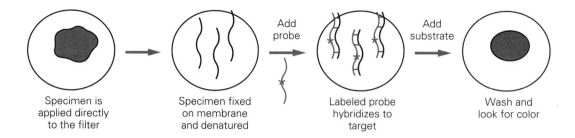

FIG. 12–2. Dot-blot hybridization assay.

However, there may be difficulty with the interpretation of weak positive reactions because there can be background interference.[5]

Sandwich hybridization is a modification of the dot-blot procedure. It was designed to overcome some of the background problems associated with the use of unpurified samples.[2] The technique uses two probes, one of which is bound to the membrane and serves to capture target sample DNA. The second probe anneals to a different site on the target DNA, and it has a label for detection. The sample nucleic acid is thus sandwiched in between the capture probe on the membrane and the signal-generating probe.[2] Because of the fact that two hybridization events must take place, specificity is increased. Sandwich hybridization assays have been developed using microtiter plates instead of membranes, which has made the procedure more adaptable to automation.[2]

To characterize DNA present in a patient sample in a more detailed fashion, enzymes called **restriction endonucleases** are often used. These enzymes cleave both strands of a double-stranded DNA at specific recognition sites that are approximately 4 to 6 base pairs long.[1] Human DNA may yield millions of unique fragments.[1] The resulting fragments are separated out on the basis of size and charge by a procedure known as **gel electrophoresis.** Digested cellular DNA from a patient blood or tissue sample is placed in wells in an agarose gel and covered with buffer. The molecules migrate through the gel under the influence of an electrical field, and they are separated on the basis of molecular weight. Smaller fragments migrate faster, while the larger fragments remain closer to the origin. The gel can either be stained with ethidium bromide and viewed under ultraviolet (UV) light to see the entire pattern of fragments, or specific nucleic acid sequences can be identified through the use of DNA probes (Fig. 12–3).

Differences in restriction patterns are referred to as **restriction fragment length polymorphisms (RFLPs).** This is caused by variations in nucleotides

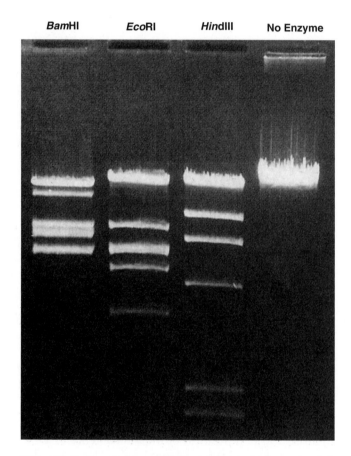

FIG. 12–3. Restriction analysis of bacteriophage lambda DNA. Three enzymes—BamH1, EcoRI, and HindIII—are used to cleave the DNA, and each produces a different pattern when the DNA is electrophoresed. Ethidium bromide is used to help visualize the DNA under UV light. (From Restriction Enzyme and DNA Kit, Carolina Biological Supply Company, Burlington, NC, with permission.)

within genes that change where the restriction enzymes cleave the DNA. When such a mutation occurs, different size pieces of DNA are obtained. Such patterns can be used to identify specific microorganisms, to establish strain relatedness, to detect polymorphisms in major histocompatibility complex (MHC) genes, or to obtain a DNA fingerprint of a particular individual.[6]

Analysis of DNA fragments using probes is typically carried out using a technique known as a Southern hybridization assay or **Southern blot,** named after its discoverer, E.M. Southern. After DNA fragments are separated out by gel electrophoresis, the pieces are denatured using alkali and transferred to a nitrocellulose or nylon membrane for the hybridization reaction to take place. The transfer is accomplished by placing the membrane on top of the gel and allowing the buffer plus DNA to wick up into it. Traditionally, this procedure takes overnight, but newer methods using vacuum and pressure systems have significantly speeded up the transfer.[2]

Once the DNA is on the nitrocellulose membrane filter, heating or using UV light to crosslink the strands onto the membrane immobilizes it. A labeled probe is then added to the membrane for hybridization to take place. Probes are typically added in excess so that as target molecules reanneal, they are more likely to attach to probes rather than the original complementary single stranded partner. The membrane is then washed, and the amount of bound probe remaining is determined by detection of the label (Fig. 12–4). Several nonradiolabeled probes, including enzyme and acridinium labels, have been developed for use, and these appear to be as sensitive as the original radiolabeled probes. They avoid the hazards associated with use of radioactivity.[7] The absence of any visible bands indicates an absence of any complementary sequences.

Southern blots have been used to determine the clonal composition of lymphocyte populations. Only when a large number of cloned cells are present do rearranged genes specific for T cell receptors or immunoglobulins appear in sufficient quantity to produce a detectable band that is different from the normal or germ-line DNA. This is typically an indicator of a lymphoid malignancy such as B cell lymphoma, chronic myelogenous leukemia, or hairy cell leukemia.[1,4] Detection of clonality, or identical DNA, can help distinguish between reactive lymphocytes seen in an inflammatory process and true malignancies. DNA testing is especially helpful in both diagnosis and classification of T cell malignancies.[4] It has had a tremendous impact on diagnosis of non-Hodgkin's lymphomas.[8] Molecular testing can also be used to monitor therapy and remission of lymphomas. If tissue from separate lymphomatous lesions are from the same original source, they usually show identical DNA rearrangements and produce identical bands on a Southern blot.[1]

In general, however, Southern blots are complex, time-consuming to perform, and require a relatively large sample.[5] Controls such as a known lambda phage DNA must be used to monitor the activity of restric-

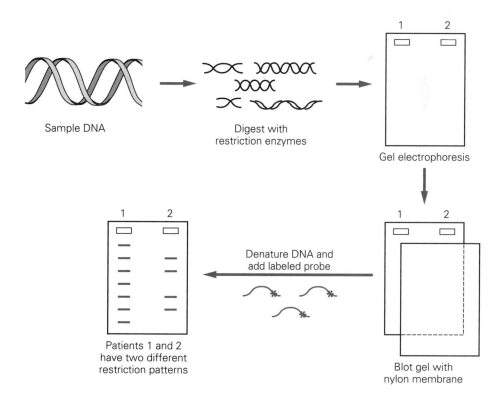

Sample DNA

Digest with restriction enzymes

Gel electrophoresis

Blot gel with nylon membrane

Denature DNA and add labeled probe

Patients 1 and 2 have two different restriction patterns

FIG. 12–4. Southern blot.

tion enzymes and provide molecular markers to evaluate electrophoretic separation.[2] For these reasons, they have limited clinical application.

Northern blots are performed in a similar manner, but in this case it is RNA that is extracted and separated. This technique is used most often to determine the level of expression of a particular messenger RNA species to see if a gene is actually being expressed.[2] Because RNA is a short, single-stranded molecule, it does not have to be digested before electrophoresis, but it has to be denatured to ensure that it is in an unfolded, linear form. Probes are then used to identify the presence of specific bands.

Solution Hybridization

Hybridization assays can also be performed in a solution phase. In this type of setting, both the target nucleic acid and the probe are free to interact in a reaction mixture, and the sensitivity tends to be higher than that of solid support hybridization.[5] It also requires a smaller amount of sample, although the sensitivity is improved when target DNA is extracted and purified.[5]

For solution hybridizations, the probe must be single-stranded and incapable of self-annealing.[4] Several unique detection methods exist. In one of these, an S1 nuclease is added to the reaction mix. This will only digest unannealed or single stranded DNA, leaving the hybrids intact. Double-stranded DNA can then be recovered by precipitation with trichloroacetic acid or by binding it to hydroxyapatite columns.[4,9]

A second and less technically difficult means of solution hybridization is the hybridization protection assay. For this assay, a chemiluminescent acridium ester is attached to a probe. After the hybridization reaction takes place, the solution is subjected to alkaline hydrolysis, which hydrolyzes the chemiluminescent ester if the probe is not attached to the target molecule. If the probe is attached to the target DNA, the ester is protected from hydrolysis. Probes that remain bound to a specific target sequence give off light when exposed to a chemical trigger such as hydrogen peroxide at the end of the assay.

Solution phase hybridization assays are fairly adaptable to automation, especially those using chemiluminescent labels. Assays can be performed in a few hours.[4] However, low positive reactions are difficult to interpret because of the possibility of cross-reacting target molecules.[9]

In Situ *Hybridization*

In situ **hybridization** represents a third type of hybridization reaction in which the target nucleic acid is found in intact cells. It provides information about the presence of specific DNA targets and their distribution in the tissues. For probes to reach the nucleic acid, they must be small enough, usually limited to 500 bases or less, to penetrate the cells in question.[4] Formalin-fixed and paraffin-embedded tissue sections are typically used for this procedure. Because preparation of tissue specimens can vary greatly in each lab, it is recommended that an endogenous control probe be used.[5] This is a probe that will react positively with all cells and is used to indicate that penetration of the sample has occurred.

Probes have typically been labeled with radioactive substances, but the trend today is toward using fluorescent or enzyme labels. If a fluorescent tag is used, the procedure is called fluorescent *in situ* hybridization, or *FISH*. After completion of the procedure, evaluation should be performed by an experienced histopathologist.[5] This technique is used to detect a number of malignancies linked to chromosomal abnormalities, such as chronic myelogenous leukemia, in which there is a translocation from chromosome 9 to chromosome 22.

DNA Chip Technology

Biochips, also called microarrays, are very small devices used to examine DNA, RNA, and other substances. These chips allow thousands of biological reactions to be performed at once.[10] Typically, a biochip consists of a small rectangular solid surface that is made of glass or silicon with short DNA or RNA probes anchored to the surface.[11] The number of probes on a biochip surface can vary from 10 to 20 up to hundreds of thousands.[10,11] Usually, the nucleic acid in the sample is amplified before applying it to the probe. After amplification, the sample is labeled with a fluorescent tag, and it is loaded onto the chip. Hybridization is allowed to take place, and the surface of the chip allows thousands of hybridization reactions all at one time. Unbound strands of the target sample are then washed away. The hybridized sample nucleic acid remaining is detected by exciting the fluorescent tags with a laser, and then determining fluorescence emission with an optical scanner[10] (Fig. 12–5). The intensity of the signal at a particular location indicates a match at a particular locus. Complete sequence matches give a bright patch of fluorescence. Single-base mismatches give a dimmer signal. These indicate a point mutation. Detection of point mutations can be used for classification of leukemias, molecular staging of tumors, and characterization of microbial agents.[12] One prime example is the determination of genes associated with drug resistance in human immunodeficiency virus (HIV) testing.

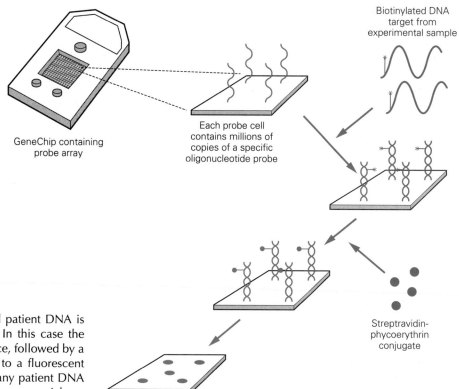

Biotinylated DNA
target from
experimental sample

Each probe cell
contains millions of
copies of a specific
oligonucleotide probe

GeneChip containing
probe array

Streptravidin-
phycoerythrin
conjugate

Fluorescence

FIG. 12–5. Analysis of HIV-I. Labeled patient DNA is placed on the biochip or microarray. In this case the label is biotin. Hybridization takes place, followed by a washing step. Strepavidin conjugated to a fluorescent dye is added. This will complex with any patient DNA present. The resulting fluorescent pattern can pick up mutations associated with drug resistance.

Identification of such genes guides the physician in selecting a proper drug regimen for a particular patient.

Drawbacks of Hybridization Techniques

In any of the previously mentioned hybridization techniques, conditions of the reaction itself may determine how sensitive and specific the technique is. Under the conditions in which most assays are conducted, two nucleic acid strands must share at least 16 to 20 consecutive bases of perfect complementarity to form a stable hybrid.[12] **Stringency,** or correct pairing, is most affected by the salt concentration, the temperature, and the concentration of destabilizing agents such as formamide or urea. Decreasing the salt concentration, increasing the temperature, and increasing the concentration of formamide or urea all help to ensure that only the most perfectly matched strands will remain paired in a stable helix. If the conditions are not carefully controlled, however, mismatches can occur, and the results will not be valid.

In addition, even under carefully controlled conditions, often the amount of nucleic acid in a patient specimen may present in very low quantity, which may be below the threshold for probe detection. The sensitivity can be increased by means of several amplification techniques. These fall into three general categories:

target amplification, probe amplification, and signal amplification. Each of these will be discussed and relevant clinical examples given.

Target Amplification

Target amplification systems are *in vitro* methods for the enzymatic replication of a target molecule to levels at which it can be readily detected.[5] This allows the target sequence to be identified and further characterized. There are numerous different types of target amplification. Examples include polymerase chain reaction (PCR), transcription mediated amplification (TMA), strand displacement amplification (SDA), and nucleic acid sequence-based amplification (NASBA) Two of these, PCR and TMA will be discussed in more detail. Of these, PCR is the best known and has the widest clinical application.[6]

Polymerase Chain Reaction

The **polymerase chain reaction (PCR)** is capable of amplifying tiny quantities of nucleic acid up to levels that can be detected by hybridization with nucleic acid probes. Kary Mullis was awarded the Nobel Prize in 1993 for the discovery of this technique. Cells, typically white blood cells, are separated out and lysed, and the double-stranded DNA is separated into single strands. **Primers,** or small segments of DNA no more than 20 to 30 nucleotides long, are added. Primers are complementary to segments of opposite strands that flank the target sequence. Only the segments of the target DNA between the primers will be replicated.

Each cycle of PCR basically consists of three steps: (1) denaturation of the target DNA to separate the two strands, (2) an annealing step in which the reaction mix is cooled to allow primers to anneal to the target sequence, and (3) an extension reaction in which the primers initiate DNA synthesis using a DNA polymerase.[5] These three steps constitute a thermal cycle.

High heat (95°C) is used to denature or dissociate double-stranded DNA, and then the reaction mix is cooled to anneal DNA strands, coupling primers to single strands. Two specific hybridization events take place, using two different oligonucleotide primers.[13] These are synthesized to be complementary to two annealing sites within the two different DNA strands. Each one initiates DNA synthesis toward the annealing site for the primer on the opposite strand. These two sites must be in a reasonable proximity to each other.[13] The usual span between primers is between 50 and 1500 nucleotide bases.[5] Annealing of primers is carried out at 55°C. Once primers have attached, a temperature of 72°C is used to allow the four nucleotide bases in solution to pair in a very specific manner and complete the strand between the primers. The DNA polymerase used adds nucleotides to the 3^1 end of each primer.

Each PCR cycle results in a doubling of target sequences, and typically the reaction is allowed to run through 30 cycles.[5,6] One cycle takes approximately 60 to 90 seconds, so the entire process is very fast. The resulting DNA fragments, referred to as the *amplicon,* are detected by using labeled nucleic acid probes. In this manner, a target sequence present at fewer than 100 copies can be detected.[14]

Originally, new DNA polymerase had to be added for each new cycle. Performing the reaction was greatly simplified when a thermostable DNA polymerase was discovered. The DNA polymerase used is from *Thermus aquaticus,* an organism that grows in hot springs in a temperature of 70°C to 75°C.[5] The enzyme, known as Taq polymerase, is able to withstand the repeated 95°C thermocycling in a PCR reaction.

PCR is an extremely sensitive technique that is used to amplify a target sequence present in low abundance. It is often used for organisms such as viruses that are hard to grow in the laboratory, and it is so sensitive that it can actually detect nonreplicating viral genomes. One of the major uses for PCR is in testing for the presence of HIV. Because HIV is an RNA virus, an initial enzyme, reverse transcriptase, must be added to convert the original RNA into DNA. This is known as reverse transcriptase PCR (RT-PCR). A blood sample of only 1 to 2 mL is sufficient to perform this test, making it ideal for testing neonates.[15] It is also useful in detecting infected individuals during the window period before antibody appears, in predicting prognosis, and in monitoring treatment.[15–18]

RT-PCR is also considered the gold standard for detection and monitoring therapy in infection with hepatitis C virus.[19] Additional uses for PCR include identification of *Mycobacterium tuberculosis* and to diagnose early initial infection with cytomegalovirus (CMV).[19]

Another important use of PCR in immunology is the identification of human leukocyte antigens (HLAs) for tissue transplantation, especially bone marrow transplantation in which the nature of the match determines the success or failure of the transplant. PCR is used to amplify HLA gene sequences so that donors and recipients can be matched at the allele level.[19,20] This is especially helpful in identification of polymorphisms at the HLA DP locus, which is specifically related to graft versus host reactivity in bone marrow transplants. HLA typing for class I antigens had traditionally been done using serologic methods, but this was not helpful in identification of HLA class II antigens. It has been reported that at least 25 percent of serologically identified class II antigens were incorrectly identified.[4] Matching of class II antigens at the allelic level has proved to increase the success rate of bone marrow transplants.[20]

HLA antigens can be identified by PCR using several different methods. *Sequence specific oligonucleotide probe hybridization (SSOPH)* creates millions of copies of HLA genes in a test tube using a generic primer for the whole region.[4,21] The amplified DNA is then tested with a series of probes. The level of resolution is controlled by the choice and number of probes used in testing.[21] Numerous probes are required for clear resolution of HLA antigens to the allele level. This is currently the most commonly used method for DNA-based typing.[21] It is used for high resolution typing by the National Marrow Donor Program registry.

A second method, called sequence specific primer typing, uses only PCR to identify specific HLA alleles. There are unique primer pairs for each gene locus, so when electrophoresis is done, presence of a band indicates that gene is there.[4] The PCR product can also be subjected to direct sequence base typing to detect exact alleles present. The latter is more complex and more expensive.

The activity of cytokines (see Chapter 6) can also be measured using PCR. Because cytokines tend to have a short half-life, identification of messenger RNA is a more sensitive method of determining cytokine production. RT-PCR is a highly sensitive method that requires only a few hours to perform and needs only a nanogram of total RNA. Measurement of cytokines is a very new field and has great potential for monitoring and treating a number of hematologic diseases.

The extreme sensitivity of PCR can be detrimental, however, because carryover from prior DNA samples may cause false-positive results. A single molecule can cause sample contamination if amplicon is aerosolized.[9] PCR also requires many manual steps, so it is time-consuming and costly. However, the availability of reagents in kit form and the lower cost of oligonucleotide probes has led to increased use of this method.[5] Although it may not be suitable for routine screening, when used as an adjunct to standard testing, PCR may be extremely helpful. It will probably play a larger role in diagnosis as further refinements are made.

False-positives can be decreased by physically separating areas for sample preparation from the amplification process itself. UV light can be used to inactivate DNA within a hood and on pipettes, test tubes, and reaction mixes.[9] Additionally, the use of negative controls is essential.

Transcription-Mediated Amplification

Transcription-mediated amplification (TMA) was the first non-PCR amplification system developed.[13] It is an isothermal RNA amplification system that uses two enzymes to drive the reaction: an RNA polymerase and a reverse transcriptase.[22] In addition, two primers are used to target a particular nucleic acid sequence. One of the primers contains a promotor sequence for RNA polymerase.

The first step is to produce a DNA template for RNA transcription by hybridizing the promotor-primer to the target rRNA at a particular site. Reverse transcriptase creates a DNA copy, called cDNA, of the target rRNA. The original RNA strand is destroyed by the RNase activity of the reverse transcriptase. A new strand of DNA is synthesized from the DNA copy, thus making a double-stranded DNA molecule. RNA polymerase recognizes the promotor sequence in the DNA template and begins transcription of up to 40 copies[13] (Fig. 12–6).

Each newly synthesized RNA molecule can serve as a template for a new round of replication. This initiates an autocatalytic cycle in which up to 10 billion RNA

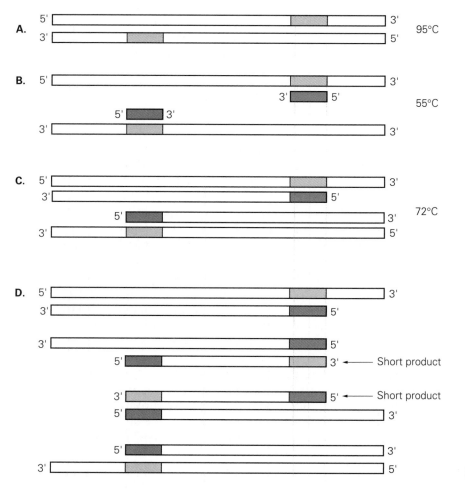

FIG. 12–6. Principles of PCR.

molecules can be transcribed from the DNA template in less than 1 hour.[4,22,23] Applications include detection of *Chlamydia trachomatis, Mycobacterium tuberculosis, Mycobacterium avium,* and HIV-1.[13,14,24,25]

Probe Amplification

Qβ Replicase

Rather than directly amplifying the target, there are several techniques that amplify the detection molecule or probe instead of the target molecule itself. Two of these are the Qβ replicase reaction and the ligase chain reaction. The **Qβ replicase reaction** uses an RNA-directed RNA polymerase that replicates the genomic RNA of a bacteriophage named Qβ. The RNA genome of Qβ is essentially the only substrate recognized by the polymerase.[13] Because a short probe can be inserted into the Qβ RNA, this becomes the system used for amplification. This short sequence probe is selected to be very specific for the target molecule of interest.

After the probe has annealed to the target, unbound probe is treated with RNase and washed away. The hybridized probe is RNase resistant. When Qβ replicase is added, the probe is enzymatically replicated to detectable levels.[13] Because occasional nonspecific hybridization may occur, this technique is subject to higher background signals than other methods.[13] However, the technique is easy to perform because all phases are carried out at room temperature, and the amount of replication approaches 10^9 in approximately 30 minutes. This system has been used for detection of *Chlamydia trachomatis* and HIV-1.[14]

Ligase Chain Reaction

DNA ligase amplification, or the **ligase chain reaction (LCR),** patented by Abbott Laboratories, represents the second main type of probe amplification technique.[26] A DNA ligase enzyme is a repairing enzyme that links preexisting DNA strands together by joining the 5' end of one to the 3' end of another strand.[1] In this case, the enzyme is used to join two pairs of oligonucleotide probes only after they have bound to the complementary target sequence, which will hold them in precise end-to-end alignment.[1] Each pair of probes must hybridize to opposite ends (3' and 5') of the target DNA molecule. Once the probes are in place, the ligase joins the two together. After this has occurred, each linked pair of probes can be made single-stranded and then act as a template for ligation

of additional probes (Fig. 12–7). The thermostable ligase enzyme from *T aquaticus* remains active throughout the thermal cycling process. This technique has been used for detection of *Borrelia burgdorferi, Mycobacteria species,* and *Neisseria gonorrhoeae.*[13]

Ligation reactions are very specific because a single base pair mismatch at the junction of oligonucleotides keeps ligation from occurring.[2] LCR is also more adaptable to automation than PCR. Disadvantages, however, include the possibility of blunt end ligation of probes without the target being present. Thus, the exact sequence of the region to be amplified must be known to help prevent false-positive results from occurring. Generally, probes used in LCR are also more expensive to produce than PCR primers.[2]

Signal Amplification

The last major type of amplification replicates the signal rather than either the target or the probe. This technique is based on the reporter group (the labeled tag) being attached in greater numbers to the probe molecule or increasing the signal intensity generated by each labeled tag.[13] Because the patient nucleic acid itself is not replicated or amplified, this type of technique is less prone to product contamination. However, the sensitivity is generally lower than for enzyme amplification methods, so it may have a more limited use in cases of low numbers of target copies.[13]

Perhaps the best known of the signal amplification methods is called **branched chain signal amplification** developed by Chiron Corporation. This technique employs several simultaneous hybridization steps. It has been compared to decorating a Christmas tree, and involves several sandwich hybridizations. In the first step, target specific oligonucleotide probes capture the target sequence to a solid support. Then a second set of target specific probes called extenders hybridize to adjoining sequences and act as binding sites for a large piece called the branched amplification multimer. Each branch has multiple side branches and is capable of binding numerous labeled oligonucleotides. In fact, as many as 3000 enzyme labels can be incorporated onto each target molecule.[13] This type of detection system is fairly sensitive, with a range of 10^3 to 10^5 target molecules.[13]

Branched chain systems are well suited to detection of nucleic acid target with sequence heterogeneity, such as hepatitis C and HIV, because if one or two of the capture or extender probes fail to hybridize, the signal-generating capacity is not lost as a result of the presence of several remaining probe complexes. Additionally, the

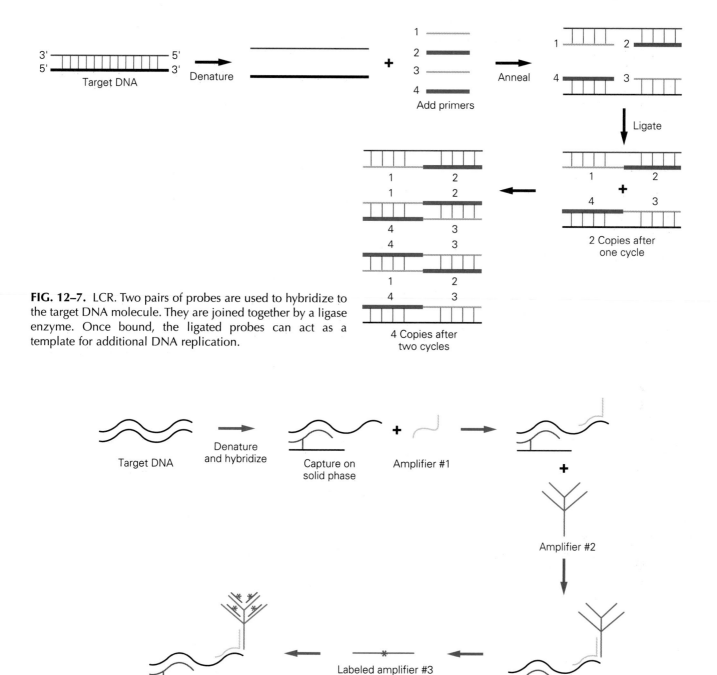

FIG. 12–7. LCR. Two pairs of probes are used to hybridize to the target DNA molecule. They are joined together by a ligase enzyme. Once bound, the ligated probes can act as a template for additional DNA replication.

FIG. 12–8. Branched chain amplification. Several different probes are used to amplify the signal rather than the target DNA itself. The first probe captures the target. Amplifier 1 binds in a different place and forms the base for amplifier 2, the branched chain. Amplifier 3 contains the signal.

need for several independent probe-target hybridization events provides a great deal of specificity. The danger of false-positive results caused by carryover of target material is decreased because the target itself is not amplified. However, nonspecific localization of reagents can result in background amplification.[2] Assays for hepatitis B and C, HIV-1, and CMV have been developed using this method.[13] A new version of the system used to identify HIV-1 is able to detect the presence of low levels of the virus.[18] It has been validated for the quantitation of viral load testing of all the subtypes. Therefore, this technique can be used for quantitation and to help monitor the therapeutic response.

Drawbacks of Amplification Systems

Amplification systems in general are subject to several potential problems. The greatest of these is the potential for false-positive results caused by contaminating nucleic acids. In the case of PCR and LCR, DNA products are the main source of contamination. For Qβ replicase and TMA, RNA products are the possible contaminants. Therefore, there is a need for employing some form of product inactivation as a part of a quality control program.[13] Separating sample preparation areas from amplification areas and the use of inactivation systems such as UV light help to alleviate contamination. Additionally, as more automation is developed for amplification, closed systems will cut down considerably on contamination and labor costs.[27]

The exquisite sensitivity of these techniques can present a problem in that very small numbers of pathogens present may not be significant. There is also the possibility that inhibiting substances in clinical specimens may affect enzymatic amplification methods and cause false-negative reactions.

Future of Molecular Diagnostic Techniques

In spite of these technical problems and the fact that nucleic acid amplification can be costly and labor-intensive, there are many instances in which rapid diagnosis may prove invaluable. For example, rapid identification of mycobacteria may actually save money by eliminating the need for unnecessary respiratory isolation for patients suspected of having tuberculosis.[13] Detection of multi-drug resistant strains of *Mycobacterium tuberculosis* may lead to more timely public health control measures. Identification of genes for antimicrobial resistance in other organisms will help in more effective treatment for severe infections.[14] In general, the increased information on slow-growing or nonculturable organisms, which can be obtained in a more rapid fashion, will have a major effect on patient management.

In addition to direct detection of microorganisms, there are numerous applications in immunology and hematology. Molecular HLA typing has revolutionized histocompatibility testing.[4] The impact on class II typing has resulted in a significant decrease in morbidity and mortality in bone marrow transplants. Hematologic diseases can also be followed more easily now, and molecular technology likely will influence treatment choices in acute leukemia cases.[4]

The problem of contamination is beginning to be addressed in numerous ways. Several closed systems have been developed so that both amplification and detection take place in the same test tube. These newer techniques are also more suitable to automation. This will bring labor costs down considerably. As diagnostic kits and reagents become more widely available, use of these techniques will increase.

The increased specificity and sensitivity of molecular testing will become the standard of practice in immunology and microbiology. Rapid turn around time plus increasing automation will bring down the cost and allow such techniques to be used in smaller hospitals in addition to the larger medical centers. Molecular techniques will not replace culture for those organisms that are easily grown and identified in the laboratory, nor will it replace hematologic procedures that are standardized and efficient. However, for esoteric organisms and diseases, molecular techniques will most likely replace serologic techniques that are subject to cross-reactivity and the unpredictability of the antibody response in individual patients.

SUMMARY

The unique characteristics of DNA and RNA make them ideal tools to use as diagnostic indicators of disease. Both are made up of nucleotides that occur in very specific sequences in different cells and microorganisms. They can be used to determine the presence of microorganisms, particular genes that would indicate cancerous or precancerous states, and much more. DNA exists as a double-stranded molecule with very specific base pair linkages: Adenine pairs with thymine, and guanine pairs with cytosine. When the DNA molecule is replicated, the strands are separated, and a new strand is created that is exactly complementary to the parent strand. This exact base pairing forms the basis for identification of unknown sequences through the use of known short nucleic acid sequences called probes. Hybridization is the pairing of a probe with a complementary DNA strand. The probe is labeled with a marker for detection. Dot-blots and sandwich hybridization techniques are used to directly identify specific sequences in patient samples.

Detailed characterization of DNA can be accomplished through the use of enzymes called restriction endonucleases that cleave DNA at specific recognition sites. Then when the DNA is electrophoresed, the resulting fragments can be separated on the basis of size. Individuals or specific microorganisms can be identified on the basis of unique patterns obtained, called RFLPs. If the resulting electrophoretic pattern is transferred to a membrane for use in hybridization, this is known as a Southern blot. Northern blots involve separation of RNA in a similar manner.

Hybridization of probes with target nucleic acids can also take place in solution or in intact cells. The hybridization protection assay is an example of the former. The label on the probe is only protected from degradation if it is attached to the target nucleic acid. If intact cells or tissue is used, this is called *in situ* hybridization.

DNA chips represent a microenvironment in which thousands of hybridization reactions are possible. Chips are used to identify particular strains of viruses such as HIV, in addition to determining resistance to particular therapeutic drugs.

If there is not enough nucleic acid in a specimen to positively identify it, amplification methods can be used to increase either the target or the detection system. Polymerase chain reaction (PCR) is the most widely used method of target amplification. Specific primers coupled with a thermostable DNA polymerase are used to make copies of the original DNA strands. Each cycle results in a doubling of a specific target sequence, and approximately 30 cycles produce millions of copies of the original molecules. This technique is used clinically to identify viruses such as hepatitis B, hepatitis C, and

HIV, and to perform HLA typing and measurement of cytokine activity.

Transcription-mediated amplification (TMA) is another target amplification method based on the use of a DNA template to make numerous RNA copies of the target sequence. *Chlamydia trachomatis, Mycobacterium tuberculosis, Mycobacterium avium,* and HIV are some examples of microorganisms identified by this method.

Probes rather than target nucleic acid can be amplified by the Qβ replicase reaction and the ligase chain reaction (LCR). Qβ replicase uses an RNA-directed RNA polymerase to replicate a small piece of RNA that contains the probe sequence. The LCR actually splices two DNA probes together to make a single strand copy of the target nucleic acid sequences.

Signal amplification is another means of detecting small amounts of target nucleic acid. The branched chain method uses a series of hybridization steps, including a capture probe, an extender probe, and a multimer probe to enhance the signal to a detectable level.

All amplification techniques are subject to false-positive reactions resulting from either contamination with previously amplified products or background reactivity. In addition, quality control procedures and laboratory standardization need to be developed. However, molecular techniques are exceedingly specific and rapid and will eventually replace serologic techniques for identification of organisms that are difficult to culture and antigens such as HLA, in which small differences must be distinguished.

Exercise: Gel Electrophoresis of DNA

PRINCIPLE

This experiment will demonstrate the use of restriction enzymes to cleave DNA from the bacteriophage lambda (48,502 base pairs in length). The resulting fragments will be separated out using gel electrophoresis. The three restriction endonucleases used are: BamHI, EcoRI, and HindIII. BamHI and HindIII are from *Haemophilus influenzae,* and EcoRI is from *Escherichia coli*. Three sample tubes of lambda DNA are prepared and incubated at 37°C with one of the enzymes in each tube. A fourth tube, the negative control, is incubated without an endonuclease.

The DNA samples are then loaded into wells of an agarose gel and electrophoresed. An electrical field applied across the gel causes the DNA fragments in the samples to migrate through the gel toward the positive electrode. The smaller DNA fragments migrate faster than the larger ones. Each enzyme will produce a different set of bands, representing different size fragments. Only one band should be produced from the control tube, in which no enzymatic digestion took place. The resulting pattern for each is called a DNA fingerprint. After electrophoresis, a compound that binds to DNA is used the make the bands visible. A Polaroid camera can be used to make a permanent record of the results.

SAMPLE PREPARATION

Dehydrated DNA is reconstituted by adding distilled or deionized water. The dehydrated DNA and enzymes used in the kit can be stored at room temperature for up to 2 years. DNA and the enzymes are not of human origin, but they should be handled using standard safety precautions.

REAGENTS, MATERIALS, AND EQUIPMENT

Kit from Carolina Biological Supply Company, which contains the following:

Vials of lambda DNA
6 vials BamHI
6 vials EcoRI
6 vials HindIII
6 vials loading dye
6 control reaction tubes

Tris-borate-ethylenediaminetetra-acetic acid (TBE) buffer concentrate
6 staining trays
15 1.5 mL tubes
Agarose (3.2 grams for 400 mL)
Floating tube rack

Additional equipment needed:

Micropipettors (0–10 μL or 0–20 μL)
Micropipet tips
Gel electrophoresis chambers and power supplies
Boiling water bath or microwave oven
Water bath at 60°C
Water bath at 37°C
White light box/UV light box with mid- or long-wavelength for viewing stained gels
0.25 N HCl and 0.25 N NaOH for decontaminating ethidium bromide staining solution

Optional equipment:
Polaroid gun camera or other camera for recording results

CAUTION

Ethidium bromide is a mutagen and a suspected carcinogen. If it is used for staining, gloves should be worn at all times, and staining should be confined to a small area of the laboratory. After staining, a funnel can be used to decant as much ethidium bromide as possible from the staining tray back into the storage container. The stain may be reused to stain 15 or more gels. Used staining solutions and gels need to be disabled first before discarding. The steps for doing so are listed in the procedure.

PROCEDURE★

A. Restriction Digest
1. To reconstitute the DNA, add 280 μL of distilled or deionized water to each of 2 tubes of DNA provided. Allow to sit for 5 minutes.
2. Hold each closed tube firmly at the top, and flick the side of the tube repeatedly to mix the contents. Do this for 1 full minute.
3. Allow tubes to stand for an additional 5 minutes. The DNA solution should look slightly opaque. It is very important that the DNA be totally dissolved.
4. Aliquot 90 μL of DNA into each of six 1.5-mL tubes to be used by each laboratory group.

★ Procedure is taken from the Teacher's Manual included with the kit called Restriction Enzyme and DNA kit from Carolina Biological Supply Company, Burlington, N.C.

5. Select four 0.2-mL tubes, each of which contains a different enzyme. The blue tube contains BamHI, the pink tube contains EcoRI, the green tube contains HindIII, and the yellow tube has no enzyme at all.
6. Add 20 μL of DNA into each of the colored tubes. Mix the DNA and enzymes by pipetting up and down several times. There should be no concentration of the blue color in the bottom of the tube if DNA and enzymes are mixed sufficiently. Use a fresh pipet tip when adding DNA into each reaction tube to prevent crosscontamination.
7. Incubate all reaction tubes for a minimum of 20 minutes at 37°C.

B. Preparation of Cast Agarose Gel
1. Prepare the TBE buffer solution by pouring the contents of the 20X TBE concentrate into a 3-L flask or carboy. Add 2850 mL of distilled or deionized water for a final volume of 3 L. Stir for 1 to 2 minutes.
2. Prepare 0.8-percent agarose solution by adding 3.2 grams of agarose to 400 mL of TBE buffer in a clean 1-L flask. Cover with aluminum foil, and heat in a boiling water bath for 10 to 20 minutes. Swirl to ensure that no undissolved agarose remains. Alternatively, prepare four individual flasks of agarose by weighing out 0.8 grams of agarose for each flask and adding it to 100 mL of buffer in a 250-mL flask. Cover flasks with parafilm, and heat one individually in a microwave until the solution becomes clear.
3. Place flasks in a 60°C water bath to cool the agarose to 60°C before pouring.
4. Seal ends of gel-casting tray with tape, or use a self-sealing tray. Insert the well-forming comb.
5. Carefully pour enough agarose solution into the casting tray to fill it to a depth of about 5 mm. The gel should cover only about one-third the height of comb teeth. While the agarose is still liquid, a pipet tip or toothpick can be used to move large bubbles or solid debris to the sides or end of tray.
6. Let gel solidify without disturbing for about 20 minutes. Gel will become cloudy as it solidifies.
7. Unseal ends of casting tray, and place the gel in the gel box for electrophoresis with the comb at the negative (black) end.
8. Fill gel box with 1X TBE buffer to a level that just covers the entire surface of the gel.
9. Gently remove comb by pulling straight up, being careful not to rip the wells.
10. Make sure that the wells are completely covered with buffer. If there are any dimples, slowly add buffer until the dimples disappear.

C. Electrophoresis
1. Add 2 μL of loading dye to each reaction tube, and mix dye with digested DNA by tapping the tube on the lab bench, or pulse with a microcentrifuge.
2. Use a micropipet to load contents of each reaction tube into a separate well in the gel. Load wells by steadying pipet with two hands. Expel any air in the micropipet tip end before loading gel. Place pipet tip through surface of buffer, and position the tip over a well. Slowly expel the mixture. The loading dye should cause the sample to sink to the bottom of the well.
3. Close the top of the electrophoresis chamber, and connect electrical leads to a power supply, anode to anode and cathode to cathode.
4. Turn on power supply, and set voltage for approximately 125 volts. Note that this voltage will allow for adequate separation on mini-gels in approximately 1 hour.
5. Allow the DNA to migrate until the bromphenol blue band from the loading dye is near the end of the gel.
6. Turn off power supply, disconnect leads from the inputs, and remove the top of the electrophoresis chamber.
7. Carefully remove casting tray, and slide gel into staining tray.
8. Flood gel with ethidium bromide solution, and allow to stain for 10 to 15 minutes. Decant stain back into the container, using a funnel.
9. Rinse gel and tray under running water to remove excess ethidium bromide solution.
10. Place on UV light box for viewing and photography.

NOTE: Another version of this kit comes with Carolina BLU dye, which avoids the hazards of working with ethidium bromide and which can be viewed with a regular light box instead of one with a UV light source.

Disabling the Gels and Used Staining Solution

1. Add one volume of 0.05 M KmnO$_4$, and mix carefully.
2. Add one volume of 0.25 N HCl, and mix carefully. Let stand at room temperature for several hours.
3. Add one volume of 0.25 N NaOH, and mix carefully.
4. Discard disabled solution down sink. Discard gels in the regular trash.

INTERPRETATION OF RESULTS:

Digestion with BamHI should produce five fragments, EcoRi should produce five fragments, and HindIII will produce six fragments. Because each enzyme recognizes a distinctive base pair sequence, a different pattern will be obtained with each enzyme, and no separation will take place in the control tube. This same technique is used with human DNA to obtain a DNA fingerprint or to look for particular mutations that result in differences in numbers of bands.

1. Which technique is based on probe amplification rather than amplification of the target in question?
   a. PCR
   b. TMA
   c. Dot-blot
   d. Branched chain amplification

2. How are DNA are RNA different?
   a. Only RNA contains uracil.
   b. Only DNA contains cytosine.
   c. DNA is less stable than RNA.
   d. RNA is usually double-stranded.

3. All of the following are true of a nucleic acid probe *except:*
   a. It is a long nucleic acid chain.
   b. It can be made up of either DNA or RNA.
   c. It is labeled with a marker for detection.
   d. It attaches to single-stranded DNA.

4. In which method does transfer of DNA fragments to a membrane take place?
   a. Dot-blot
   b. Southern blot
   c. Hybridization protection assay
   d. LCR

5. All of the following would be advantages of nucleic acid amplification techniques *except:*
   a. Detection of nonviable organisms
   b. Extreme sensitivity
   c. Early detection of disease
   d. Low cost

6. Which best describes the principle of DNA chip technology?
   a. Probes are mixed with the sample and filtered onto a chip.
   b. Chips contain multiple copies of one unique probe.
   c. The sample is labeled with a fluorescent tag.
   d. Hybridization is detected by the presence of radioactivity.

7. A hybridization reaction involves which of the following?
   a. Binding of two complementary DNA strands
   b. Cleaving of DNA into smaller segments
   c. Separating DNA strands by heating
   d. Increasing the number of DNA copies

8. Which best describes the PCR?
   a. Two probes are joined by a ligating enzyme.
   b. RNA copies of the original DNA are made.
   c. Extender probes are used to detect a positive reaction.
   d. Primers are used to make multiple DNA copies.

9. When DNA strands are annealed, what does this mean?
   a. Single strands join to form a double helix.
   b. Strands are separated by heating.
   c. An RNA copy is made.
   d. Protein is made from the DNA strands.

10. What is the function of restriction endonucleases?
    a. They splice short DNA pieces together.
    b. They cleave DNA at specific sites.
    c. They make RNA copies of DNA.
    d. They make DNA copies from RNA.

11. To what does *in situ* hybridization refer?
    a. Nucleic acid probes react with intact cells.
    b. Probes are protected from degradation if hybridized.
    c. RNA polymerase copies messenger RNA.
    d. Hybridization takes place in solution.

12. What is PCR used for in clinical settings?
    a. Detection of early HIV infection
    b. Determination of specific HLA antigens
    c. Measurement of cytokines
    d. All of the above

References

1. Parslow, TG: Molecular genetic techniques for clinical analysis of the immune system. In Stites, DP, Terr, AI, and Parslow, TG (eds): Medical Immunology, ed. 9. Appleton & Lange, Stamford, Conn., 1997, pp 309–318.
2. Unger, ER, Piper, MA, and Border, BG: Nucleic acid techniques. In Burtis, CA, and Ashwood, ER (ed): Tietz Fundamentals of Clinical Chemistry, ed. 5. WB Saunders, Philadelphia, 2001, pp 195–212.
3. Wisecarver, J: The ABCs of DNA. Lab Med 28:48, 1997.
4. Podzorski, RP, KuKuruga, DL, and Long, PM: Introduction to molecular methodology. In Rose, NR, De MacArio, EC, and Folds, JD, et al (eds): Manual of Clinical Laboratory Immunology, ed. 5. American Society for Microbiology, Washington, D.C., 1997, pp 77–107.
5. Tenover, FC, and Unger, ER: Nucleic acid probes for detection and identification of infectious agents. In Persing, DH, Smith, TF, and Tenover, FC, et al (eds): Diagnostic Molecular Microbiology: Principles and Applications. American Society for Microbiology, Washington, D.C., 1993, pp 3–25.
6. Forbes, BA, Sahm, DF, and Weissfeld, AS: Bailey and Scott's Diagnostic Microbiology, ed. 10. Mosby, St. Louis, 1998, pp 188–207.
7. Whetsell, AJ, Drew, JB, and Milman, G, et al: Comparison of three

nonradioisotopic polymerase chain reaction-based methods for detection of human immunodeficiency virus type 1. J Clin Microbiol 30:845, 1992.

8. Hansen, CA: Clinical applications of molecular biology in diagnostic hematology. Lab Med 24:562, 1993.

9. Unger, ER, and Piper, MA: Molecular diagnostics: Basic principles and techniques. In Henry, JB (ed): Clinical Diagnosis and Management by Laboratory Methods, ed. 20. WB Saunders, Philadelphia, 2001, pp 1275–1295.

10. Friedrich, MJ: New chip on the block. Lab Med 30:180, 1999.

11. Check, W: Clinical microbiology eyes nucleic acid-based technologies. ASM News 64:84, 1998.

12. Schrenzel, J, Hibbs, JR, and Persing, DH: Hybridization array technologies. In Henry, JB (ed): Clinical Diagnosis and Management by Laboratory Methods, ed. 20. WB Saunders, Philadelphia, 2001, pp 1296–1302.

13. Persing, DH: In vitro nucleic acid amplification techniques. In Persing, DH, Smith, TF, and Tenover, FC, et al (eds): Diagnostic Molecular Microbiology: Principles and Applications. American Society for Microbiology, Washington, D.C., 1993, pp 51–87.

14. Mitchell, PS, and Persing, DH: Current trends in molecular microbiology. Lab Med 30:263, 1999.

15. Schochetman, G: Diagnosis of HIV infection. Clin Chim Acta 211:1, 1992.

16. http://www.roche-diagnostics.com/ba_rmd/pcr_applications.html#1, accessed September 2, 2002.

17. Weikersheimer, PB: Viral load testing for HIV: Beyond the CD4 count. Lab Med 30:102, 1999.

18. http://www.aidsmap.com/publications/factsheets/fs11c.htm, accessed August 31, 2002.

19. Eisenbrey, AB: Choosing appropriate methodologies on the clinical environment: Immunological techniques versus molecular methods. In Rose, NR, De MacArio, EC, and Folds, JD, et al (eds): Manual of Clinical Laboratory Immunology, ed. 5. American Society for Microbiology, Washington, D.C., 1997, pp 108–115.

20. Perkins, HA: HLA typing for transplantation of stem cells form unrelated donors. Lab Med 28:451, 1997.

21. http://www.nmdpresearch.org/HLA/hla_typing_resources.html, accessed September 2, 2002.

22. Hill, CS: Molecular diagnostics for infectious diseases. Journal of Clinical Ligand Assay 19:43,1996.

23. New directions in molecular diagnostic testing. Gen-Probe Inc, San Diego, pp 1–12.

24. http://www.gen-probe.com/productfaq.html, accessed August 27, 2002.

25. Nelson, NC: Molecular tools for building nucleic acid IVDs. IVD Technology, March/April 1997.

26. http://www.abbottdiagnostics.com/systems_tests/system.cfm?syscat_id=6&sys_id=29&path=1, accessed August 10,2002.

27. http://www.clontech.com/index.shtml, accessed July 31, 2002.

Immune Disorders

Hypersensitivity

Learning Objectives

After completing this chapter, the reader will be able to:
1. Define hypersensitivity, atopy, and allergen.
2. Discuss the key immunologic reactant involved in immediate hypersensitivity.
3. Describe the changes that take place in IgE-coated mast cells and basophils when binding with a specific antigen occurs.
4. Relate clinical manifestations of immediate hypersensitivity to specific mediators released from mast cells and basophils.
5. Describe anaphylaxis.
6. Discuss the advantages and disadvantages of skin testing for immediate hypersensitivity.
7. Compare the radioallergosorbent test (RAST) and radioimmunosorbent test (RIST) regarding detection methods, sensitivity, and the significance of the diagnostic findings.
8. Discuss how cellular damage occurs in type II hypersensitivity.
9. Give examples of type II hypersensitivity reactions.
10. Explain the significance of a positive direct antiglobulin test.
11. Distinguish between type II and type III hypersensitivity reactions on the basis of the nature of the antigen involved and mechanisms of cellular injury.
12. Discuss the Arthus reaction and serum sickness as examples of type III hypersensitivity reactions.
13. Relate how type IV sensitivity differs from the other three types of hypersensitivity reactions.
14. Explain the nature of the immunologic reaction in contact dermatitis and hypersensitivity pneumonitis.

Key Terms

Anaphylaxis
Arthus reaction
Atopy
Cold autoagglutinins
Contact dematitis
Delayed hypersensitivity
Eosinophil chemotactic factor
  of anaphylaxis (ECF-A)
Goodpasture's syndrome

Hemolytic disease of the
  newborn (HDN)
Histamine
Hypersensitivity
Hyposensitization
Immediate
  hypersensitivity
Neutrophil chemotactic
  factor

Passive cutaneous
  anaphylaxis
Radioallergosorbent test
  (RAST)
Radioimmunosorbent test
  (RIST)
Serum sickness
Warm autoimmune
  hemolytic anemia

In previous chapters, the immune response has been described as a defense mechanism by which the body rids itself of potentially harmful antigens. In some cases, however, this process can end up causing damage to the host. When this type of reaction occurs, it is termed hypersensitivity. **Hypersensitivity** can be defined as a heightened state of immune responsiveness. Typically, it is an exaggerated response to an innocuous antigen that results in gross tissue changes that are deleterious to the host. British immunologists P. G. H. Gell and R. R. A. Coombs devised a classification system for such reactions based on four different categories. In type I reactions, cell-bound antibody reacts with antigen to release physiologically active substances. Type II reactions are those in which free antibody reacts with antigen associated with cell surfaces, while in type III hypersensitivity, antibody reacts with soluble antigen to form complexes that precipitate in the tissues. In these latter two types, complement plays a major role in producing tissue damage. Type IV hypersensitivity differs from the other three because sensitized T cells rather than antibody are responsible for the symptoms that develop. Figure 13–1 gives a illustrative comparison of the four main types of hypersensitivity.

Although some disease manifestations may overlap among these categories, knowledge of the general characteristics of each will help in understanding the immune processes that trigger such tissue damage. Types I through III have previously been referred to as **immediate hypersensitivity** because symptoms develop within a few minutes to a few hours. Type IV hypersensitivity has been called **delayed hypersensitivity** because its manifestations are not seen until 24 to 48 hours after contact with antigen. For each of the four main types of reactions, the nature of the immune reactants is discussed, examples are given, and relevant testing is reviewed. Refer to Table 13–1 for a summary of the main characteristics that distinguish each class.

Type I Hypersensitivity

The distinguishing feature of type I hypersensitivity is the short time lag, usually seconds to minutes, between exposure to antigen and the onset of clinical symptoms. The key reactant present in type I or immediate sensitivity reactions is IgE. Antigens that trigger formation of IgE are called atopic antigens, or allergens.[1] **Atopy** refers to an inherited tendency to respond to naturally occurring inhaled and ingested allergens with continued production of IgE.[1,2] Most allergens are

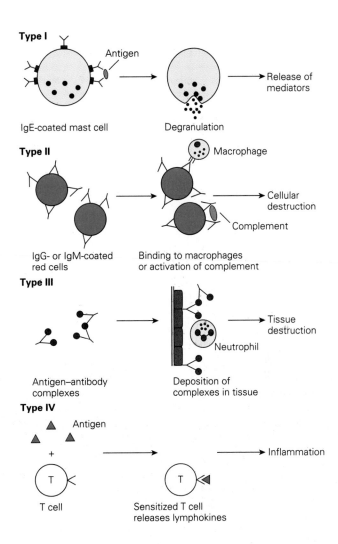

FIG. 13–1. Comparison of hypersensitivity reactions for types I to IV. *(Type I)* Antigen-specific IgE is bound to mast cells. Antigen bridges adjacent antibody molecules, causing disruption of the cell membrane with release of mediators. *(Type II)* Antibody is directed against cellular antigens. Complement is activated, and target cells are destroyed. *(Type III)* Soluble antigens combine with antibody to form immune complexes. These are deposited in tissues. Complement activation and exocytosis cause tissue damage. *(Type IV)* T cells become sensitized to antigen and release lymphokines on second exposure to that antigen. A localized inflammatory reaction occurs.

small proteins or protein-bound substances with a molecular weight of between 15,000 and 40,000 D.[1] Typically, patients who exhibit allergic or immediate hypersensitivity reactions usually produce a large

TABLE 13–1. Comparison of Hypersensitivity Reactions

	Type I	Type II	Type III	Type IV
Immune mediator	IgE	IgG	IgG or IgM	T cells
Antigen	Heterologous	Autologous or heterologous	Autologous or heterologous	Autologous or heterologous
Complement involvement	No	Yes	Yes	No
Immune mechanism	Release of mediators from mast cells and basophils	Cytolysis due to antibody and complement	Deposits of antigen–antibody complexes	Release of cytokines
Examples	Anaphylaxis, hay fever, food allergies, asthma	Transfusion reactions, autoimmune hemolytic anemia, HDN	Serum sickness, Arthus reaction, lupus erythematosus	Contact dermatitis, tuberculin test, pneumonitis

HDN = Hemolytic disease of the newborn.

amount of IgE in response to a small concentration of antigen. IgE levels appear to depend on the interaction of both genetic and environment factors.

Carl Wilhelm Prausnitz and Heinz Küstner were the first researchers to show that a serum factor was responsible for type I reactions. Serum from Küstner, who was allergic to fish, was injected into Prausnitz. A later exposure to fish antigen at the same site resulted in an allergic skin reaction.[3] This type of reaction is known as **passive cutaneous anaphylaxis.** It occurs when serum is transferred from an allergic individual to a nonallergic individual, and then the second individual is challenged with specific antigen. Although this experiment was conducted in 1921, it was not until 1967 that the serum factor responsible, namely IgE, was identified. Characteristics of IgE are described in Chapter 5.

Triggering of Type I Reactions by IgE

IgE is primarily synthesized in the lymphoid tissue of the respiratory and gastrointestinal tracts. Normal levels range from approximately 0.1 to 0.4 μg/mL.[1] The regulation of IgE production appears to be a function of a subset of T cells called type 2 helper cells (Th2).[4] The normal immune response to microorganisms and possible allergens is a function of type 1 helper cells (Th1), which produce interferon-gamma (IFN-γ). IFN-γ, along with interleukin-12 and interleukin-18, which are produced by macrophages, may actually suppress production of IgE type antibodies.[4] However, in people with allergies, Th2 cells respond instead and produce interleukin-4 (IL-4), interleukin-5 (IL-5), interleukin-9 (IL-9), and interleukin-13 (IL-13) (see Chapter 6). IL-4 and IL-13 are responsible for the final differentiation that occurs in B cells, initiating the transcription of the gene that codes for the epsilon-heavy chain of immunoglobulin molecules belonging to the

IgE class.[4] IL-5 and IL-9 are involved in the development of eosinophils, while IL-4 and IL-9 promote development of mast cells. IL-4, IL-9, and IL-13 all act to stimulate overproduction of mucus, a characteristic of most allergic reactions.

Although actual antibody synthesis is regulated by the action of cytokines, the tendency to respond to specific allergens appears to be linked to inheritance of certain major histocompatibility complex (MHC) genes. Various human leukocyte antigen (HLA) class II molecules, especially HLA-DR and HLA-DQ, seem to be associated with a high response to individual allergens.[3,5] HLA-D molecules are known to play a role in antigen presentation (see Chapter 4), and thus individuals who possess particular HLA molecules are more likely to respond to certain allergens.[3,5]

In addition, individuals who are prone to allergies exhibit certain variations in the gene that codes for receptors for IgE found on several types of cells.[4] These so-called high-affinity receptors, named Fcε-RI receptors, bind the fragment crystallizable (Fc) region of the epsilon-heavy chain and are found on basophils and mast cells. A single cell may have between 40,000 and 500,000 such receptors.[5] Other cells, such as monocytes, eosinophils, Langerhans cells, and dendritic cells, also have receptors for IgE, but their concentration is low.[6] Hence, these cells play a minor role in allergic reactions.[3] Binding of IgE to cell membranes increases the half-life of IgE from 2 or 3 days up to at least 10 days. Once bound, IgE serves as an antigen receptor on mast cells and basophils. Crosslinking of antibody molecules triggers release of mediators from these cells. Figure 13–2 depicts this reaction.

Role of Mast Cells and Basophils

Mast cells are derived from precursors in the bone marrow that migrate to specific tissue sites to mature.

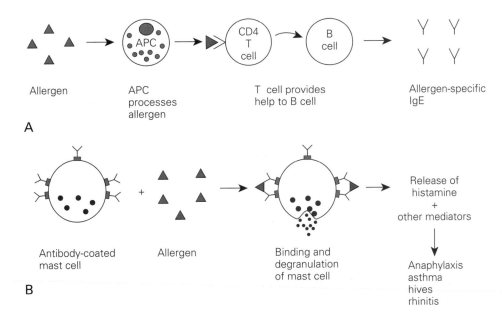

FIG. 13–2. Type I hypersensitivity. *(A)* Sensitization. Formation of antigen-specific IgE that attaches to mast cells. *(B)* Activation. Re-exposure to specific antigen with subsequent degranulation of mast cells and release of mediators. (APC = antigen-processing cell.)

Although they are found throughout the body, they are most prominent in the skin, the upper and lower respiratory tract, and the gastrointestinal tract.[7,8] In most organs, mast cells tend to be concentrated around the small blood vessels, the lymphatics, the nerves, and the glandular tissue.[8] These cells contain numerous cytoplasmic granules that are enclosed by a bilayered membrane. Histamine, one of the granular constituents, is found in ten times greater supply per cell than in eosinophils.[5]

There appear to be two different populations of mast cells in humans, based on the presence or absence of certain proteolytic enzymes, notably tryptase and chymase.[8] Mast cells found in the skin and connective tissue have both enzymes, while those in the alveoli, bronchial and bronchiolar regions, and mucosa of the small bowel contain only tryptase. Both types of cells are triggered in the same manner, however. They both release a variety of cytokines that enhance the allergic response.[1]

Basophils represent approximately 1 percent of the white blood cells in peripheral blood. They have a half-life of about 3 days. They contain histamine-rich granules as well as high-affinity receptors for IgE, just as in mast cells. They respond to chemotactic stimulation and tend to accumulate in the tissues during an inflammatory reaction. In the presence of IgE, the number of receptors has been found to increase, indicating a possible mechanism of upregulation during an allergic reaction.[5,6]

Mediators Released from Granules

Preformed Mediators

Crosslinking of surface-bound IgE by a specific allergen causes changes in the cell membrane that resul in the release of mediators from the cytoplasmic granules. These preformed mediators include histamine, eosinophil chemotactic factor of anaphylaxis (ECF-A), neutrophil chemotactic factor, and proteolytic enzymes.[1,3,8] Release of these substances is responsible for the early phase symptoms seen in allergic reactions, which occur within 30 to 60 minutes after exposure to the allergen. The effect of each of these mediators is discussed and a summary is presented in Table 13–2.

Histamine, a major component of mast cell granules, is a vasoactive amine with a molecular weight of 111. Its effects, which appear within 30 to 60 seconds after release, are dependent on activation of specific receptors found on cells in various types of tissue. Activation of H_1 receptors results in contraction of smooth muscle in bronchioles, blood vessels, and the intestines.[1,3,9] In addition, there is increased capillary permeability, altered cardiac contractility, and increased mucous gland secretion in the upper respiratory tract.[1,8] Binding to H_2 receptors increases gastric acid secretion, airway mucus production, and permeability of capillaries and venules.[8] H_3 receptors are found only on neural tissue, and the effects are more limited.

In the skin, histamine is responsible for local

TABLE 13–2. Mediators of Immediate Hypersensitivity

	Mediator	Structure	Actions
Preformed	Histamine	MW 111	Smooth muscle contraction, vasodilation, increased vascular permeability
	ECF-A	MW 380–2000	Chemotactic for eosinophils
	Neutrophil chemotactic factor	MW 600,000	Chemotactic for neutrophils
	Tryptase	MW 130,000	Converts C3 to C3b
Newly synthesized	PGD$_2$	Arachidonic acid derivative	Vasodilation, increased vascular permeability
	PGE$_2$, PGF$_2$, PGI	Arachidonic acid derivative	Vasodilation
	LTB$_4$	Arachidonic acid derivative	Chemotactic for neutrophils, eosinophils
	LTC$_4$, LTD$_4$, LTE$_4$	Arachidonic acid derivatives	Increased vascular permeability, bronchoconstriction, mucus secretion
	Platelet activating factor	MW 300–500	Platelet aggregation

MW = Molecular weight; ECF-A = eosinophil chemotactic factor of anaphylaxis; PGD = prostaglandin; LT = leukotriene.

erythema or redness and wheal and flare formation.[8] Contraction of the smooth muscle in the bronchioles may result in airflow obstruction. Increased vascular permeability may cause hypotension or shock. Depending on the route by which an individual is exposed to the triggering allergen, one or more of these effects may be seen.

Eosinophil chemotactic factor of anaphylaxis (ECF-A) is another preformed factor released from granules. This attracts eosinophils to the area, as well as inducing expression of eosinophil receptors for C3b.[8] Eosinophils have granules that contain histaminase and phospholipase D. These degrade histamine and platelet-activating factor (PAF) released from mast cells and basophils, so that eosinophils act as an internal negative control mechanism.[3]

A second chemotactic factor, **neutrophil chemotactic factor,** is less well characterized than ECF-A. It appears to be a heat-stable molecule with a molecular weight of approximately 600,000 that acts as an attractant for neutrophils.[3,8]

One of the proteolytic enzymes released is *tryptase.* Tryptase cleaves kininogen to generate bradykinin, which induces prolonged smooth muscle contraction, increases vascular permeability, and increases secretory activity.[1,8] Complement split products are also released when C3 is converted to C3a and C3b.

Newly Synthesized Mediators

In addition to immediate release of preformed mediators, mast cells and basophils are triggered to synthesize certain other reactants from the breakdown of phospholipids in the cell membrane. These products are responsible for a late-phase allergic reaction seen within 6 to 8 hours after exposure to antigen. Newly formed mediators include PAF; prostaglandin (PG) D$_2$; and leukotrienes B$_4$, C$_4$, D$_4$, and E$_4$ (leukotriene [LT] B$_4$, LTC$_4$, LTD$_4$, LTE$_4$).[3,4,8,9] *Prostaglandins* as well as *leukotrienes* are derived from arachidonic acid, a membrane lipid, by two separate metabolic pathways. In one pathway, the enzyme 5-lipoxygenase cleaves arachidonic acid to generate leukotrienes. The other pathway uses cyclooxygenase, which results in prostaglandin production.

PGD$_2$ is the major product of the cyclooxygenase pathway. When released by mast cells, it mimics the effects of histamine, causing bronchial constriction.[9] In skin reactions, PGD$_2$ triggers wheal and flare formation. Thus the overall effect is to enhance and potentiate the action of histamine.

Leukotrienes, resulting from the 5-lipoxygenase pathway of arachidonic acid metabolism, are also responsible for late-phase symptoms of immediate sensitivity. Leukotrienes C$_4$, D$_4$, and E$_4$ were originally collectively named the *slow-reacting substances of anaphylaxis (SRS-A).* LTC$_4$ and LTD$_4$ are 100 times more potent than histamine in causing increased vascular permeability, bronchoconstriction, and increased mucus secretion in small airways.[1,4,9] In the intestines, leukotrienes induce smooth muscle contraction.[8] Systemically, they may produce hypotension as a result of diminished cardiac muscle contractility and lessened blood flow.

LTB$_4$ is a potent chemotactic factor for neutrophils and eosinophils.[10] The appearance of eosinophils is especially important as a negative feedback control mechanism. Eosinophils release histaminase, which degrades histamine, and phospholipase D, which degrades PAF. Additionally, superoxides created in both eosinophils and neutrophils cause the breakdown of leukotrienes.

PAF is a phospholipid released by monocytes, macrophages, neutrophils, and eosinophils as well as by mast cells and basophils. The effects of PAF include platelet aggregation, chemotaxis of eosinophils and neutrophils, increased vascular permeability, and contraction of smooth muscle in the lungs and intestines.[3,5,8]

Clinical Manifestations of Immediate Hypersensitivity

The clinical manifestations caused by release of both preformed and newly synthesized mediators from mast cells and basophils vary from a localized skin reaction to a systemic response known as anaphylaxis. Symptoms depend on such variables as route of exposure, dosage, and frequency of exposure. If an allergen is inhaled, it is most likely to cause respiratory symptoms such as asthma or rhinitis. Ingestion of an allergen may result in gastrointestinal symptoms, and injection into the bloodstream can trigger a systemic response.

Anaphylaxis is the most severe type of allergic response because it is an acute reaction with simultaneous involvement of multiple organs. It may be fatal if not treated promptly. Coined by biologists Paul-Jules Portier and Charles Robert Richet in 1902, the term literally means "without protection." Anaphylactic reactions are typically triggered by glycoproteins or large polypeptides. Smaller molecules, such as penicillin, are haptens that may become immunogenic by combining with host cells or proteins. Typical agents that induce anaphylaxis include venom from bees, wasps, and hornets; drugs such as penicillin; and foods such as shellfish, peanuts, or dairy products.[1,11] Additionally, latex sensitivity is now a significant cause of anaphylaxis among health-care workers as well as in patients who have had multiple surgery procedures, such as children with spina bifida.[11,12]

Clinical signs begin within minutes after antigenic challenge and may include bronchospasm and laryngeal edema, vascular congestion, skin manifestations such as urticaria (hives) and angioedema, diarrhea and/or vomiting, and intractable shock because of the effect on blood vessels and smooth muscle of the circulatory system.[3] The severity of the reaction depends on the number of previous exposures to the antigen with consequent buildup of IgE on mast cells and basophils. Massive release of reactants, especially histamine, from the granules is responsible for the ensuing symptoms. Death may result from asphyxiation due to upper airway edema and congestion, irreversible shock, or a combination of these symptoms.[11]

Rhinitis is the most common form of atopy, or allergy. It affects between 5 and 22 percent of the population, or approximately 23 million people in the United States alone.[13] Symptoms include paroxysmal sneezing; rhinorrhea, or runny nose; nasal congestion; and itching of the nose and eyes.[2,14,15] Although the condition itself is merely annoying, complications such as sinusitis, otitis media (ear infection), eustachian tube dysfunction, and sleep disturbances may result. Pollen, mold spores, animal dander, and particulate matter from house dust mites are examples of airborne foreign particles that act directly on the mast cells in the conjunctiva and respiratory mucous membranes to trigger rhinitis.

Particles no larger than 2 to 4 μm in diameter may reach the lower respiratory tract to cause asthma. *Asthma* is derived from the Greek word for panting or breathlessness. It can be defined clinically as recurrent airflow obstruction that leads to intermittent sneezing, breathlessness, and occasionally, a cough with sputum production.[9] The airflow obstruction is due to bronchial smooth muscle contraction, mucosal edema, and heavy mucus secretion. All of these changes lead to an increase in airway resistance, making it difficult for inspired air to leave the lungs. This trapped air creates the sense of breathlessness.

Food allergies are another example of type I immediate hypersensitivity reactions. Some of the most common food allergies involve cow's milk, peanuts, and eggs.[15] Symptoms limited to the gastrointestinal tract include cramping, vomiting, and diarrhea, while spread of antigen through the bloodstream may cause hives and angioedema on the skin, as well as asthma or rhinitis.[1,11] Eczema, an itchy red skin rash, may be caused by food allergens as well as exposure to house dust mites.[15]

Treatment of Immediate Hypersensitivity

Drugs used to treat immediate hypersensitivity vary with the severity of the reaction. Localized allergic reactions, such as hay fever, hives, or rhinitis, can be treated easily with antihistamines. Asthma is often treated with a combination of therapeutic reagents including antihistamines and bronchodilators, followed by corticosteroids.[3] Systemic reactions require the use of epinephrine to quickly reverse symptoms.[11]

Another approach to treatment involves **hyposensitization.** Very small quantities of sensitizing antigen are injected into the patient with the idea of building up IgG antibodies. These so-called blocking antibodies circulate in the blood and combine with antigen before it can reach IgE-coated cells. In addition, it appears that T cell–mediated suppression occurs, thus decreasing synthesis of IgE.[15] This is most effective for antigens that would enter the circulation, such as insect venom.

Recent research with a recombinant anti-IgE antibody holds much promise. This antibody combines with IgE at the same site that IgE would normally use to bind to receptors on mast cells. Blocking of this site does not allow IgE to bind to mast cells, thus helping to alleviate allergic symptoms.[16,17] This approach has been successful in treating moderate to severe asthma.[13]

Testing for Immediate Hypersensitivity

In Vivo Skin Tests

Testing for allergies or immediate hypersensitivity can be categorized as *in vivo* or *in vitro* methods. *In vivo* methods involve direct skin testing. Cutaneous and intradermal tests are the two skin tests most often used. In *cutaneous testing,* or a *prick test,* a small drop of material is injected into the skin at a single point. After 20 minutes, the spot is examined, and the reaction is recorded. Reactions are usually graded from negative to 4+, with the latter representing formation of a wheal with erythema. A negative saline control and a positive control of histamine should always be included.[18] Cutaneous testing uses a 1000-fold higher concentration than intradermal tests, but a lesser amount of antigen is used, thus decreasing the chances of an anaphylactic response.[5,19]

Intradermal tests use a greater amount of antigen and are more sensitive than cutaneous testing. However, they are usually only performed if prick tests are negative and allergy is still suspected. An extremity, such as an arm, to which a tourniquet can be applied, is used to stop an unexpected systemic reaction.[7] A 1-mL tuberculin syringe is used to administer 0.02 mL of test solution between layers of the skin. After 15 minutes, the site is inspected for erythema and wheal formation. A 5- to 10- millimeter wheal is considered a positive test.[5] If there is no reaction, the site is reinspected at 30 minutes. If there is still no reaction, the test is considered to be negative.

Skin testing is relatively simple, is inexpensive, and lends itself to screening for a number of allergens. However, there is the danger that a systemic reaction can be triggered, or a new sensitivity may develop.[20] In addition, it may not be suitable for certain patient populations, such as young children.

In Vitro Tests: Total IgE

Principles of RIST. *In vitro* tests involve measurement of either total IgE or antigen-specific IgE. These are less sensitive than skin testing but usually are less traumatic to the patient. The first test developed for the measurement of total IgE was the competitive **radio-immunosorbent test (RIST).** The RIST uses radiolabeled IgE to compete with patient IgE for binding sites on a solid phase coated with anti-IgE. Competitive RISTs are expensive to perform because they require human radiolabeled IgE, so indirect RIST has largely been replaced by noncompetitive solid-phase immunoassays.[21]

In noncompetitive solid-phase immunoassay, antihuman IgE is bound to a solid phase such as a paper disk or microtiter well. Patient serum is added and allowed to react, and then a radiolabeled anti-IgE is added to detect the bound patient IgE. The second anti-IgE antibody recognizes a different epitope than that recognized by the first antibody. The resulting "sandwich" of solid-phase anti-IgE, serum IgE, and radiolabeled anti-IgE is washed, and the radioactivity is measured. In this case, the amount of label detected is directly proportional to the IgE content of the serum (Fig. 13–3). Standards that have a known concentration of IgE are run along with patient samples, and the radioactivity levels are compared. Although the second incubation doubles the time of the assay, the sensitivity of this type of testing is excellent, and the results are minimally affected by the presence of nonspecific serum factors.[21]

This same type of noncompetitive assay has been modified to make use of enzyme labels rather than radioactivity. This eliminates the health hazard of working with radioactivity, and the expense is considerably less.

Interpretation of RIST.   Total IgE values are reported in International Units (IU) per milliliter. One IU is equal to a concentration of 2.4 ng of protein per milliliter. IgE concentration varies with age, sex, and smoking history of the patient as well as family history of allergy.[18] Levels also vary as a function of exposure to allergens. In infants, serum levels of IgE of more than 20 IU/mL are indicative of allergic disease,[5] while after the age of 14 years, IgE levels of greater than 333 IU are considered to be abnormally elevated.[21] A cutoff point of 100 IU, however, is frequently used in testing to identify individuals with allergic tendencies. Although two-thirds of the adults who have allergic symptoms would fall into this category, the other one-third might be incorrectly diagnosed.[18] Additionally, IgE levels may be elevated due to other conditions, such as helminth infections, Wiskott–Aldrich syndrome, DiGeorge syndrome, and hyper-IgE syndrome.[5,18] Thus, total IgE levels must be interpreted in light of the patient's personal and family history, and they should not be regarded as an absolute predictor of allergy. Although measurement of total IgE levels can be a useful screening tool, allergen-specific IgE is more helpful in actual treatment of the patient.[20]

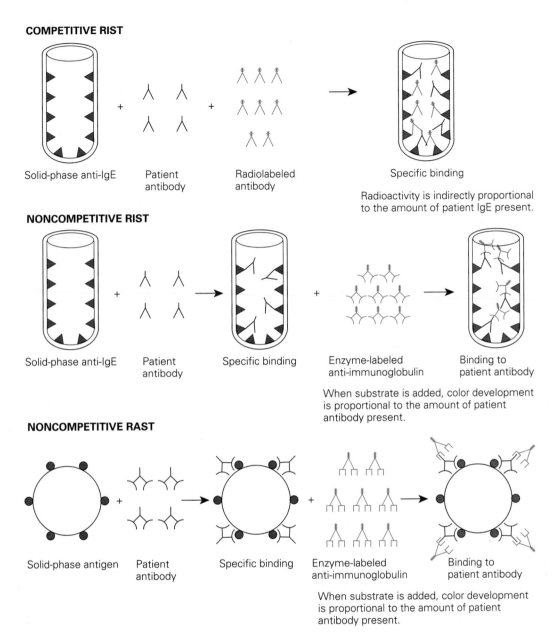

FIG. 13–3. Comparison of RIST and RAST. RIST measures total IgE by competitive and noncompetitive methods. In both cases, patient IgE is the antigen that is reacted with anti-IgE. Noncompetitive RAST measures antigen-specific IgE by using solid-phase antigen to capture patient antibody. Then a second antibody, enzyme-labeled anti-IgE immunoglobulin, is added. This combines with any bound IgE to produce a visible reaction in the presence of substrate.

Antigen-Specific IgE Testing

Principles of RAST. The **radioallergosorbent test (RAST)** was introduced in 1966 and remains the method of choice for serologic determination of antigen–specific IgE.[21] It is safer to perform than skin testing and easier on some patients, especially children or apprehensive adults, but it is not as sensitive as the direct skin tests.[21] It is especially useful in the detection of allergies to common allergens such as ragweed, trees, grasses, molds, animal dander, milk, and egg albumin.

The RAST is a noncompetitive solid–phase immunoassay in which the solid phase is coated with specific allergen and reacted with patient serum. A carbohydrate solid phase, such as paper cellulose disks, agarose beads, or microcrystalline cellulose particles, seems to work better than polystyrene microtiter wells or tubes.[21] After washing to remove unbound antibody, a labeled anti-IgE is added. Traditional RAST used a radioactive label, while newer tests use an enzyme or fluorometric label.[22] A second incubation occurs, and then, after a washing step, the amount of radioactivity or enzyme activity in the sample is measured. The amount of label detected is directly proportional to the amount of specific IgE in the patient's serum. Controls and standards are run in parallel with patient serum. Figure 13–3 shows a comparison of the RAST and RIST.

Interpretation of RAST.   There is as yet no universally accepted method for defining sensitivity to any given allergen.[5] Thus careful interpretation of RAST results should be made because 10 to 25 percent of patients with positive skin tests were found to have negative RAST results.[18] A study of testing from several commercial laboratories showed that results were not always comparable or reproducible.[23] IgG, IgM, or IgA may compete with IgE and falsely lower test results.[18,21] If carefully designed, however, RAST can come close to matching the sensitivity of skin testing.[21]

Type II Hypersensitivity

The reactants responsible for type II hypersensitivity, or cytotoxic hypersensitivity, are IgG and IgM. They are triggered by antigens found on cell surfaces. These antigens may be altered self-antigens or heteroantigens. Antibody coats cellular surfaces and promotes phagocytosis by both opsonization and activation of the complement cascade. Macrophages, neutrophils, and eosinophils have Fc receptors that bind to antibody, thus enhancing phagocytosis. Natural killer (NK) cells also have Fc receptors, and if these link to cellular antigens, cytotoxicity results. If the complement cascade is activated, complement can trigger cellular destruction in two ways: (1) by coating cells with C3b, thus facilitating phagocytosis through interaction with specific receptors on phagocytic cells, or (2) by complement-generated lysis if the cascade goes to completion. Hence, complement plays a central role in the cellular damage that typifies type II reactions.

Transfusion Reactions

Transfusion reactions are examples of cellular destruction that result from antibody combining with heteroantigens. There are more than 25 different blood group systems, with many antigenic variants in each.[24] Some antigens are stronger than others and are more likely to stimulate antibody production. Major groups

involved in transfusion reactions include the ABO, Rh, Kell, Duffy, and Kidd systems.[24,25] Certain antibodies are produced naturally with no prior exposure to red blood cells, while other antibodies are only produced after contact with cells carrying that antigen.

The ABO blood group is of primary importance in considering transfusions. Anti-A and anti-B antibodies are so-called naturally occurring antibodies, probably triggered by contact with identical antigenic determinants on microorganisms. Individuals do not form such antibodies to their own red blood cells. Thus, an individual who has type A blood has anti-B in the serum, and a person with type B blood has anti-A antibodies. An individual with type O blood has both anti-A and anti-B in the serum because O cells have neither of these two antigens.

If a patient is given blood for which antibodies are already present, a transfusion reaction occurs. This can range from acute massive intravascular hemolysis to an undetected decrease in red blood cell survival. The extent of the reaction depends on the following factors: (1) the temperature at which the antibody is most active, (2) the plasma concentration of the antibody, (3) the particular immunoglobulin class, (4) the extent of complement activation, (5) the density of the antigen on the red blood cell, and (6) the number of red blood cells transfused.[25] It is most important to detect antibodies that react at 37°C. If a reaction only occurs below 30°C, it can be disregarded because such antigen–antibody complexes tend to dissociate at 37°C.

Acute hemolytic transfusion reactions may occur within minutes or hours after transfusion of incompatible blood. In this case, the individual has been exposed to the antigen before and has preformed antibodies to it. Reactions that begin immediately are most often associated with ABO blood group incompatibilities, and antibodies are of the IgM class.[25] As soon as cells bearing that antigen are introduced into the patient, intravascular hemolysis occurs because of complement activation, and it results in the release of hemoglobin and vasoactive and procoagulant substances into the plasma. This may induce disseminated intravascular coagulation (DIC), vascular collapse, and renal failure. Symptoms in the patient may include fever, chills, nausea, lower back pain, shock, and hemoglobin in the urine.[1]

Delayed hemolytic reactions occur 4 to 10 days following a transfusion and are caused by a secondary response to the antigen. The type of antibody responsible is IgG. Antigens most involved in delayed reactions include those in the Rh, Kell, Duffy, and Kidd blood groups.[1,25] Rh and Kell antigens may also be involved in immediate transfusion reactions. In a delayed reaction, antibody-coated red blood cells are removed extravascularly in the spleen or in the liver, and the patient may experience a mild fever, low hemoglobin, mild jaundice, and anemia.

Hemolytic Disease of the Newborn

Hemolytic disease of the newborn (HDN) appears in infants whose mothers have been exposed to blood-group antigens on the baby's cells that differ from their own. The mother makes IgG antibodies in response, and these cross the placenta to cause destruction of fetal red cells. Severe HDN is called *erythroblastosis fetalis*. The most common antigen involved is the D antigen, a member of the Rh blood group.

Exposure usually occurs during the birth process, where fetal cells leak into the mother's circulation. Typically the first child is unaffected, but the second and later children have an increased risk of the disease. Approximately 8 percent of women who are Rh-negative produce anti-D after the first pregnancy, and up to 23 percent show antibody production after multiple pregnancies.[26] The extent of the fetal-maternal bleed influences whether antibodies will be produced.

Depending on the degree of antibody production in the mother, the fetus may be aborted, stillborn, or born with evidence of hemolytic disease as indicated by jaundice. As red blood cells are lysed and free hemoglobin released, this is converted to bilirubin, which builds up in the plasma. Bilirubin levels above 20 mg/dL are associated with deposition in tissue such as the brain and result in a condition known as kernicterus. Treatment for severe HDN involves an exchange transfusion to replace antibody-coated red cells. If serum antibody titrations during the pregnancy indicate a high level of circulating antibody, intrauterine transfusions can be performed.[27]

To prevent the consequences of HDN, all women should be screened at the onset of pregnancy. If they are Rh-negative, they should be tested for the presence of anti-D antibodies on a monthly basis. In current practice, anti-D immune globulin is administered prophylactically at 28 weeks of gestation and within 72 hours following delivery.[27] It is assumed that the immune globulin inhibits production of antibody by combining with and destroying the D+ red blood cells, thus preventing them from being antigenic (Fig. 13–4). This practice has reduced the number of women who form anti-D antibodies from 7 to 8 percent to a little over 1 percent.[26]

Autoimmune Hemolytic Anemia

Autoimmune hemolytic anemia is an example of a type II hypersensitivity reaction directed against self-antigens because individuals with this disease form antibodies to their own red blood cells. Symptoms include malaise, lightheadedness, weakness, and possibly mild jaundice.[28] Such antibodies can be categorized into two groups: warm reactive antibodies, which react at 37°C, and cold reactive antibodies, which react only below 30°C.

Cold autoagglutinins, representing approximately 30 percent of all immune hemolytic anemias, typically are found in older persons who are in their fifties and sixties.[29] These are thought to be triggered by antigens on microorganisms because antibodies have been known to occur following Mycoplasma pneumonia, infectious mononucleosis, cytomegaloviris infection, and the mumps.[26] Cold autoagglutinins have also been seen in such diseases as chronic lymphocytic leukemia, non-Hodgkin's lymphoma, or connective tissue diseases such as systemic lupus erythematosus.[26] In children, such antibodies have been associated with virus and respiratory infections.

These cold-reacting antibodies belong to the IgM class, and most are specific for the Ii blood groups on red cells.[26,28] Reactions are only seen in the patient if that individual is exposed to the cold and the temperature in the peripheral circulation falls below 30°C. Peripheral necrosis may result. Although complement activation begins in the cold, it can proceed at body temperature. If the entire complement sequence is activated, intravascular hemolysis may occur.[28] If red blood cells become coated with C3b, this helps macrophages to bind, and these cells are rapidly cleared in the liver, further decreasing the number of circulating red blood cells. A simple treatment is to keep the patient warm, especially the hands and feet, to prevent complement activation.

Warm autoimmune hemolytic anemia is characterized by formation of IgG antibody, which reacts most strongly at 37°C. This is the most common type of immune hemolytic anemia. Some of these antibodies may occur with other autoimmune diseases; with virus or respiratory infections, such as infectious mononucleosis, cytomegalovirus, or chronic active hepatitis; or with immunoproliferative diseases such as chronic lymphocytic leukemia and lymphomas.[26] Certain drugs are adsorbed onto red blood cells and are capable of stimulating antibody production. Examples include acetaminophen, penicillins, cephalosporin, rifampin, sulfonamides, methyldopa, and procainamide.[1,26,30] Often, however, the underlying cause of antibody production is unknown, so this is referred to as idiopathic autoimmune hemolytic anemia. Typically, the patient exhibits symptoms of anemia because of clearance of antibody-coated red blood cells by the liver and spleen. Intravascular hemolysis can also

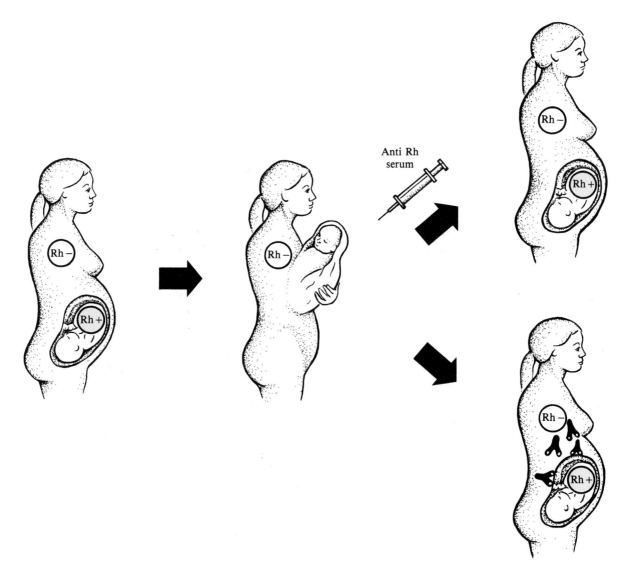

FIG. 13–4. Passive immunization to prevent hemolytic disease of the newborn. An Rh-negative mother is exposed to Rh antigens during pregnancy with an Rh-positive fetus. If passively immunized with anti-Rh sera at 7 months and on delivery, the maternal anti-Rh immune response is suppressed. A subsequent pregnancy *(upper right)* is uncomplicated by HDN. If passive immunization is not practiced, the mother may develop anti-Rh antibodies, and a second Rh-positive fetus is likely to exhibit destruction of red blood cells characteristic of HDN. (From Barrett, JT: Textbook of Immunology, ed. 5. Mosby, St. Louis, 1988 p 339, with permission.)

occur when complement is activated. Patients with warm autoimmune hemolytic anemia are usually treated with corticosteroids or splenectomy in more serious cases.[29]

Autoimmune Thrombocytopenic Purpura

Autoimmune or idiopathic thrombocytopenic purpura (ITP) is another example of a type II reaction involving destruction of self-antigens. This disease is characterized by increased platelet destruction or shortened platelet survival and the presence of antibody bound to platelets. It can be classified as acute, intermittent, or chronic, depending on the severity and frequency of the symptoms. Acute autoimmune thrombocytopenic purpura occurs mainly in children following an upper respiratory viral illness.[31] The disease lasts an average of 1 to 2 months. Intermittent ITP may occur in a child or an adult. It is characterized by episodes in which the platelet count drops, followed by periods in which the count is normal. Chronic ITP is seen in adults, and it may last for years or indefinitely.[31,32]

ITP can be drug induced by the following: quinidine, quinine, sulfonamides, *p*-aminosalicylic acid, phenytoin, cephalothin, digitoxin, aspirin, and rifampin.[26,32] The drug acts as a hapten and adheres to the surface of the platelets. This type of ITP is reversed when the drug is withdrawn.

The thrombocytopenia results from antibody-coated platelets that are destroyed by phagocytosis, especially in the spleen. Destruction is directly related to the quantity of bound antibody. When the platelet count goes below 30,000 to 50,000 cells/μL, capillary bleeding results.[26] Generally this is manifested as tiny pinpoint hemorrhages or petechiae on skin or mucosal surfaces. The classic treatment is removal of the spleen, the site of destruction of damaged platelets. Most children, however, have spontaneous remission, and splenectomy is seldom necessary.

Type II Reactions Involving Tissue Antigens

All the reactions that have been discussed so far deal with individual cells that are destroyed when a specific antigen–antibody combination takes place. Some type II reactions involve destruction of tissues because of combination with antibody. **Goodpasture's syndrome** is an example of such a disease (see Chapter 14 for details). The antibody produced during the course of this disease is one that reacts with basement membrane protein. Usually the glomeruli in the kidney and pulmonary alveolar membranes are affected.[33] Antibody binds to glomerular and alveolar capillaries, triggering the complement cascade, which provokes inflammation.[34] Treatment usually involves the use of corticosteroids or other drugs to suppress the immune response.

Other examples of reactions to tissue antigens include some of the autoimmune diseases such as Hashimoto's disease, myasthenia gravis, and insulin-dependent diabetes mellitus. Immunologic manifestations and detection of these diseases are presented in Chapter 14.

Testing for Type II Hypersensitivity

As discussed in Chapter 10, the discovery of the antiglobulin test by Coombs in 1945 made possible the detection of antibody or complement on red blood cells. Direct antiglobulin test (DAT) is performed to detect transfusion reactions, hemolytic disease of the newborn, and autoimmune hemolytic anemia. Refer to the exercise at the end of the chapter for details. Polyspecific antihuman globulin is a mixture of antibodies to IgG and complement components such as C3d. If the test is positive, then it should be repeated using monospecific anti-IgG and anti-C3d to deter-

mine which of these is present.[30] If an autoimmune hemolytic anemia is caused by IgM antibody, only the test for complement component C3d would be positive (see Fig. 10–4 in Chapter 10).

The indirect Coombs' test is used in the crossmatching of blood to prevent a transfusion reaction. It is used either to determine the presence of a particular antibody in a patient or to type patient red blood cells for specific blood group antigens. This is a two-step process, in which red blood cells and antibody are allowed to combine at 37°C, and then the cells are carefully washed to remove any unbound antibody. Antihuman globulin is added to cause a visible reaction if antibody has been specifically bound. Any negative tests are confirmed by quality control cells, which are coated with antibody. Refer to Chapter 10 for additional details on indirect antiglobulin testing.

Idiopathic thrombocytopenic purpura can be diagnosed by means of a platelet agglutination test. Patient serum that has been heated to 56°C to destroy complement is added to an aliquot of platelet-rich plasma. This is followed by overnight incubation at 5°C. In 65 percent of the cases of ITP, patient serum will test positive by this method.[30]

Diagnosis of Goodpasture's syndrome is usually accomplished by using direct fluorescence.[34] Standard histologic slides are made from a frozen section of a biopsy specimen. These are overlaid with fluorescent-labeled antihuman IgG. An evenly bound linear deposition of IgG in glomerular basement membrane is indicative of Goodpasture's syndrome.

Type III Hypersensitivity

Type III hypersensitivity reactions are similar to type II reactions in that IgG or IgM is involved and in that destruction is complement mediated. However, in the case of type III diseases, the antigen is a soluble one. When soluble antigen combines with antibody, complexes are formed that precipitate out of the serum. These complexes deposit in the tissues and bind complement, causing damage to the particular tissue. Deposition of antigen–antibody complexes is influenced by the relative concentration of both components. If a large excess of antigen is present, sites on antibody molecules become filled before crosslinks can be formed. In antibody excess, a lattice cannot be formed because of the relative scarcity of antigenic determinant sites. The small complexes that result in either of the preceding cases remain suspended or may pass directly into the urine. Precipitating complexes, on the other hand, occur in mild antigen excess, and these are the ones most likely to deposit in the tissues. Sites in which this typically occurs include the glomerular basement membrane, vascular endothelium, joint linings, and pulmonary alveolar membranes.[1]

Complement binds to these complexes in the tissues, causing the release of mediators that increase vasodilation and vasopermeability, attract macrophages and neutrophils, and enhance binding of phagocytic cells by means of C3b deposited in the tissues. If the target cells are large and cannot be engulfed for phagocytosis to take place, granule and lysosome contents are released by a process known as *exocytosis.* This results in the damage to host tissue that is typified by type III reactions. Long-term changes include loss of tissue elements that cannot regenerate and accumulation of scar tissue.

Arthus Reaction

The classic example of a type III reaction is the **Arthus reaction,** demonstrated by Maurice Arthus in 1903. Using rabbits that had been immunized to produce an abundance of circulating antibodies, Arthus showed that when these rabbits were challenged with an intradermal injection of the antigen, a localized inflammatory reaction resulted. This reaction, characterized by erythema and edema, peaks within 3 to 8 hours and is followed by a hemorrhagic necrotic lesion that ulcerates.[35] The inflammatory response is caused by antigen–antibody combination and subsequent formation of immune complexes that deposit in small dermal blood vessels. Complement is fixed, attracting neutrophils and causing aggregation of platelets. Neutrophils release toxic products such as oxygen-containing free radicals and proteolytic enzymes.[35] Activation of complement is essential for the Arthus reaction because the C3a and C5a generated activate mast cells to release permeability factors, with the consequent localization of immune complexes along the endothelial cell basement membrane. The Arthus reaction is rare in humans (Fig. 13–5). One example, however, occurs in the lungs and is caused by fungal spores, especially those of *Aspergillus fumigatus.*[35]

Serum Sickness

Serum sickness is a type III reaction that is seen in humans, although not as frequently as it used to be. **Serum sickness** results from passive immunization with animal serum, usually horse or bovine serum, used to treat such infections as diphtheria, tetanus, and gangrene. Approximately 50 percent of the individuals who receive a single injection develop the disease.[35] Vaccines and bee stings may also trigger this type of reaction. Generalized symptoms appear about 1 to 2 weeks after injection of the animal serum and include

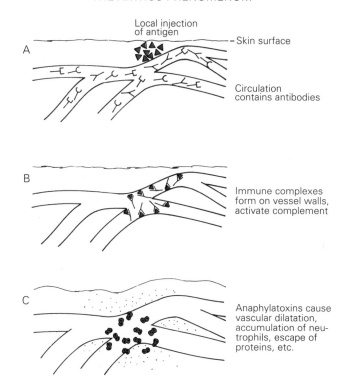

FIG. 13–5. The Arthus phenomenon. *(A)* Antigen is injected into the skin of an individual who has circulating antibody of that specificity. *(B)* Immune complexes are formed and deposit on the walls of blood vessels, activating complement. *(C)* Complement fragments cause dilation and increased permeability of blood vessels, edema, and accumulation of neutrophils. (From Widmann, FK: An Introduction to Clinical Immunology. FA Davis, 1989, p 228, with permission.)

headache, fever, nausea, vomiting, joint pain, rashes, and lymphadenopathy. Recovery takes between 7 and 30 days.[1,35]

In this disease, the sensitizing and the shocking dose of antigen are one and the same because antibodies develop while antigen is still present. High levels of antibody form immune complexes that deposit in the tissues. Usually this is a benign and self-limiting disease, but previous exposure to animal serum can cause cardiovascular collapse on re-exposure.[35] Antibiotic use has diminished the need for this type of therapy.

Autoimmune Diseases

Type III hypersensitivity reactions can be triggered by autologous antigens as well as by heterologous ones. Several of the autoimmune diseases fall into this category. Systemic lupus erythematosus (SLE) and rheumatoid arthritis are two such examples. In SLE, antibodies are directed against constituents such as deoxyribonucleic acid (DNA) and nucleohistones, which are found in most cells of the body. Immune complex deposition involves multiple organs, but the main damage occurs to the glomerular basement membrane in the kidney.

In rheumatoid arthritis, an antibody called rheumatoid factor is directed against IgG. Immune complex deposition occurs in the membranes of inflamed joints. Complement enhances tissue destruction in both diseases. See Chapter 14 for a more detailed discussion of these two diseases.

Testing for Type III Hypersensitivity

In specific diseases such as SLE and rheumatoid arthritis, the presence of antibody can be detected by agglutination reactions using antigen-coated carrier particles such as red blood cells or latex particles. Fluorescent staining of tissue sections has also been used as a means of determining deposition of immune complexes in the tissues. The staining pattern seen, as well as the particular tissue affected, helps to identify the disease and determine its severity.

A more general method of determining immune complex diseases is by measurement of complement levels. Decreased levels of individual components or decreased functioning of the pathway may be indicative of antigen–antibody combination. The results must be interpreted with regard to other clinical findings, however. Refer to Chapter 7 for a discussion of complement testing.

Type IV Hypersensitivity

Type IV, or delayed, hypersensitivity differs from the other three types of hypersensitivity in that sensitized T cells, usually a subpopulation of Th1 cells, play the major role in its manifestations. Antibody and complement are not directly involved. Symptoms usually take several hours to develop, reach a peak 48 to 72 hours after exposure to antigen, and then regress over several days.[1,36] The reaction cannot be transferred from one animal to another by means of serum, but only through transfer of T lymphocytes. T helper cells are activated and release cytokines, including IL-2, IFN-γ, and tumor necrosis factor-beta (TNF-β) that recruit macrophages and neutrophils, produce edema, promote fibrin deposition, and generally enhance an inflammatory response.[1] Cytotoxic T cells are also recruited, and they bind with antigen-coated target cells to cause tissue destruction. Allergic skin reactions to bacteria, viruses, fungi, and environmental antigens such as poison ivy typify this type of hypersensitivity.

Contact Dermatitis

Contact dermatitis is a form of delayed hypersensitivity that accounts for a significant number of all occupationally acquired illnesses. This reaction is usually due to low-molecular-weight compounds that touch the skin. The most common causes include poison ivy, poison oak, and poison sumac, all of which give off pentadecylcatechol in the plant sap and on the leaves. Over 50 percent of the population of the United States exhibits clinical symptoms on exposure to these compounds.[37] Other common compounds that produce allergic skin manifestations include nickel, rubber, dyes and fabric finishes, cosmetics, and medications applied to the skin, such as topical anesthetics, antiseptics, and antibiotics.[12] In addition, latex allergy has been reported to affect between 3.8 and 17 percent of all health-care workers in the United States.[12] Most of these substances probably function as haptens that bind to glycoproteins on skin cells. The *Langerhans cell*, a skin macrophage, functions as the antigen-presenting cell at the site of antigen contact.[36,37] It appears that Langerhans cells may migrate to regional lymph nodes and generate sensitized T cells there. This sensitization process takes several days, but once it occurs, its effects last for years.[37]

After repeat exposure to the antigen, a skin eruption characterized by erythema, swelling, and the formation of papules appears in anywhere from 6 hours to several days after the exposure.[36,37] The papules may become vesicular, with blistering, peeling, and weeping. There is usually itching at the site (Fig. 13–6). The dermatitis is first limited to skin sites exposed to the antigen, but then it spreads out to adjoining areas.

Simple redness may fade of its own accord within several days. If the area is small and localized, a topic steroid may be used for treatment. Otherwise, systemic corticosteroids may be administered. The patient also needs to avoid contact with the offending allergen.

Hypersensitivity Pneumonitis

Recent evidence shows that hypersensitivity pneumonitis is mediated predominantly by sensitized T lymphocytes that respond to inhaled allergens.[37] IgG and IgM antibodies are formed, but these are thought to play only a minor part. This is an allergic disease of the lung parenchyma, characterized by inflammation of the alveoli and interstitial spaces. It is caused by chronic inhalation of a wide variety of antigens, and it is most often seen in men between the ages of 30 and 50 years.[37,38] Depending on the occupation and the particular antigen, the disease goes by several names, including farmer's lung, pigeon breeder's disease, and

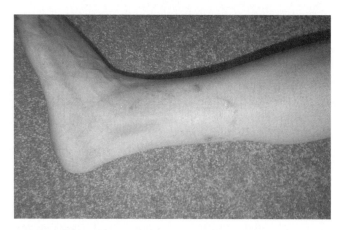

FIG. 13–6. Contact hypersensitivity. Formation of papules after exposure to poison ivy.

humidifier lung disease. The reaction is most likely due to microorganisms, especially bacterial and fungal spores, that individuals are exposed to from working with moldy hay, pigeon droppings, compost, moldy tobacco, infested flour, and moldy cheese, to name just a few examples. Symptoms include a dry cough, shortness of breath, fever, weight loss, and general malaise, which may begin within 4 to 8 hours after exposure to a high dose of the offending allergen.[37,38] Alveolar macrophages and lymphocytes trigger a chronic condition characterized by interstitial fibrosis with alveolar inflammation. Systemic corticosteroid therapy is used for treatment.[37]

Tuberculin-Type Hypersensitivity

Testing for exposure to tuberculosis is a classic example of a delayed hypersensitivity reaction. This is based on the principle that soluble antigens from *Mycobacterium tuberculosis* induce a reaction in people who have or have had tuberculosis. When challenged with antigen intradermally, previously sensitized individuals develop an area of erythema and induration at the site of the injection. This is the result of infiltration of T lymphocytes and macrophages into the area. The blood vessels become lined with mononuclear cells, and the reaction reaches a peak by 72 hours after exposure.

The tuberculin skin test uses a *Mycobacterium tuberculosis* antigen prepared by making a purified filtrate from the cell wall of the organism. This purified protein derivative (PPD) is injected under the skin, and the reaction is read at 48 to 72 hours. For a test to be considered positive, the lesion at the reaction site must be at least 10 mm in diameter.[7] A positive test indicates that the individual has previously been exposed to

Mycobacterium tuberculosis or a related organism at some time, but it does not necessarily mean there is a presently active case.

Testing for Delayed Hypersensitivity

Skin tests for delayed hypersensitivity are performed in much the same manner as testing for the presence of IgE. Typically, 0.1 mL of the antigen is injected intradermally, using a syringe and a fine needle.[7] The test site is read at 48 and 72 hours for the presence of induration. The reactions can be graded on a scale of 1 to 4, with induration of 1 to 5 mm representing a 1+ and reactions greater than 20 mm a 4+.[7] Antigens typically used for testing are *Candida albicans,* diphtheria toxoid, tetanus toxoid, tuberculin, and fungal antigens such as trichophyton and histoplasmin.[39]

A patch test can also be performed to determine the cause of a persistent dermatitis. This must be done when the patient is free of symptoms, or at least has a clear test site.[39] A nonabsorbent adhesive patch containing the suspected allergen is applied to the skin, and the skin is checked for a reaction over the next 48 hours. Redness with papules and/or tiny blisters is considered a positive test.[37]

The extent of lymphocyte activation or stimulation by specific antigens can also be determined. This has been found to be especially helpful in diagnosis of hypersensitivity lung diseases.[40] Proliferation assays are performed by isolating patient mononuclear cells from peripheral blood using density gradient centrifugation with Ficoll-Hypaque. Cell suspensions are then placed in individual wells in microtiter plates along with culture media. The cultures are stimulated with different concentrations of several antigens, one to each well.[40] Cultures are incubated for approximately 6 days at 37°C, followed by exposure to radioactive thymidine for an additional 18 hours. The amount of radioactive thymidine incorporated into the DNA is an indicator of lymphocyte responsiveness to a particular antigen.

Antigen-induced proliferation depends on previous sensitization of lymphocytes to the antigen being tested, and this usually involves a small percentage of the test population.[7] Although this is technically a more difficult test to perform, it is often a more sensitive indicator of cellular hypersensitivity than skin testing.[7]

SUMMARY

Hypersensitivity reactions are exaggerated reactions to antigens that are typically not harmful. Usually there is destruction of host tissue in the process of attempting to destroy the antigen. Gell and Coombs devised a system of classification for such reactions based on immune mediators and the nature of the triggering antigen. Type I hypersensitivity, or immediate hypersensitivity, is manifested within minutes of exposure to antigen. The principle mediator is IgE, which does not remain free in the serum, but binds to mast cells and basophils. When cell-bound antibody binds antigen, the resulting degranulation of the effector cells releases mediators that enhance the inflammatory response. Preformed mediators that are released include histamine, eosinophil chemotactic factor of anaphylaxis, neutrophil chemotactic factor, and proteolytic enzymes such as tryptase. Together, these factors are responsible for contraction of smooth muscle in the bronchioles, blood vessels, and intestines; increased capillary permeability; increased concentration of eosinophils and neutrophils in the area; and decreased coagulability of blood. Newly synthesized mediators, such as prostaglandins, leukotrienes, and PAF, potentiate the effects of histamine and other preformed mediators.

Clinical manifestations of immediate hypersensitivity vary from localized wheal and flare skin reactions, or rhinitis, to systemic anaphylactic reactions, which can be life threatening. Tests to determine the potential for incurring such reactions include both *in vitro* and *in vivo* methods. The noncompetitive RIST measures total IgE by using radiolabeled anti-IgE that binds to patient's IgE on solid phase. RAST is a noncompetitive or capture method to determine antibody to specific allergens. *In vivo* skin tests such as the prick or intradermal tests are done by exposing the patient directly to a very small amount of allergen injected under the skin. A positive test produces a wheal and flare reaction.

The reactants responsible for type II hypersensitivity are IgG and IgM. They react with antigens located on cellular surfaces and trigger activation of the complement cascade. Target cells are damaged or destroyed by the opsonizing effect of antibody or complement components, or by complement-generated lysis if the cascade goes to completion. Examples of type II reactions due to exogenous antigens include autoimmune hemolytic anemia, transfusion reactions, and HDN.

The DAT is used to screen for transfusion reactions, autoimmune hemolytic anemia, and hemolytic disease of the newborn. Washed patient red blood cells are combined with antihuman globulin and observed for agglutination, indicating the presence of IgG or complement components on the cells.

Thrombocytopenic purpura and Goodpasture's syndrome are additional examples of type II reactions directed against self-antigens. In thrombocytopenic purpura, platelets are damaged or destroyed. Goodpasture's syndrome is the result of antibody that reacts with the basement membrane of the glomerulus. Complement is activated, causing tissue damage and eventual loss of renal function.

In type III hypersensitivity reactions, IgG, IgM, and complement are also involved, but the reaction is directed against soluble rather than cellular antigens. If mild antigen excess occurs, the antigen–antibody complexes precipitate out and deposit in the tissues. The sites most affected are the basement membrane in the kidneys, linings of blood vessels, and joint linings. When complement binds to these complexes, phagocytic cells are attracted to the area. If the target cells cannot be engulfed, a reverse phagocytic process called exocytosis takes place. The Arthus reaction, characterized by deposition of antigen–antibody complexes in the blood vessels, is a classic example of a type III reaction. Other examples include serum sickness and autoimmune diseases such as SLE and rheumatoid arthritis. Specific tests can be performed to determine the nature of the antibody involved.

Type IV, or delayed, hypersensitivity differs from the other three categories in that antibody and complement do not play a major role. Activation of T cells with the subsequent release of cytokines is responsible for the tissue damage seen in this type of reaction. Contact dermatitis resulting from exposure to poison ivy, poison oak, or a metal such as nickel is an example of haptens triggering a reaction to self-antigens. Skin testing and lymphocyte activation are used to determine sensitivity to particular antigens.

All four types of hypersensitivity represent defense mechanisms that stimulate an inflammatory response to cope with and react to antigen that is seen as foreign. In many cases, the antigen is not harmful, but the response to it results in tissue damage. This necessitates treatment to limit the damage.

Case Studies

1. A 13-year-old male had a number of absences from school in the spring due to cold symptoms that included head congestion and cough. He had been on antibiotics twice, but he seemed to go from one cold to the next. A complete blood cell (CBC) count showed no overall increase in white blood cells, but a mild eosinophilia was present. Because he had no fever or other signs of infection, his physician suggested that a total IgE screening test be run. The total IgE value was 250 IU/mL, which was within high normal limits.

Questions

   a. What would account for the eosinophilia noted?

   b. What conclusions can be drawn from the total IgE value?

   c. What other tests might be indicated?

2. A 55-year-old male went to his physician complaining about feeling tired and run down. Two months previously, he had pneumonia and was concerned that he might not have completely recovered. He indicated that his symptoms only become noticeable if he goes out in the cold. A CBC count was performed, showing that his white cell count was within normal limits, but his red cell count was just below normal. A DAT performed on red blood cells was weakly positive after incubating at room temperature for 5 minutes. When the DAT was repeated with monospecific reagents, the tube with anti-C3d was the only one positive.

Questions

   a. What does a positive DAT indicate?

   b. What is the most likely class of the antibody causing the reaction?

   c. Why was the DAT positive only with anti-C3d when monospecific reagents were used?

Exercise: Direct Antiglobulin Test

PRINCIPLE

The direct antiglobulin test (DAT) is used to detect *in vivo* coating of red blood cells with antibody, usually IgG, or complement degradation products such as C3d or C3dg. Presence of complement products indicates that antigen–antibody combination triggered the complement pathway and produced split products. DAT testing helps to diagnose autoimmune hemolytic anemia, HDN, transfusion reactions, or other type II hypersensitivity reactions.

SAMPLE PREPARATION

Collect blood by venipuncture using aseptic technique and avoiding hemolysis. Use ethylenediaminetetra-acetic acid (EDTA) as the anticoagulant.

REAGENTS, MATERIALS, AND EQUIPMENT

   Polyspecific antihuman globulin reagent (AHG)
   Bovine albumin, 22 percent
   12 × 75 mm disposable glass test tubes
   Disposable plastic blood bank pipettes

PROCEDURE

1. Prepare a 2- to 5-percent suspension of patient red cells by using saline.
2. Prepare a 6-percent suspension of bovine albumin by diluting the 22-percent suspension. To make 10 ml of a 6-percent suspension, add 2.7 mL of 22-percent bovine albumin to 7.3 mL of saline.
3. Place one drop of the red cell suspension in each of two labeled test tubes.
4. Fill each tube with saline, and centrifuge in a blood bank centrifuge for approximately 1 minute.
5. Decant tube, add saline to completely resuspend the cell button, and recentrifuge. Repeat this procedure three more times for a total of four washes.
6. Completely decant the final wash, and immediately add one or two drops of polyspecific AHG (as specified by the manufacturer) to one tube. Add one or two drops of 6-percent bovine albumin to the other tube.
7. Mix and centrifuge for approximately 30 seconds.
8. Dislodge the button from the bottom of the tube by gently tilting back and forth until no cells remain at the bottom of the tube.
9. Examine the tube carefully for agglutination by tilting back and forth and looking for clumps.
10. Leave any nonreactive tests for 5 minutes at room temperature, and then centrifuge and read again.
11. Add one drop of IgG-coated red cells to any nonreactive tube.
12. Centrifuge and examine the cells for agglutination. Any previously negative tube should be positive when the control cells are added.

INTERPRETATION

This test represents a screening test for the presence of immunoglobulin, namely either IgG or IgM on red cells. It also detects breakdown products of complement activation, namely C3d, indicating that complement activation has taken place. C3d is a breakdown product of C3b, the most abundant complement component. If C3d is present, this indicates that antigen–antibody combination must have taken place to initiate the complement cascade.

In either case, a positive test would indicate that red cells have been coated *in vivo* and that a type II hypersensitivity reaction has occurred. Typically, coating with antibody usually causes an immediate reaction, while if only complement products are present, the reaction may need to be incubated and reread in 5 minutes.

A negative result is confirmed by the use of check cells or control cells. These red cells have been coated with IgG by the manufacturer. When antibody-coated cells are added to a tube that is negative, the antihuman globulin that is still present and not bound will bind to the control cells. When centrifuged, a tube with control cells should show at least a 2+ agglutination. This ensures that the patient cells have been properly washed to get rid of any residual immunoglobulins in the serum. It also confirms that reactive AHG was added.

A positive DAT would be found in the case of autoimmune hemolytic anemia, in which the patient produces an antibody to his or her own red cells. In the case of a transfusion reaction, a positive DAT indicates that the patient had preformed antibody to the red cells that were transfused. If cord blood cells are tested and found to be positive, this is an indicator of HDN, in which the mother's antibodies have coated the baby's red cells.

Positive results with polyspecific antiglobulin can be followed up by repeating the entire procedure with monospecific reagents (i.e., one that is specific for IgG, and one that reacts with C3d). A reaction with only anti-C3d indicates that the antibody triggering the reaction is likely of the IgM class.

1. Which of the following characterizes hypersensitivity reactions?
   a. Immune responsiveness is depressed.
   b. Antibody is involved in all reactions.
   c. Either self-antigen or heterologous antigen may be involved.
   d. The antigen triggering the reaction is a harmful one.

2. Which of the following is associated with an increase in IgE production?
   a. Transfusion reaction
   b. Activation of Th1 cells
   c. Reaction to poison ivy
   d. HDN

3. Which of the following would cause a false-negative result in a DAT test?
   a. Incubating longer than 5 minutes
   b. Not washing red cells thoroughly
   c. Using EDTA anticoagulated blood
   d. Presence of IgG on red cells

4. All of the following are associated with type I hypersensitivity *except:*
   a. Release of preformed mediators from mast cells
   b. Activation of complement
   c. Cell-bound antibody bridged by antigen
   d. An inherited tendency to respond to allergens

5. Which newly synthesized mediator has a mode of action similar to that of histamine?
   a. LTB_4
   b. Heparin
   c. ECF-A
   d. PGD_2

6. Which of the following is associated with anaphylaxis?
   a. Buildup of IgE on mast cells
   b. Activation of complement
   c. Increase in cytotoxic T cells
   d. Large amount of circulating IgG

7. To determine if a patient is allergic to rye grass, the best test to perform is:
   a. RAST
   b. RIST
   c. DAT
   d. Complement fixation

8. Which condition would result in HDN?
   a. Buildup of IgE on mother's cells
   b. Sensitization of cytotoxic T cells
   c. Exposure to antigen found on both mother and baby red cells
   d. Prior exposure to foreign red cell antigen

9. What is the immune mechanism involved in type III hypersensitivity reactions?
   a. Cellular antigens are involved.
   b. Deposition of immune complexes occurs in antibody excess.
   c. Only heterologous antigens are involved.
   d. Tissue damage results from exocytosis.

10. What is the immune phenomenon associated with the Arthus reaction?
    a. Tissue destruction by cytotoxic T cells
    b. Removal of antibody-coated red blood cells
    c. Deposition of immune complexes in blood vessels
    d. Release of histamine from mast cells

11. Contact dermatitis can be characterized by all of the following *except:*
    a. Formation of antigen–antibody complexes
    b. Generation of sensitized T cells
    c. Langerhans cells acting as antigen-presenting cells
    d. Complexing of a hapten to self-antigen

12. Which of the following conclusions can be drawn about a patient whose total IgE level is determined to be 150 IU/mL?
    a. The patient definitely has allergic tendencies.
    b. The patient may be subject to anaphylactic shock.
    c. Further antigen-specific testing should be done.
    d. The patient will never have an allergic reaction.

References

1. Goldsby, RA, Kindt, TJ, and Osborne, BA: Hypersensitive Reactions. In Goldsby, RA, Kindt, TJ, Osborne, BA: Kuby Immunology. WH Freeman and Company, New York, 2000, pp 395–421.
2. Terr, AI: The atopic diseases. In Stites, DP, Terr, AI, and Parslow, TG (eds): Medical Immunology, ed. 9. Appleton & Lange, East Norwalk, Conn., 1997, pp 389–408.
3. Goust, JM: Immediate hypersensitivity. Immunol Ser 58:343, 1993.
4. Kay, AB: Allergy and allergic diseases, Part I. N Engl J Med 344:30–37, 2001.
5. Homberger, HA: Allergic diseases. In Henry, JB (ed): Clinical Diagnosis and Management by Laboratory Methods, ed. 20. WB Saunders, Philadelphia, 2001, pp 1016–1027.

6. Kinet, JP: The high-affinity IgE receptor (FceRI): From physiology to pathology. Ann Rev Immunol 17:931–972, 1999.

7. Terr, AI: Mechanisms of hypersensitivity. In Stites, DP, Terr, AI, and Parslow, TG (eds): Medical Immunology, ed. 9. Appleton & Lange, East Norwalk, Conn., 1997, pp 376–388.

8. Tharp, MD: IgE and immediate hypersensitivity. Dermatological Clinics of North America 8:619, 1990.

9. Kaliner, M, and Lemanske, R: Rhinitis and asthma. JAMA 268:2807, 1992.

10. Lewis, RA, Austen, KF, and Soberman, R: Leukotrienes and other products of the 5-lipoxygenase pathway. N Engl J Med 323:645, 1990.

11. Terr, AI: Anaphylaxis and urticaria. In Stites, DP, Terr, AI, and Parslow, TG (eds): Medical Immunology, ed. 9. Appleton & Lange, East Norwalk, Conn., 1997, pp 409–418.

12. Zak, HN, Kaste, LM, Schwarzenberger, K, et al: Health-care workers and latex allergy. Archives of Environmental Health 55:336–347, 2000.

13. Berger, WE: Monoclonal anti-IgE antibody: A novel therapy for allergic airways disease. Ann Allergy, Asthma, Immunol 88:152–160, 2002.

14. Naclerio, RM: Allergic rhinitis. N Engl J Med 325:860, 1992.

15. Kay, AB: Allergy and allergic diseases, Part II. N Engl J Med 344:109–113, 2001.

16. Hughes, ATD: Anti-IgE antibody may help treat some asthma patients. JAMA 284:2859–90, 2000.

17. Milgrom, H, Fick, RB Jr., Su, JQ, et al: Treatment of allergic asthma with monoclonal anti-IgE antibody. N Engl J Med 341(26):1966–1973, 1999.

18. Lopez, M, Fleisher, T, and deShazo, RD: Use and interpretation of diagnostic immunologic laboratory tests. JAMA 268:2970, 1992.

19. Norman, PS, and Peebles, RS: In vivo diagnostic allergy testing methods. In Rose, NR, et al (eds): Manual of Clinical Laboratory Immunology, ed. 5. ASM Press, Washington, D.C., 1997, pp 875–880.

20. Stevens, CD: Current status of in vitro allergy testing. Tech Sample 1998.

21. Hamilton, RG, and Adkinson, Jr, NF: Immunological tests for diagnosis and management of human allergic disease: Total and allergen-specific IgE and allergen-specific IgG. In Rose, NR, et al (eds): Manual of Clinical Laboratory Immunology, ed. 5. ASM Press, Washington, D.C., 1997, pp 881–892.

22. Nolte, H, and DuBuske, LM: Performance characteristics of a new automated enzyme immunoassay for the measurement of allergen-specific IgE. Ann Allergy Asthma Immunol 79:27–34, 1997.

23. Szeinbach, SL, Barnes, JH, Sullivan, TJ, et al: Precision and accuracy of commercial laboratories' ability to classify positive and/or negative allergen-specific IgE results. Ann Allergy, Asthma, Immunol. 86:373–381, 2001.

24. Garratty, G, Dzik, W, Issitt, PD, et al: Terminology for blood group antigens and genes—historical origins and guidelines in the new millennium. Transfusion 40:477–489, 2000.

25. Beadling, WV, Cooling, L, and Henry, JB: Immunohematology. In Henry, JB (ed): Clinical Diagnosis and Management by Laboratory Methods, ed. 20. WB Saunders, Philadelphia, 2001, pp 660–717.

26. Wells, JV, and Isbister, JP: Hematologic diseases. In Stites, DP, Terr, AI, and Parslow, TG (eds): Medical Immunology, ed. 9. Appleton & Lange, East Norwalk, Conn., 1997, pp 493–512.

27. Boral, LI, Weiss, ED, and Henry, JB: Transfusion medicine. In Henry, JB (ed): Clinical Diagnosis and Management by Laboratory Methods, ed. 20. WB Saunders, Philadelphia, 2001, pp 717–775.

28. Elghetany, MT, and FR Davey: Erythrocytic disorders. In Henry, JB (ed): Clinical Diagnosis and Management by Laboratory Methods, ed. 20. WB Saunders, Philadelphia, 2001, pp 542–585.

29. Smith, LA. Autoimmune hemolytic anemias: Characteristics and classification. Clin Lab Sci 12(2):110–113, 1999.

30. Petz, LD: Autoimmune hemolytic anemias. In Rose, NR, et al (eds): Manual of Clinical Laboratory Immunology, ed. 5. ASM Press, Washington, D.C., 1997, pp 1018–1025.

31. Kickler, TS: Autoimmune thrombocytopenia. In Rose, NR, et al (eds): Manual of Clinical Laboratory Immunology, ed. 5. ASM Press, Washington, D.C., 1997, pp 1026–1030.

32. Miller, JM: Blood platelets. In Henry, JB (ed): Clinical Diagnosis and Management by Laboratory Methods, ed. 20. WB Saunders, Philadelphia, 2001, pp 623–641.

33. Fieselmann, JF, and Richerson, HB: Respiratory diseases. In Stites, DP, Terr, AI, and Parslow, TG (eds): Medical Immunology, ed. 9. Appleton & Lange, East Norwalk, Conn., 1997, pp 599–612.

34. Goldsby, RA, Kindt, TJ, and Osborne, BA: Autoimmunity. In Goldsby, RA, Kindt, TJ, Osborne, BA: Kuby Immunology. WH Freeman, New York, 2000, pp 497–516.

35. Terr, AI: Immune-complex allergic disease. In Stites, DP, Terr, AI, and Parslow, TG (eds): Medical Immunology, ed. 9. Appleton & Lange, East Norwalk, Conn., 1997, pp 419–424.

36. Roitt, I, Brostoff, J, and Male, D (eds): Immunology, ed. 4. Mosby, London, 1996, pp 25.1–25.12.

37. Terr, AI: Cell-mediated hypersensitivity diseases. In Stites, DP, Terr, AI, and Parslow, TG (eds): Medical Immunology, ed. 9. Appleton & Lange, East Norwalk, Conn., 1997, pp 425–432.

38. Merrill, W: Hypersensitivity pneumonitis: Just think about it. Chest, 2001.

39. Klimas, N: Delayed hypersensitivity skin testing. In Rose, NR, et al (eds): Manual of Clinical Laboratory Immunology, ed. 5. ASM Press, Washington, D.C., 1997, pp 276–280.

40. Kurup, VP, and Fink, JN: Immunological tests for evaluation of hypersensitivity pneumonitis and allergic bronchopulmonary aspergillosis. In Rose, NR, et al (eds): Manual of Clinical Laboratory Immunology, ed. 5. ASM Press, Washington, D.C., 1997, pp 908–915.

chapter 14

Autoimmunity

Learning Objectives

After finishing this chapter, the reader will be able to:

1. Describe the factors that contribute to the development of autoimmunity.
2. Distinguish organ-specific and systemic autoimmune diseases, giving an example of each.
3. Describe the effects of systemic lupus erythematosus (SLE) on the body.
4. Discuss the immunologic mechanisms known for SLE.
5. List four types of autoantibodies found in lupus, and describe the pattern seen with each in immunofluorescence testing.
6. Differentiate screening tests from antibody-specific tests for lupus.
7. Discuss the symptoms of rheumatoid arthritis (RA).
8. Describe characteristics of the key antibody found in RA.
9. Discuss screening tests for rheumatoid factor (RF), explaining the limitations of current testing procedures.
10. Differentiate Hashimoto's thyroiditis and Graves' disease on the basis of laboratory findings and immune mechanisms.
11. List the main antibodies tested for in Graves' and Hashimoto's diseases, and describe testing procedures.
12. Relate genetic susceptibility to the development of insulin-dependent diabetes mellitus.
13. Explain immunologic mechanisms known to cause destruction of β cells in type I diabetes mellitus.
14. Discuss the immunologic findings in multiple sclerosis (MS), myasthenia gravis (MG), and Goodpasture's syndrome.

Key Terms

Antinuclear antibody (ANA)	Molecular mimicry	Thyroid-stimulating hormone (TSH)
Autoimmune disease	Multiple sclerosis (MS)	Thyroid-stimulating immunoglobulin (TSI)
Fluorescent antinuclear antibody (FANA) testing	Myasthenia gravis (MG)	
	Rheumatoid arthritis (RA)	Thyrotoxicosis
Graves' disease	Rheumatoid factor (RF)	Type I diabetes mellitus
Hashimoto's thyroiditis	Systemic lupus erythematosus (SLE)	

Autoimmune diseases are conditions in which damage to organs or tissues results from the presence of autoantibody or autoreactive cells. Such diseases affect 5 to 7 percent of the population and are thought to be caused by the loss or breakdown of self-tolerance.[1] In the early 1900s, Ehrlich described this phenomenon as "horror autotoxicus," literally meaning fear of self-poisoning. Thus, it was recognized early on that under normal circumstances, the immune response was held in check so that self-antigens were not destroyed.

Self-tolerance is believed to be brought about by several mechanisms, including clonal deletion of relevant effector cells, and active regulation by T cells. As described in Chapter 3, during the maturation process of T cells, the great majority of undifferentiated lymphocytes that are processed through the thymus do not survive. It is thought that this is where potentially self-reactive T cell clones are destroyed. Some T cells that can react to self-antigen do leave the thymus, but tolerance is maintained by a balance between the T helper cell type 1 (Th1) and T helper cell type 2 (Th2) populations.[1] In animal models of autoimmune disease, the Th1 cells have been implicated as primary mediators of autoimmune disease because they release proinflammatory cytokines.[1] The reaction to foreign antigens is typically a Th2 response, and the accompanying cytokines do not cause the same type of destruction as Th1 cells.

In addition to the T cells, the major histocompatability complex (MHC) products influence antigen recognition or nonrecognition by determining the type of peptides that can be presented to the T cells. There is a close fit between an antigenic peptide and the groove of an individual MHC molecule, as discussed in Chapter 4. Therefore, inheritance of a gene coding for a specific MHC molecule may make an individual more susceptible to a particular autoimmune disease. In addition, the expression of class II molecules on cells where they are not normally found may result in the presentation of self-antigens for which no tolerance has been established.[2] In several of the diseases presented in this chapter, there are examples of host cells that exhibit class II molecules on their surfaces after an inflammatory response. Links between inheritance of certain MHC genes and the tendency to develop particular autoimmune diseases is discussed.

In addition to the role played by MHC molecules, several other mechanisms are thought be contribute to autoimmunity. These are release of sequestered antigens, molecular mimicry, and polyclonal B cell activation. Antigens that are protected from encountering the circulation are not exposed to potentially reactive lymphocytes. Examples of these are myelin basic protein, normally sequestered by the blood–brain barrier, and sperm. Trauma to the tissue by means of an accident or infection may introduce such antigens to the general circulation. In the case of sperm, vasectomy can induce autoantibody formation.

Molecular mimicry refers to the fact that many individual viral or bacterial agents contain antigens that closely resemble self-antigens. Exposure to such foreign antigens may trigger antibody production that in turn reacts with similar self-antigens. Examples are poliovirus VP2 and acetylcholine (ACH) receptors, measles virus P3 and myelin basic protein, and papilloma virus E2 and insulin receptors.[1] Further examples will be discussed with individual diseases.

The last major factor is polyclonal B cell activation. Many gram-negative bacteria, and several viruses such as cytomegalovirus and Epstein-Barr virus (EBV) are all polyclonal activators, inducing proliferation of a number of clones of B cells that express IgM in the absence of T helper (Th) cells.[1] In this process, B cells that may be reactive to self-antigens can be activated.

Besides the factors mentioned previously, a number of others must be taken into account in the etiology of autoimmune diseases. Some of these are defects in the immune system, the influence of hormones, and environmental conditions. Defects in natural killer cells, in the secretion of cytokines, in phagocytosis, and in complement components all may contribute to the loss of self-tolerance. Hormones, especially estrogens, may also play a role because they are known to affect cytokine production and may influence which T cells, either Th1 or Th2, are more active in a particular response.[3] This explains in part why women are more prone to autoimmune diseases. Thus, there is not one cause but many contributing factors that are responsible for the pathologic conditions known as autoimmune disease.

Autoimmune diseases can be classified as systemic or organ-specific. There is often a good bit of overlap between the two because some diseases that start out as organ-specific later affect other organs. A listing of some of the more important autoimmune diseases is given in Table 14–1. Many of the key diseases for which serologic testing is available are discussed in this chapter.

TABLE 14–1. Spectrum of Autoimmune Diseases

Specificity	Disease	Target Tissue
Organ-Specific	Hashimoto's thyroiditis	Thyroid
	Graves' disease	Thyroid
	Pernicious anemia cells	Gastric parietal
	Addison's disease	Adrenal glands
	Type I diabetes mellitus	Pancreas
	MG	Nerve-muscle synapses
	MS	Myelin sheath of nerves
	Autoimmune hemolytic anemia	Red blood cells
	Idiopathic thrombocytopenic purpura	Platelets
	Goodpasture's syndrome	Kidney, lungs
	RA	Joints, lungs, skin
	Scleroderma	Skin, gut, lungs, kidney
Systemic	SLE	Skin, joints, kidney, brain, heart, lungs

MG = Myasthenia gravis; MS = multiple sclerosis; RA = rheumatoid arthritis; SLE = systemic lupus erythematosus.

Systemic Lupus Erythematosus

Systemic lupus erythematosus (SLE) represents the prototype of human autoimmune diseases. It is a chronic systemic inflammatory disease marked by alternating exacerbations and remissions, affecting approximately 1 in every 2000 individuals. Incidence of the disease has tripled over the last 4 decades.[4] The peak age of onset is usually between 20 and 40 years of age. Women are much more likely than men to be stricken, by a margin of approximately 10 to 1.[1,5] It is also more common in African Americans and Hispanics than in whites.[5]

The immune response is directed against a broad range of target antigens, and it appears that both genetic and environmental factors play a role. In whites, there is a strong association with human leukocyte antigen (HLA) DR3 or DR2.[6,7] In addition to the HLA region, there are at least 13 other chromosomal regions that demonstrate a link to lupus.[6] Environmental factors include exposure to ultraviolet light, certain medications, and exposure to infectious agents.[8] Hormones are also important because they may influence the regulation of transcription of genes that are central to the expression of SLE.[8]

Clinical Signs

The clinical signs are extremely diverse, and nonspecific symptoms such as fatigue, weight loss, malaise, fever, and anorexia are often the first to appear. Joint involvement seems to be the most frequently reported manifestation because over 90 percent of patients with SLE are subject to polyarthralgias or arthritis.[5,7] Typically, the arthritis is symmetric and involves the small joints of the hands, wrists, and knees.

After joint involvement, the next most common signs are skin manifestations. An erythematous rash may appear on any area of the body exposed to ultraviolet light.[5,7] Less common, but perhaps more dramatic, is the appearance of the classic butterfly rash across the nose and cheeks. This is what is responsible for the name lupus, derived from the Latin term meaning wolflike. This rash appears in only about 30 to 40 percent of all patients (Fig. 14–1). In discoid lupus, skin lesions have central atrophy and scarring.

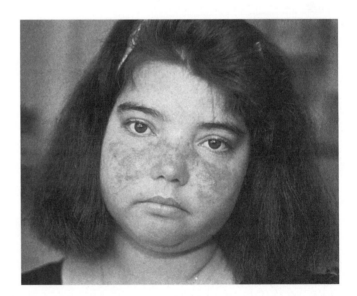

FIG. 14–1. Butterfly rash in SLE. Characteristic rash over the cheekbones and forehead is diagnostic of SLE. The disease often begins in young adulthood and may eventually involve many organ systems. (From Steinman, L: Autoimmune disease. Sci Am 269:107, 1993, with permission.)

One half to two thirds of all patients exhibit evidence of renal involvement. There are several types of lesions, but the most dangerous is diffuse proliferative glomerulonephritis, in which there is cellular proliferation in at least 50 percent of the glomeruli.[5,7] Other conditions may include deposition of immune complexes in the subendothelial tissue and thickening of the basement membrane itself. All of these can lead to renal failure, the most frequent cause of death in patients with SLE.

Other systemic effects may include cardiac involvement with pericarditis, tachycardia, or ventricular enlargement; pleurisy with chest pain; neuropsychiatric manifestations such as seizures, mild cognitive dysfunction, psychoses, or depression; or hematologic abnormalities such as anemia, leukopenia, thrombocytopenia, or lymphopenia.[5,7,9,10]

Immunologic Findings

The first clue in the mystery of lupus was the discovery of the LE cell by Malcolm Hargraves in 1948. The LE cell is a neutrophil that has engulfed the antibody-coated nucleus of another neutrophil. This phenomenon, which mainly appears *in vitro*, occurs when cells are damaged and release nuclear material. Nine years after the LE cell was discovered, the first anti-deoxyribonucleic acid (DNA) antibody was identified.[11] Now it is known that SLE is associated with more than 25 autoantibodies. Some of the more common ones are listed in Table 14–2.

The large number of possible autoantibodies reflects a generalized dysregulation of the immune system.[12] Dysfunctional processing in the routine nonimmunologic clearing of cellular debris may be key to the pathogenesis of SLE.[12] Abnormal apoptosis, or programmed cell death, of certain types of cells may occur, releasing excess amounts of cellular constituents such as DNA and ribonucleic acid (RNA). Individuals who inherit certain HLA genes are more likely to respond to such self-antigens. Constant presence of antigenic material triggers polyclonal activation of B cells, one of the main immunologic characteristics in lupus. There is an accompanying alteration in the function of both Th1 and Th2 helper cells, resulting in enhanced production of certain cytokines that contribute to up-regulation of antibody production by B cells.[13] In particular, increased production of interleukin-10 (IL-10), which normally serves an immunosuppressive role, correlates with increased antibody production and with disease activity. IL-10 appears to trigger an increase in antibodies directed against DNA and stimulate production of platelet-activating factor.[7,14,15] Platelet-activating factor is a secondary mediator of infection and can cause vascular injury.[15]

Once immune complexes are formed, they cannot be cleared as well from the circulation because of other possible deficiencies. These include defects in complement receptors on phagocytic cells, defects in receptors for the fragment crystallizable (Fc) portion of immunoglobulins, or deficiencies of early complement

TABLE 14–2. Common Antinuclear Antibodies

Autoantibody	Characteristics of Antigen	Immunofluorescent Pattern	Disease Association
Anti–ds-DNA	Specific for ds-DNA	Peripheral/homogeneous	Only in SLE
Anti–ss-DNA	Related to purines and pyrimidines	Not detected on routine screen	SLE, many other diseases
Anti-histone	Different classes of histones	Homogeneous/peripheral	Drug-induced SLE, other diseases
Anti-DNP	DNA-histone complex	Homogeneous	SLE, drug-induced SLE
Anti-Sm	Extractable nuclear antigen (RNA component)	Speckled	Diagnostic for SLE
Anti-RNP	Proteins complexed with nuclear RNA	Speckled	SLE, mixed connective tissue diseases
Anti-SS-aRo	Proteins complexed to RNA	Speckled or negative	SLE, Sjögren's syndrome, others
Anti-SS-bLa	Phosphoprotein complexed to RNA polymerase	Speckled	SLE, Sjögren's syndrome, others
Anti-nucleolar	RNA polymerase, nucleolar protein	Nucleolar	SLE, scleroderma
Anti-Scl-70	DNA topoisomerase I	Atypical speckled	Scleroderma
Anti–Jo-1	Histidyl-t RNA synthetase	? Cytoplasmic	Polymyositis

Adapted from Fritzler, MJ: Immunofluorescent antinuclear antibody tests. In Rose, NR, De MacArio, EC, Folds, JD, et al (eds): Manual of Clinical Laboratory Immunology, ed. 5. American Society for Microbiology, Washington, D.C., 1997.
DNA = Deoxyribonucleic acid; SLE = systemic lupus erythematosus; DNP = deoxyribonucleoprotein; RNA = ribonucleic acid; RNP = ribonucleoprotein.

components such as C1q, C2, or C4.[6,8] Accumulation of IgG seems to be the most pathogenic because it forms complexes of an intermediate size that become deposited in the glomerular basement membrane. In addition, DNA as one of the main antigens has an affinity for the basement membrane, thus enhancing the likelihood of deposition of such complexes.[9] Accumulation of immune complexes with activation of the complement cascade is responsible for the damage to the kidney seen with this disease.

Drug-induced lupus differs from the more chronic form of the disease in that symptoms usually disappear once the drug is discontinued. Typically, this is a milder form of the disease, usually manifested as arthritis or rashes.[7] The most common drugs implicated are procainamide, hydralazine, chlorpromazine, isoniazid, quinidine, anticonvulsants such as methyldopa, and possibly oral contraceptives.[5]

Laboratory Diagnosis of Systemic Lupus Erythematosus

Typically the first test done when SLE is suspected is a screening test for **antinuclear antibodies (ANA). Fluorescent antinuclear antibody (FANA) testing** is the most widely used and accepted test.[5,16] This is an extremely sensitive test and relatively easy to perform, but it has low diagnostic specificity because many of the antibodies are associated with other autoimmune diseases.[16] Mouse kidney or human epithelial HEp-2 cells are fixed to a slide and allowed to react with patient serum. After careful washing to remove all unreacted antibody, an antihuman immunoglobulin with a fluorescent tag or an enzyme label such as horseradish peroxidase is added. Approximately 2 percent of healthy individuals and up to 75 percent of elderly individuals test positive.[16,17] Conversely, up to 5 percent of SLE patients test negative, so this test cannot be used to absolutely rule out SLE. If FANA testing is positive at dilutions of 1:4 and 1:16, then further dilutions of 1:64 and 1:256 should be prepared and the test repeated.[16] Patients with SLE usually have high titers of high affinity antibody against specific antigens. Profile testing for individual antibodies could be done as a follow-up. A diagram of the possible fluorescent patterns is shown in Figure 14–2 (see also Color Plate 10). Some of the individual antinuclear antibodies and other categories of antibodies are discussed below.

Antinuclear Antibodies

FANA Testing
Double-stranded DNA (ds-DNA) antibodies are the most specific for SLE because they are seen only in

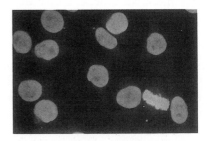
Homogeneous pattern

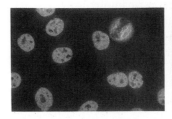 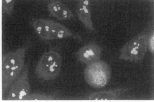
Speckled pattern   Nucleolar pattern

FIG. 14–2. Patterns of immunofluorescent staining for antinuclear antibodies. Examples of predominant staining patterns obtained are homogeneous—staining of the entire nucleus, discrete speckled pattern—staining of centromeres, speckled pattern—staining throughout the nucleus, and nucleolar pattern—staining of the nucleolus. (From Sack, KE, and Fye, KH: Rheumatic diseases. In Stites, DP, Terr, AI, and Parslow, TG (eds): Manual of Clinical Laboratory Immunology, ed 4. American Society of Microbiology, Washington, D.C., 1992, with permission.) Color Plate 10.

patients with lupus, and levels correlate with disease activity.[9,11,16] Although they are found in only 50 to 70 percent of patients, the presence of these antibodies is considered diagnostic for SLE, especially when they are found in combination with low levels of complement component C3. Antibodies to ds-DNA typically produce a peripheral or a homogeneous staining pattern on indirect immunofluorescence (IIF).[16]

In testing for antibodies to ds-DNA, a purified antigen preparation that is free from single-stranded DNA (ss-DNA) must be used, as antibodies to ss-DNA are also found in lupus, RA, malignancies, chronic active hepatitis, biliary cirrhosis, and bacterial and parasitic infections.[7] One particularly sensitive assay for ds-DNA is an immunofluorescent test using *Crithidia luciliae*, a hemoflagellate, as the substrate. This trypanosome has circular ds-DNA in the kinetoplast. A positive test is indicated by a brightly stained kinetoplast with a dilution of 1:10 or greater of patient serum.[18] This test has a high degree of specificity, although it is less sensitive than other FANA tests.[18,19] Other assays that can be used to detect ds-DNA include immunodiffusion, radioimmunoassay (RIA), and enzyme immunoassay (EIA) tests.[19]

A second major antibody found in lupus patients is *antihistone antibody*. Histone is a nucleoprotein that is a major constituent of chromatin. It can be detected in almost all patients with drug-induced lupus. About 70 percent of other patients with SLE have elevated levels of antihistone antibodies, but the titers are usually fairly low.[5,19] Presence of antihistone antibody alone or combined with antibody to ss-DNA supports the diagnosis of drug-induced lupus.[7,9] Antihistone antibodies are also found in rheumatoid arthritis (RA) and primary biliary cirrhosis, but the levels are usually lower. High levels of antihistone antibodies tend to be associated with the more active and severe forms of SLE.[19] Antihistone antibodies are typically detected by immunofluorescent assays, immunoblotting, and EIA. On IIF, either a homogeneous pattern, representing fluorescence of the entire nucleus, is seen, or staining of the periphery occurs.[16]

Antibodies are also stimulated by DNA complexed to histone, known as *deoxyribonucleoprotein (DNP).* Immunofluorescent patterns are similar to those discussed previously. Latex particles coated with DNP are used in a simple slide agglutination test for SLE.

Antibody to a preparation of extractable nuclear antigen was first described in a patient named Smith, hence the name *anti-Sm antibody*. Extractable nuclear antigens represent a family of small nuclear proteins that are associated with uridine-rich RNA. The anti-Sm antibody is specific for lupus because it is not found in other autoimmune diseases. However, it is only found in between 15 and 30 percent of patients with this disease.[5,9] This antibody produces a coarsely speckled pattern of nuclear fluorescence on IIF. It can also be measured by immunodiffusion, immunoblotting, immunoprecipitation, and EIA.[16]

SS-A/Ro and SS-B/La antigens also belong to the family of extractable nuclear antigens. SS-A/Ro antigen is a RNA complexed to one of two proteins with molecular weights of 60kD or 52kD, and antibody to it appears in approximately 30 percent of patients with SLE.[9] This antibody is most often found in patients who have cutaneous manifestations of SLE, especially photosensitivity dermatitis.[9] Anti-Ro/SSA has been found to bind to cell surface antigens on neutrophils and can cause a mild neutropenia, often seen in patients with SLE.[10] SS-B/La antigen is a phosphoprotein that appears to be bound to products of RNA III polymerase.[9] Anti-SS-B/La is found in only 10 to 15 percent of patients with SLE, and all of these have anti-SS-A/Ro.[5] Both SS-A/Ro and SS-B/La antibodies are highly prevalent in patients with other autoimmune

diseases, notably scleroderma and Sjögren's syndrome.[5] To detect the presence of these antibodies on IIF, human tissue culture cells such as HEp-2 (human epithelial) must be used, because SS-A/Ro and SS-B/La antigens are not found in mouse or rat liver and kidney. A finely speckled pattern is evident. These can also be detected by immunoprecipitation, immunoblotting, and EIA.[16]

An antibody that produces a coarsely speckled IIF pattern is *anti-nRNP antibody*. Ribonucleoprotein (RNP) is protein complexed to a particular type of nuclear RNA called U1-nRNP (U for uridine-rich). Although it is detected in about 30 to 40 percent of patients with SLE, it is also found at a high titer in individuals with mixed connective tissue disease and other autoimmune diseases.[7,9] Anti-nRNP can be measured by immunoblotting, immunoprecipitation, EIA, and IIF.[16]

Staining of the nucleolus in IIF indicates antibody to *fibrillarin,* a dense component of the nucleolus. This is indicated by clumpy nucleolar fluorescence.[16] This pattern is associated with other autoimmune diseases such as scleroderma and polymyositis.[18]

Other Assays for ANA

ANAs can also be detected by immunodiffusion. Typically, immunodiffusion is used to determine the immunologic specificity of a positive FANA test. Such testing is valuable in identification of specific disease states and in ruling out those normal patients who exhibit a positive FANA test. Ouchterlony double diffusion detects antibody to several of the small nuclear ribonucleoproteins, or extractable nuclear antigens (ENA). These include antibodies to the following antigens: Sm, nRNP, SS-A/Ro, SS-B/La, Scl-70 (DNA topoisomerase I), and Jo-1 (antigens found in dermatopolymyositis).[20] Table 14–2 shows the source of these antigens and associations with specific diseases. A positive reaction is indicated by immunoprecipitation lines of serologic identity (Fig. 14–3). (Refer to Chapter 9 for a description of the principles of Ouchterlony immunodiffusion.) Although this type of testing is not as sensitive as some other techniques, it is highly specific.[20]

Immunoblotting techniques separate out antigens by means of polyacrylamide gel electrophoresis. The pattern is then electrotransferred to a nitrocellulose sheet, which is incubated with dilutions of patient serum. Either radiolabeled or enzyme labeled antibody conjugates are then used to visualize individual bands. This technique has been found to be reliable, sensitive, and specific, and has begun to be used more widely.[21]

EIA has also come into wider use for detection of anti–ds-DNA, antihistone antibodies, and anti–SS-A

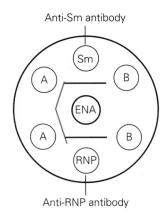

Anti-Sm antibody

Anti-RNP antibody

FIG. 14–3. Extractable nuclear antibody (ENA) immunodiffusion pattern. A mixture of extractable nuclear antigens, including RNP, Sm, and other soluble nuclear antigens, is placed in a central well in an agarose gel. Sm antibody and RNP antibody are run as positive controls, and patient samples are placed between the controls. The pattern of precipitin lines formed indicates the antibodies present in patient serum. The arc of serologic identity formed between Sm and patient A indicates that serum A contains anti-Sm antibodies. The arc of partial identity formed between serum A and RNP occurs because RNP is always found complexed to Sm antigen. RNP antibodies are not present. Serum B contains neither Sm nor RNP antibody.

and anti–SS-B. It is particularly good for detection of the later two antibodies.[22] EIA testing is quantitative, is less subjective, and lends itself well to automation.[22] However, IIF is still considered the "gold" standard.

Antiphospholipid Antibodies

Antiphospholipid antibodies have been found in up to 60 percent of patients with lupus, and these are heterogeneous in nature.[9,23] They appear to be of at least two types: *anticardiolipin* and an antibody known as the *lupus anticoagulant*. Both types bind negatively charged phospholipids, but patients who test positive for one do not always have elevated levels of the other.[24] Presence of anticardiolipin antibodies causes false-positive results for syphilis. The lupus anticoagulant was so named because it produces prolonged activated partial thromboplastin time (APT) and prothrombin time (PT). This is also found in patients without SLE. Ironically, patients with this antibody have an increased risk of clotting and spontaneous abortion, resulting from the fact that the lupus anticoagulant binds to a clotting inhibitor *in vivo*.[24] *In vitro*, it binds to clotting factors Xa and Va, phospholipid, and calcium to prolong clotting time in coagulation testing. In the body, the antibody is believed to bind to the phospholipid

membrane of endothelial cells in close proximity to protein C, thus preventing activation of the protein C molecule. Protein C is a natural inhibitor of clotting. Platelet function may be affected also. In addition to determining the PT and APT, there are several EIAs for anticardiolipin antibodies that are sensitive and relatively simple to perform.[23,25]

Treatment

If fever or arthritis is the primary symptom, a high dose of aspirin or other anti-inflammatory drug may bring relief. For skin manifestations, antimalarials, such as hydroxychloroquine or chloroquine, and topical steroids are often prescribed.[5] Systemic corticosteroids are used for acute fulminant lupus, lupus nephritis, or central nervous system complications because these suppress the immune response and lower antibody titers.[5,7] Other drugs used include cyclophosphamide, azathioprine, methotrexate, and chlorambucil, but all of these may have serious side effects such as bone marrow suppression, and they must be monitored closely. A new approach for patients whose symptoms cannot be controlled by other means involves autologous stem cell harvesting and reinfusion after the patient undergoes intensive chemotherapy.[26] Results indicate that long term remission may be possible using this method. Overall, the present 5-year survival rate approaches 90 percent.[5]

Rheumatoid Arthritis

Rheumatoid arthritis (RA) is another example of a systemic autoimmune disorder. It affects between 1 and 3 percent of people in the United States.[7,27] Women are three times as likely to be affected as men. Typically it strikes individuals between the ages of 30 and 50, although it may occur at any age.[1,7,27] In addition to a decline in functional ability, it has been shown that the median life expectancy is shortened by 7 years in men and 3 years in women.[27] Progress of the disease varies because there may be spontaneous remissions or an increasingly active disease that results in joint deformity and disability.

As in SLE, there appears to be an association of RA with certain of the MHC class II genes. These genes code for the two chains, α and β, that make up the HLA class II antigens (see Chapter 4). The strongest association appears with the DR1 and DR4 genes.[28] These occur in 70 percent of patients with RA. All of the alleles involved appear to code for a similar amino acid sequence at positions 67 to 74 in the β chain.[29] This "shared epitope" on the HLA class II β chain may act to facilitate antigen presentation to Th cells and to B cells.

Clinical Signs

Diagnosis of RA is based on the 1987 criteria established by the American College of Rheumatology.[30] Key symptoms are morning stiffness around the joints lasting at least 1 hour; swelling of the soft tissue around three or more joints; swelling of the proximal interphalangeal, metacarpophalangeal, or wrist joints; symmetric arthritis; subcutaneous nodules; a positive test for rheumatoid factor (RF); and radiographic evidence of erosions in the joints of the hands, the wrists, or both. At least four of these must be present for 6 weeks or more for the diagnosis to be made.

Typically the patient experiences nonspecific symptoms such as malaise, fever, weight loss, and transient joint pain that begins in the small joints of the hands and feet. Morning stiffness and joint pain usually improve during the day. Joint involvement progresses to the larger joints in a symmetric fashion, often affecting the knees, hips, elbows, shoulders, and cervical spine. The joint pain experienced leads to muscle spasm, which, because of the consequent limitation of motion, results in permanent joint deformity[7] (Fig. 14–4). About 25 percent of patients have nodules over the bones. These consist of necrotic areas surrounded by large mononuclear cells with an outer zone of granulation tissue containing plasma cells and lymphocytes.[7] Nodules can also be found in the myocardium, pericardium, heart valves, pleura, lungs, spleen, and larynx. Other systemic symptoms may include anemia, formation of subcutaneous nodules, pericarditis, lymphadenopathy, splenomegaly, interstitial lung disease, or vasculitis.

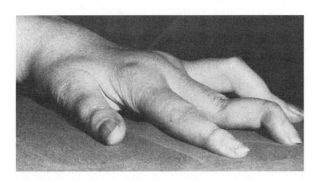

FIG. 14–4. Joint deformity in RA. Swan neck deformity of the middle finger in RA. This results from hyperextension of the proximal interphalangeal joints and flexion of distal interphalangeal joints. (Courtesy of SmithKline Beecham, Clinical Laboratories, Philadelphia.)

For many years there has been a search for an infectious agent or agents may be involved in the etiology of RA. A number of agents, including mycobacteria, rubella, cytomegalovirus, herpes simplex, EBV, mycobacteria, and mycoplasma have been proposed as possible triggering antigens. New evidence indicates that certain proteins found in such agents share a certain homology in an amino acid sequence that is similar to antigens found in the joints.[31] T cells found in individuals with RA appear to target this sequence. Thus, molecular mimicry may set off the autoimmune response.[7] Eighty percent of patients with RA have been found to have circulating antibody to specific EB viral antigens, but no other definite link has been established.[32]

Immunologic Findings

The main immunologic finding in RA is the presence of an antibody called the **rheumatoid factor (RF),** found in approximately 80 percent of patients with the disease.[7] It is most often of the IgM class and is directed against the Fc portion of IgG. IgM antibodies combine with IgG, and these immune complexes become deposited in the joints, resulting in a type III (or immune complex) hypersensitivity reaction. The complement protein C1 binds to the immune complexes, triggering activation of the classical complement cascade. During this process, C3a, C5a, and C5b67 are generated, all of which act as chemotactic factors for neutrophils. Neutrophils accumulate in large numbers at the site of deposition of immune complexes. Tissue damage results from the release of hydrolytic enzymes such as acid hydrolases, myeloperoxidase, lysozyme, and proteases by neutrophils as they attempt to phagocytose the immune complexes.[1] In addition, C3a, C4a, and C5a cause localized mast cell degranulation, resulting in the release histamine and chemotactic factors that increase vascular permeability and attract macrophages and neutrophils. The continual presence of macrophages may lead to the chronic inflammation usually observed that damages the synovium itself. The proliferation of cells that line the synovium, such as fibroblasts, macrophages, and lymphocytes results in formation of a *pannus,* an organized mass of cells that grows into the joint space and invades the cartilage.[33]

Other targets of autoantibodies associated with RA include collagen, human cartilage glycoprotein called HCgp39, p205 antigen present in the synovial membrane, p68 antigen present in the endoplasmic reticulum, and glucose-6-phosphate isomerase present in almost all cytoplasmic membranes.[31,34] In addition, low titers of antinuclear antibodies are present in about 40 percent of patients.[35] The pattern most identified is the speckled pattern directed against ribonucleoprotein. The significance of this group of autoantibodies remains unclear because they do not appear to be directly related to pathogenesis.

In addition to the presence of autoantibodies, there is increasing evidence that cytokines play a major role in chronic inflammation. Cytokines found in synovial fluid include interleukin-1 (IL-1), interleukin-6 (IL-6), interleukin-8 (IL-8), granulocyte-monocyte colony stimulating factor (GM-CSF) and tumor necrosis factor-alpha (TNF-α).[29,36,37] Interaction among antigen-presenting cells, T lymphocytes, and B lymphocytes leads to activation of macrophages. Macrophages release IL-1 and TNF-α, which drives the process of tissue destruction.[38] Prostaglandins and proteases produced by fibroblasts also act to erode and destroy bone and cartilage.[29] In addition, collagenase and other tissue-degrading enzymes are released from synoviocytes and chondrocytes that line the joint cavity.

Laboratory Diagnosis of Rheumatoid Arthritis

Diagnosis of RA is made on the basis of a combination of clinical manifestations, radiographic findings, and laboratory testing. Because RF is the most common autoantibody found, this is the antibody that is most often tested for to aid in making the initial diagnosis. Two types of agglutination tests for RF have been developed: one using sheep red blood cells coated with IgG and the other using latex particles coated with the same antigen. Because the latex test has a greater sensitivity, this is the predominant agglutination test used. Agglutination tests, however, only detect the IgM isotype, found in approximately 80 percent of patients. Thus, a negative result does not rule out the presence of RA. Conversely, a positive test result is not specific for RA because RF can be found in other diseases such as syphilis, SLE, chronic active hepatitis, tuberculosis, leprosy, infectious mononucleosis, and Sjörgren's syndrome.[7,29]

Testing for two other antibody classes of RF, IgG or IgA, tends to be more specific. These two isotypes are rarely found in other disease states, which may help in making a differential diagnosis.[39] The elevation of IgA early in the disease appears to be associated with a poorer prognosis, such as development of bone erosions and systemic manifestations.[40] Testing for IgG and IgA isotypes requires the use of EIA techniques, however, and is much more time consuming than slide agglutination tests. More recently developed

nephelometric assays can test for the presence of all three isotypes. These are based on increases in light scattering as immune complexes accumulate, and the sensitivity is somewhat better than manual agglutination methods.[41] Both EIA and nephelometric methods are helpful in confirming low titer obtained in manual agglutination methods, and because they are automated, they have largely replaced manual methods for detection of RF.

Testing for other autoantibodies may also be helpful in making a differential diagnosis. Autoantibodies that are specific to RA include anti-p68, anti-p205, anti-gp39, and anticollagen.[31] Once the diagnosis is made, however, the most helpful tests used to follow progress of the disease are general indicators of inflammation such as measurement of erythrocyte sedimentation rate, C-reactive protein (CRP), and complement components. Typically, CRP and sedimentation rates are elevated, and the level of complement components is normal or increased, indicating increased synthesis. Although not specific, following the inflammatory response is a more sensitive measure of disease activity than is a change in RF levels.[35]

Treatment

Traditional therapy for RA has included anti-inflammatory drugs such as salicylates and ibuprofen to control local swelling and pain. The discovery that joint destruction occurs early on during the disease has prompted more aggressive treatment. *Disease-modifying antirheumatic drugs (DMARDS)* are now prescribed if disease activity persists after 4 to 6 weeks of treatment with nonsteroidal anti-inflammatory drugs.[33,42] Such drugs include methotrexate, hydroxychloro-quine, sulfasalazine, cyclosporin, and penicillamine.[43] Corticosteroids such as prednisone cannot be used long-term, but they are given in short oral courses for disease flare-ups. These agents appear to halt the inflammatory response and slow the progression of joint erosion.

A recent development involves treatment with biological agents that block the activity of TNF-α. Agents that act against TNF-α are classified into two different categories: monoclonal antibody to TNF-α (infliximab) and TNF-α receptors fused to an IgG molecule (etanercept). Both specifically target and neutralize TNF-α, and they have shown very promising results in halting joint damage without producing major side effects.[29,40,42,44-46] A third new agent, leflunomide, is an inhibitor of an enzyme called dihydro-orotate dehydrogenase. It apparently helps to halt the immune response by affecting lymphocyte function.[42]

Hashimoto's Thyroiditis

Hashimoto's thyroiditis and Graves' disease are examples of organic-specific autoimmune diseases. Although these conditions have distinctly different symptoms, they do share some antibodies in common, and both interfere with functioning of the thyroid. The thyroid gland is located in the anterior region of the neck and is normally between 12 and 20 grams in size.[47] It consists of units called *follicles* that are spherical in shape and lined with cuboidal epithelial cells. Follicles are filled with material called colloid. The primary constituent of colloid is *thyroglobulin,* a large iodinated glycoprotein, which is the precursor of the thyroid hormones *triiodothyronine (T3)* and *thyroxine (T4).*

Under normal conditions, *thyrotropin-releasing hormone (TRH)* is secreted by the hypothalamus to initiate the process that eventually causes release of hormones from the thyroid. TRH acts on the pituitary to induce release of **thyroid-stimulating hormone (TSH).** TSH, in turn, binds to receptors on the cell membrane of the thyroid gland, causing thyroglobulin to be broken down into secretable T3 and T4. Production of autoantibodies interferes with this process and causes under- or overactivity of the thyroid.

Hashimoto's thyroiditis, also known as chronic autoimmune thyroiditis, is most often seen in middle-aged women, although it may occur anywhere from childhood up to about 70 years of age.[1,48] Patients develop a combination of *goiter,* or enlarged thyroid, hypothyroidism, and thyroid autoantibodies. The goiter is large and rubbery, and immune destruction of the thyroid gland occurs. Symptoms of hypothyroidism include dry skin, decreased sweating, puffy face with edematous eyelids, pallor with a yellow tinge, weight gain, and dry and brittle hair.[47]

A genetic predisposition has been postulated because the condition is more common in families in which another member has autoimmune thyroid disease. An association with HLA antigens DR4 and DR5 has been reported, but this is not consistent among different ethnic populations.[2] HLA-DR antigens are in fact expressed on the surface of thyroid epithelial cells during the progress of the disease. Certain other genes, notably DQA1 and DQB1, seem to confer resistance because Hashimoto's thyroiditis is far less prevalent among individuals with either of these genes.[49]

Immunologic Findings

Within the thyroid gland itself, lymphocytic infiltration is evident, with the development of germinal centers that almost completely replace the normal glandular architecture of the thyroid.[2,47] Cellular types present include activated T and B cells (with T cells predominating), macrophages, and plasma cells.[2] Autoantibody is found in 80 percent or more of patients. The disease is thus characterized by both a cellular and a humoral response, although it is believed that thyroid follicular destruction is predominantly T cell mediated.[47] This immune response progressively destroys the thyroid gland.

Laboratory Testing

The two major autoantibodies present are antibodies to thyroglobulin and to *thyroid peroxidase.*[2] Antibodies to the latter are directed against a 105kD fraction of the thyroid epithelial cell cytoplasm, and they are found in approximately 90 to 95 percent of patients with the disease.[47] They seem to correlate most closely with disease activity. Antibodies to thyroglobulin can be detected in titers greater than 1:1000 in 80 percent of patients with Hashimoto's thyroiditis.[48] Other antibodies present include colloid antibody (CA2) and TSH-binding inhibitory immunoglobulin (TBII). Antibody activity contributes to the destruction of thyroid cells.

Antibodies to peroxidase can be measured by IIF, but they are now typically measured by particle agglutination assays or EIA.[2,48] Antibodies to thyroglobulin can be demonstrated by indirect immunofluorescent assays, passive agglutination, and EIA.[48,50] Passive hemagglutination using tanned red blood cells is the most commonly used test. Indirect immunofluorescent testing is less sensitive than passive hemagglutination, but it can detect nonagglutinating antibody.[50] Indirect immunofluorescent assays use methanol-fixed monkey cryostat tissue sections as substrate.[48] Thyroglobulin antibodies will create a floccular or puffy staining pattern. Antibody to CA2 produces a diffuse or ground-glass appearance. Peroxidase antibodies produce staining of the cytoplasm and not the nucleus of thyroid cells.

Because antithyroglobulin antibodies are not found in all patients, a negative test result, therefore, does not necessarily rule out the disease. Healthy individuals may have a low titer of antithyroglobulin antibody, but in patients with Hashimoto's thyroiditis, the titer is considerably higher, so differentiation can be made in this manner.

Treatment

Treatment for Hashimoto's disease consists of thyroid hormone replacement therapy. TSH levels should be monitored throughout treatment.[47]

Graves' Disease

Graves' disease is a second autoimmune disease affecting the thyroid, but in contrast to Hashimoto's thyroiditis, Graves' disease is characterized by hyperthyroidism. It is, in fact, the most common cause of hyperthyroidism, affecting approximately 0.5 percent of the population.[2] It is also the most prevalent autoimmune disorder in the United States today.[51] Women exhibit greater susceptibility by a margin of about 7 to 1, and they most often present with the disease between the ages of 30 and 40.[2,48]

As with Hashimoto's thyroiditis, the tendency of Graves' disease to occur in families indicates some sort of genetic linkage. In whites, the disease has been associated with the HLA antigens DR3 and DQA1*0501, while inheritance of HLA DRB1*0701 seems to confer resistance.[51] The disease also appears to be associated with polymorphisms in the CTLA-4 gene, which codes for an antigen found on cytotoxic T cells.[51] This antigen may cause cytotoxic T cells to be inactivated, allowing the response to self-antigens to occur.

Clinical Signs

The disease is manifested as **thyrotoxicosis** with a diffusely enlarged goiter that is soft instead of rubbery. Clinical symptoms include nervousness, insomnia, depression, weight loss, heat intolerance, sweating, rapid heartbeat, palpitations, breathlessness, fatigue, cardiac dysrhythmias, and restlessness.[51] Another sign present in approximately 50 percent of patients is exophthalmus, in which hypertrophy of the eye muscles and increased connective tissue in the orbit cause the eyeball to bulge out so that the patient has a large-eyed staring expression. There is evidence that orbital fibroblasts express TSH receptor-like proteins that are affected by thyroid-stimulating immunoglobulin just as the thyroid is.[52] Thus, Graves' disease is now seen as a multiorgan autoimmune disorder, causing both hyperthyroidism and ophthalmopathy, and localized edema in the lower legs.

Immunologic Findings

The thyroid shows uniform hyperplasia with a patchy lymphocyte infiltrate.[2] The follicles themselves have little colloid but are filled with hyperplastic epithelium. A large number of these cells express HLA-DR antigens on their surface in response to interferon (IFN)-γ produced by infiltrating T cells.[51] This allows presentation of self-antigens such as the thyrotropin receptor to activated T cells. B cells, in turn, are stimulated to produce antibody.

While there are a number of unique autoantibodies present, the most significant is TSH receptor antibody (TSHRab) often referred to as **thyroid-stimulating immunoglobulin (TSI).**[48] Antigen–antibody combination mimics the normal action of TSH and results in stimulation of the receptor with the release of thyroid hormones to produce the symptoms of hyperthyroidism. These have been shown to stimulate production of thyroid hormones by increasing cyclic adenosine monophosphate (AMP) levels after binding to receptors.[48,50,51]

In addition to TSI, 75 percent of patients with Graves' disease also produce antibody to thyroid peroxidase, the same antibody seen in patients with Hashimoto's thyroiditis.[51,52] A third autoantibody found in a number of patients is a thyrotropin receptor–blocking antibody that may coexist with thyroid-stimulating antibody.[48,50,52] Depending upon the relative activity of blocking and stimulating autoantibodies, symptoms in the patient may vary from hyperthyroidism to euthyroidism to hypothyroidism.[52] This may confound patient diagnosis.

Laboratory Diagnosis

A key laboratory finding in Graves' disease is elevated levels of total and free triiodothyronine (T3) and thyroxine (T4), the thyroid hormones. In addition, TSH levels are low because of antibody stimulation of the thyroid. Increased uptake of radioactive iodine also helps to confirm the diagnosis.[2,53]

Measurement of thyroid antibodies is done only when results of these assays are unclear. Tests for thyroid-stimulating antibodies are of two types: bioassays and binding assays. Bioassays require fresh animal or human thyroid tissue and thus are difficult to perform.[50,51] Binding assays are based on competition between labeled TSH and patient autoantibodies for binding to thyrotropin receptors. Approximately 80 percent of patients with Graves' hyperthyroidism test positive by this method.[51]

Thyroid peroxidase antibodies are found in approximately 75 percent of patients with Graves' disease.[51] These are detected by relatively simple procedures, as mentioned earlier. The presence of these antibodies indicates an autoimmune process affecting the thyroid, and thyroxine levels can then be used to differentiate Graves' from Hashimoto's disease.

Treatment

Several different protocols are used in the treatment of Graves' disease. In the United States, the first line of treatment involves radioactive iodine, which emits beta particles that are locally destructive within an area of a few millimeters. This is given for a period of 1 to 2 years, and it results in a 30 to 50 percent long-term remission rate.[52] Some patients, however, become hypothyroidal within 5 years, so continued monitoring is essential. In Europe, the patient is first placed on antithyroid medications such as methimazole, carbimazole, or propylthiouracil with beta blockers as adjuvant therapy.[52] Surgery to remove part of the thyroid may also be considered as an alternative.

Type I Diabetes Mellitus

Type I diabetes mellitus is now regarded as a chronic autoimmune disease that occurs in a genetically susceptible individual as a result of environmental factors.[54] It is characterized by insufficient insulin production caused by selective destruction of the beta cells of the pancreas. Beta cells are located in the pancreas in clusters called the islets of Langerhans. Type I diabetes affects 0.5 percent of whites and usually appears in an individual before the age of 30.[2] Unlike other autoimmune endocrine diseases, hormone replacement cannot be given orally, and chronic vascular complications result in major morbidity and mortality.

Family studies indicate that there is an inherited genetic susceptibility to the disease, probably attributable to multiple genes. Approximately 90 percent of white diabetics carry the HLA-DR3 or DR4 gene.[2] There appears to be an increased risk when both of these genes are present. However, recent research indicates that the true susceptibility genes for type I diabetes mellitus may occur in the HLA-DQ region, especially in the coding of the DQ β chain. As discussed in Chapter 4, HLA antigens are made up of two separate protein chains, α and β. Both of these chains are involved in antigen recognition. Within the β chain, substitutions for the amino acid, 57, aspartic acid, are associated with increasing risk for diabetes. This amino acid position is adjacent to the antigen-binding groove and may affect the structure and function of the binding site.[2,55] This correlation is strongest with haplotypes DQA1*0301/DQB1*0302, and DQA1*0501/DQB1*0201.[56,57] About 90 percent of the Caucasian population with type I diabetes mellitus have DQB1*0302 and/or DQB1*0201 compared with less than 40 percent in the normal population.[58] Several other genetic loci, including DQA1*0102 and DQB1*0602, seem to afford protection from the disease.

Environmental influences include the possibility of viral infections and early exposure to cow's milk.

Studies have attempted to link mumps virus, rubella virus, cytomegalovirus, influenza virus, and Coxsackie B4 virus with diabetes, but most research is inconclusive. It has been shown, however, that there is molecular homology between Coxsackie viral protein P2-C and the enzyme glutamic acid decarboxylase (GAD), to which antibodies are formed in type I diabetes mellitus.[2] Antibody production could possibly be initiated as a result of **molecular mimicry,** with a virus as the stimulating antigen triggering antibody production against a self-antigen.

Immunopathology

Progressive inflammation of the islets of Langerhans in the pancreas leads to fibrosis and destruction of most of the beta cells. The subclinical period may last for years, and only when 80 percent or more of the beta cells are destroyed does hyperglycemia become evident. Immunohistochemical staining of inflamed islets shows a preponderance of CD8 lymphocytes, along with plasma cells and macrophages. B cells themselves may act as antigen-presenting cells, stimulating activation of CD4 lymphocytes.[59] A shift to a Th1 response causes production of certain cytokines, including TNF-α, IFN-γ, and IL-1. The generalized inflammation that results is responsible for the destruction of beta cells. Although islet autoantibodies trigger the immune response, they do not appear to play a direct role in cell destruction. This is substantiated by the fact that antibodies are found in individuals who have no evidence of disease. Cell death is likely caused by apoptosis and attack by cytotoxic lymphocytes.[56]

It is apparent that autoantibody production precedes the development of type I diabetes mellitus by up to several years. Autoantibodies are present in prediabetic individuals (i.e., those who are being monitored because they have a high risk of developing diabetes) and in newly diagnosed patients.[60] Antibody production diminishes with time, however. Among the antibodies found are the following: antibodies to two tyrosine phosphataselike transmembrane proteins called IA-2 (ICA 512) and IA-2βA (phogrin), anti-insulin antibodies, antibodies to the enzyme GAD, and antibodies to various islet cell proteins, called islet cell antibodies (ICAs).[48,56,61]

Laboratory Testing

Although type I diabetes mellitus is usually diagnosed by the prime characteristic of hyperglycemia, it may be useful to have serologic tests to screen for diabetes before beta-cell destruction occurs to the extent necessary to cause symptoms. Antibodies to islet cells have traditionally been detected by IIF using frozen sections of human pancreas.[48] ICAs have been reported in the sera of greater than 75 percent of patients newly diagnosed with type I diabetes mellitus.[50,56] However, such assays are rather cumbersome to perform. Antibodies to insulin itself can be detected using RIA or EIA methods.[46] RIA and EIA are also used to detect anti-GAD antibodies and anti–IA-2 antibodies.[50] Combined screening for IA-2A and GAD antibodies appears to have the most sensitivity and best positive predictive value for type I diabetes mellitus in high-risk populations.[50,62]

Treatment

The use of injected insulin has been the mainstay of therapy for diabetes. New trials, however, center around the use of immunosuppressive agents. Cyclosporin A, azathioprine, and prednisone have all been used to inhibit the immune response.[2] All have potentially toxic side effects. Immunotherapy aimed at providing overstimulation to the immune system, thus triggering a Th2 instead of a Th1 response, has been used in mice with some success and may have potential for the future.[63] Limited trials in humans using a small peptide self-antigen called a heat shock protein for immunization indicate that beta-cell destruction can be halted in this manner.[64] Use of growth factors or transplantation of beta islet cells may also be of use in the future.

Other Diseases

Other organ-specific diseases that appear to have an autoimmune etiology include multiple sclerosis (MS), myasthenia gravis (MG), and Goodpasture's syndrome. MS and MG are disorders of the nervous system, while Goodpasture's syndrome is responsible for glomerulonephritis. Each of these are discussed briefly. Table 14–3 lists additional diseases for which there appears to be an autoimmune cause.

Multiple Sclerosis

Multiple sclerosis (MS) is an inflammatory autoimmune disorder of the central nervous system, affecting approximately 350,000 Americans and 2.5 million individuals worldwide.[65,66] It is characterized by the formation of lesions called plaques in the white matter of the brain and spinal cord, resulting in the progressive destruction of the myelin sheath of axons. Plaques vary in size from 1 or 2 mm up to several centimeters.[65] As is the case for most other autoimmune diseases, a combination of genetic and environmental factors is responsible for development of this condition. Although there are probably a number of independent loci, MS is most closely associated with inheritance of HLA molecules coded for by class II alleles called DRB1*1501, DRB5*0101, and DQB1*0602.[65,67] It has been theorized that the inflammatory response is triggered by molecular mimicry, in which viral or other

TABLE 14–3. Other Autoimmune Diseases

Disease	Organ or Tissue	Immunologic Manifestations
Addison's disease	Adrenal glands	Antibody to adrenal cells
Autoimmune hemolytic anemia	Red blood cells	Antibody to red blood cells
Autoimmune thrombocytopenic purpura	Platelets	Antiplatelet antibody
Crohn's disease	Intestines	Inflammatory infiltrate of T and B cells: mechanism unknown
Disseminated encephalomyelitis	Central nervous system	Sensitized T cells
Pernicious anemia	Stomach	Parietal cell antibody, intrinisic factor antibody
Poststreptococcal glomerulonephritis	Kidney	Streptococcal antibodies that cross-react with kidney tissue
Rheumatic fever	Heart	Streptococcal antibodies that cross-react with heart tissue
Scleroderma	Connective tissue	Antinuclear antibodies: anti-Scl-70, anticentromere antibody
Sjögren's syndrome	Eyes, mouth	Antinuclear antibodies, RA factor antisalivary duct antibodies, antilacrimal gland antibodies
Sarcoidosis	Multisystem granulomas, pulmonary manifestations	Activation of T lymphocytes

RA = Rheumatoid arthritis.

foreign peptides are presented in the groove of specific HLA class II molecules to T cells. Once initiated, the immune response becomes directed against self-antigens that are indistinguishable from the original foreign antigen.[66] Recent studies indicate that patients with MS have four times the blood concentration of antibody to EBV as was found in a control population.[68] Other viruses possibly implicated are measles, herpes simplex, varicella, rubella, influenza C, human herpes virus-6, and some parainfluenza viruses.[65]

Damage to the tissue of the central nervous system can cause visual disturbances, weakness or diminished dexterity in one or more limbs, locomotor incoordination, and numerous sensory abnormalities such as tingling or "pins and needles" that runs down the spine or extremities and flashes of light seen on eye movement.[66] The disease is most often seen in young and middle-aged adults, and it is twice as common in women as in men. Fifty percent of patients alternate between remissions and relapses for many years, while the remainder follow a chronic progressive course.[48,65]

Within the plaques, T cells and macrophages predominate, and they are believed to orchestrate demyelination.[65] Antibody binds to the myelin membrane and may initiate the immune response, stimulating macrophages and specialized phagocytes called microglial cells.[66] The cascade of immunologic events results in acute inflammation, injury to axons and glia, structural repair with recovery of some function, and then postinflammatory neurodegeneration.[66] Activated T cells must penetrate into the central nervous system to begin the response. They may do so by inducing changes in the endothelium that allows them to penetrate the blood–brain barrier, while vessel walls remain intact.[65] Cytokines IL-1, TNF-α, and IFN-γ have been thought to be central to the pathogenesis observed. However, treatment aimed at neutralizing the Th1 response has not been particularly successful. Therefore, other cytokines characterized by a Th2 response, including interleukin-4 (IL-4), interleukin-5 (IL-5), and IL-10, may play a pathogenic role.[65]

Immunoglobulin is increased in the spinal fluid in approximately 90 percent of patients with MS, producing two or more distinct bands on protein electrophoresis that are not seen in the serum.[69,70] While there is not one specific antibody that is diagnostic for MS, a large percentage of patients produce antibody directed against a myelin basic protein peptide.[71] Other antibodies are directed against components of oligodendrocytes and against myelin membranes, but the majority of antibodies have yet to be identified.[66] A measure of the IgG index, comparing the amount of IgG in spinal fluid to that of serum, may be useful in making a diagnosis even though it is not specific for MS. Magnetic resonance imaging that shows damage at two or more individual sites in the central nervous system is also used to aid in diagnosis.

Many healthy individuals have antibodies that bind with low affinity, but antibody with high-affinity binding is only found in disease states. There is no one specific therapy, but newer treatment for relapsing-remitting MS centers around three drugs, IFN-β1b, IFN-β1a, and glatiramer-actatae.[65,66] These are believed to work by causing down regulation of MHC molecules on antigen-presenting cells and down regulating production of proinflammatory cytokines. Acute exacerbations are treated with prednisolone. Other immunosuppressive drugs that appear to lessen the severity of symptoms include azathioprine, methotrexate, and cyclophosphamide.[72]

Myasthenia Gravis

Myasthenia gravis (MG) is a neuromuscular disorder characterized by weakness and fatigability of skeletal muscles. It occurs in 0.25 to 2 people per 100,000 annually, and the incidence appears to be increasing, especially in individuals over the age of 60.[73] Antibody-mediated damage to the acetylcholine receptors in skeletal muscle leads to this progressive muscle weakness. Early signs are drooping of the eyelids and the inability to retract the corners of the mouth, often resulting in a snarling appearance.[73,74] Other symptoms may include difficulty in speech, chewing, and swallowing, and inability to maintain support of the trunk, the neck, or the head.[48] If respiratory muscle weakness occurs, it can be life threatening.[73] Onset of symptoms can be acute, or they may develop and worsen over time.

MG is often associated with the presence of other autoimmune diseases, such as SLE, RA, pernicious anemia, and thyroiditis. Early onset disease, which is usually defined as occurring before the age of 40, appears to be linked to two HLA antigens, B8 and DR3.[73] In this age group, the disease is seen more frequently in women. Late-onset MG, presenting in patients older than the age of 40, is linked to HLA antigens B7 and DR2 and is more likely to appear in men.[73] MG can also be associated with thymoma, a tumor of the thymus. In this case there are no clear links to particular HLA antigens. Approximately 80 to 85 percent of patients have *antibody to ACH receptors*, and this may be the main contributor to the pathogenesis of the disease.[74] Normally, ACH is released from nerve endings to generate an action potential that causes the muscle fiber to contract. It is believed that when the antibody combines with the receptor site, binding of ACH is blocked, and the receptors are destroyed because of the action of antibody and complement (Fig. 14–5). In the 15 percent of patients lacking this antibody, other antibodies are present, including anti–muscle-specific kinase (MUSK).[73]

RIA procedures can be used to detect antibody, based on assays that block the binding of receptors by anti-ACH receptor (ACHR) antibody. A radio-labeled snake venom called α-bungarotoxin is used to bind irreversibly to ACHRs and then precipitation of receptors caused by combination with antibody is measured.[48]

Anticholinesterase agents are used as the main treatment therapy. Thymectomy is beneficial to some patients with early-onset disease, but there is some question about its overall benefits.[75]

Goodpasture's Syndrome

Goodpasture's syndrome is characterized by the presence of autoantibody to glomerular, renal tubular, and alveolar basement membranes, resulting primarily in injury to the glomerulus that can rapidly progress to renal failure.[76] This rare disorder occurs with an annual incidence of approximately 0.5 per million.[77] Between 50 and 70 percent of patients also exhibit pulmonary hemorrhage resulting from interaction of antibody

with basement membranes found in lung tissue. In contrast with other autoimmune diseases, Goodpasture's syndrome is more likely to occur in young males between the ages of 15 and 40.[77,78] Often, it follows a viral infection.

Severe necrosis of the glomerulus is triggered by an antibody that has specificity for the noncollagenous region of the alpha 3 chain of type IV collagen.[77,78] This autoantibody reacts with collagen in the glomerular or alveolar basement membranes. Immune deposits accumulate, and complement fixation causes injury because of the release of oxygen species and proteolytic enzymes. These immune reactants progressively destroy the renal tubular, glomerular, and pulmonary alveolar basement membranes.[79] Signs of renal involvement include gross or microscopic hematuria, proteinuria, a decreased 24-hour creatinine clearance, and an increase in blood urea and serum creatinine levels.[79] Pulmonary symptoms include hemorrhage, dyspnea, weakness, fatigue, and cough.[79]

This syndrome differs from glomerulonephritis as a result of the nonspecific accumulation of circulating immune complexes found in other autoimmune diseases because specific antibasement antibodies can be demonstrated by formation of a smooth linear ribbonlike pattern on direct immunofluorescent assay of glomerular basement membrane from patients with the disease.[76,77] Greater than 90 percent of patients with Goodpasture's nephritis test positive for presence of this antibody. Although little is known about the circumstances that trigger the autoimmune response, 80 percent of patients carry the HLA-DR15 or DR4 alleles, indicating a genetic predisposition. This is the case in most other autoimmune diseases.

Circulating antibodies can be detected by RIA, EIA, and IIF assay. The IIF assay, long held as the standard, is often hard to interpret and has a high percentage of false-positive and false-negative results.[80] A Western blot technique has been developed, which separates out basement membrane antigens by polyacrylamide gel electrophoresis followed by transfer to nitrocellulose paper for immunoblotting. This is often used as a confirmatory test because it appears to be the most sensitive and the most specific immunoassay.[80] About 20 percent of patients also have low titers of ANAs, which usually exhibit the perinuclear staining pattern. Current treatment strategies focus on removal of circulating antibodies by plasmapheresis or dialysis, or use of immunosuppressive agents such as glucocorticoids, cyclophosphamide, and azathioprine.[77] The sooner therapy is initiated, the more likely it is that renal failure can be prevented.

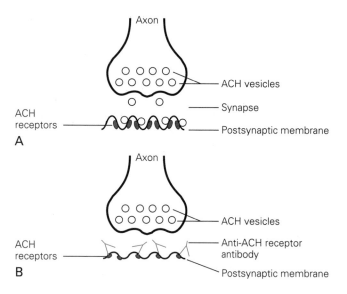

FIG. 14–5. Mechanism of immunologic injury in MG. *(A)* Normal nerve impulse transmission. ACH is released from the axon and taken up by receptors on the postsynaptic membrane. *(B)* In MG, antibodies to the ACH receptors are formed, blocking transmission of nerve impulses.

SUMMARY

Autoimmune diseases result from a loss of self-tolerance, a delicate balance set up in the body to restrict the activity of T and B lymphocytes. A combination of genetic and environmental factors may work together to allow reactions to self-antigens to occur. Self-antigens become recognized in conjunction with certain MHC antigens, and it is here that genetic factors come into play. The shape of particular class II MHC molecules allows recognition to take place. Molecular mimicry in which foreign viral or bacterial agents resemble self-antigens may trigger antibodies that in turn react with self-antigens. Such agents may also act as polyclonal activators, turning on a number of clones of B cells. Each clone of B cells would be capable of manufacturing a different type of antibody. Thus, environmental factors play a role also.

Autoimmune diseases can be classified as organ-specific or systemic, depending on whether tissue destruction is localized or affects multiple organs. SLE and RA are examples of systemic diseases, while Hashimoto's thyroiditis, Graves' disease, type I diabetes mellitus, MS, MG, and Goodpasture's syndrome are considered organ-specific diseases.

SLE is a chronic inflammatory disease characterized by joint involvement, an erythematous rash that appears on exposure to sunlight, and deposition of immune complexes in the kidney to cause glomerulonephritis. Autoantibodies include anti–ds-DNA, anti-DNP, anti-histone, anti-Sm, anti-nRNP, anticytoplasmic, antinucleolar, and antiphospholipid antibodies. Each of these exhibits specific staining patterns in the fluorescent antibody screening test for this disease.

RA affects the synovial lining of joints; necrotic areas are surrounded by granulation tissue that eventually leads to disintegration of the joint. The main immunologic finding is the presence of an antibody called RF. RF is typically a 19S antibody directed against IgG. A number of other autoantibodies contribute to the inflammation observed in the joints. Diagnosis of RA is made on the basis of both clinical manifestations and a positive RF test result.

Hashimoto's thyroiditis is an organ-specific condition that affects the thyroid gland and causes it to be enlarged and rubbery. Lymphocyte infiltration in the thyroid with the presence of antithyroglobulin antibody leads to gradual destruction of the thyroid. Clinical symptoms are consistent with hypothyroidism. Laboratory assays focus on detection of two major antibodies, antithyroglobulin and antiperoxidase, which are measured by RIA, IIF, and agglutination.

The hyperthyroidism that is evident in Graves' disease produces symptoms such as nervousness, insomnia, weight loss, heat intolerance, sweating, rapid heartbeat, cardiac dysrhythmias, and bulging eyeballs. TSHRab, or TSI, stimulates receptors, causing continuous release of thyroid hormones. Elevated levels of thyroid hormones are the key laboratory findings, and testing for autoantibodies is done only when results of hormone assays are unclear.

Type I diabetes mellitus is now considered to be an autoimmune disease. Genetic susceptibility appears to lie within the DQ region of the MHC group. Viral infections may provide the trigger for the autoimmune response. The progressive destruction of beta cells in the pancreas results in a lack of insulin production and symptoms of hyperglycemia. Antibodies to two transmembrane proteins, ICA 512 and IA-2βA; to the enzyme GAD; and to insulin can be detected by means of RIA or EIA. These can be important predictors of disease in high-risk populations.

MS is characterized by visual disturbances, weakness in the extremities, locomotor incoordination, and sensory abnormalities. T cells initiate a chain of events that include both antibody and cytokine production that progressively destroys the myelin sheath of axons and damages oligodendrocytes, causing lesions called plaques. Antibodies directed against myelin basic protein and against myelin oligodendrocyte glycoprotein are produced, but these are not diagnostic because they are not present in all cases of disease. Protein electrophoresis of cerebrospinal fluid that shows two or more bands not present in serum is helpful in making a diagnosis. The IgG index, a measure of the ratio of antibody in the spinal fluid to that in the serum, may also be useful.

Another disease affecting the nervous system is MG. Extreme muscle weakness results from the presence of antibody to ACH receptors. By combining with the receptor site, antibody blocks the binding of ACH, and the receptors are destroyed as a result of activation of complement. RIA procedures can be used to detect antibody, based on binding assays with ACH receptors.

Goodpasture's syndrome is characterized by severe necrosis of the glomerulus triggered by an antibody that reacts with glycoprotein in the glomerular basement membrane. The result is glomerulonephritis, in which immune deposits accumulate and complement fixation causes injury to the tissue, eventually producing renal failure. This antibody can also react with basement membrane in lung tissue, producing pulmonary hemorrhage. Antibasement antibody is usually detected by IIF, RIA, or EIA.

These examples represent a sampling of the autoimmune diseases for which some of the responsible immunologic mechanisms have been discovered. There is a common thread in all of the diseases covered in this chapter: All are the result of a combination of genetic and environmental factors. It appears that the MHC antigens recognized by T cells are a key factor in whether a response will be mounted to a particular self-antigen. Small changes in amino acid sequences change the shape of the receptor and allow self-antigen to be recognized. Environmental factors, probably in the nature of viral or bacterial infections, trigger an inflammatory response that polyclonally activates T and B cells. As more is learned about the mechanisms that trigger autoimmune responses, it may be possible to specifically turn off those responses without affecting the rest of the immune system.

Case Studies

1. A 25-year-old female consulted her physician because she had been experiencing symptoms of weight loss, joint pain in the hands, and extreme fatigue. Her laboratory results were as follows: RA slide test positive at 1:10; ANA slide test positive at 1:40; red blood cell count 3.5×10^{12} per L (normal is $4.1–5.1 \times 10^{12}$ per L); white blood cell count 5.8×10^{9} per L (normal is $4.5—11 \times 10^{9}$ per L).

Questions

   a. What is a possible explanation for positive results on both the RA test and the ANA test?
   b. What is the most likely cause of the decreased red blood cell count?
   c. What further testing would help the physician distinguish between RA and SLE?

2. A 40-year-old female went to her doctor because she was feeling tired all the time. She had gained about 10 pounds in the last few months and exhibited some facial puffiness. Her thyroid gland was enlarged and rubbery. Laboratory results indicated a normal red and white blood cell count, but her T4 level was decreased, and an assay for antithyroglobulin antibody was positive.

Questions

   a. What do these results likely indicate?
   b. What effect do antithyroglobulin antibodies have on thyroid function?
   c. How can this condition be differentiated from Graves' disease?

Exercise: Rapid Slide Test for Antinucleoprotein Antibody Found in Systemic Lupus Erythematosus

PRINCIPLE

Antibodies to DNP, a histone associated with DNA, are found in over 90 percent of patients with SLE. They are the most common antinuclear antibodies encountered in lupus. Although they are not specific for lupus, testing for their presence is a helpful screening procedure. In this test system, latex particles are coated with DNP extracted from calf thymus. When combined with patient serum containing antibody to DNP, visible agglutination occurs.

SPECIMEN COLLECTION

Collect blood by venipuncture, using aseptic technique and avoiding hemolysis. Hemolyzed or contaminated serum may give erroneous results and should not be used. Allow the blood to clot for at least 10 minutes at room temperature. Serum should be removed and refrigerated if not tested immediately. Specimens can be kept at 2°C to 8°C for up to 72 hours. If longer storage is required, the sample may be frozen and tested at a later time. Avoid repeated freezing and thawing. Plasma should not be used for this procedure.

REAGENTS, MATERIALS, AND EQUIPMENT

Reagent test kit such as Seradyn SLE or Immunoscan SLE, which contains the following:

SLE test reagent–latex particles coated with DNP
SLE positive control
SLE negative control
Glass agglutination slide
Capillary pipets
Applicator sticks

Other materials required but not provided:

Serologic pipets or automatic pipets and tips
Timer
Physiologic saline (0.85 or 0.9 percent sodium chloride)
Disposable test tubes (12 × 75 mm)
Test tube rack

CAUTION

The reagent test kit contains sodium azide. Azides are reported to react with lead to form compounds that may detonate on percussion. When disposing of solutions containing sodium azide, flush with large volumes of water to minimize the buildup of metal azide compounds.

Sera used for controls have been found to be negative when tested for hepatitis B surface antigen and HIV by FDA required test. However, the controls should be handled with the same precautions as those used in handling human sera.

PROCEDURE★

Qualitative Test

1. Bring all reagents and test samples to room temperature before use.
2. Gently mix the SLE test reagent to disperse and suspend the latex particles in the buffer. Avoid vigorous shaking.
3. Thoroughly clean a glass slide before use. The slide should be washed with detergent, rinsed with deionized water, and dried with a lint-free tissue.
4. Using a capillary pipet provided, place 1 drop (50 μL) of patient specimen in one section of the glass slide. Hold the capillary perpendicular to the slide to deliver a full drop of specimen.
5. Place 1 drop of positive control in the left section of the slide and 1 drop of negative control in the right section by inverting the appropriate dropper vial and squeezing out 1 drop onto the test slide.
6. Using the dropper, add 1 drop of the SLE reagent to each of the divisions containing specimen and controls.
7. Mix each section with a disposable applicator stick, spreading each mixture over the entire section. Use a clean applicator stick for each section.
8. Tilt the slide slowly back and forth for 3 minutes. Read immediately for agglutination under direct light.
9. Positive specimens should be diluted and retested.

Quantitative Test

1. Bring all reagents and test samples to room temperature before use.
2. Using physiologic saline, dilute specimens 1:2, 1:4, 1:8, 1:16, 1:32, or as needed.
3. Gently mix the SLE test reagent to disperse and suspend the latex particles in the buffer. Avoid vigorous shaking.
4. Using a capillary pipet provided, place 1 drop (50 μL) of each dilution on successive fields of the reaction slide. Hold the capillary perpendicular to the slide to deliver a full drop of specimen each time.
5. Place 1 drop of positive control in the left section of the slide and 1 drop of negative control in the right section by inverting the appropriate dropper vial and squeezing out 1 drop onto the test slide.

★Package Insert from Seradyn Seratest for SLE, Remel, Lenexa, KS 66215.

6. Mix each section with a disposable applicator stick, spreading each mixture over the entire section. Use a clean applicator stick for each section.

7. Tilt the slide slowly back and forth for 3 minutes. Read immediately for agglutination under direct light.

RESULTS AND INTERPRETATION

The negative control should give a smooth or slightly granular suspension with no agglutination, while the positive control should form a visible agglutination reaction distinctly different from the slight granularity observed with the negative control. This test will be positive for over 90 percent of patients with untreated SLE. However, it may also be positive with other diseases such as RA, scleroderma, chronic liver disease, and progressive systemic sclerosis. Antinuclear antibodies can also be found in about 10 percent of the normal healthy population, but typically the titer is too low in individuals under the age of 60 to produce a positive agglutination test. A positive reaction in this test indicates that the level of antinuclear antibody is in the range commonly found in SLE. This is a screening test, and clinical manifestations and laboratory results must be taken into account when a diagnosis is made.

 # Exercise: Slide Agglutination Test for the Detection of Rheumatoid Factor

PRINCIPLE

RF is an IgM antibody directed against IgG. It is found in 70 to 80 percent of patients with RA. Passive agglutination can be employed to test for the presence of the antibody, using a carrier particle such as sheep erythrocytes sensitized with IgG. When patient serum containing RF is mixed with the sensitized reagent cells, visible agglutination occurs.

SPECIMEN COLLECTION

Collect blood by venipuncture, using aseptic technique and avoiding hemolysis. Allow the blood to clot for at least 10 minutes at room temperature. Loosen the clot with a wooden applicator stick, and centrifuge at 1000 g for 10 minutes, or until the supernatant is free of cells. Serum should be removed and tested immediately. Specimens may be kept refrigerated for up to 24 hours. For longer storage, freeze specimens at −20°C. Avoid repeated freezing and thawing. Plasma should not be used.

REAGENTS, MATERIALS, AND EQUIPMENT

Reagent test kit such as Rheumaton Kit, which contains the following:

Stabilized sheep erythrocytes sensitized with rabbit gamma globulin
Positive control

Negative control
Calibrated capillary tubes with rubber bulbs
Glass slide

Other materials needed:

Disposable stirrers
Distilled water or isotonic saline
Test tubes, 12 × 75 mm
Centrifuge capable of 1000 g
Serologic pipets or automatic pipets and tips
Timer

CAUTION

The reagent test kit contains sodium azide. Azides are reported to react with lead to form compounds that may detonate on percussion. When disposing of solutions containing sodium azide, flush with large volumes of water to minimize the buildup of metal azide compounds.

Sera used for controls have been found to be negative when tested for hepatitis B surface antigen and HIV by FDA required test. However, the controls should be handled with the same precautions as those used in handling human sera.

PROCEDURE*

1. Bring all reagents and test samples to room temperature before use.

---

* Adapted from the package insert for the Rheumaton Test produced by Wampole Laboratories, Division of Carter-Wallace, Inc., Cranbury, NJ 08512.

2. Fill a capillary to the mark with patient serum, and empty it into the center of the middle section of the slide.
3. Place 1 drop of positive control in the left section of the slide and 1 drop of negative control in the right section.
4. Add 1 drop of well-shaken reagent to each section of the slide.
5. Mix with a disposable stirrer, spreading each mixture over the entire section. Use a clean disposable stirrer for each mixture.
6. Rock the slide gently with a rotary motion for 2 minutes and immediately observe for agglutination. If the test is positive for agglutination, dilute the specimen 1:10 with distilled water or isotonic saline, and repeat the test.

Quantitative Procedure

If a titer is desired, the following procedure can be used:
1. Label eight 12 × 75-mm test tubes 1 through 8 and place in a test tube rack.
2. Add 1.8 mL of saline to tube 1 and 1.0 mL of saline to tubes 2 through 8.
3. Add 0.2 mL of specimen to tube 1, mix, and transfer 1.0 mL of this mixture to tube 2. Mix the contents of tube 2 and transfer 1.0 mL of this mixture to tube 3. Continue serially diluting in this manner through tube 8. Starting with a 1:10 dilution in the first tube, the dilution in the final tube will be 1:1280.
4. Test each dilution as described in the qualitative procedure. The last dilution to show positive agglutination is reported as the titer.

RESULTS AND INTERPRETATION

Positive specimens show readily visible agglutination, while negative specimens show no agglutination or a finely granular pattern. If agglutination is positive in only the undiluted specimen, this represents a very low titer that might be present in a variety of other diseases. Some of these other diseases are SLE, endocarditis, tuberculosis, syphilis, viral infections, and diseases of the liver, lung, or kidney. In addition, low titer can be found in approximately 1 percent of healthy individuals. Thus, a positive test is not specific for RA.

Conversely, a negative test does not rule out RA because approximately 25 percent of patients with the disease test negative for RF. The results of this simple screening test for RA must be interpreted in the light of clinical symptoms.

Review Questions

1. All of the following may contribute to autoimmunity *except:*
   a. Clonal deletion of self-reactive T cells
   b. Molecular mimicry
   c. New expression of class II MHC antigens
   d. Polyclonal activation of B cells

2. Which of the following would be considered an organ-specific autoimmune disease?
   a. SLE
   b. RA
   c. Hashimoto's thyroiditis
   d. Goodpasture's syndrome

3. SLE can be distinguished from RA on the basis of which of the following?
   a. Joint pain
   b. Presence of antinuclear antibodies
   c. Immune complex formation with activation of complement
   d. Deposition of immune complexes in the kidney

4. Autoantibody production in SLE may be triggered by all of the following *except:*
   a. Abnormal apoptosis of old cells
   b. Presence of certain HLA genes
   c. Accumulation of cellular debris
   d. Activation of Th2 cells

5. A homogeneous pattern of staining of the nucleus on IIF may be caused by which of the following antibodies?
   a. Anti-Sm antibody
   b. Anti-SSA/Ro antibody
   c. Antihistone antibody
   d. Anti–double-stranded DNA

6. Which of the following is characteristic of RA?
   a. Association with certain HLA-DR genes
   b. Joint involvement that is symmetric
   c. Presence of antibody against IgG
   d. All of the above

7. Which of the following best describes the slide agglutination test for RF?
   a. It is specific for RA.
   b. A negative test rules out the possibility of RA.
   c. It is a sensitive screening tool.
   d. It detects IgG made against IgM.

8. Hashimoto's thyroiditis can best be differentiated from Graves' disease on the basis of which of the following?
   a. Decrease in thyroid hormone levels
   b. Presence of thyroid peroxidase antibodies
   c. Enlargement of the thyroid
   d. Presence of lymphocytes in the thyroid

9. Which of the following would be considered a significant finding in Graves' disease?
   a. Increased TSH levels
   b. TSI
   c. Decreased T3 and T4
   d. Antithyroglobulin antibody

10. Immunologic findings in type I diabetes mellitus include all of the following *except:*
    a. Presence of CD8 T cells in the islets of Langerhans
    b. Antibody to colloid
    c. Antibody to insulin
    d. Antibody to GAD

11. Destruction of the myelin sheath of axons caused by the presence of antibody is characteristic of which disease?
    a. MS
    b. MG
    c. Graves' disease
    d. Goodpasture's syndrome

12. Blood was drawn from a 25-year-old woman with suspected SLE. A FANA screen was performed, and a speckled pattern resulted. Which of the following actions should be taken next?
    a. Report out as diagnostic for SLE.
    b. Report out as drug-induced lupus.
    c. Perform an antibody profile.
    d. Repeat the test.

References

1. Goldsby, RA, Kindt, TJ, and Osborne, BA: Kuby Immunology, ed. 4. WH Freeman, New York, 2000, pp 497–516.
2. Baker, JR: Endocrine diseases. In Stites, DP, Terr, AI, and Parslow, TG (eds): Medical Immunology, ed. 9. Appleton & Lange, Stamford, Conn., 1997, pp 480–492.
3. Whitacre, CC, Blankenhorn, E, and Brinley, Jr, FJ, et al: Sex differences

in autoimmune disease: Focus on multiple schlerosis. Science Magazine. Available at http://www.sciencemag.org/feature/data/983519.shl. Accessed July 20, 2002.

4. Ruiz-Irastorza, G, Khamashta, MA, and Castellino, G, et al: Systemic lupus erythematosus. Lancet 357:1027–1032, 2001.

5. Hahn, BH: Systemic lupus erythematosus. In Braunwald, E, Fauci, AS, and Kasper, DL, et al (eds): Harrison's Principles of Internal Medicine, ed. 15. McGraw-Hill, New York, 2001, pp 1922–1928.

6. Lindqvist, AK, and Alarcon-Riquelme, ME: The genetics of systemic lupus erythematosus. Scand J Immunol 50:562–571, 1999.

7. Sack, KE, and Fye, KH: Rheumatic diseases. In Stites, DP, Terr, AI, and Parslow, TG (eds): Medical Immunology, ed. 9. Appleton & Lange, Stamford, Conn., 1997, pp 456–479.

8. Tsokos, GC: Systemic lupus erythematosus. A disease with a complex pathogenesis. Lancet 358:ps65, 2001.

9. Von Mühlen, CA, and Nakamura, RM: Clinical and laboratory evaluation of systemic rheumatic diseases. In Henry, JB (ed.): Clinical Diagnosis and Management by Laboratory Methods, ed. 20. WB Saunders, Philadelphia, 2001, pp 974–989.

10. Kurien, BT, Newland, J, and Paczkowski, C, et al: Association of neutropenia in systemic lupus erythematosus (SLE) with anti-Ro and binding of an immunologically cross-reactive neutrophil membrane antigen. Clin Exp Immunol 120:209–217, 2000.

11. Buskila, D, and Shoenfeld, Y: Anti-DNA antibodies. In Lahita, RG (ed): Systemic Lupus Erythematosus, ed. 2. Churchill Livingstone, New York, 1992, pp 205–236.

12. Kimberly, RP: Prospects for autoimmune disease: Research advances in systemic lupus erythematosus. JAMA 285:650–652, 2001.

13. Csiszar, A, Nagy, G, and Gergely, P, et al: Increased interferon-gamma (IFN-gamma), IL-10 and decreased IL-4 mRNA expression in peripheral blood mononuclear cells (PBMC) from patients with systemic lupus erythematosus. Clin Exp Immunol 122:464–470, 2000.

14. Tyrrell-Price, J, Lydyard, PM, and Isenberg, DA: The effect of interleukin-10 and of interleukin-12 on the in vitro production of anti-double-stranded DNA antibodies from patients with systemic lupus erythematosus. Clin Exp Immunol 124:118–125, 2001.

15. Bussolati, B, Rollino, C, and Mariano, F, et al: IL-10 stimulates production of platelet-activating factor by monocytes of patients with active systemic lupus erythematosus (SLE). Clin Exp Immunol 122:471–476, 2000.

16. Fritzler, MJ: Immunofluorescent antinuclear antibody tests. In Rose, NR, De MacArio, EC, and Folds, JD, et al (eds): Manual of Clinical Laboratory Immunology, ed. 5. American Society for Microbiology, Washington, DC, 1997, pp 920–927.

17. Ulvestad, E, Kanestrom, A, and Madland, TM, et al: Evaluation of diagnostic tests for antinuclear antibodies in rheumatological practice. Scand J Immunol 52:309–315, 2000.

18. Ballou, SP: Crithidia luciliae immunofluorescence test for antibodies to DNA. In Rose, NR, and De MacArio, EC (eds): Manual of Clinical Laboratory Immunology, ed. 4. American Society for Microbiology, Washington, D.C., 1992, pp 730–734.

19. Rubin, RL: Enzyme-linked immunosorbent assays for antibodies to native DNA, histones, and (H2A-H2B)-DNA. In Rose, NR, De MacArio, EC, and Folds, JD, et al (eds): Manual of Clinical Laboratory Immunology, ed. 5. American Society for Microbiology, Washington, D.C., 1997, pp 935–941.

20. Wilson, MR, and Sanders, RD: Immunodiffusion assays for antibodies to small nuclear ribonuclear proteins and other cellular antigens. In Rose, NR, and De MacArio, EC (eds): Manual of Clinical Laboratory Immunology, ed. 4. American Society for Microbiology, Washington, D.C., 1992, pp 741–746.

21. Chan, EKL, and Pollard, KM: Detection of autoantibodies to ribonucleoprotein particles by immunoblotting. In Rose, NR, De MacArio, EC, and Folds, JD, et al (eds): Manual of Clinical Laboratory

Immunology, ed. 5. American Society for Microbiology, Washington, D.C., 1997, pp 928–934.

22. Blomberg, S, Ronnblom, L, and Wallgren, AC, et al: Anti-SSA/Ro antibody determination by enzyme-linked immunosorbent assay as a supplement to standard immunofluorescence in antinuclear antibody screening. Scand J Immunol 51:612–617, 2000.

23. Gharvi, AE, and Lockshin, MD: Antiphospholipid antibodies. In Rose, NR, De MacArio, EC, and Folds, JD, et al (eds): Manual of Clinical Laboratory Immunology, ed. 5. American Society for Microbiology, Washington, D.C., 1997, pp 949–953.

24. Feinstein, DI, and Francis, RB: The lupus anticoagulant and anticardiolipin antibodies. In Wallace, DJ, and Hahn, BH (eds): Dubois' Lupus Erythematosus, ed. 4. Lea & Febiger, Philadelphia, 1993, pp 246–253.

25. Asherson, RA, and Cervera, R: Anticardiolipin antibodies, chronic biologic false-positive tests for syphilis and other antiphospholipid antibodies. In Wallace, DJ, and Hahn, BH (eds): Dubois' Lupus Erythematosus, ed. 4. Lea & Febiger, Philadelphia, 1993, pp 233–245.

26. Traynor, AE, Schroeder, J, and Rosa, RM, et al: Treatment of severe systemic lupus erythematosus with high-dose chemotherapy and haemopoietic stem-cell transplantation: A phase I study. Lancet 356:701–707, 2000.

27. Gremillion, RB, and van Vollenhoven, RF: Rheumatoid arthritis. Designing and implementing a treatment plan. Postgrad Med 103:103, 1998.

28. Van Jaarsveld, CH, Otten, HG, and Jacobs, JW, et al: Association of HLA-DR with susceptibility to and clinical expression of rheumatoid arthritis: Re-evaluation by means of genomic tissue typing. Br J Rheumatol 37:411–416, 1998.

29. Lipsky, PE: Rheumatoid arthritis. In Braunwald, E, Fauci, AS, and Kasper, DL, et al (eds): Harrison's Principles of Internal Medicine, ed. 15. McGraw-Hill, New York, 2001, pp 1929–1937.

30. Arnett, FC, Edworthy, SM, and Bloch, DA, et al: The American Rheumatism Association 1987 revised criteria for the classification of rheumatoid arthritis. Arthritis Rheum 31:315, 1988.

31. Blass, S, Engel, JM, and Burmester, GR: The immunologic homunculus in rheumatoid arthritis. Arthritis Rheum 42:2499–2506, 1999.

32. Sewell, KL, and Trentham, DE: Pathogenesis of rheumatoid arthritis. Lancet 341:283, 1993.

33. Cohen, P: Systemic autoimmunity. In Paul, WE (ed): Fundamental Immunology, ed. 4. Lippincott Williams & Wilkins, Philadelphia, 1999, pp 1067–1088.

34. Senior, K: Researchers describe autoimmune mechanism for rheumatoid arthritis. Lancet 359:1040, 2002.

35. Ward, MM: Laboratory testing for systemic rheumatic diseases. Postgrad Med 103:93–100, 1998.

36. Bathon, JM: Rheumatoid arthritis: Pathophysiology. Johns Hopkins Arthritis Center. Published by the faculty of Johns Hopkins University Division of Rheumatology. Available at http://www.hopkins arthritis.som.jhmi.edu/rheumatoid/rheum_clin_path.html. Accessed June 14, 2002.

37. Koopman, WJ: Prospects for autoimmune disease: Research advances in rheumatoid arthritis. JAMA 285:648–650, 2001.

38. Arend, WP, and Dayer, JM: Inhibition of the production and effects of interleukin-1 and tumor necrosis factor alpha in rheumatoid arthritis. Arthritis Rheum 38:151–160, 1995.

39. Swedler, W, Wallman, J, and Froelich, CJ, et al: Routine measurement of IgM, IgG, and IgA rheumatoid factors: High sensitivity, specificity, and predictive value for rheumatoid arthritis. J Rheumatol 24:1037–1044, 1997.

40. Maini, R, St. Clair, EW, and Breedveld, F, et al: Infliximab (chimeric antitumour necrosis factor alpha monoclonal antibody) versus placebo in rheumatoid arthritis patients receiving concomitant methotrexate: A randomised phase III trial. ATTRACT Study Group. Lancet 354:1932–1939, 1999.

41. Wener, MH, and Mannik, M: Rheumatoid factors. In Rose, NR, De MacArio, EC, and Folds, JD, et al (eds): Manual of Clinical Laboratory Immunology, ed. 5. American Society for Microbiology, Washington, D.C., 1997, pp 942–948.

42. Lee, DM, and Weinblatt, ME: Rheumatoid arthritis. Lancet 358:903–911, 2001.

43. Brooks, PM: Clinical management of rheumatoid arthritis. Lancet 341:286, 1993.

44. Furst, DE, Keystone, EC, and Breedveld, FC, et al: Updated consensus statement on tumour necrosis factor blocking agents for the treatment of rheumatoid arthritis and other rheumatic diseases. Ann Rheum Dis 60 (suppl III):2–5, 2001.

45. Moreland, LW, Cohen, SB, and Baumgartner, SW, et al: Long-term safety and efficacy of etanercept in patients with rheumatoid arthritis. J Rheumatol 28:1238–44, 2001.

46. Day, R: Adverse reactions to TNF-alpha inhibitors in rheumatoid arthritis. Lancet 359:540–541, 2002.

47. Jameson, JL, and Weetman, AP: Disorders of the thyroid gland. In Braunwald, E, Fauci, AS, and Kasper, DL, et al (eds): Harrison's Principles of Internal Medicine, ed. 15. McGraw-Hill, New York, 2001, pp 2060–2082.

48. Bylund, DJ, and Nakamura, RM: Organ-specific autoimmune diseases. In Henry, JB, (ed.): Clinical Diagnosis and Management by Laboratory Methods, ed. 20. WB Saunders, Philadelphia, 2001, pp 1000–1015.

49. Tamai, H, Kimura, A, and Dong, RP, et al: Resistance to autoimmune thyroid disease is associated with HLA-DQ. J Clin Endocrinol Metab 78:94, 1994.

50. Bigazzi, PE, Burek, CL, and Rose NL, et al: Endocrinopathies. In Rose, NR, De MacArio, EC, and Folds, JD, et al (eds): Manual of Clinical Laboratory Immunology, ed. 5. American Society for Microbiology, Washington, D.C., 1997, pp 972–982.

51. Weetman, AP: Graves' disease. N Engl J Med 343:1236–1248, 2000.

52. McKenna, TJ: Graves' disease. Lancet 357:1793–1796, 2001.

53. Maugendre, D, and Massart, C: Clinical value of a new TSH binding inhibitory activity assay using human TSH receptors in the follow-up of antithyroid drug treated Graves' disease. Comparison with thyroid stimulating antibody bioassay. Clin Endocrinol 54:89–96, 2001.

54. Nakamura, RM: Human autoimmune diseases: progress in clinical laboratory tests. MLO 32:32–45, 2000.

55. Sanjeevi, CB, Lybrand, TP, and DeWeese, C, et al: Polymorphic amino acid variations in HLA-DQ are associated with systematic physical property changes and occurrence of IDDM. Members of the Swedish Childhood Diabetes Study. Diabetes 44:125–131, 1995.

56. Powers, AC: Diabetes mellitus. In Braunwald, E, Fauci, AS, and Kasper, DL, et al (eds): Harrison's Principles of Internal Medicine, ed. 15. McGraw-Hill, New York, 2001, pp 2109–2143.

57. Van der Auwera, B, Van Waeyenberge, C, and Schuit, F, et al: DRB1*0403 protects against IDDM in Caucasians with the high risk heterozygous DQA1*0301-DQB1*0302/DQA1*0501-DQB1*0201 genotype. Belgian Diabetes Registry. Diabetes 44:527–530, 1995.

58. Sabbah, E, Savola, K, and Kulmala, P, et al: Disease-associated autoantibodies and HLA-DQB1 genotypes in children with newly diagnosed insulin-dependent diabetes mellitus (IDDM). The Childhood Diabetes in Finland Study Group. Clin Exp Immunol 116:78–83, 1999.

59. Falcone, M, Lee, J, and Patstone, G, et al: B lymphocytes are crucial antigen-presenting cells in the pathogenic autoimmune response to GAD65 antigen in nonobese diabetic mice. J Immunol 161:1163–1168, 1998.

60. De Aizpurua, HJ, Wilson, YM, and Harrison, LC: Glutamic acid decarboxylase autoantibodies in preclinical insulin-dependent diabetes. Proc Natl Acad Sci USA 89:9841, 1992.

61. Bonifacio, E, Lampasona, V, and Bingley, PJ: IA-2 (islet cell antigen 512) is the primary target of humoral autoimmunity against type 1 diabetes-associated tyrosine phosphatase autoantigens. J Immunol 161:2648–2654, 1998.

62. Kulmala, P, Savola, K, and Petersen, JS, et al: Prediction of insulin-dependent diabetes mellitus in siblings of children with diabetes. A population-based study. The Childhood Diabetes in Finland Study Group. J Clin Invest 101:327–336, 1998.

63. Rowe, PM: Treating type 1 diabetes by regulating autoimmunity. Lancet 352:966, 1998.

64. Raz, I, Elias, D, and Avron, A, et al: Beta-cell function in new-onset type 1 diabetes and immunomodulation with a heat-shock protein peptide (DiaPep277): A randomised, double-blind, phase II trial. Lancet 358:1749–53, 2001.

65. Hauser, SL, and Goodkin, DE: Multiple sclerosis and other demyelinating diseases. In Braunwald, E, Fauci, AS, and Kasper, DL, et al (eds): Harrison's Principles of Internal Medicine, ed. 15. McGraw-Hill, New York, 2001, pp 2452–2461.

66. Compston, A, and Coles, A: Multiple sclerosis. Lancet 359:1221–1231, 2002.

67. Baranzini, SE, Oksenberg, JR, and Hauser, SL: New insights into the genetics of multiple sclerosis. J Rehabil Res Dev 39:201–209, 2002.

68. Ascherio A, Munger, KL, and Lennette, ET, et al: Epstein-Barr virus antibodies and risk of multiple sclerosis : A prospective study. JAMA 286:3083–3088, 2001.

69. Keren, DF: Clinical indications for electrophoresis and immunofixation. In Rose, NR, De MacArio, EC, and Folds, JD, et al (eds): Manual of Clinical Laboratory Immunology, ed. 5. American Society for Microbiology, Washington, D.C., 1997, pp 65–74.

70. Kyle, RA, and Katzmann, JA: Immunochemical characterization of immunoglobulins. In Rose, NR, De MacArio, EC, and Folds, JD, et al (eds): Manual of Clinical Laboratory Immunology, ed. 5. American Society for Microbiology, Washington, D.C., 1997, pp 156–176.

71. Prat, E, and Martin, R: The immunopathogenesis of multiple sclerosis. J Rehabil Res Dev 39:187–199, 2002.

72. Tullman, MJ, Lublin, FD, and Miller, AE: Immunotherapy of multiple sclerosis—Current practice and future directions. J Rehabil Res Dev 39:273–285, 2002.

73. Vincent, A, Palace, J, and Hilton-Jones, D: Myasthenia gravis. Lancet 357:2122–2128, 2001.

74. Drachman, DB: Myasthenia gravis and other diseases of the neuromuscular junction. In Braunwald, E, Fauci, AS, and Kasper, DL, et al (eds): Harrison's Principles of Internal Medicine, ed. 15. McGraw-Hill, New York, 2001, pp 2515–2520.

75. Werneck, LC, Cunha, FM, and Scola, RH: Myasthenia gravis: A retrospective study comparing thymectomy to conservative treatment. Acta Neurol Scand 101:41–46, 2000.

76. Wilson, CB, Feng, L, and Ward, DM: Renal diseases. In Stites, DP, Terr, AI, and Parslow, TG (eds): Medical Immunology, ed. 9. Appleton & Lange, Stamford, Conn., 1997, pp 549–563.

77. Brady, HR, O'Meara, YM, and Brady, BM: The major glomerulopathies. In Braunwald, E, Fauci, AS, and Kasper, DL, et al (eds): Harrison's Principles of Internal Medicine, ed. 15. McGraw-Hill, New York, 2001, pp 1580–1590.

78. Salama, AD, Levy, JB, and Lightstone, L, et al: Goodpasture's disease. Lancet 358:917–920, 2001.

79. Fieselmann, JF, and Richerson, HB: Respiratory diseases. In Stites, DP, Terr, AI, and Parslow, TG (eds): Medical Immunology, ed. 9. Appleton & Lange, Stamford, Conn., 1997, pp 599–612.

80. Collins, AB, and Colvin, RB: Kidney and lung disease mediated by glomerular basement membrane antibodies: Detection by western blot analysis. In Rose, NR, De MacArio, EC, and Folds, JD, et al (eds): Manual of Clinical Laboratory Immunology, ed. 5. American Society for Microbiology, Washington, D.C., 1997, pp 1008–1012.

chapter 15

Immunoproliferative Diseases

Maureane Hoffman, MD, PhD

Learning Objectives

After finishing the chapter, the reader will be able to:

1. Recall the organization and development of the cellular and humoral arms of the immune system.
2. Understand how surface antigens (CD antigens) reflect the differentiation of hematopoietic cells.
3. Relate the clonal hypothesis of malignancy.
4. Describe how uncontrolled proliferation of lymphoid cells and overproduction of antibody can lead to clinical manifestations.
5. Contrast leukemias and lymphomas.
6. Differentiate multiple myeloma, Waldenström's macroglobulinemia, and polyclonal gammopathies.
7. Discuss how laboratory tests can be used to diagnose and follow the progression of multiple myeloma and related disorders.
8. Discuss how laboratory tests are used to diagnose and classify leukemias and lymphomas.

Key Terms

Cluster designation (CD)	Leukemia	Waldenström's
Cryoglobulins	Monoclonal gammopathy	macroglobulinemia
Flow cytometry	Multiple myeloma	
Hodgkin's lymphoma (HL)	Oncogene	
Non-Hodgkin's lymphoma	Paraprotein	
(NHL)	Plasma cell dyscrasias	

This chapter focuses on malignancies of the immune system, particularly cells of the lymphoid lineage. The lymphoid malignancies are broadly classed into leukemias and lymphomas. In **leukemias,** the malignant cells are primarily present in the bone marrow and peripheral blood. In lymphomas, the malignant cells arise in lymphoid tissues, such as lymph nodes, tonsils, or spleen. There can be an overlap between the sites affected by leukemias and lymphomas, especially when the malignancy is far advanced. However, it is generally most useful to classify the malignancy according to the site where it first arose, rather than the sites it can ultimately involve.

The plasma cell dyscrasias primarily include multiple myeloma and Waldenström's macroglobulinemia. These commonly involve the bone marrow, lymphoid organs, and other nonlymphoid sites. They are usually considered biologically distinct and not classified as either leukemias or lymphomas. However, plasma cells may be found in the blood late in the course of myeloma. This phenomenon is sometimes referred to as plasma cell leukemia.

The chapter will also deal with the means by which lymphoid malignancies can be diagnosed and monitored by the clinical laboratory. This chapter is not intended as a comprehensive treatment of hematopoietic malignancy, but rather as an introduction to the conditions most commonly evaluated in the clinical laboratory. Benign hyperactivity or inappropriate activity of the immune system (autoimmunity) is discussed in Chapter 14.

Concepts of Malignant Transformation

Malignancy is characterized by an excess accumulation of cells. In some cases this is because of rapid proliferation of the cells (i.e., excess production). In other cases, the cells proliferate at a normal rate, but fail to undergo apoptosis and die appropriately. Cells of the immune system, especially lymphoid cells, normally respond to a stimulus by proliferating. Thus, malignancy may reflect an initially normal process in which regulatory steps have failed. The failure of cellular regulation may be triggered by a viral infection or other persistent proliferative stimulus. However, it is generally accepted that malignant transformation requires the development of chromosomal abnormalities (mutations). In addition to a failure of growth regulation, the mutations generally result in arrest of maturation. This means that the malignant cells do not develop into properly functioning mature cells, but are "stuck" at some earlier stage of differentiation.

Malignant and premalignant proliferation of cells can occur at any stage in the differentiation of the lymphoid lineages. Despite suffering from abnormal regulation, the malignant cells generally retain some or all of the morphologic and functional characteristics of their normal counterpart, for example, their characteristic cell surface antigens or secretion of immunoglobulin. These characteristics are used to classify lymphoid malignancies.

From your knowledge of normal immune function, you can recognize that the cells of the immune system are at great risk for malignant transformation. This is because the features that characterize the development of malignancy are also a normal part of the immune response: an antigenic stimulus results in proliferation of lymphoid cells as well as a high rate of mutation during gene rearrangement and affinity maturation.

Based largely on animal experiments, a dysregulative theory of lymphoma was developed some 15 years ago. The basic concept of this theory was that lymphomas arise when persistent immunostimulation coincides with some kind of immune deficiency. The persistent stimulation provokes persistent proliferation and mutation in lymphoid precursors. The immune deficiency can play two roles. First, the presence of an ineffective immune response can ensure persistent stimulation by failing to clear an infection. Second, the immune system is responsible for surveillance against malignancy. Because it is not possible to prevent cells from ever undergoing malignant transformation, the immune system attacks and removes those cells that escape proper regulation. It is now clear that patients with an immunodeficiency have a much higher rate of malignancy, especially lymphoid malignancy, than individuals with a normally functioning immune system.

The immune system is naturally diverse and heterogeneous in preparation for its encounters with a wide range of potential pathogens. However, malignancies are thought to arise from the excessive proliferation of a single genetically identical line, or clone, of cells. That is, all of the malignant cells arose from a single mutant parent cell. The mutation gives the affected cell a survival advantage. It either proliferates uncontrollably or fails to die appropriately, thus producing a large number of similarly malignant offspring. Normal immune responses are polyclonal (i.e., cells with different features such as antigen specificity all proliferate in response to an immune stimulus). Therefore, malignancy can often be diagnosed when a population of cells is found to be more uniform than normal. For example, because each B cell only secretes one type of immunoglobulin, the persistent presence of a large amount of a single type of immunoglobulin suggests malignancy. By contrast, an increase in the amount of total immunoglobulin, without an increase in any one specific clone, is characteristic of benign reactive immunoproliferation. Similarly, it is nearly always diagnostic of malignancy when the lymphocytic cells in the blood, bone marrow, or lymphoid tissues consist primarily of a uniform population of cells.

Many of the genes involved in regulation of cell growth and proliferation were originally identified because they are the normal cellular counterparts of viral products that stimulate host-cell proliferation and eventual malignant transformation. These viral products are called viral **oncogenes,** and the corresponding host genes are called proto-oncogenes. One such proto-oncogene, c-myc, plays an important role in the transition of lymphocytes from a resting state into the cell cycle. Thus, c-myc levels rise early in the process of normal lymphocyte activation, and a fall in c-myc levels is linked to a return to a nonproliferative state. A failure of regulation of c-myc levels is seen in some malignancies of lymphocytic cells.[1] One example is Burkitt's lymphoma, a B cell malignancy associated with Epstein-Barr virus (EBV) infection. In this case, a gene translocation involving the c-myc locus and the immunoglobulin μ heavy chain alters regulation of c-myc levels. The high c-myc levels drive the affected cells to continually proliferate.

Most cases of follicular lymphoma have a t(14;18) gene translocation.[2] This results in a rearranged and constitutively overexpressed gene called bcl-2. The bcl-2 gene tells the body to produce an inner mitochondrial membrane protein that blocks programmed cell death (apoptosis). This means that the cells affected by this translocation do not die normally. Thus, even though the malignant clone may not be proliferating at an excessive rate, an excessive number of the cells accumulate in the body because their survival is enhanced compared to normal cells. Many cases of small noncleaved cell lymphomas including Burkitt's also have a gene translocation—the myc gene, t(8;14). Most mantle cell lymphomas rearrange the bcl-1 gene, t(11;14).

The specific mutation(s) leading to malignant transformation are not known for most malignancies. However, more are being identified every day. This knowledge suggests that we may someday be able to treat malignancies by administering drugs that specifically target the abnormal protein that is produced by the mutant gene in a specific malignancy.

Lymphomas

Overall, the lymphomas are divided into **Hodgkin's lymphoma (HL)** and **non-Hodgkin's lymphoma (NHL).** The classification of NHL has frustrated pathologists and clinicians alike for decades, and many classification schemes have been proposed. The oldest classification scheme is the Rappaport classification, which was developed before lymphoid cells were divided into B cells and T cells. It is based solely on morphologic features by light microscopy. From this scheme comes the following terms that are still heard occasionally.

> Well-differentiated lymphocytic lymphoma (WDLL) = small lymphocytic lymphoma
> Poorly differentiated lymphocytic lymphoma (PDL) = follicular center cell lymphoma with primarily small-cleaved cells.
> Histiocytic lymphoma = large-cell lymphoma

In 1974 the Lukes and Collins scheme was introduced, which was the first to consider the B or T cell lineage in classifying lymphomas. By the 1980s, a number of different schemes were in use. Based on a study designed to determine which classifications had prognostic and clinical significance, investigators at the National Cancer Institute reviewed lymphomas classified by the existing schemes. None of the schemes clearly emerged as superior. Therefore, they developed yet another scheme, the Working Formulation. This was devised to translate among the many schemes being used, and it became the standard scheme. It, too, was based on the evaluation of the light microscopic appearance of lymph node architecture and the cytology of the malignant cells. It also did not consider the B or T cell lineage of the process. It did, however, classify the lymphomas into low-, intermediate-, and high-grade processes, based on the aggressiveness of the untreated lymphoma.

By the 1990s most investigators and clinicians were using immunologic, cytogenetic, and molecular techniques to assist in lymphoma classification. Advances in understanding basic lymphocyte biology had led to major rethinking of the use of a classification scheme based solely on morphology. In 1994 a group of hematopathologists, the International Lymphoma Study Group, proposed a consensus list of lymphomas, the Revised European-American Lymphoma (REAL)

<table>
<tr><td>

TABLE 15–1. Hodgkin's Lymphoma

I. Nodular lymphocyte predominance Hodgkin's
   lymphoma
II. Classical Hodgkin's lymphoma
   a. Nodular sclerosis Hodgkin's lymphoma
   b. Lymphocyte-rich classical Hodgkin's lymphoma
   c. Mixed cellularity Hodgkin's lymphoma
   d. Lymphocyte depletion Hodgkin's lymphoma

</td></tr>
</table>

TABLE 15–2. Non-Hodgkin's Lymphomas

B Cell Neoplasms
I. Precursor B cell neoplasm
   a. Precursor B lymphoblastic leukemia/lymphoma
II. Mature (peripheral) B cell neoplasms
   a. B cell chronic lymphocytic leukemia/small
      lymphocytic lymphoma
   b. B cell prolymphocytic leukemia
   c. Lymphoplasmacytic lymphoma
   d. Splenic marginal zone B cell lymphoma
   e. Hairy cell leukemia
   f. Plasma cell myeloma/plasmacytoma
   g. Extranodal marginal zone B cell lymphoma of
      mucosa-associated lymphoid tissue
   h. Nodal marginal zone lymphoma
   i. Follicle center lymphoma, follicular,
   j. Mantle cell lymphoma
   k. Diffuse large-cell B cell lymphoma
   l. Burkitt's lymphoma/Burkitt's cell leukemia
T Cell and NK Cell Neoplasms
I. Precursor T cell neoplasm
   a. Precursor T lymphoblastic lymphoma/leukemia
II. Mature (peripheral) T cell and NK cell neoplasms
   a. T cell prolymphocytic leukemia
   b. T cell granular lymphocytic leukemia
   c. Aggressive NK cell leukemia
   d. Adult T cell lymphoma/leukemia (HTLV1+)
   e. Extranodal NK/T cell lymphoma, nasal type
   f. Enteropathy-type T cell lymphoma
   g. Hepatosplenic gamma-delta T cell lymphoma
   h. Subcutaneous panniculitislike T cell lymphoma
   i. Mycosis fungoides/Sezary's syndrome
   j. Anaplastic large-cell lymphoma, T/null cell, primary
      cutaneous type
   k. Peripheral T cell lymphoma, not otherwise
      characterized
   l. Angioimmunoblastic T cell lymphoma
   m. Anaplastic large-cell lymphoma, T/null cell, primary
      systemic type

NK = Natural killer.

classification. This list sets forth the diagnostic features of lymphomas that the group members consider to be widely recognized and clearly diagnosable by contemporary techniques.[3]

The REAL approach represents a new paradigm in lymphoma classification. The recognized lymphomas are distinct biologic entities defined by clinicopathologic and immunogenetic features. The classification is based on the principle that a classification is a list of "real" disease entities, which are defined by a combination of morphology, immunophenotype, genetic features, and clinical features. The relative importance of each of these features varies among diseases, and there is no one gold standard. In some tumors, morphology is paramount; in others, it is immunophenotype, a specific genetic abnormality, or clinical features. The REAL scheme divides NHL into neoplasms of precursor cells and neoplasms of mature cells of B, T, or natural killer (NK) cell lineage. An individual entity can exhibit a range of morphologic appearances and a range of clinical behavior. The REAL classification was validated by a major multi-institutional study involving 1378 cases (The Non-Hodgkin's Lymphoma Classification Project), showing that it is both reproducible and clinically relevant. This REAL scheme is the basis for the most recent classification scheme adopted by the World Health Organization (WHO) and will probably be the standard classification scheme in use in the near future.[4] The REAL classification scheme is detailed in Tables 15-1 and 15-2.

Hodgkin's Lymphoma

Hodgkin's lymphoma (HL) is a highly treatable and often curable lymphoma that occurs both in young adults and in the elderly.[5] It is characterized by the presence of Reed-Sternberg (RS) cells in affected lymph nodes and lymphoid organs. RS cells are typically large with a bilobed nucleus and two prominent nucleoli. This makes the cell look like an owl's eyes. There are also variants of RS cells that do not have this typical appearance. The REAL/WHO classification recognizes a basic distinction between lymphocyte predominance HL (LP-HL) and classic HL, reflecting the differences in clinical presentation and behavior, morphology, phenotype, and molecular features.

Classic HL is subdivided into four types: lymphocyte rich, nodular sclerosing, mixed cellularity, and lymphocyte depleted. Although the origin of the RS cells has long been a matter of debate, a consensus has now been reached that the malignant RS cells are of B cell lineage. However, most of the cells in affected lymph nodes are reactive and appear to represent a host immune response to the malignant cells. The more intense the immune response, the better the prognosis. The lymphocyte predominant form has the best prognosis, but only represents about 5 percent of the cases of HL and tends to occur in young males. Nodular sclerosing HL is the most common subtype, representing about 65 percent of cases. It is characterized by infiltration of a mixture of normal macrophages, lymphocytes, and granulocytes in affected tissues along with small numbers of RS cells. There is also marked fibrosis, dividing affected lymph nodes into nodules. Mixed cellularity HL also has a mixed infiltrate of normal cells, but with less fibrosis and greater numbers of RS cells. It accounts for about 25 percent of cases. Lymphocyte-depleted HL has diffuse fibrosis, few infiltrating normal cells, and a worse prognosis than the other subtypes of HL. The laboratory generally has little role in the diagnosis or monitoring of HL.

HL is unusual among human malignancies in that its epidemiology suggests an infectious etiology. Histochemical stains demonstrate EBV in approximately 40 percent of all HLs, suggesting a role in tumorigenesis and the potential for EBV-targeted therapy.[6]

Non-Hodgkin's Lymphoma

Non-Hodgkin's lymphoma (NHL) includes a wide range of neoplasms. Overall, B cell lymphomas represent the majority (about 85 percent in the United States) of NHL cases. The most common of these is diffuse large B cell lymphoma. The next most common type is follicular lymphoma. Marginal zone B cell (including those of mucus-associated lymphoid tissue [MALT], peripheral T cell, small B lymphocytic, and mantle cell lymphoma each constitute between 5 and 10 percent of lymphoma cases. Some of these entities tend to be slowly progressive and compatible with long-term survival, while others are typically highly aggressive and rapidly fatal if not treated. The various B cell lymphoma types can be divided into three broad groups for prognostic purposes: (1) the low-risk group includes chronic lymphocytic leukemia/lymphoma (CLL), follicular lymphomas, and MALT lymphomas; (2) the intermediate-risk group includes diffuse large B cell lymphoma and Burkitt's lymphoma; and (3) the high-risk group includes mantle cell lymphoma and lymphoblastic lymphoma. With respect to clinical prognosis, T/NK cell lymphomas fell into three groups: (1) relatively low-risk group comprising anaplastic large-cell lymphoma, angioimmunoblastic T cell lymphoma, mycosis fungoides, and lymphoblastic lymphoma; (2) relatively intermediate-risk group comprising NK/T cell lymphoma and unspecified lymphoma; and (3) extremely high-risk group comprising acute T cell leukemia.

Reflecting the stepwise process of oncogenesis, a lymphoma may progressively develop a more aggressive phenotype over the course of the disease, a process referred to as *lymphoma progression*. Changes in lymphoma morphology frequently indicate alterations in the clinical and biologic behavior of the disease.[7]

Lymphomas can usually be identified as having a B cell origin by three characteristics: (1) surface immunoglobulin, which is found on no other cell type, (2) other cell surface proteins such as CD19 that are both sensitive and specific for B cells, and (3) rearranged immunoglobulin genes. In almost all cases, both the surface immunoglobulin and the rearranged immunoglobulin genes have features of clonality.

Some lymphomas, such as small lymphocytic lymphoma (also called chronic lymphocytic lymphoma/leukemia), originate from small lymphocytes that are quietly awaiting their first encounter with antigen. These lymphomas are indolent but inexorable diseases that are compatible with survival for up to a decade. They progress to prolymphocytic leukemia in 10 to 30 percent of cases and to large-cell lymphoma or other aggressive lymphoid malignancies in 10 to 15 percent of cases.

Other B cell lymphomas, such as diffuse large-cell lymphoma or lymphoblastic lymphoma, derive from rapidly dividing cells. Lymphoid cells undergo proliferation at two stages in their development: an early cycle as they first emerge from the bone marrow and a later cycle in response to antigen exposure. Thus, rapidly proliferative lymphomas can correspond to either early or late stages of normal development. These lymphomas behave aggressively, and if untreated, they may kill their victims in less than a year.

The T cell lymphomas are more difficult to characterize than B cell lymphomas because in cases that are morphologically not clearly malignant, there is no easy way to assay their clonality comparable to testing for monotypic light-chain expression in B cell cases. There are also a number of T cell syndromes that progress stealthily from atypical but nonclonal proliferations into clonal malignancies. In cases that are not clearly malignant based on their morphology, two ancillary methods of establishing clonality are available. The first is to use molecular techniques to look for a clonal rearrangement of the T cell receptor gene. In benign populations, each cell exhibits a slightly different rearrangement, but in malignant proliferations, the population of cells uniformly expresses the same rearrangement. A second method is to demonstrate by flow cytometry that the suspicious population of T cells uniformly fails to express an antigen that is normally expressed on all T cells.

Lymphocytic Leukemias

Leukemias are generally classified as either acute or chronic. Chronic leukemias are usually slowly progressive and compatible with extended survival. However, they are generally not curable with chemotherapy. By contrast, acute leukemias are generally much more rapidly progressive, but have a higher response rate to therapy.

Acute Lymphocytic Leukemia

Acute lymphocytic leukemia (ALL) is characterized by the presence of very poorly differentiated precursor cells (blast cells) in the bone marrow and peripheral blood. These cells can also infiltrate soft tissues, leading to organ dysfunction. ALL is usually seen in children and is the most common form of leukemia in this age group. ALL is also a very treatable disease, with a cure rate of 60 to 70 percent in children. The cure rate is lower in adults with ALL.

ALL is divided into three types by the French-American-British (FAB) classification scheme. These types are termed L1, L2, and L3 and are based on the cytologic characteristics of the leukemic blasts. ALL can also be divided on the basis of immunologic markers into T cell, B cell, and non-B, non-T cell–derived types. The non-B, non-T type can be further divided based on whether or not the malignant cells express the "common ALL antigen" (CALLA). About 70 percent of childhood ALL is of the non-B, non-T, CALLA-positive type, and about 20 percent is T cell–derived. B cell ALL is rare. The immunologic classification of ALL has the advantage that it is better correlated with prognosis than is the FAB classification. Thus, CALLA-positive ALL has the best prognosis, followed by CALLA-negative, T cell, and B cell ALL.

Chronic Lymphoid Leukemic Disorders

The chronic lymphoid leukemias are a group of diseases that are almost exclusively of B cell origin. They include classic chronic lymphocytic leukemia/lymphoma, prolymphocytic leukemia, and hairy cell leukemia.

Chronic Lymphocytic Leukemia/Lymphoma

CLL is a common hematopoietic malignancy that involves the expansion of a clone of B cells that have the appearance of small mature lymphocytes. In about 5 percent of cases the malignant clone is T cell derived. The cytologically normal lymphocytes accumulate in the bone marrow and blood as well as in the spleen, lymph nodes, and other organs. In most cases, the malignant cells express weak surface immunoglobulin that is restricted to one light chain (evidence of the clonal nature of the process). CLL primarily occurs in patients over 45 years of age with a 2:1 male predomi-

nance. Patients usually present with an increase in the blood lymphocyte count, which may be an incidental finding on a routine physical examination. As the malignant lymphocytes continue to accumulate, replacement of normal elements in the bone marrow leads to anemia and thrombocytopenia. Lymph node enlargement is prominent early in the disease. CLL is compatible with a long survival. Palliative therapy is used to control some of the symptoms of the disease.

Prolymphocytic Leukemia

PLL is a variant of CLL that is composed of larger cells with round to oval nuclei and a coarser chromatin pattern. The blood lymphocyte count can be very high, often over 100,000/µL. PLL carries a much worse prognosis than typical CLL.

Hairy Cell Leukemia

Hairy cell leukemia is a rare, slowly progressive disease characterized by infiltration of the bone marrow and spleen by leukemic cells, without involvement of lymph nodes. It has a 4:1 male predominance and is seen in adults over 20 years of age. Patients usually present with cytopenias because of marrow infiltration, but the blood lymphocyte count is usually not very high. However, the splenomegaly may be striking. The malignant lymphocytes are round with a very bland cytologic appearance. They often have irregular "hairy" cytoplasmic projections from their surfaces, most easily visible on a wet-mounted preparation. The malignant cells may express surface immunoglobulin with restricted light-chain expression. They characteristically contain tartrate-resistant acid phosphatase (TRAP) in their cytoplasm, which can be identified by histochemical staining.

Plasma Cell Dyscrasias

The **plasma cell dyscrasias** include several related syndromes: multiple myeloma, Waldenström's macroglobulinemia, light-chain disease, heavy-chain disease, and monoclonal gammopathy of undetermined significance. They all share the characteristic overproduction of a single immunoglobulin component, called a **paraprotein** or myeloma protein, by a clone of lymphoid cells. Diagnosis and monitoring of the plasma cell dyscrasias depends heavily on detecting and quantitating the paraprotein. Laboratory evaluation of this type of lymphoproliferative process is common, with screening and confirmatory tests being performed in most clinical laboratories.

Multiple Myeloma

Multiple myeloma is a malignancy of mature plasma cells.[8] It is the most serious and common of the plasma cell dyscrasias. It is usually diagnosed in persons between 40 and 70 years of age, and blacks are twice as likely as whites to be affected. Men are nearly twice as likely as women to develop myeloma. Patients with multiple myeloma typically have excess plasma cells in the bone marrow, a monoclonal immunoglobulin component in the plasma and/or urine, and lytic bone lesions. The plasma cells infiltrating the marrow may be morphologically normal or may show atypical or even bizarre cytologic features. The level of normal immunoglobulin is often decreased in proportion to the amount of abnormal immunoglobulin present in the serum.

The immunoglobulin produced by the malignant clone can be of any type, with IgG being the most common, followed by IgA, IgM, and light chains only. Only rarely do myelomas produce IgD, IgE, or heavy chains only. Very rarely, two or more distinct paraproteins are produced, or a clinically typical myeloma may produce no secretory product.

An important feature supporting the diagnosis of multiple myeloma is the presence of Bence Jones protein in the urine. Bence Jones protein is the name given to free immunoglobulin light chains (κ or λ) excreted in the urine. About half of patients with myeloma excrete excessive amounts of protein in the urine. Very often the production of heavy and light chains by the malignant plasma cells are not well synchronized, and an excess of light chains may be produced. In about 10 percent of cases, the myeloma cells exclusively produce light chains. The light chains are rapidly excreted in the urine and can be detected by specific techniques, such as immunoelectrophoresis, or nonspecific techniques, such as heat precipitation (see Exercise: Detection of Urinary Bence Jones Proteins at the end of the chapter).

The clinical manifestations of multiple myeloma are primarily hematologic, immunologic, and skeletal. Hematologic problems are related to the failure of the bone marrow to produce a normal number of hematopoietic cells because myeloma cells progressively replace them. This leads to anemia, thrombocytopenia, and neutropenia. When immunoglobulin levels in the blood are sufficiently high, the presence of rouleaux may be seen on examination of the peripheral blood smear. The excess production of the abnormal immunoglobulin (paraprotein) is accompanied by a progressive decrease in the normal immunoglobulins. This leads to a deficiency of normal antibody responses and a tendency to infectious complications. Myeloma tends to preferentially involve bone and forms multiple lytic lesions, often leading to bone pain and pathologic fractures. Hypercalcemia is very common because the myeloma promotes bone resorption. In advanced disease the hypercalcemia itself can reach life-threatening levels.

The type and severity of clinical manifestations depend on the type of immunoglobulin component produced. Up to 15 percent of patients with multiple myeloma develop light-chain deposition disease or amyloidosis. These two are related disorders in which free light chains or fragments of immunoglobulin are deposited in the tissues. Amyloid fibers stain with the dye Congo red and show apple-green birefringence when viewed under a polarizing microscope. Light chains can be identified in tissue sections by immunofluorescence or immunohistochemical staining with specific antibodies.

The deposition of antibody-derived material results in organ dysfunction. The kidneys are most often affected, but every tissue in the body can develop the deposition of amyloid. Cardiomyopathy, peripheral neuropathy, hepatosplenomegaly, and ecchymoses are the most common manifestations.

Patients with myeloma can develop either acute or chronic renal failure. As many as two-thirds of myeloma patients exhibit some degree of renal insufficiency. Patients with myelomas that produce light chains or IgD are much more likely to develop renal failure than those with other types. The light chains can damage the kidneys by precipitating in the tubules and causing intrarenal obstruction.

Hyperviscosity can develop when the level of paraprotein in the serum is high. Because viscosity depends on the size of the molecule in solution, and IgM is the largest of the immunoglobulins, hyperviscosity is most often seen with IgM-producing tumors. Hyperviscosity syndrome is also sometimes seen with an IgG3-producing myeloma because IgG3 is the largest of the IgG subclasses.

The presence of the paraprotein can interfere with normal hemostasis in several different ways. When coupled with thrombocytopenia because of marrow replacement, hemorrhage is a very likely complication of multiple myeloma.

Waldenström's Macroglobulinemia

Waldenström's macroglobulinemia is a malignant proliferation of IgM-producing lymphocytes. The malignant cells are more immature than plasma cells and have a microscopic appearance somewhere between that of small lymphocytes and plasma cells.

These plasmacytoid lymphocytes infiltrate the bone marrow, spleen, and lymph nodes.

Some IgM paraproteins behave as **cryoglobulins.** That is, they precipitate at cold temperatures and so can occlude small vessels in the patient's extremities in cold weather. Occlusion of small vessels can lead to the development of skin sores or even necrosis of portions of the fingers or toes. Cryoglobulins can be detected when a blood or plasma sample is refrigerated in the clinical laboratory. The precipitate that forms at low temperature dissolves upon rewarming. Some IgM paraproteins have specificity for i or I antigens and will agglutinate red blood cells in the cold. Patients with such paraproteins may have a cold agglutinin–mediated hemolytic anemia and exhibit increased hemolysis associated with cold exposure. Some patients exhibit stable production of a monoclonal IgM with cold agglutinin activity, but no infiltration of the marrow or lymphoid tissues by plasmacytoid lymphocytes. These patients are considered to have cold agglutinin syndrome, a benign monoclonal macroglobulinemia, and not Waldenström's macroglobulinemia.

The clinical symptoms of Waldenström's macroglobulinemia are often related to anemia, bleeding, or hyperviscosity. Bence Jones proteinuria, lytic bone lesions, and hypercalcemia are rare. The median length of survival for patients with Waldenström's macroglobulinemia is longer than with multiple myeloma (5 years versus 3 years).

The Role of the Laboratory in Evaluating Immunoproliferative Diseases

The laboratory is involved in three major ways in evaluating lymphoproliferative disorders. First, the laboratory very commonly assesses the immunophenotype of hematopoietic cells in the blood, bone marrow, or lymphoid tissues by flow cytometry. This is done by detecting the antigens on the surface of the cells that are characteristic of a specific lineage and stage of differentiation. This technology serves as an excellent complement to microscope-based traditional diagnostic methods and adds distinctive capabilities that are unmatched by any other diagnostic methods. Examples of applications include the detection of clonal cells in B cell lymphoma, the recognition of antigenic expression anomalies in B or T cell malignancies, the identification of malignant plasma cells, and the rapid measurement of cell cycle fractions.

The second and probably most straightforward role of the laboratory is in evaluating the amount and char-acteristics of immunoglobulins. Because the B cell lineage develops into plasma cells that produce antibody, malignancies of certain B cells are associated with excessive or abnormal antibody production. The amount and characteristics of plasma or urine immunoglobulin can be used to diagnose and evaluate the plasma cell dyscrasias.

Third, the laboratory is increasingly involved in the assessment of genetic and chromosomal abnormalities in hematopoietic malignancies. Although this is mostly done in large referral centers or reference laboratories, genetic techniques are moving progressively closer to routine practice.

Immunophenotyping by Flow Cytometry

Analysis of cell surface marker expression is commonly used in the diagnosis and classification of leukemias and lymphomas.[9] Because the malignant cells express markers that often correspond to those of their normal precursors, insight into the lineage of origin and stage of maturation can often be determined by this technique.

Researchers in many laboratories painstakingly identified many lymphoid surface antigens and developed antibodies to them. Not surprisingly, antibodies from different laboratories and bearing different names were often found to detect the same antigen/molecule. At that point, the antigen would be assigned a **cluster designation,** or **CD** number, meaning that a known cluster of antibodies recognized this antigen. Here are a few of the most commonly used markers:

All lymphoid cells: CD45, also called leukocyte common antigen.
B cells: Almost all of are reactive for CD19, CD20, and CD22. Certain low-grade B cell lymphomas are reactive for two markers otherwise found on T cells: CD5 and CD43. Follicular lymphomas and lymphoblastic lymphomas are frequently CD10+.
T cells: Almost all T cells express CD2, CD3, CD5, and CD7. Most T cells are also positive for either CD4 (helper cells) or CD8 (suppressor cells or cytotoxic cells).
NK cells: Usually express CD16, CD56, or CD57.

The presence of these antigens on the surface of hematopoietic cells is often detected by **flow cytometry** as follows. Samples of potentially neoplastic cells are incubated with antibody preparations specific for relevant antigens. In many cases, the antibodies are directly labeled with a fluorescent tag. Thus, cells that express a particular antigen are bound by the antibody and become fluorescent. The cell suspension is passed through the flow cytometer in which the cells flow single file through a laser beam. Based on the way the cells scatter the laser light, their size and granularity can be determined. In addition, the laser excites the fluorescent tag, and those cells that fluoresce can be detected. This allows the antigenic profile, or phenotype, of the cell population to be determined.

Flow cytometry is ideal for fluids in which cells are naturally suspended, but it is also useful in lymphoid tissues, from which single-cell suspensions can be easily obtained. The advantages of flow cytometry are largely based on its ability to analyze very rapidly, even in small samples, multiple-cell properties simultaneously, including size, granularity, surface and intracellular antigens, and deoxyribonucleic acid (DNA) content. The quantitative nature of the data produced, both with regard to cell population distributions and to expression of individual cell antigens, offers objective criteria for interpretation of results.

Evaluation of Immunoglobulins

As discussed in Chapter 5, the basic immunoglobulin unit consists of two identical heavy chains and two identical light chains, covalently linked by disulfide bonds. The structure of the heavy chain defines the class of the antibody (e.g., IgG, IgM). The two types of light chains (κ and λ) can each occur in combination with any of the types of heavy chains. The heavy and light chains each contain constant and variable regions. The constant regions contain the sites of immunoglobulin binding to cellular receptors and sites involved in complement fixation. The variable regions are responsible for the antigen specificity of the antibody. The immunoglobulins in plasma are heterogeneous in structure because they recognize a variety of different antigens. The variability in their amino acid sequences means that they also vary slightly in their physical characteristics, such as molecular weight and charge.

The antibody-producing plasma cell is produced by maturation of B cells through several stages. Each cell in the B cell lineage only recognizes a single antigenic site or epitope. An early B cell precursor is stimulated to proliferate and mature when it encounters an antigen that it recognizes. When a foreign molecule enters the body, the many different epitopes on it each stimulate a B cell response, leading to the production of an array of different antibodies in the normal response. However, in a malignant disorder, the clonal proliferation of transformed plasma cells leads to overproduction of a single immunoglobulin. This is called a **monoclonal gammopathy.**

Quantitative measurement of serum or urine immunoglobulins is used in the workup of some lymphoproliferative disorders. However, the evaluation of a patient for the possibility of a monoclonal gammopathy requires the qualitative as well as quantitative analysis of immunoglobulins.[10] The initial tests used to screen for the presence of a monoclonal gammopathy are serum immunoglobulin levels and serum protein electrophoresis. A high clinical index of suspicion, abnormal results on immunoglobulin levels, or findings suggestive of a monoclonal component on serum protein electrophoresis will prompt additional testing.

Serum Protein Electrophoresis

Serum protein electrophoresis (SPE) is a technique in which molecules are separated on the basis of their size and electrical charge. SPE allows reproducible separation of the major plasma proteins. The SPE is traditionally divided into four regions: albumin, as well as alpha, beta, and gamma globulins. IgG, IgM, IgD, and IgE migrate in the gamma globulin region, while IgA migrates as a broad band in the beta and gamma regions. A stylized drawing showing the distribution of proteins in normal serum is shown in Figure 15–1, *panel A.* As can be seen, immunoglobulins normally show a range of mobilities. The SPE pattern for a polyclonal increase in serum immunoglobulins and a monoclonal gammopathy are shown in *panels B* and *C* of Figure 15–1. Polyclonal increases in serum immunoglobulins are seen in a variety of disorders, including infections, autoimmune disorders, liver disease, and some immunodeficiency states (hyper-IgE with recurrent infections, hyper-IgM syndrome). Additional evaluation of serum immunoglobulin is performed if the SPE shows a monoclonal component, if there is a significant quantitative abnormality of serum immunoglobulins, or if the clinical picture strongly suggests a plasma cell dyscrasia. Myeloma in which only light chains are produced may not be detected on SPE because the light chains are rapidly cleared in the urine.

Therefore, additional studies on a random or 24-hour urine sample may be indicated even in the presence of a normal SPE.

Immunoelectrophoresis

The next step in evaluating a monoclonal gammopathy is generally immunoelectrophoresis (IEP). IEP allows the identification of specific heavy-chain and light-chain components of a monoclonal immunoglobulin in a semiquantitative fashion. IEP is a two-step process. First, the serum (or urine) proteins are separated by electrophoresis. Second, the separated proteins are

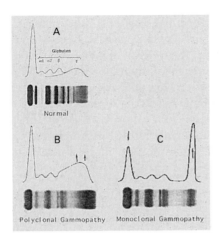

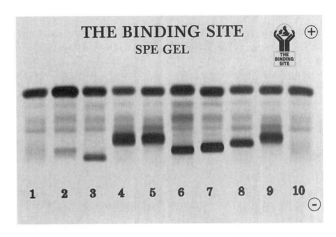

FIG. 15–1. Serum protein electrophoresis of normal and abnormal samples. The lower portion of each panel is a representation of a stained agarose electrophoresis gel. The intensity of staining corresponds to the amount of protein in each region of the gel. In the upper portion of each panel is a densitometer tracing of a gel similar to the one beneath it. In the upper panel showing a normal serum sample, the largest peak is albumin. The globulin regions are as indicated.

FIG. 15–2. Agarose gel immunofixation electrophoresis of serum. The same patient sample is placed on all six lanes and electrophoresed. Following electrophoresis, antisera are added to each lane as follows: lane 1—antitotal serum protein; lane 2—anti-IgG; lane 3—anti-IgA; lane 4—anti-IgM; lane 5—anti-κ; and lane 6—anti-λ. The patient is exhibiting a monoclonal IgM λ immunoglobulin. (Courtesy of The Binding Site Ltd., Birmingham, UK.) See Color Plate 11.

reacted with specific antibodies. Generally, specific antibodies to α, γ, and μ heavy chains and κ and λ light chains are placed in troughs cut into the electrophoresis gel. The antibody and the electrophoresed proteins are then allowed to diffuse throughout the gel toward one another. Where an antibody–antigen reaction occurs, the complex precipitates. Uncomplexed proteins are removed by washing, and the remaining antigen–antibody complexes are visualized by staining. The shape, thickness, and intensity of the precipitin arcs that form reflect the concentration of the immunoglobulin proteins. IEP is a standard technique for characterizing monoclonal immunoglobulins; however, it has certain limitations. It takes quite a bit of experience to interpret IEF results, and the turnaround time is rather long (1 to 2 days). For an accurate analysis, patient samples must always be analyzed along with normal plasma samples for comparison.

Immunofixation Electrophoresis

Another method of characterizing monoclonal gammopathies is immunofixation electrophoresis (IFE). In IFE, serum samples are electrophoresed, just as for SPE, and then specific antibody is applied directly to the separating gel. The antibody–antigen complexes form and are visualized by staining as in IEP. Areas of diffuse staining indicate polyclonal immunoglobulins, while monoclonal bands produce narrow, intensely stained bands (see Fig. 15–2). IFE is much faster than IEP, has

much greater sensitivity, and is the most accurate for typing paraproteins; however, IFE is also more labor intensive and expensive, and most paraproteins can be adequately typed by IEP. Thus, it is reasonable to first evaluate paraproteins detected on SPE by IEP. If the monoclonal component cannot be typed, IFE should then be performed.

Evaluation of Genetic and Chromosomal Abnormalities

The majority of B cell lymphomas and some T cell lymphomas are characterized by specific chromosome translocations. Often these translocations can be detected by cytogenetic techniques. Like all cells, malignant lymphoid cells can be made to proliferate *in vitro*, and their metaphase chromosomes can be examined for grossly visible abnormalities that correspond to characteristic translocations. Many of the translocations involve the immunoglobulin or T cell receptor loci with various partner chromosomes and lead to abnormal proto-oncogene expression. Other characteristic translocations result in the production of a novel fusion protein. The detection of translocations is of particular value in diagnosis and in the detection of minimal residual disease. Aneuploidy and deletion of specific chromosome regions are common secondary chromosome events that are rarely specific to a particular type of lymphoma but provide valuable prognostic information.

Traditional cytogenetic evaluation has been expanded by a technique known as fluorescence in situ hybridization (FISH). FISH is a technique to directly identify a specific region of DNA in a cell. FISH involves the preparation of short sequences of single-stranded DNA, called probes, which are complementary to the DNA sequences of interest. These probes bind to the complementary chromosomal DNA and, because they are labeled with fluorescent tags, allow one to see the location of those sequences of DNA. The probes can be used on chromosomes, interphase nuclei, or tissue biopsies. FISH is rapid and quite sensitive and does not require cell culture. However, it only provides information about the specific probe being tested. For example, FISH can be used to examine chromosome preparations to determine whether two gene markers that are normally on different chromosomes have been translocated to be adjacent to one another on the same chromosome.

Lymphoid malignancies can also be evaluated by molecular genetic techniques. These techniques are usually geared toward finding clonal rearrangements of the immunoglobulin gene in B cell malignancies or of the T cell receptor gene in T cell malignancies. These rearrangements are too subtle to be detected by conventional cytogenetics.

As a result of progress on the human genome project, approximately 19,000 genes have been identified and tens of thousands more tentatively identified as fragments of genes. Most of these genes are only partially characterized, and the functions of the vast majority are as yet unknown. It is likely that many genes that might be useful for diagnosis and/or prognostication of human malignancies have yet to be recognized. The advent of cDNA microarray technol-ogy now allows the efficient measurement of expression for almost every gene in the human genome in a single overnight hybridization experiment. This genomic scale approach has begun to reveal novel molecular-based subclasses of many malignancies, including lymphoma and leukemia.[11] In several instances, gene microarray analysis has already identi-fied genes that appear to be useful for predicting clini-cal behavior. It is likely that additional molecular techniques will find their way into routine clinical practice in the near future.

SUMMARY

Malignancies of lymphocytes, both lymphomas and leukemias, are commonly encountered in clinical prac-tice. The classification of these disorders depends on the identification of their cell of origin. The B or T cell derivation of a lymphoid malignancy is often deter-mined in the laboratory by flow cytometry. Some disorders of B cells result in abnormal immunoglobulin secretion. Multiple myeloma is a malignancy of plasma cells that is characterized by production of a mono-clonal immunoglobulin or paraprotein. The paraprotein may be of any immunoglobulin class or may be an immunoglobulin heavy or light chain. Waldenström's macroglobulinemia is a malignancy of plasmacytoid lymphocytes that produces an IgM paraprotein. Identification and quantification of the paraprotein are central to the diagnosis and monitoring of these conditions. SPE is used to detect the presence of a para-protein, which is then characterized by immuno-electrophoresis or immunofixation electrophoresis. Evaluation of genetic and chromosomal abnormalities is a rapidly evolving area of laboratory practice.

Exercise: Detection of Urinary Bence Jones Proteins

PRINCIPLE

Reagent test strips used to screen for proteinuria are generally not sensitive to immunoglobulin or free light chains. Therefore, other techniques are required to detect Bence Jones proteins in the urine. One time-honored method exploits the unique heat solubility properties of these proteins. Bence Jones proteins precipitate at temperatures between 40°C and 60°C and redissolve again at around 100°C. This approach can generally detect levels of protein down to about 30 mg/dL.

SPECIMEN COLLECTION

A 24-hour or random urine specimen is collected into a clean container. The sample may be stored in a refrigerator to prevent bacterial growth.

REAGENTS, MATERIALS, AND EQUIPMENT

  Acetate buffer, 2 mol/L, pH 4.9
  Test tubes
  Boiling water bath

NOTE: For acetate buffer, add 4.1 mL of glacial acetic acid to 17.5 g of sodium acetate trihydrate, and then add water to give a total volume of 100 mL.

PROCEDURE

1. Place 4 mL of clear urine in a test tube. Add 1 mL of acetate buffer and mix.
2. Heat for 15 minutes at 56°C in a water bath or heating block. The development of turbidity is indicative of Bence Jones proteins.
3. If the sample has become turbid, transfer the test tube to a boiling water bath for 3 minutes. The turbidity should decrease if it is because of the presence of Bence Jones proteins, which redissolve at 100°C.
4. If the turbidity of the sample increases after boiling, it is because of albumin and globulins. Filter the test sample immediately on removing from the boiling water bath. If Bence Jones proteins are present, the sample will become cloudy as it cools, then clear again as it reaches room temperature. If the precipitate is quite heavy at 56°C, it may not dissolve easily on boiling. It is best to repeat the test with a diluted urine specimen.

COMMENTS

This is simply a screening test for detection of Bence Jones proteinuria. The best method of detecting Bence Jones proteins is protein electrophoresis followed by immunoelectrophoresis. See the exercise in Chapter 16.

Review Questions

1. In general, a myeloma secreting which type of paraprotein is most likely to cause renal failure?
   a. IgG
   b. κ light chains
   c. IgM
   d. μ heavy chains

2. Which of the following would be the best indicator of a malignant clone?
   a. Overall increase in antibody production
   b. Increase in IgG and IgM only
   c. Increase in antibody directed against a specific epitope
   d. Decrease in overall antibody production

3. Which is not a feature of malignancy?
   a. Chromosomal mutations
   b. Rapid proliferation
   c. Excess apoptosis
   d. Clonal proliferation

4. Which feature is not commonly used to classify lymphoid neoplasms?
   a. Morphology/cytology of the malignant cells
   b. Presence of gene translocations
   c. Cell of origin
   d. Exposure of the patient to carcinogens

5. Hodgkin's lymphoma is characterized by:
   a. The presence of Reed-Sternberg cells in lymph nodes
   b. Excess immunoglobulin production
   c. Incurable, rapidly progressive course
   d. Proliferation of T cells

6. Chronic leukemias are characterized by:
   a. Rapidly progressive course
   b. Curable with chemotherapy
   c. Usually occur in children
   d. Usually of B cell origin
   e. a, b, and c

7. Acute leukemias are characterized by:
   a. Rapidly progressive course
   b. Curable with chemotherapy
   c. Usually occur in children
   d. Usually of B cell origin
   e. a, b, and c

References

1. Potter, M: Pathogenetic mechanisms in B-cell non-Hodgkin's lymphomas in humans. Cancer Res 52:5522s, 1992.
2. Falini, B, and Mason, DY: Proteins encoded by genes involved in chromosomal alterations in lymphoma and leukemia: Clinical value of their detection by immunocytochemistry. Blood 99(2): 409–426, 2002.
3. Harris, NH, Jaffe, ES, Stein, H, et al: A revised European-American classification of lymphoid neoplasms: A proposal from International Study Group. Blood 87:1361, 1994.
4. Harris, ML, Jaffe, ES, Diebold, J, et al: The World Health Organization classification of hematological malignancies. Report of the Clinical Advisory Committee meeting, Airline House, Virginia, November 1997. Mod Pathol 13:193, 2000.
5. Pileri, SA, Ascani, S, Leoncini, L, et al: Hodgkin's lymphoma: The pathologist's viewpoint. J Clin Pathol 55(3):162–176, 2002.
6. Jaffett, RF: Viruses and Hodgkin's lymphoma. Ann Oncol 13 Suppl 1:23–29, 2002.
7. Muller-Hermelink, HK, Zettl, A, Pfeifer, W, et al: Pathology of lymphoma progression. Histopathology 38(4):285–306, 2001.
8. Osserman, EF: Plasma-cell myeloma, II. Clinical aspects. N Engl J Med 261:952, 1959.
9. Stetler-Stevenson, M, and Braylan, RC: Flow cytometric analysis of lymphomas and lymphoproliferative disorders. Semin Hematol 38(2):111–123, 2001.
10. Guinan, JEC, Kenny, DF, and Gatenby, PA: Detection and typing of paraproteins: Comparison of different methods in a routine diagnostic laboratory. Pathology 21:35, 1989.
11. Rosenwald, A, and Staudt, LM. Clinical translation of gene expression profiling in lymphomas and leukemias. Semin Oncol 29(3):258–263, 2002.

chapter 16

Immunodeficiency Diseases

Maureane Hoffman, MD, PhD, and Christine Stevens

Learning Objectives

After finishing the chapter, the reader will be able to:

1. Recall the organization and development of the cellular and humoral arms of the immune system.
2. Explain how a defect in the B cell, T cell, myeloid, or complement systems can lead to typical clinical manifestations.
3. Discuss how laboratory tests can be used to diagnose and monitor the different types of congenital immunodeficiency syndromes.
4. Distinguish common variable immunodeficiency from Bruton's X-linked agammaglobulinemia.
5. Discuss the manifestations of the DiGeorge anomaly, purine-nucleoside phosphorylase (PNP) deficiency, severe combined immunodeficiency (SCID), Wiskott-Aldrich syndrome (WAS), and ataxia-telangiectasia (AT).
6. Recognize the association between immunodeficiency states and the risk of developing malignancy.
7. Explain the significance of loss of neutrophil function to host defenses.

Key Terms

Ataxia-telangiectasia (AT)
Bruton's
  agammaglobulinemia
Chronic granulomatous
  disease (CGD)
Common variable
  immunodeficiency (CVI)

DiGeorge anomaly
Oxidative burst
Purine-nucleoside
  phosphorylase (PNP)
  deficiency
Severe combined
  immunodeficiency (SCID)

Transient
  hypogammaglobulinemia
Wiskott-Aldrich syndrome
  (WAS)

The immune system is a diverse and complicated network of many biochemical and cellular components. The components of the immune system include (1) the T cell system (cellular immunity, T cells, and their cytokines), (2) the B cell system (humoral immunity, B cells, and immunoglobulins), (3) the phagocytic system (mononuclear phagocytes and granulocytes), and (4) the complement system. A simplified rendition of the organization of cellular components of the immune system is shown in Figure 16–1. The organization, development, and function of the immune system have been discussed in greater detail in Chapters 3, 5, and 6. This chapter focuses on dysfunction of the immune system, with emphasis on the lymphoid lineage, and the means by which dysfunctional states can be diagnosed and monitored by the clinical laboratory. This chapter is not intended as a comprehensive treatment of abnormalities of the immune system, but rather as an introduction to the conditions most commonly evaluated in the clinical laboratory.

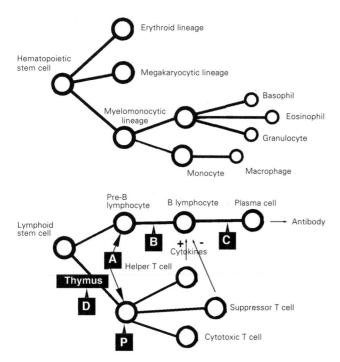

FIG. 16–1. Cells of the immune system. The figure shows the developmental relationships between cellular components of the immune system. The letters indicate the stages at which a defect occurs in some of the congenital immunodeficiency syndromes. *A,* adenosine deaminase deficiency; *B,* Bruton's agammaglobulinemia; *C,* common variable immunodeficiency; *D,* DiGeorge anomaly; and *P,* PNP deficiency.

Immunodeficiency Diseases

General Observations

The components of the immune system play unique, but overlapping, roles in the host defense process. Therefore, defects in any one of the cellular or soluble components result in distinct clinical manifestations. However, because the components of the immune system interact extensively through many regulatory loops, a defect in one arm of the system may affect other aspects of immune function as well. In many cases, it appears that deficiency of one component of the system is accompanied by hyperactivity of other components. This may be because persistent infections continuously stimulate the remaining immune cells. In addition, the deficient component may normally exert regulatory control over other components of the immune system—control that is lacking in the deficiency state. For instance, as illustrated in Figure 16–1, T cell subsets each secrete cytokines that regulate the development of B cells into plasma cells. A defect in T cell function removes or unbalances this regulatory

loop. Whatever the mechanism, many partial immunodeficiency states are associated with allergic or autoimmune manifestations.

With the exception of IgA deficiency, primary immunodeficiency syndromes are rare, with a combined incidence of about 2 in 10,000 live births.[1,2] Several of the most important immunodeficiency syndromes show X-linked inheritance and, therefore, affect primarily males. Others show primarily autosomal recessive inheritance. In spite of their rarity, it is important to consider the possibility of primary immunodeficiency in children with recurrent infections because early detection and treatment can help prevent the development of serious, long-term tissue damage or overwhelming sepsis. Early diagnosis can also provide the opportunity for appropriate genetic counseling, carrier detection, and prenatal diagnosis for other family members.[3]

More than 50 different congenital forms of immunodeficiency have been reported, including defects in lymphoid cells, phagocytic cells, and complement proteins.[4] The molecular mechanisms have been determined for some of these deficiencies. In most cases, patients with congenital immunodeficiency states present in childhood with recurrent infections or failure to thrive. The types of infection can give important clues to the type of immunodeficiency present. In general, defects in humoral immunity (antibody production) result in pyogenic bacterial infections, particularly of the upper and lower respiratory tract. Recurrent sinusitis and otitis media are common. The clinical course of infections with viral agents is not significantly different from that in normal hosts, with the exception of hepatitis B, which may have a fulminant course in agammaglobulinemic patients. Defects in T cell–mediated immunity result in recurrent infections with intracellular pathogens such as viruses, fungi, and intracellular bacteria, and patients with these defects almost always develop mucocutaneous candidiasis. They are also prone to disseminated viral infections, especially with latent viruses such as herpes simplex, varicella zoster, and cytomegalovirus. T cells also play a crucial role in tumor surveillance. Age-adjusted rates of malignancy in patients with immunodeficiency disease are 10 to 200 times greater than the expected rates.[4] Most of the malignancies are lymphoid and may be related to persistent stimulation of the remaining immune cells, coupled with defective immune regulation.

The phagocytic system is part of the nonspecific immune response and includes neutrophils and mononuclear phagocytes. Neutrophils are the first line of defense against invading organisms and are also important effector cells in antibody-mediated killing.

Defects in neutrophil function are usually reflected in recurrent pyogenic bacterial infections. Macrophages within the liver and spleen are in contact with the blood and are responsible for clearing circulating microorganisms. Splenectomy is associated with an increased risk of overwhelming bacterial infection accompanied by septicemia. Tissue macrophages are present in all tissues and also play an important role in processing and presenting antigens to T cells in combination with class II major histocompatibility complex (MHC) molecules, to initiate a specific immune response.

The complement system, as discussed in Chapter 7, is activated to produce biologically active molecules that enhance inflammation and promote lysis of cells and microorganisms. Deficiency of complement components results in recurrent bacterial infections and autoimmune-type manifestations. The severity of the syndrome varies with the particular complement component that is deficient. Specific defects of each of the components of the immune system are described in the following sections.

Deficiencies of the B Cell System (Agammaglobulinemias)

Immunoglobulins migrate in the "gamma region" of the serum protein electrophoretic profile (discussed in Chapter 5). Therefore, deficiencies of immunoglobulins have been termed agammaglobulinemias. The mechanisms of the agammaglobulinemias include genetic defects in B cell maturation or defective interactions between B and T cells. A wide range of immunoglobulin deficiency states have been reported and involve virtually all combinations of immunoglobulins and all degrees of severity. In some cases, only a single isotype of one immunoglobulin class is deficient, while all of the other isotypes are normal. Only the more common and well-characterized syndromes are described here and are summarized in Table 16–1.

In evaluating immunoglobulin deficiency states, it is important to remember that blood levels of immunoglobulins change with age. The blood level of IgG at birth is about the same as the adult level, reflecting transfer of maternal IgG across the placenta. The IgG level drops over the first 2 or 3 months of life as maternal antibody is catabolized. Levels of IgA and IgM are very low at birth. The concentrations of all immunoglobulins gradually rise when the infant begins to produce antibodies at a few months of age, in response to environmental stimuli. IgM reaches normal adult levels first, around 1 year of age, followed by IgG at about 5 to 6 years of age. In some normal children, IgA levels do not reach normal adult values until adolescence. Therefore, it is important to compare a child's immunoglobulin level with normal controls of the same age.

Transient Hypogammaglobulinemia of Infancy

All infants experience low levels of immunoglobulins at approximately 5 to 6 months of age, but in some babies the low levels persist for a longer time. Because these children do not begin synthesizing immunoglobulin promptly, they can experience severe pyogenic sinopulmonary and skin infections as protective maternal IgG is cleared. Cell-mediated immunity is normal, and there may be normal levels of IgA and IgM.[5] IgG appears to be the most affected, dropping to approximately 350mg/dL.[6] Immunoglobulin levels usually normalize spontaneously, usually by 9 to 15 months of age. The mechanism of this **transient hypogammaglobulinemia** is not known, but it may be related to a delayed maturation of one or more components of the immune system, possibly T helper cells.[6]

TABLE 16–1. Characteristics of Selected Defects of the B Cell System

Condition	Deficiency	Level of Defect	Presentation
Transient hypogammaglobulinemia of infancy	All antibodies; especially IgG	Slow development of helper function in some patients	2–6 months; resolves by 2 years
IgA deficiency	IgA; some with reduced IgG2 also	IgA-B cell differentiation	Often asymptomatic
X-linked agammaglobulinemia	All antibody isotypes reduced	Pre-B cell differentiation	Infancy
Common variable immunodeficiency	Reduced antibody; many different combinations	B cell; excess T suppression	Usually 20–30 years of age
Isolated IgG subclass deficiency	Reduced IgG1, IgG2, IgG3, or IgG4	Defect of isotype differentiation	Variable with the class and degree of deficiency
Immunodeficiency with hyperimmunoglobulin M	Reduced IgG, IgA, IgE, with elevated IgM	B cell switching	Infancy

X-Linked Bruton's Agammaglobulinemia

Bruton's agammaglobulinemia, first described in 1952, is X-chromosome–linked, so this syndrome affects males almost exclusively. Patients with X-linked agammaglobulinemia lack circulating mature B cells and exhibit a deficiency or lack of immunoglobulins of all classes.[5] Furthermore, they have no plasma cells in their lymphoid tissues. They do have pre-B cells in their bone marrow.[7,8] Because of the lack of B cells, the tonsils and adenoids are small or entirely absent, and lymph nodes lack normal germinal centers. T cells are normal in number and function. About half of the patients have a family history of the syndrome. They develop recurrent bacterial infections beginning in infancy, as maternal antibody is cleared. They most commonly develop sinopulmonary infections caused by encapsulated organisms such as streptococci, meningococci, and *Haemophilus influenzae.* Other infections seen include bacterial otitis media, bronchitis, pneumonia, meningitis, and dermatitis.[6] Some patients also have a susceptibility to certain types of viral infections, including vaccine-associated poliomyelitis. In general, live virus vaccines should be avoided in immunodeficient patients.

X-linked hypogammaglobulinemia results from arrested differentiation at the pre–B cell stage, leading to a complete absence of B cells and plasma cells.[7,9] The underlying genetic mechanism is a deficiency of an enzyme called the Bruton tyrosine kinase (Btk) in B cell progenitor cells.[1,9] Lack of the enzyme apparently causes a failure of Vh gene rearrangement. As discussed in Chapter 5, during B cell maturation, there is a rearrangement of V, D, and J segments to create functioning genes that code for immunoglobulin heavy and light chains. The syndrome can be effectively treated by administration of intramuscular or intravenous immunoglobulin preparations and vigorous antimicrobial treatment of infections. The syndrome can be differentiated from transient hypogammaglobulinemia of infancy by the abnormal histology of lymphoid tissues and by its persistence beyond 2 years of age.

IgA Deficiency

Selective IgA deficiency is the most common congenital immunodeficiency, occurring in about 1 in 600 persons of European descent.[5,6] Most patients with a deficiency of IgA are asymptomatic. Those with symptoms usually have infections of the respiratory and gastrointestinal tract and an increased tendency to autoimmune diseases such as systemic lupus erythematosus, rheumatoid arthritis, and thyroiditis. Allergic disorders and malignancy are also more common.[5] About 20 percent of the IgA-deficient patients who develop infections also have an IgG2 subclass defi-

ciency. If the serum IgA is less than 5 mg/mL, the deficiency is considered severe. If the IgA level is two standard deviations below the age-adjusted mean but greater than 5 mg/mL, the deficiency is partial. Although the genetic defect has not been established, it is hypothesized that lack of IgA is caused by impaired differentiation of lymphocytes to become IgA-producing plasma cells.[6]

Anti-IgA antibodies are produced by 30 to 40 percent of patients with severe IgA deficiency. These antibodies can cause anaphylactic reactions when blood products containing IgA are transfused.[7] Because many patients with severe Ig deficiency have no other symptoms, the IgA deficiency may not be detected until the patient experiences a transfusion reaction resulting from the presence of anti-IgA antibodies. Products for transfusion to known IgA-deficient patients should be collected from IgA-deficient donors, or cellular products should be washed to remove as much donor plasma as possible.

Most gamma globulin preparations contain significant amounts of IgA. However, replacement IgA therapy is not useful because the half-life of IgA is short (around 7 days) and intravenously or intramuscularly administered IgA is not transported to its normal site of secretion at mucosal surfaces. Furthermore, administration of IgA-containing products can induce the development of anti-IgA antibodies or provoke anaphylaxis in patients who already have antibodies.

Common Variable Immunodeficiency

Common variable immunodeficiency (CVI) is a heterogeneous group of disorders with a prevalence of about 1 in 25,000.[8] Patients usually begin to have symptoms in their 20s and 30s, but age at onset ranges from 7 to 71 years of age. The disorder can be congenital or acquired, or familial or sporadic, and it occurs with equal frequency in men and women. CVI is characterized by hypogammaglobulinemia that leads to recurrent bacterial infections, particularly sinusitis and pneumonia. In addition, up to 20 percent of CVI patients develop herpes zoster (shingles), a much higher incidence than in immunologically normal young adults. There is usually a deficiency of both IgA and IgG, but selective IgG deficiency may occur. CVI is often associated with a spruelike syndrome characterized by malabsorption and diarrhea. CVI is also associated with an increased risk of lymphoproliferative disorders, gastric carcinomas, and autoimmune disorders.[10] The most common autoimmune manifestations of CVI are immune thrombocytopenia and autoimmune hemolytic anemia. Other symptoms may include lymphadenopathy, splenomegaly, and intestinal hyperplasia.[6]

CVI is diagnosed by demonstrating a low serum IgG level in patients with recurrent bacterial infections. Additionally, blood group isohemagglutinins, or the so-called naturally occurring antibodies, are typically absent or low.[6] In contrast to X-linked agammaglobulinemia, most patients with CVI have normal numbers of mature B cells. However, these B cells do not differentiate normally into immunoglobulin-producing plasma cells. Three major types of cellular defects have been found in CVI patients. In some cases, T cells or their products appear to suppress differentiation of B cells into plasma cells. Secondly, T cells may fail to provide adequate help to support terminal differentiation of B cells. Finally, there appears to be a primary defect in the B cell line in some patients.

CVI can usually be effectively treated with intramuscular or intravenous immunoglobulin preparations. However, because of their low levels of secretory IgA, patients are still susceptible to respiratory and gastrointestinal infections, and the clinician should be vigilant for these infections and treat them vigorously with antibiotics.

Isolated IgG Subclass Deficiency

Patients can have an isolated deficiency of any one of the four IgG subclasses. Most IgG antibodies directed against protein antigens are of the IgG1 and IgG3 subclasses, while most IgG antibodies against carbohydrate antigens are IgG2. A selective deficiency of IgG2 can result in impaired responses to polysaccharide antigens, which cause recurrent infections with polysaccharide-encapsulated bacteria such as *Streptococcus pneumoniae* and *Hemophilus influenzae*. About 70 percent of the total IgG is normally IgG1, 20 percent IgG2, 6 percent IgG3, and 4 percent IgG4. Therefore, a deficiency of a single subclass may not result in a total IgG level below the normal range. The syndrome may be caused by a regulatory defect that prevents normal B cell differentiation.[5] Levels of the different subclasses should be measured if the total IgG level is normal but the clinical picture suggests immunoglobulin deficiency.[11]

Deficiencies of Cellular Immunity

Defects in cell-mediated immunity can result from abnormalities at many different stages of T cell development. Many different molecular defects can result in a similar clinical picture (as in severe combined immunodeficiency [SCID]). In some cases a primary defect in cell-mediated immunity can also have secondary effects on humoral immunity. This is because T cells provide helper functions that are necessary for normal B cell development and differentiation. Some of the more common defects of cellular and combined cellular and humoral immunity are summarized in Table 16–2.

In general, defects in cellular immunity are more difficult to manage than defects in humoral immunity. When immunoglobulin production is deficient, replacement therapy is often very effective. However, there is usually no soluble product that can be administered to treat a deficiency of cell-mediated immunity. Transplantation of immunologically intact cells, usually in the form of allogenic bone marrow transplantation, is often required to reconstitute immune function.

Patients with severe defects in cell-mediated immunity may develop graft-versus-host (GvH) disease. Transfused lymphocytes are normally destroyed by the T cell system of the recipient. However, a severe defect in the T cell system allows the donor lymphocytes to survive, proliferate, and attack the tissues of the recipient as foreign. GvH disease can occur in any patient

TABLE 16–2. Characteristics of Selected Defects of the T Cell System and Combined Defects			
Condition	**Deficiency**	**Level of Defect**	**Presentation**
DiGeorge anomaly	T cells; some secondary effects on antibody production	Embryologic development of the thymus	Neonatal, with hypocalcemia or cardiac defects if severe; incomplete forms may present later with infection
PNP deficiency	T cells; some secondary effects on antibody production	PNP, purine metabolism	Infancy
SCID	Both T and B cells	ADA, purine metabolism; HLA expression; RAG1/2; JAK3	Infancy
WAS	Reduced IgM and T-cell defect	CD43 expression	Usually infancy; mild variants occur
AT	Reduced IgG2, IgA, IgE, and T lymphocytes	DNA instability	Infancy
Reticular dysgenesis	All leukocytes	Stem cell defect	Neonatal
PNP = Purine-nucleoside phosphorylase; SCID = severe combined immunodeficiency; ADA = adenosine deaminase; HLA = human leukocyte antigen; WAS = Wiskott-Aldrich syndrome; AT = ataxia-telangiectasia.			

with a severe defect in cell-mediated immunity (e.g., in bone marrow transplant recipients) and can be fatal. Irradiation of cell-containing blood products (platelet concentrates, packed red blood cells, and whole blood) before transfusion destroys the ability of the donor lymphocytes to proliferate and prevents development of GvH disease in immunodeficient recipients. It should be noted that a defect in humoral immunity does not predispose to GvH disease.

GvH disease also occurs in patients who have received a bone marrow transplant as therapy for a congenital immune deficiency. The closer the match between the genetic constitution of the patient and the graft donor, the less severe the GvH disease is likely to be. Thus, although bone marrow transplantation can potentially cure the immune defect, it can also have serious, lifelong complications of its own.

DiGeorge Anomaly

DiGeorge anomaly is a developmental abnormality of the third and fourth pharyngeal pouches that affects thymic development. All organs derived from these embryonic structures can be affected. Associated abnormalities include mental retardation, absence of ossification of the hyoid bone, cardiac anomalies, abnormal facial development, and thymic hypoplasia.[9,12] The severity and extent of the developmental defect can be quite variable. Many patients with a partial DiGeorge anomaly have only a minimal thymic defect and, thus, near normal immune function. However, about 20 percent of children with a defect of the third and fourth pharyngeal pouches have a severe and persistent decrease in T cell numbers.[11] These children tend to have severe, recurrent viral and fungal infections. Severely affected children usually present in the neonatal period with tetany (caused by hypocalcemia resulting from hypoparathyroidism) or manifestations of cardiac defects. The possibility of immune deficiency can be overlooked if the association between the presenting abnormality and a possible thymic defect is not recognized.

The immunodeficiency associated with the DiGeorge anomaly is a quantitative defect in thymocytes. Not enough mature T cells are made, but those that are present are functionally normal. The immunodeficiency of DiGeorge syndrome can be treated with fetal thymus transplantation. Bone marrow transplantation has also been successful in some patients, as has administration of thymic hormones.

Purine Nucleoside Phosphorylase Deficiency

One immunodeficiency state for which a specific enzymatic basis has been defined is **purine-nucleoside phosphorylase (PNP) deficiency.** PNP deficiency is

a rare autosomal recessive trait.[11] The condition presents in infancy with recurrent or chronic pulmonary infections, oral or cutaneous candidiasis, diarrhea, skin infections, urinary tract infections, and failure to thrive. PNP deficiency affects an enzyme involved in the metabolism of purines. It produces a moderate to severe defect in cell-mediated immunity, with normal or only mildly impaired humoral immunity.[11] The number of T cells progressively decreases because of the accumulation of deoxyguanosine triphosphate, a toxic purine metabolite. The levels of immunoglobulins are generally normal or increased. About two thirds of PNP-deficient patients also have neurologic disorders, but no characteristic physical abnormalities have been described. Because of the relatively selective defect in cell-mediated immunity, PNP deficiency can be confused with neonatal human immunodeficiency virus (HIV) infection. The two conditions can usually be distinguished by specific tests for anti-HIV antibody (if the infant is old enough to be producing antibody) and by assays for PNP activity.

Combined Deficiencies of Cellular and Humoral Immunity

Defects in both humoral (B cell) and cell-mediated (T cell) immunity can be caused by a defect that affects development of both types of lymphocytes or a defective interaction between the two limbs of the immune system. Because helper T cell functions are necessary for normal differentiation and antibody secretion by B cells, a severe defect of T cell function will have effects on immunoglobulin levels as well.

Severe Combined Immunodeficiency

The most serious of the congenital immune deficiencies is **severe combined immunodeficiency (SCID).** It is actually a group of related diseases that all affect T and B cell function but with differing causes. X-linked SCID is the most common form of the disease, accounting for approximately 46 percent of the cases in the United States today.[1] This occurs with a frequency of about 1 in 50,000 births.[7] The abnormal gene involved codes for a protein chain called the gamma chain that is common to receptors for interleukins-2, 4, 7, 9, and 15. Normal signaling cannot occur in cells with defective receptors, thus halting natural maturation.[1,7] T cells, B cells, and natural killer (NK) cells are all affected. T cells are usually absent, while B cells are present and often found in increased numbers. No antibody production or lymphocyte proliferative response follows an antigen challenge in such cases, however.

An autosomal recessive form of SCID, affecting both males and females, has also been identified. In this case, the defect is lack of a specific intracellular kinase called Jak 3.[7] Lymphocytes are unable to transmit signals from interleukins-2 and 4.[1,11] These patients have B cells, but T cells are lacking, and symptoms are similar to the X-linked form of the disease.

About 15 to 20 percent of the patients with SCID have an adenosine deaminase (ADA) deficiency. Like PNP deficiency, ADA deficiency affects an enzyme involved in the metabolism of purines. In ADA deficiency, toxic metabolites of purines accumulate in lymphoid cells and impair proliferation of both B and T cells. As in PNP deficiency, there is a progressive decrease in lymphocyte numbers. A number of different mutations have been found to lead to ADA deficiency, and the degree of immunodeficiency correlates with the degree of ADA deficiency. Patients with only mildly reduced ADA activity may have only a slight impairment of immune function.

Other molecular defects have been identified as causes of SCID. Infants with a lack of both T and B cells but with functioning NK cells were found to have a mutation in a recombinase activating gene (RAG1 or RAG2). These genes cause a profound lymphocytopenia because of the inability of T and B cells to rearrange deoxyribonucleic acid (DNA) necessary to produce functional immunoglobulins or T cell receptors.[11] Defective expression of human leukocyte antigen (HLA) class II antigens, normally found on B cells, also impairs the immune response.[9] A newly identified molecular defect is a mutation in the gene encoding a common leukocyte protein called CD45. It is a transmembrane phosphatase that regulates signal transduction of T and B cell receptors.[11]

Patients with SCID generally present early in infancy with infection by nearly any type of organism. Oral candidal infections, pneumonia, and diarrhea are the most common manifestations. The administration of live vaccines can cause severe illness. Unless immune reconstitution can be achieved by bone marrow transplantation or by specifically replacing a deficient enzyme, patients with SCID die before they are 2 years old.

ADA deficiency is a special case because it presents a good opportunity for enzyme replacement therapy or somatic cell gene therapy. Although the ADA is normally located within cells, its deficiency can be treated by maintaining high plasma levels of ADA.[13] Red blood cell transfusion has been used in some patients to raise ADA to near normal levels. However, bovine ADA conjugated with polyethylene glycol (PEG) has a longer half-life than native ADA and can be used to raise the ADA level up to three times higher than normal. This treatment increases T cell production and specific antibody responses. Side effects of ADA–PEG administration appear to be minimal. However, this therapy is very expensive (about $250,000/year), and is primarily used in patients for whom a suitable bone marrow donor cannot be found or for those patients who are too sick to undergo marrow transplantation. Studies are currently underway to attempt to treat ADA deficiency by transfecting a normal ADA gene into patients' T cells or stem cells. These cells could then be reinfused into the patient. Theoretically, the gene therapy approach could be curative, but many obstacles remain to be overcome.

Wiskott-Aldrich Syndrome

Wiskott-Aldrich syndrome (WAS) is a rare X-linked recessive syndrome that probably affects six patients a year in the United States.[14] It is defined by the triad of immunodeficiency, eczema, and thrombocytopenia. WAS is usually lethal in childhood because of infection, hemorrhage, or malignancy. Milder variants have also been described, such as an X-linked form of thrombocytopenia.

The laboratory features of WAS include a decrease in platelet number and size with a prolonged bleeding time. The bone marrow contains a normal or somewhat increased number of megakaryocytes. There are abnormalities in both the cellular and humoral arms of the immune system, related to a general defect in antigen processing. This is manifest as a severe deficiency of the naturally occurring antibodies to blood group antigens (isohemagglutinins). Patients with WAS can have a variety of different patterns of immunoglobulin levels, but they usually have low levels of IgM, normal levels of IgA and IgG, and increased levels of IgE.[5] Absence of isohemagglutinins (IgM antibodies against ABO blood group antigens) is the most consistent laboratory finding in WAS and is often used diagnostically. These patients also have persistently increased levels of serum alpha-fetoprotein, which can also be a useful diagnostic feature.

The primary molecular defect in the syndrome appears to be an abnormality of the integral membrane protein CD43.[11] The gene responsible for the defect is called the WASp gene, and it is involved in the regulation of protein glycosylation.[11] Abnormalities cause defective actin polymerization and affect its signal transduction in lymphocytes and platelets.[15,16]

Platelets have a shortened half-life, and T lymphocytes are affected also, although B lymphocytes appear to function normally.[5] Splenectomy can be very valuable in controlling the thrombocytopenia. Current treatment for this immunodeficiency is bone marrow transplantation or cord blood stem cells from an HLA identical sibling.[17]

Ataxia-Telangiectasia

Ataxia-telangiectasia (AT) is a rare autosomal recessive syndrome characterized by cerebellar ataxia and telangiectasias, especially on the earlobes and conjunctiva. Blood vessels in the sclera of the eyes may be dilated, and there may also be a reddish butterfly area on the face and ears. Ninety-five percent of patients exhibit increased levels of serum alpha fetoprotein.[11] The incidence is between 1:10,000 to 1:100,000, although as much as 1 percent of the population is heterozygous for the gene.[5] Abnormal genes produce a combined defect of both humoral and cellular immunity.[5] Antibody response to antigens, especially polysaccharides, is blunted. The levels of IgG2, IgA, and IgE are often low or absent, although the pattern can be quite variable. In addition, the number of circulating T cells is often decreased. Death usually occurs in early adult life from either pulmonary disease or malignancy.[1]

Patients with AT have a defect in a gene that is apparently essential to the recombination process for genes in the immunoglobulin superfamily. This abnormality results in a defective kinase involved in DNA repair and in cell cycle control.[7] Rearrangement of T cell receptor and immunoglobulin genes does not occur normally.[11] Patients' lymphocytes often exhibit chromosomal breaks and other abnormalities involving the T cell receptor genes in T cells and immunoglobulin genes in B cells. These are sites of high levels of chromosomal recombination, and errors that occur during gene rearrangements may not be repaired properly. The syndrome is associated with an even greater risk of lymphoid malignancy than other immunodeficiency syndromes, presumably because the failure to properly repair DNA damage leads to accumulation of mutations. The only effective therapy for AT is allogenic bone marrow transplantation.

Defects of Neutrophil Function

Neutrophils play a crucial role in the immediate and nonspecific response to invading organisms by responding before specific antibody and cell-mediated immune response can be mounted. In addition, neutrophils are even more effective at ingesting and killing organisms coated with specific antibody and thus continue to play an important role in host defense even after a specific immune response is established. To destroy invading organisms, neutrophils must adhere to vascular endothelial lining cells, migrate through the capillary wall to a site of infection, and ingest and kill the microbes.

Defects affecting each of these steps have been described, each leading to an increased susceptibility to pyogenic infections.

Chronic Granulomatous Disease

Chronic granulomatous disease (CGD) is a group of disorders inherited as either an X-linked or autosomal recessive gene that affects neutrophil microbicidal function. The X-linked disease accounts for 70 percent of the cases, and it tends to be more severe.[18] Symptoms of CGD include recurrent suppurative infections, pneumonia, osteomyelitis, draining adenopathy, liver abscesses, dermatitis, and hypergammaglobulinemia. Typically, catalase-positive organisms such as *Staphylococcus aureus, Burkholderia cepacia,* and *Chromobacteria violaceum* are involved.[5] Infections usually begin before 1 year of age, and the syndrome is often fatal in childhood.

CGD is the most common and best characterized of the neutrophil abnormalities. Several specific molecular defects have been described in this syndrome, all of which result in the inability of the patient's neutrophils to produce the reactive forms of oxygen necessary for normal bacterial killing. There are three different autosomal recessive genes involved, and all of these affect subunits of nicotinamide adenine dinucleotide phosphate (NADPH) oxidase.[7,18] Normally, neutrophil stimulation leads to the production of reactive oxygen molecules, such as hydrogen peroxide (H_2O_2), by NADPH oxidase on the plasma membrane.[2] The plasma membrane enfolds an organism as it is phagocytized, and hydrogen peroxide is generated in close proximity to the target microbe. Neutrophil granules fuse with, and release their contents into, the forming phagosome. Hydrogen peroxide is then used by the granule enzyme myeloperoxidase to generate the potent microbicidal agent hypochlorous acid.

The process of generating partially reduced forms of oxygen by stimulated neutrophils was first detected as an increase in oxygen consumption. Therefore, this response was originally termed the neutrophil "respiratory burst." A more correct term is **oxidative burst.** A genetic defect in any of the several components of the NADPH oxidase system can result in the CGD phenotype by making the neutrophil incapable of generating an oxidative burst.[19]

CGD is usually diagnosed by measuring the ability of a patient's neutrophils to reduce the dye nitroblue tetrazolium (NBT). NBT reduction is caused by the production of hydrogen peroxide and other reactive forms of oxygen. Reduction converts the nearly colorless NBT into a blue precipitate that can be assessed visually on a microscope slide. Newer techniques use a dye that can be oxidized by reactive oxygen compounds to a fluorescent form. The intensity of the fluorescence of each individual neutrophil can be quantitated by flow cytometry. This technique is more objective and quantitative than the traditional NBT technique and deserves to be used more widely.

Although therapy with granulocyte transfusions may allow resolution of an acute infectious episode, it is impossible to provide enough granulocytes to treat the condition on a chronic basis. Administration of cytokines, such as interferon, may increase the oxidative burst activity in some patients. Continuous use of antibiotics can greatly reduce the occurrence of severe infections.[7] Bone marrow transplantation or use of peripheral blood stem cells may result in a permanent cure.[20]

Other Microbicidal Defects

Several other recognized defects can result in impaired neutrophil microbicidal activity. Neutrophil glucose-6-phosphate dehydrogenase deficiency leads to an inability to generate enough NADPH to supply reducing equivalents to the NADPH oxidase system. This leads to a defect in hydrogen peroxide production and a clinical picture similar to that of CGD. Myeloperoxidase deficiency is relatively common, occurring in about one in 3000 persons in the United States. Deficient patients may have recurrent candidal infections. Defects of neutrophil secondary granules have been described also. However, the molecular nature of the defects is unknown.

Leukocyte Adhesion Deficiency

Even if microbicidal activity is normal, neutrophils cannot perform their functions properly if they fail to leave the vasculature and migrate to a site of incipient infection. Adhesion receptors on leukocytes and their counter-receptors on endothelial cells and extracellular matrix play important roles in these activities. In leukocyte adhesion deficiency (LAD) a protein (CD18) that is a component of adhesion receptors on neutrophils and monocytes (with CD11b or CD11c) and on T cells (with CD11a) is defective.[21] The CD18 deficiency is transmitted with autosomal recessive inheritance and has variable expression. This defect leads to abnormal adhesion, motility, aggregation, chemotaxis, and endocytosis by the affected leukocytes.[18] The defects are clinically manifest as delayed wound healing, chronic skin infections, intestinal and respiratory tract infections, and periodontitis. A defect in CD18 can be diagnosed by detecting a decreased amount of the CD11/18 antigen on patient leukocytes by flow cytometry.

The CD11/18 protein is not the only neutrophil molecule involved in adhesion, motility, and phagocytosis. Recently, another type of adhesion molecule deficiency (LAD II) has been characterized. A carbohydrate molecule involved in adhesive interactions, CD15s, or sialyl Lewis X, was found to be deficient.[18,21,22]

Laboratory Evaluation of Immune Dysfunction

It is important in performing diagnostic testing for immunodeficiency that the results for a patient be compared with appropriate age-matched controls. In tests of cellular function, the patient's cells need to be tested in parallel with cells from a normal control. If an abnormal test result is obtained, it should be confirmed by repeat testing.

Screening Tests

Screening tests used for the initial evaluation of suspected immunodeficiency states are summarized in Table 16–3. Most of these tests can be performed routinely in any hospital laboratory. The evaluation of possible immunodeficiency starts with a complete blood count and white blood cell differential, which may reveal a reduced lymphocyte count. Thrombocytopenia with small platelets can be detected in WAS.

Measurement of the levels of serum IgG, IgM, and IgA and levels of the subclasses of IgG are used to screen for defects in antibody production. Assay for

TABLE 16–3. Screening Tests for Immunodeficiencies

Suspected Disorder	Tests
All immuno-deficiencies	Complete blood cell count, white blood cell differential count
Humoral immunity	Serum IgG, IgA, IgM levels, IgG subclass levels, isohemagglutinin titers (IgM), IgG antibody response to protein and polysaccharide antigens
Cell-mediated immunity	Delayed hypersensitivity skin tests (i.e., candida, diphtheria, tetanus, PPD)
	Chest X-ray (thymus shadow)
Phagocyte defect	NBT test
	IgE level (hyper-IgE syndrome)
Complement	CH$_{50}$ (classical pathway)
	Serum C3 level

PPD = Purified protein derivative; NBT = nitroblue tetrazolium.

isohemagglutinins is easily performed by the transfusion service. By the age of 2, a child should have naturally occurring IgM antibodies against ABO blood group antigens. The absence of these antibodies suggests an abnormal IgM response.

An overall assessment of antibody-mediated immunity can be made by measuring antibody responses to antigens to which the population is exposed normally or following vaccination. This can be easily done by measuring the titer of the specific antibody produced in response to immunization with a commercial vaccine such as diphtheria/tetanus. In an unimmunized child, the development of tetanus or diphtheria antibodies is determined 2 weeks after immunization. In a previously immunized patient, the response to a booster injection can be evaluated. A wide range of other protein and polysaccharide antigens can also be used in these tests.

Delayed-hypersensitivity–type skin reactions can be used to screen for defects in cell-mediated immunity. These tests are generally performed by the clinician and not by laboratory personnel. Delayed cutaneous hypersensitivity is a localized cell-mediated reaction to a specific antigen. The prototype is the tuberculin skin test. An antigen to which most of the population has been exposed, such as candida, mumps, or tetanus toxoid, is injected intradermally. The presence of induration 48 to 72 hours later indicates a cell-mediated immune response. A negative test result in young infants is not informative because they may not have been previously exposed to the test antigen.

Defects in neutrophil oxidative burst activity have traditionally been evaluated by NBT assay. Newer tests based on flow cytometry are now being adopted, and these will likely be more reliable.

Confirmatory Tests

If the screening tests detect an abnormality, or the clinical suspicion is high, more specialized testing will probably be necessary to precisely identify an immune abnormality. Some of the tests used for confirming an immunodeficiency state are summarized in Table 16–4.

Enumeration of classes of lymphocytes in the peripheral blood is performed by flow cytometry. Even though types of lymphocytes cannot be distinguished morphologically, they exhibit different patterns of antigen or surface immunoglobulin expression that correlate with functional characteristics. For flow cytometric evaluation, antibodies to antigens specific for different types of lymphocytes are labeled with a fluorescent probe. These antigens are generally referred to by cluster of differentiation (CD) number. The antibodies

TABLE 16–4. Specialized Confirmatory Tests for Immunodeficiencies	
Suspected Disorder	**Tests**
Humoral immunity	B cell counts (total and IgM, IgD, IgG, IgA-bearing)
	B cell proliferation in vitro
	Histology of lymphoid tissues
Cell-mediated immunity	T cell counts (total and helper-supressor subsets)
	T cell functions *in vitro*
	Enzyme assays (ADA, PNP)
Phagocyte defect	Leukocyte adhesion molecule analysis (CD11a, CD11b, CD11c, CD18)
	Phagocytosis and bacterial killing assays
	Chemotaxis assay
	Enzyme assays (myeloperoxidase, glucose-6-phosphate dehydrogenase, components of NADPH oxidase)
Complement	Other specific component assays

NADPH = Nicotinamide adenine dinucleotide phosphate.

are allowed to react with peripheral blood mononuclear cells. The flow cytometer is used to count the cells that are labeled with each fluorescent antibody. Lymphocytes can then be assigned to specific types based on antigen expression: B cells (CD19), T cells (CD3), T helper cells (CD3/CD4), cytoxic T cells (CD3/CD8), and NK cells (CD16 or CD56). Flow cytometry is objective and quite reliable. It allows detection of those defects that result in a decrease in one or more types of lymphocytes, such as DiGeorge anomaly.

T cell function can be measured by assessing the ability of isolated T cells to proliferate in response to an antigenic stimulus or to nonspecific mitogens in culture. Activated T cells also secrete cytokines, which can be assayed. Unfortunately, the *in vitro* functional assays can be quite unreliable and require a high degree of experience to perform. It can also be difficult to determine a normal range of responses for such tests.

Evaluation of Immunoglobulins

Quantitative measurement of serum or urine immunoglobulins is used in the workup of both immunodeficiency states and some lymphoproliferative disorders. Serum protein electrophoresis can be quantitative if the total serum protein is determined and the results are read using a densitometer.

Serum Protein Electrophoresis

Serum protein electrophoresis (SPE) is a technique in which molecules are separated on the basis of their size and electrical charge. SPE allows reproducible separation of the major plasma proteins. See Chapter 5 for details. The serum protein electrophoretic profile is traditionally divided into five regions: albumin and alpha-1, alpha-2, beta, and gamma globulins. IgG, IgM, IgD, and IgE migrate in the gamma globulin region, while IgA migrates as a broad band in the beta and gamma regions. Immunoglobulins normally show a range of mobilities. Additional evaluation of serum immunoglobulin is performed if the SPE shows a monoclonal component, or if there is a significant quantitative abnormality of serum immunoglobulins.

Immunofixation Electrophoresis

Another method of characterizing immune deficiencies is immunofixation electrophoresis (IFE). In IFE, serum samples are electrophoresed, just as for SPE, and then specific antibody is applied directly to the separating gel. The antibody–antigen complexes form and are visualized by staining. Polyclonal immunoglobulins are indicated by areas of diffuse staining, while monoclonal bands produce narrow, intensely stained bands (refer to Fig. 15–2). Lack of bands indicates immunodeficiencies of one or more immunoglobulin classes. IFE is labor intensive and expensive, although it is fairly fast.

Bone Marrow Biopsy

A bone marrow aspirate and biopsy is indicated in any evaluation of monoclonal gammopathy or immunodeficiency state. It is important in establishing the diagnosis of such disorders and for excluding other diseases.

SUMMARY

The immune system consists of a network of interconnected components. Defects in the development and regulation of individual portions of the immune system are recognized as causes of clinically distinct syndromes. Defects in antibody-mediated immunity lead to recurrent infections with pyogenic bacteria, particularly of the respiratory tract. Defects in T cell–mediated immunity generally lead to recurrent infections with intracellular pathogens. Primary defects in T cell function can also lead to secondary abnormalities in antibody

production and an increased risk of malignancy. Defects in phagocyte function generally lead to pyogenic bacterial infections, often of the skin. The clinical manifestations of these deficiency states have led to a better understanding of the normal roles of the different components of the immune system.

Immunodeficiency states run the gamut from quite mild to lethal. It is important to diagnose immunodeficiency states early in life because effective therapies are available for many of them. Failure to begin therapy as soon as possible can result in permanent organ damage or death caused by infection. The diagnosis must be suspected clinically and is evaluated by serologic analysis, first by screening tests measuring leukocyte counts and immunoglobulin levels, then by specialized laboratory testing. Prenatal diagnosis and carrier detection is possible for some familial immunodeficiency syndromes.

Case Studies

1. A 7-month-old male child was diagnosed with bacterial meningitis. Previously he had been hospitalized with bacterial pneumonia. Laboratory testing results were as follows: red cell count: normal; white cell count: $22 \times 10^9/L$ (normal is 5-$24 \times 10^9/L$); differential: 70-percent neutrophils, 15-percent monocytes, 5-percent eosinophils, and 10-percent lymphocytes; and SPE: no gamma band present.

Questions

   a. What possible conditions do these results indicate?
   b. How are these conditions inherited?
   c. What type of further testing do you recommend?

2. A 3-year-old female child appeared to be developmentally slow. She had several facial anomalies, including a small jaw and ears that were set farther back than usual. She seemed prone to infections, especially yeast infections. Laboratory testing results were as follows: red cell count was normal; white cell count was low normal; and a differential white cell count indicated a decrease in lymphocytes. Flow cytometry results demonstrated that the decrease in lymphocyte population was caused by low numbers of T cells. SPE showed a weak gamma band present.

Questions

   a. What immunodeficiency do you suspect?
   b. Are the facial anomalies linked to the immunologic findings?
   c. What kinds of treatment are possible?

Exercise: Immunoelectrophoresis

PRINCIPLE

Electrophoresis to separate out serum protein bands is combined with immunodiffusion, which allows antigen–antibody reactions to occur to identify specific components of each band. This technique is useful in identification of immunodeficiencies, increased immunoglobulin production (gammopathies), and other serum protein deficiencies.

SAMPLE PREPARATION

Obtain serum from whole blood by using a clot tube. Centrifuge and remove the supernatant. Discard any samples that appear to be hemolyzed. Serum is stable for up to 5 days if the specimen is refrigerated. Avoid freezing samples because it tends to denature protein.

REAGENTS, MATERIALS, AND EQUIPMENT

Corning Electrophoresis System (or equivalent), which includes:
A cell base with cover and a power supply (90 V, DC)
Universal agarose film
Universal pH adjusted buffer
Amido black stain
Goat antihuman serum
Stir-stain dishes
5-percent acetic acid
Microliter pipette
Incubator/oven or drying oven
Optional:
Goat antihuman IgG, IgM, IgA
Goat antihuman κ and λ

SOLUTIONS

1. Buffer preparation: The Universal barbital buffer kit contains 17.7 g of sodium barbital, 2.6 g of barbital, 1.0 g of sodium chloride, and 0.7 g of ethylene diamine tetra–acetic acid (EDTA). Empty the contents of the vial into a clean 2-L volumetric flask about half-filled with deionized water. Rinse the vial, and empty into the flask. Dilute to volume, and mix by stirring with a magnetic stirrer until the powder is completely dissolved. If stored in the refrigerator, the buffer is stable for up to 4 months. Check for any signs of contamination. The buffer must be at room temperature before using.
2. 5-percent acetic acid: Add 50 mL of glacial acetic acid to 950 mL of deionized water. Stir to mix.
3. Amido black stain: Empty dry powder from one vial into a 1-L flask. Bring the volume up to 1 L with 5-percent acetic acid. Cover the flask, and mix by inversion. If stored in an airtight container at room temperature, the stain is stable for up to 3 months.

PROCEDURE

1. Fill each side of the electrophoresis chamber with 95 mL of universal barbital buffer.
2. Connect the filled cell base to the power supply.
3. Gently peel the agarose film from the hard plastic backing.
4. Apply 1.0 mL of sample (serum, urine, or cerebrospinal fluid) and normal controls not directly into the well but centered on the anode side of each well.
5. Insert the film into the cassette holder of the cell cover with the agarose side out. Be sure to match the anode (1) side of the film with the anode side of the cell cover.
6. Place the cell cover on the base and electrophorese for approximately 35 minutes. A light on the unit will indicate that current is flowing.
7. Following electrophoresis, remove the cell cover, and drain without inverting. Grasp the film by the edges, and remove from the cassette holder.
8. Add antisera to troughs on the agarose film. Use two applications of 20 mL each, for a total of 40 mL.
9. Add a piece of sta-Moist paper to a stir-stain dish containing about 50 mL of deionized water.
10. Place the film in the chamber, and seal the chamber tightly with the cover.
11. Allow diffusion to take place for 48 hours at room temperature.
12. Following diffusion, place the film in 0.85-percent saline, and rinse by stirring for 6 hours or overnight.
13. Remove excess moisture, and place the film back in the drying oven until completely dry.
14. Observe for abnormalities in the precipitin bands.

INTERPRETATION

Immunoelectrophoresis is a two-step process in which serum proteins are first separated into five main bands on the basis of electrical charge and then further identified by precipitation with specific antiserum. After electrophoretic migration has occurred, antibody is placed in a well parallel to the separated proteins. Diffusion of antihuman globulin from the well occurs, and precipitin bands form where specific antigen–antibody combination takes place. Bands from patient samples are compared to those of normal serum. Lack of a band indicates a deficiency, while increased precipitation occurs with abnormal antibody production such as that seen in multiple myeloma or monoclonal gammopathies. Results must be interpreted on the basis that this is a semiquantitative screening technique, and further testing may be indicated if abnormalities are seen.

Review Questions

1. Patients with which immunodeficiency syndrome should receive irradiated blood products to protect against the development of GvH disease?
   a. Bruton's agammaglobulinemia
   b. Severe IgA deficiency
   c. SCID
   d. CGD

2. T cell subset enumeration by flow cytometry would be most useful in making the diagnosis of which disorder?
   a. Bruton's agammaglobulinemia
   b. Severe IgA deficiency
   c. SCID
   d. Multiple myeloma

3. What clinical manifestations would be seen in a patient with myeloperoxidase deficiency?
   a. Defective T cell function
   b. Inability to produce IgG
   c. Defective NK cell function
   d. Defective neutrophil function

4. Defects in which arm of the immune system are most commonly associated with severe illness after administration of live virus vaccines?
   a. Cell-mediated immunity
   b. Humoral immunity
   c. Complement
   d. Phagocytic cells

5. Which of the following statements applies to Bruton's X-linked agammaglobulinemia?
   a. It typically appears in females.
   b. There is a lack of circulating mature B cells.
   c. T cells are abnormal.
   d. There is a lack of pre-B cells in the bone marrow.

6. DiGeorge anomaly may be characterized by all of the following *except*:
   a. Autosomal recessive inheritance
   b. Cardiac abnormalities
   c. Parathyroid hypoplasia
   d. Decreased number of mature T cells

7. A 3-year-old boy is hospitalized because of recurrent bouts of pneumonia. Laboratory tests are run, and the following findings are noted: prolonged bleeding time, decreased platelet count, increased level of serum alpha-fetoprotein, and a deficiency of naturally occurring isohemagglutinins. Based on these results, which is the most likely diagnosis?
   a. PNP deficiency
   b. Selective IgA deficiency
   c. SCID
   d. WAS

8. Which of the following are associated with AT?
   a. Inherited as an autosomal recessive
   b. Defect in both cellular and humoral immunity
   c. Chromosomal breaks in lymphocytes
   d. All of the above

References

1. Buckley, RH: Primary immunodeficiency diseases due to defects in lymphocytes. N Engl J Med 343:1313–1324, 2000.
2. Cunningham-Rundles, C: Immunodeficiency diseases: Introduction. In Rose, NR, De MacArio, EC, and Folds, JD, et al (eds): Manual of Clinical Laboratory Immunology, ed. 5. American Society for Microbiology, Washington, D.C., 1997, pp 813–814.
3. Puck, JM: Prenatal diagnosis and genetic analysis of X-linked immunodeficiency disorders. Pediatr Res 33(suppl):S29, 1993.
4. Primary immunodeficiency diseases. Report of a WHO scientific group. Immunodefic Rev 3:195, 1992.
5. Cooper, MD, and Schroeder, HW, Jr: Primary immune deficiency diseases. In Braunwald, E, Fauci, AS, and Kasper, DL, et al (eds): Harrison's Principles of Internal Medicine, ed. 15. McGraw-Hill, New York, 2001, pp 1843–1851.
6. Ammann, AJ, and Stiehm, ER: Mechanisms of immunodeficiency. In Stites, DP, Terr, AI, and Parslow, TG (eds): Medical Immunology, ed. 9. Appleton & Lange, Stamford, Conn., 1997, pp 327–331.
7. Puck, JM: Primary immunodeficiency diseases. JAMA 278:1835–1841, 1997.
8. Fischer, A: Primary immunodeficiency diseases: An experimental model for molecular medicine. Lancet 357:1863–1869, 2001.
9. Kinnon, C, and Levinsky, RJ: Genetics of inherited immunodeficiency diseases and diagnostic techniques. In Rose, NR, De MacArio, EC, and Folds, JD, et al (eds): Manual of Clinical Laboratory Immunology, ed. 5. American Society for Microbiology, Washington, D.C., 1997, pp 815–823.
10. Sicherer, SH, and Winkelstein, JA: Primary immunodeficiency diseases in adults. JAMA 279:58–61, 1998.
11. Primary immunodeficiency diseases. Report of an IUIS Scientific Committee. International Union of Immunological Societies. Clin Exp Immunol 118(Suppl 1):1–28, 1999.
12. Kirkpatrick, JA, Jr., and DiGeorge, AM: Congenital absence of the thymus. Am J Roentgenol Radium Ther Nucl Med 103:32–37, 1968.

13. Hilman, BC, and Sorensen, RU: Management options: SCIDS with adenosine deaminase deficiency. Ann Allergy 72:395, 1994.

14. Peacocke, M, and Siminovitch, KA: Wiskott-Aldrich syndrome: New molecular and biochemical insights. J Am Acad Dermatol 27:507, 1992.

15. Cannon, JL, and Burkhardt, JK: The regulation of actin remodeling during T-cell-APC conjugate formation. Immunol Rev 186:90–99, 2002.

16. Orange, JS, Ramesh, N, and Remold-O'Donnell, E, et al: Wiskott-Aldrich syndrome protein is required for NK cell cytotoxicity and colocalizes with actin to NK cell-activating immunologic synapses. Proc Natl Acad Sci USA 99:11351–11356, 2002.

17. Filipovich, AH et al: Allogenic bone marrow transplantation (BMT) for Wiscott-Aldrich syndrome (WAS): Comparison of outcomes by donor type. J Allergy Clin Immunol 99(suppl):S102, 1997.

18. Lekstrom-Himes, JA, and Gallin, JI: Immunodeficiency diseases caused by defects in phagocytes. N Engl J Med 343:1703–1714, 2000.

19. Holland, SM, and Gallin, JI: Disorders of granulocytes and monocytes. In Braunwald, E, Fauci, AS, and Kasper, DL, et al (eds): Harrison's Principles of Internal Medicine, ed. 15. McGraw-Hill, New York, 2001, pp 366–374.

20. Ott, MG, Merget-Millitzer, H, and Ottmann, OG, et al: Mobilization and transduction of CD34+ peripheral blood stem cells in patients with X-linked chronic granulomatous disease. J Hematother Stem Cell Res 11:683–694, 2002.

21. Etzioni, A, Harlan, JM, and Pollack, S, et al: Leukocyte adhesion deficiency (LAD) II: A new adhesion defect due to absence of sialyl Lewis X, the ligand for selectins. Immunodeficiency 4:307, 1993.

22. Holland, SM: Neutropenia and neutrophil defects. In Rose, NR, De MacArio, EC, and Folds, JD, et al (eds): Manual of Clinical Laboratory Immunology, ed. 5. American Society for Microbiology, Washington, D.C., 1997, pp 855–863.

chapter 17

Transplantation Immunology

Eugene R. Heise, PhD, Diplo. (ABHI)

Learning Objectives

After completing this chapter, the reader will be able to:
1. List the immunologic barriers to graft acceptance.
2. Distinguish between direct and indirect allorecognition.
3. Discuss the mechanisms of graft rejection.
4. Explain the clinical functions of histocompatibility laboratories.
5. Describe the pre- and post-transplant laboratory methods in general use.
6. Identify risk factors for host-versus-graft (HvG) and graft-versus-host (GvH) reactions.
7. State how immunosuppressive agents promote graft survival.

Key Terms

Acute rejection
Acute GvHD
Allograft
Autograft
Chronic GvHD
Chronic rejection
Codominant
Complement-dependent
  cytotoxicity (CDC)
Cytolytic T cells
  (CTL)

Direct allorecognition
  pathway
Early or accelerated rejection
Genotype
Graft-versus-host response
  (GvHR)
Haplotype
Histocompatibility antigens
Histocompatibility tests
HLA genotype
HLA phenotype

Host-versus-graft response
  (HvGR)
Hyperacute rejection
Indirect allorecognition
  pathway
Linkage disequilibrium
Mixed leukocyte reaction
  (MLR)
One-way MLR
Syngraft
Xenograft

Immune defense systems evolved to protect the host from infectious organisms and host-derived tumor cells. In turn, pathogens and cancer cells have developed strategies to evade destruction by innate and adaptive immune mechanisms. Human leukocyte antigen (HLA) molecules are encoded by the major histocompatibility complex (MHC), located on chromosome 6 in the distal portion of the p21.3 band (as discussed in Chapter 4). The HLA system is the most important immunologic barrier to the survival of transplanted organs and tissues. HLA molecules play a key roll in both adaptive and natural immunity, including the transplant rejection response. Cells of the immune system express HLA molecules on their cell membranes where they present fragments of self and nonself proteins for recognition by antigen-specific T lymphocytes. The antigen receptors on each T cell recognize a portion of a self-MHC molecule together with a bound peptide fragment of a potential antigen. In organ transplantation, foreign HLA molecules of the graft serve as ligands (targets) for T cell receptors in the recipient, initiating an inflammatory response that leads to loss of graft function, which, if untreated, results in rejection of the graft. Thus, the transplant rejection response uses the same immune mechanisms that normally protect the individual against infectious disease and cancers that are recognized by the immune system.

This chapter discusses the immunologic and genetic principles of clinical transplantation. Pretransplant donor–recipient matching and post-transplant monitoring of the antigraft response are described. Graft outcomes, immune intervention, and immunologic considerations applicable to particular organ or tissue grafts are examined.

Histocompatibility Antigens

The HLA system consists of a cluster of linked gene loci (see Chapter 4). Compared to most other genes, HLA loci may be occupied by one of the multiple forms (alleles) of the gene that are present in the population. Within a family, however, the genetics of HLA are usually predictable: one maternal and one paternal HLA gene cluster is transmitted to each child as a **haplotype** (haploid genotype). The two parental haplotypes comprise the **genotype** of the individual. Most individuals are heterozygous (i.e., inherit two different alleles at each HLA locus) because of the extensive polymorphism that characterizes the HLA system at the population level. In less than 1 percent of families, a genetic crossover occurs during meiosis in the egg or sperm that results in a recombinant haplotype inherited by a child. HLA gene expression is **codominant** because both alleles at a given HLA locus are expressed. Individuals who inherit identical alleles at a locus are homozygous and exhibit a gene dose effect (i.e., produce twice the number of identical allele products on the cell surface compared to a locus that is heterozygous).

HLA molecules are cell-surface hetero-dimer proteins, consisting of one α chain and one β chain.[1] The cell membrane distal domain forms a cleft that is normally occupied with a peptide derived from a potential antigen or self-protein salvaged from protein turnover. Two different HLA classes (class I, II) are distinguishable in their biochemical structure, tissue regulation, and expression. HLA protein chains form loops of about 90 amino acids that resemble immunoglobulin domains. HLA class I and class II molecules are essential for immune activation of the two T lymphocyte classes that express either CD8$^+$ or CD4$^+$ coreceptors.

The biologic function of HLA molecules is to bind peptide fragments of degraded proteins and to transport the HLA:antigen peptide complex to the cell membrane for recognition by clonally derived T cells. The antigen receptors on a T cell are specific for sites on a particular HLA molecule and the HLA-bound peptide, which is derived from processed antigen. Peptide loading on HLA class I and class II molecules takes place in different cellular compartments to sample proteins from both extracellular and intracellular sources. Lymphocyte-dependent immune responses must be effective against extracellular pathogens and their products, as well as intracellular pathogens that propagate in the cytosol or in intracellular organelles. The B cell/antibody limb of immunity is highly effective against extracellular agents, but is largely ineffective against intracellular pathogens. In contrast, the T cell form of recognition permits T cells to kill host cells harboring antigens in intracellular organelles. This dual pathway provides information to T cells about antigens regardless of antigen location and initiates the appropriate response to eliminate antigen. The pathways are summarized in Table 17–1.

HLA class I molecules are expressed on most nucleated cells and are targets for **cytolytic T cells (CTLs),** or CD8 cells. CTLs accumulate in trans-

TABLE 17–1. MHC-Restricted Pathways of Antigen Recognition and Effector Responses

T Cell Subset	Antigen Source	Processing Cell Compartment	Peptides Bind to MHC	Effect on PC or Target Cell
CD4	Extracellular	Vesicle	Class II	Activate B cells
CD4	Intracellular	Vesicle	Class II	Activate accessory cells
CD8	Intracellular	Cytosol	Class I	Activate cytolytic T cells

MHC = Major histocompatibility complex.

planted organs that undergo cell-mediated rejection. Constitutive expression of class II molecules is mainly limited to antigen-presenting cells in which they display peptides derived from extracellular proteins to helper T lymphocytes. HLA class II positive cells (i.e., accessory cells required for T cell activation) and B lymphocytes, in turn, regulate the T cell response, induce inflammatory responses, and induce antibody formation. In the allogeneic response, T cells of the recipient can either react directly with donor HLA molecules or indirectly with the processed donor-HLA-derived peptides presented by the recipient's HLA molecules. Molecules and cells of the immune system attack donor organs or tissues that express HLA polymorphisms different from those of the recipient. Interestingly, the precursor frequency of T cells that respond to allogeneic HLA antigens is 10 to 100 times greater than that of T cells specific to conventional antigens.[2] This high precursor frequency, in part, is responsible for the intensity of the direct allograft response.

Many human genes are monomorphic and encode the same gene product in every individual. As indicated earlier, other genes are polymorphic because of multiple alleles encoding variant molecular forms. Every polymorphic protein is potentially antigenic if introduced into an individual that lacks the same allele because self-tolerance mechanisms delete only those T cells with receptors that react with proteins that are recognized as self-derived.[3] Polymorphisms that elicit a transplant response are termed **histocompatibility antigens.** Such antigens are classified as major or minor histocompatibility antigens, depending on their immunogenicity and the type of immune response that is induced.

Major Histocompatibility Antigens

In humans, deoxyribonucleic acid (DNA)-based typing methods can distinguish more than 800 class I and class II alleles encoded by 13 HLA loci that code for classical histocompatibility genes.[4] Additional genes in the HLA region are involved in antigen processing, peptide loading, and other immunologic functions. Class I HLA-A, -B, -C loci and class II HLA-DR, -DP, -DQ

encode six molecules per haplotype. Among class II loci, each DR1, 8, and 10 haplotype encodes one DRA:DRB1 dimer. All other DR haplotypes specify a second dimer from DRA and either the DRB3, DRB4, or DRB5 locus. Thus, depending on the DR genotype, either two or four different DR molecules are expressed. Taken together, the number of different HLA-A, -B, -C, -DR, -DP, -DQ genotypes is enormous. Transplant recipients with rare genotypes are unlikely to find an unrelated donor with a complete HLA match. It is believed that the coexistence of humans with pathogenic microorganisms is responsible for HLA diversity and for strategies that pathogens have developed to disable the immune system of the host. During fetal development and childhood, the HLA genotype influences the final T cell receptor repertoire in the individual. It is very likely that the varying frequencies of HLA alleles in different ethnic populations reflect selective pressure by pathogenic microorganisms for functional antigen-presenting HLA molecules. Certain HLA haplotype combinations are maintained through **linkage disequilibrium** between closely linked HLA loci. Some linkage disequilibria are characteristic of particular ethnic groups. The allele frequencies reflect the human migration patterns in agreement with information from anthropology and linguistics.

Minor Histocompatibility Antigens

Non-MHC transplantation antigens are termed minor histocompatibility (mH) antigens, which is somewhat of a misnomer because mH incompatibilities are not necessarily weak or minor.[5] The existence of mH antigens in humans initially was inferred from the observation that without immunosuppression, grafts exchanged between HLA-identical siblings were rejected, although survival was long, compared to HLA-mismatched sibling transplants. MH antigens are important in chronic rejection of organ grafts and can cause graft-versus-host disease (GvHD) following bone marrow transplantation from HLA-identical sibling donors. MH antigens consist of polymorphic proteins present in intracellular compartments (nucleus, cytosol, mitochondria, vesicles). One such mH antigen consists of sequences encoded by the SMCY gene on the Y chromosome. SMCY peptides are presented to T cells by HLA-A2 and B7 in individuals with either of those phenotypes. To be detected as an mH antigen, a protein probably has to generate at least two peptide fragments to generate both T cell help (HLA class II restricted) and cytotoxic T cells (HLA class I restricted).[6] Clinical mH typing is not in general use in organ transplantation because few human mH peptide sequences are defined; mH incompatibilities generally have a small effect in recipients who receive adequate immunosuppression.

Blood Group Antigens as Histocompatibility Antigens

Of the major and minor blood group systems, only the ABO system constitutes a barrier to transplantation. The ABO system is unique because anti-A, and anti-B antibodies occur naturally in individuals lacking the corresponding A or B antigens. These physiologic IgM antibodies seem to be induced by A and B blood group crossreacting epitopes present on bacteria or food products. Group-A, and -B antigens are histocompatibility antigens because they are expressed on endothelia and some epithelia in which they serve as targets of natural antibodies. Blood groups are not classified as mH antigens because rejection does not depend on T cell help. Crossing the ABO blood group barrier in vascular organ transplants generally results in hyperacute rejection.[7] Under certain circumstances, organs from donors of the A2 subtype can be transplanted into recipients of the O or B blood type. Pigs are prime candidates as xenogeneic organ donors because of the anatomic and functional similarities to corresponding human vascularized organs. A **xenograft** refers to tissue or organs transferred from one species to an individual of another species. Porcine endothelial cells that line blood vessels express galactose side chains (Gal epitope). Humans have mutations in the gene that encodes the enzyme that places galactose on cell surface glycoproteins and do not make the Gal epitope. The interaction between the natural antigalactose IgM and complement with Gal epitopes on pig cells results in rejection of pig xenografts transplanted to humans. An approach to this problem is to prevent formation of the Gal epitope by using transgenic technology to eliminate (knock out) the 1,3-galactosyltransferase gene.

Allograft Recognition

An **allograft** is tissue or organs transferred from one individual to another individual of the same species. Most clinical transplantation involves this type of graft.

A **syngraft** refers to the transfer of tissues and organs between genetically identical individuals such as identical twins. An **autograft** involves tissue removed from one area of the body and reintroduced elsewhere in the same individual. The latter are more successful because of HLA antigens on the transplanted tissue.

If, however, HLA antigens are not identical, a vigorous rejection response may occur. This is caused by the manner in which MHC molecules expressed on the donor cells are initially recognized by T lymphocytes of the recipient. The higher the density of class I molecules, the greater will be the strength of the host immune response. MHC class II molecules, found on antigen-presenting cells such as dendritic and endothelial cells, also elicit an immune response. Class II molecules are normally found in a relatively high number and are capable of activating CD4+ T cells. In some cell types, class II expression is actually induced by inflammatory cytokines, particularly interferon-gamma (IFN-γ).

Additional factors that determine the strength of an allogenic immune response include the following: high natural affinity of T cell receptors for MHC molecules; large number of peptide-MHC combinations that are recognized as nonself; and the potential for molecular mimicry involving crossreactions between self–MHC–peptide combination and allo–MHC–peptide combination.

Recognition Pathways

When allograft-donor HLA molecules activate an immune response, two different pathways of immune recognition are involved, depending on whether the antigen-presenting cells (APCs) are derived from the donor graft or from the graft recipient.[9] In the **direct allorecognition pathway,** recipient T cells recognize intact HLA molecules on donor APCs. The direct pathway predominates in the early post-transplant period and elicits a strong CTL response, requiring only interleukin-2 (IL-2) to activate MHC class I–restricted precursor CTLs into CD8+ effector CTLs. As with conventional antigen recognition, the **indirect allorecognition pathway** involves the presentation of processed donor HLA peptides bound to HLA class II molecules on recipient APCs, usually dendritic cells.[10] Activated APCs migrate from vascularized grafts to regional lymph nodes or the spleen, where naïve T cells normally encounter APCs and are primed for immune responses. Donor-derived HLA peptides are then recognized by recipient CD4+ T lymphocytes. In this way, T cells provide help to B lymphocytes for production of antidonor HLA antibodies. The indirect pathway predominates in most acute rejections and in chronic rejection.

The Mixed Leukocyte Reaction

The **mixed leukocyte reaction (MLR)** is considered an *in vitro* model of direct T cell recognition of alloantigens. The MLR measures the proliferation of responder CD8$^+$ CTLs to disparate class I antigens on stimulator mononuclear cells. HLA class II antigens on dendritic cells can be used as potent stimulators of CD4$^+$ T cells. Although B cells and macrophages exhibit class II antigens, they are weak stimulators of CD4+ T cells.[10] In clinical laboratories, MLR assays now are used mostly to evaluate cellular immune deficiencies. DNA-level HLA typing can accurately predict MLR responsiveness and has largely replaced MLR testing in the clinical transplant setting.

When a functional endpoint is desired, however, stimulator cells are prepared from peripheral blood mononuclear cells from one individual that are rendered incapable of proliferation by irradiation or treatment with a DNA inhibitor (mitomycin). In a **one-way MLR,** stimulator cells are cocultured for 5 to 7 days with untreated responder cell populations from another individual. CD4$^+$ responder T cells from immunocompetent donors will proliferate if HLA class II–disparate antigens are present on stimulator cells. If only class I–disparate HLA antigens are recognized, mainly CD8$^+$ cytotoxic cells will proliferate. The proliferative response ceases after 10 to 12 days during which the number of responding cells doubles several times each day. After about 2 weeks in culture, third-party cells sharing one or more HLA alleles with the original stimulator cells can be added to elicit a rapid proliferative response. This recall response peaks in 3 to 5 days, analogous to accelerated rejection. With suitable controls and data analysis, a negative MLR proliferation assay indicates HLA class II allele identity between the stimulator cells and responder cells. An HLA antigen dose effect is often observed in that 2-haplotype mismatched stimulator/responder combinations generally result in a proliferative response twice as large as a 1-haplotype mismatched combination.

Allograft Rejection

The goal of clinical transplantation is to replace a diseased or missing organ or tissue with a persisting functional graft. The need to understand and influence the immune response acting against foreign tissues has fostered rapid advances in immunobiology, immunogenetics, and immunosuppressive therapy. Analysis of allograft rejection mechanisms has contributed greatly to our present understanding of antigen recognition, immune regulation, and both antibody-mediated and cell-mediated cytolytic mechanisms.

Immune recognition of nonself histocompatibility antigens on solid organ grafts usually induces alloimmune mechanism(s) that attempt to reject the graft in the **host-versus-graft (HvG)** direction. The factors that determine allograft acceptance or rejection depend on the type of organ or tissue. If the transplanted organ or tissue contains considerable numbers of lymphoid cells, there is a strong likelihood of a **graft-versus-host response (GvHR).**[11] A GvHR occurs when mature T cells from the graft react with alloantigens of a immunocompromised host unable to eliminate the cytolytic cells of donor origin. GvHR is a major complication of bone marrow transplantation but may also occur in the setting of particular organ transplants. Four main types of rejection responses have been characterized.

Hyperacute and Accelerated Rejection Caused by Antibodies

Hyperacute rejection occurs within minutes to hours after joining of graft and host blood vessels in recipients. Preformed circulating antibodies against donor endothelium ABO, HLA, or endothelial-specific alloantigens are responsible for the reaction (Fig. 17–1). Hyperacute rejection is typically caused by naturally occurring anti-ABO blood group antibodies and anti-donor HLA antibodies. Kidney and heart transplants are susceptible, but liver transplants often survive hyperacute rejection. Skin grafts survive until about a week after transplantation when the donor and recipient blood vessels establish communication. This rapid and powerful type of rejection is rarely encountered in clinical transplantation today because of routine HLA antibody screening, donor lymphocyte/recipient serum crossmatching, and the use of blood group ABO-compatible donors. Allogeneic transplantation in the presence of preformed antibodies can be attempted after removal of antidonor antibodies by plasmapheresis. Alloantibodies bound to graft endothelium result in activation of complement system, release of von Willebrand factor, endothelial cell membrane injury, and exposure of basement membrane proteins. This sequence promotes platelet aggregation at the site of injury, thrombosis, and a rapid inflammatory reaction. Once the complement and coagulation cascades are activated, there is no treatment available to prevent endothelial cell activation, intravascular thrombosis, neutrophil infiltration, necrosis, and organ shutdown.

Early rejection or accelerated rejection results from a second exposure to incompatible tissue antigens. It begins within the first 5 days posttransplant and is characterized by necrosis of donor arterioles with intravascular thrombosis without lymphocyte infiltration. As in hyperacute rejection, antibody binding to

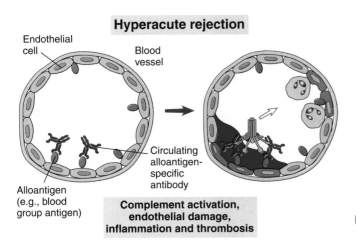

FIG. 17–1. In hyperacute rejection, preformed antibodies reactive with vascular endothelium activate complement and trigger rapid intravascular thrombosis and necrosis of the vessel wall. (From Abbas, Lichtman, & Pober: Cellular and Molecular Immunology, WB Saunders, 1991, with permission.)

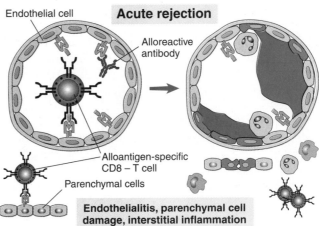

FIG. 17–2. In acute cellular rejection, CD8$^+$ T lymphocytes react with alloantigens on endothelial cells and parenchymal cells to mediate damage. Alloantibodies formed after engraftment may also contribute to vascular injury. (From Abbas, Lichtman, & Pober: Cellular and Molecular Immunology, WB Saunders, 1991, with permission.)

antigens on the donor vascular epithelium initiates the process. The endothelial changes occur more slowly, possibly because of the low levels of antibody, resulting in a type II endothelial activation. Components of the innate immune system, such as natural killer (NK) cells, may be involved in endothelial activation. T cell activation is not evident in accelerated rejection.

Acute Rejection Mediated by T Lymphocytes

Acute rejection is initiated by vascular and parenchymal tissue injury and is characterized by cellular infiltrates consisting mainly of CD8$^+$ T cells and mononuclear phagocytes (Fig. 17–2). Acute rejection episodes decrease in frequency after the first 3 months post-transplant, but the time and severity of rejection is unpredictable. HLA class II disparate grafts generally elicit dense cellular infiltrates, as compared to class I–only disparate grafts. Cellular rejection episodes are most effectively treated by increased doses of immunosuppressive drugs or with lymphocyte depleting approaches. Cell infiltrates consist of CD4$^+$ and CD8$^+$ T cells, NK cells, and macrophages. Cytotoxic T cells reactive with donor HLA class I antigens are markedly increased in cellular infiltrates of biopsy specimens of rejecting grafts. Experimental studies indicate that both cytotoxic and IL-2 producing CD4$^+$ and CD8$^+$ T cells are present in the polyclonal T cell infiltrates. The earlier view that a delayed-type hypersensitivity (DTH) response was responsible for graft

rejection does not account for the precise selectivity of effector mechanisms that destroy donor cells but spare the adjacent host cells.

Chronic Rejection Mediated by B and T Lymphocytes

The greatest risk of graft loss during the first year post-transplant is from an acute rejection. Subsequently the loss of transplanted organs continues at a uniform rate of 3 to 5 percent per year, despite continuous immunosuppressive therapy. HLA matching and improved immunosuppressive therapies have reduced the risk of early graft loss but not the risk of late graft loss from chronic rejection. Predisposing factors leading to chronic rejection include blood vessel injuries from prolonged ischemia, reperfusion, acute rejection episodes, and the toxicity of immunosuppressive agents. **Chronic rejection** occurs through a process of graft arteriosclerosis characterized by progressive fibrosis and scarring of arteries with narrowing of the lumen from proliferation of intimal smooth muscle cells (Fig. 17–3). Immunologic mechanisms are thought to be a component in most cases of chronic rejection, although no single mechanism has been identified. A chronic DTH has been proposed by which alloactivated T lymphocytes induce macrophages to secrete smooth muscle cell growth factors. Studies in experimental animals indicate that T cells can produce the lesion in response to either incompatible HLA or mH antigens. INF-γ, a macrophage activator, is involved in development of the

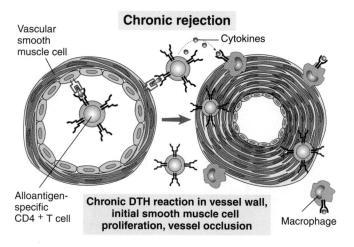

Chronic rejection

Vascular smooth muscle cell

Cytokines

Alloantigen-specific CD4 + T cell

Chronic DTH reaction in vessel wall, initial smooth muscle cell proliferation, vessel occlusion

Macrophage

FIG. 17–3. In chronic rejection with a graft arteriosclerosis, injury to the vessel wall leads to intimal smooth muscle proliferation and luminal occlusion. This lesion may be caused by a chronic delayed-type hypersensitivity (DTH) reaction to alloantigens in the vessel wall. (From Abbas, Lichtman, & Pober: Cellular and Molecular Immunology, WB Saunders, 1991, with permission.)

lesion. The fibrosis seen in chronic rejection may also result from the secretion of platelet-derived growth factor by activated macrophages, accounting for fibroblast proliferation and collagen synthesis. Wound healing after cell necrosis caused by acute rejection or alloantibodies may also lead to chronic rejection. The manifestations of chronic rejection vary somewhat between kidney, lung, heart, and liver transplants.

Graft-Versus-Host Disease

A graft antihost condition occurs when transplanted allogeneic lymphoid cells react against alloantigens of the recipient (host). **Acute GvHD** produces skin rashes, diarrhea, and an increased susceptibility to infection ranging from mild to lethal in severity. Recipients of bone marrow, small intestine, and lung transplants are at greatest risk of GvHD because these tissues contain significant numbers of T cells. Acute GvHD involves three steps.[13] First, pretransplant immunosuppression or cytoablative treatment activates host tissues to secrete inflammatory cytokines, which increases the expression of adhesion and HLA molecules. Next, activated $CD4^+/CD8^+$ T cells secrete type 1 cytokines (IL-2, INF-γ). Then, mononuclear cells that have been primed by type 1 cytokines are triggered by bacterial endotoxin to secret the inflammatory cytokines tumor necrosis factor (TNF)-α and IL-1. Cytokine-activated CTL and NK cells then destroy host

tissues. Lymphokine-activated natural killer (LAK) cells may play a role because they can lyse normal cell types, regardless of HLA genotype.[14] The primary targets of systemic acute GvHD are epithelia of the skin, gastrointestinal tract, liver, and the lymphoid system. The incidence and severity of acute GvHD is related to HLA and non-HLA incompatibilities between the donor and the host. Infection, rather than recipient organ failure, is the primary cause of weight loss and death. Removal of T cells from human marrow reduces the incidence of GvHD but also reduces the efficiency of engraftment. Acute GvHD is likely to occur in most patients, despite the use of immunosuppressive agents, such as methotrexate and cyclosporine. T cell depletion from unrelated donor marrows can reduce the severity of GvHD. Gamma-irradiation of cellular blood products is an effective method of preventing GvHD. To reduce the incidence and severity of GvHD, allele-level HLA typing is used in donor selection, and matching criteria are more stringent than for vascular organ transplantation.

Chronic GvHD resembles autoimmune connective tissue disease, with involvement of skin, eyes, mouth, and other mucosal surfaces, leading to fibrosis and atrophy. Chronic GvHD can develop in patients without prior acute GvHD and may respond to treatment, or it may be severe, debilitating, and persist for more than a year.

Organ and Tissue Transplants

Survival of most organ and tissue grafts requires pharmacologic and biologic immunosuppression to prevent destruction of the graft by HvG responses. Except for liver, vascular organ graft survival benefits from HLA matching. Kidneys and hearts contain little lymphoid tissue and rarely place the recipient at risk of GvHD, except when the host is genetically tolerant of donor HLA antigens and lacks the ability to respond in the HvGD direction. Acute GvHD commonly occurs in recipients of allogeneic bone marrow, intestine, and occasionally liver and heart transplantation or following surgery of any kind requiring blood transfusions that contain viable leukocytes.[15] The risk of transplant failure from rejection or other causes varies from one organ or tissue to another. Several different types of transplants are discussed here.

Corneal Transplants

The natural absence of blood and lymphatic vessels provides relative immunologic privilege to the eye by reducing the risk of sensitization to donor HLA alloantigens. Corneal transplants into noninflamed, nonvascularized corneal beds lack dendritic cells and have a very low incidence of rejection. However, corneal grafts transplanted to diseased eyes that are vascularized will have increased numbers of dendritic cells and are at increased risk of rejection.[16] Recipient dendritic cells migrate into the corneal transplant, triggering the indirect recognition pathway in corneal graft rejection.[17] HLA-A, -B matching appears to be beneficial to long-term corneal graft success, but HLA matching and crossmatching is rarely performed in human corneal transplantation. Multiple minor incompatibilities play a significant role in corneal rejection in rodent models, but whether they do so in humans is unknown.

Liver, Heart, and Lung Transplants

Liver, heart, and lung transplants are subject to allograft dysfunction from many nonimmunologic factors in addition to immune-mediated responses. In liver transplantation, hyperacute rejection occurs in ABO-incompatible transplants. Graft survival at 1 year is significantly better in ABO-identical grafts than in ABO-compatible grafts, and both do better than ABO-incompatible liver transplants. Acute rejection episodes are common and target the bile ducts and vascular endothelium, which express both HLA class I and II antigens; hepatocytes may be targeted later.[18] A correlation between HLA matching and liver allograft survival is not confirmed in large studies. Consequently, prospective HLA matching is not routinely performed in cadaveric liver transplantation. Some transplant centers perform prospective histocompatibility testing in cases of living donors and highly sensitized recipients. A positive flow cytometric crossmatch is associated with reduced first and second liver graft survival.[19] Irreversible chronic rejection of liver grafts is characterized by obliterative vasculopathy and loss of bile ducts. Chronic rejection is less frequent in liver transplantation as compared to other vascular organ transplants.

In cardiac transplantation, it is not often possible to take advantage of HLA matching because of the short ischemic time that heart tissue can tolerate. A positive prospective anti-HLA class I or class II donor-specific crossmatch is considered a contraindication to heart transplantation. Transplantable hearts are allocated to the most ill patients that are ABO identical or ABO compatible. Permissible mismatches may include blood types A_2 or A_2B organs transplanted to blood group B or O recipients. HLA typing and crossmatching are usually performed retrospectively. At some centers, post-transplant monitoring of antibodies by flow cytometry has been shown to correlate with earlier time to first rejection.

Renal Transplantation

Kidney transplantation is the treatment of choice for most patients with end-stage renal disease, and it is the organ most often transplanted. Introduction of new multi-immunosuppressive drug therapies over the past 15 years has steadily increased short-term (1 year) survival of kidney grafts from both living and cadaveric donor transplants, but has had little or no effect on long-term outcomes.[20]

An acute rejection episode is the strongest risk factor for chronic rejection and long-term graft loss. Immunosuppression-induced elevated cholesterol and triglyceride levels also increase the risk of chronic rejection. Evidence now indicates that mycophenylate mofetil (MMF) protects against the development of chronic renal allograft failure.[21] HLA matching has a significant beneficial effect on kidney graft outcome and patient survival. Close matching is particularly important in second and subsequent transplants because patients become highly sensitized to HLA antigens.[22]

Prospective renal transplant compatibility evaluation requires four laboratory tests: donor-recipient ABO blood group, HLA phenotype, HLA-specific antibody analysis, and serologic donor-recipient crossmatch. HLA-A, -B, and -DR typing is mandatory for unrelated donor matching; HLA-C, -DQ, -DP typing is optional. DNA-level allele typing is rapidly replacing serologic HLA typing for renal transplantation. HLA typing of the immediate family members permits assignment of the segregating haplotypes, if indicated. The need to detect low antibody titers requires techniques with high sensitivity that correlate with clinical findings.

Musculoskeletal Transplants

Allogeneic bone, cartilage, and soft tissue (cartilage and ligament) grafts are used to replace diseased or injured host tissue and often serve both mechanical and biologic functions. Graft material is tested for the presence of infectious agents and is preserved by −70°C freezing or by freeze-drying and sterilization with ethylene oxide or irradiation. Large bone grafts are commonly used to reconstruct joints in limb-sparing procedures following tumor resection. Cortical bone grafts usually lack viable cells when transplanted. Replacement bone often fails to unite with the patient's bone due to limited incorporation of the allograft into host bone, but rejection is difficult to identify and is inferred from bone resorption.[23] When viable cells are not part of the graft, the cells that form new bone are derived from host tissues, and new bone formation is delayed.[24] In animal models, the outcome of bone grafts is correlated with the method of bone graft preservation and the degree of genetic disparity between donor and recipient. Generally, allogeneic musculoskeletal tissues have not performed as well as autologous tissue. The cells of all musculoskeletal tissues express HLA class I antigens, and a subset of human osteoblasts expresses HLA class II antigens. Marrow cells are the principal source of MHC class I and II antigens in fresh allogeneic bone. Gamma radiation and inflammatory mediators induce HLA expression in bone. Bone sterilization and preservation significantly reduces the risk of HLA sensitization and rejection. Sensitization to HLA antigens often occurs in recipients of frozen osseous and osteochondral allografts as a consequence of prior exposure via blood transfusions. However, the clinical significance of anti-donor HLA alloantibodies and cell-mediated immunity to the incorporation of bone allografts requires further study.

Marrow/Stem Cell Transplantation

In general, the purpose of bone marrow transplantation is to replace malignant or genetically defective hematopoietic stem cells with healthy, functional stem cells and to allow cancer patients to survive after destruction of the malignant cells. In the case of certain cancers, immunocompetent cells can kill residual malignant cells (graft-versus-leukemia effect). Unlike vascular organ transplant recipients, allogeneic hematopoietic stem and bone marrow recipients do not require continuous long-term immunosuppressive therapy once a state of mutual GvH and HvG tolerance becomes established.[24] Donor-specific tolerance is required for permanent marrow graft survival. Acute GvHD has been associated with the development of CTLs that recognize even a single amino acid difference in an HLA class I allele between the marrow donor and recipient. The major risk of marrow transplantation is the development of GvHD, which does not occur when the donor and recipient are HLA identical at the allele level, using DNA-based typing. Risk factors for acute GvHD and failure of engraftment include mismatched HLA-A, -B, -DRB1, -DQB1 alleles as determined by DNA-level typing.[25] In the United States, the National Marrow Donor Program assists in the search for HLA allele–matched unrelated donors.[26] Donor-reactive HLA-specific antibodies are at risk for failure of marrow engraftment. After bone marrow transplantation, patients may require multiple blood transfusions and develop HLA-specific antibod-

ies that cause refractoriness to random platelet transfusion.[27]

Platelet Transfusion

Multiple transfusions of platelets from random donors can induce alloantibodies to HLA class I antigens or, less often, to platelet-specific polymorphisms. HLA sensitization occurs in about half of multitransfused patients with bone marrow failure. When this occurs, the alloimmune status and the anti-HLA-A, -B specificities are determined. The most effective treatment is HLA-matched platelet transfusion. The increasing use of leukocyte-depleted blood and blood-products should reduce the overall risk of platelet refractoriness. Antibodies in multitransfused patients are often multispecific and of the IgM and IgG isotypes.[27]

Histocompatibility Testing

Laboratories with sensitive, rapid, and reproducible immunogenetic **histocompatibility tests** of good predictive value are key components of successful clinical transplantation programs. These laboratories also contribute to the large data sets needed to evaluate immunologic and genetic risk factors in transplantation and the allocation of organs and tissues for transplantation. They work closely with the Organ Procurement and Transplantation Network (OPTN) and the United Network for Organ Sharing (UNOS) as well as other national and international agencies.

Histocompatibility (HLA) laboratories have three main functions in clinical organ transplantation:

1. Prevent hyperacute or acute rejection due to pre-existing or induced donor-reactive antibodies.
2. Improve overall graft survival rates by minimizing the number of HLA incompatibilities between donors and recipients through better matching.
3. Monitor HLA sensitization status before and after transplantation.

The classical procedure for both HLA typing and HLA antibody analysis is based on antibody-mediated, **complement-dependent cytotoxicity (CDC)**.[28] The CDC format is versatile because it can be used with antisera of known HLA specificity for HLA phenotyping or with target cells of known HLA phenotypes to determine the specificity of HLA antibodies (Fig. 17-4). CDC is a functional assay because the end point is antibody-mediated and complement-dependent lymphocyte lysis. However, the CDC assay is rather insensitive, a drawback for antibody screening and crossmatching. CDC tests can be subjective when

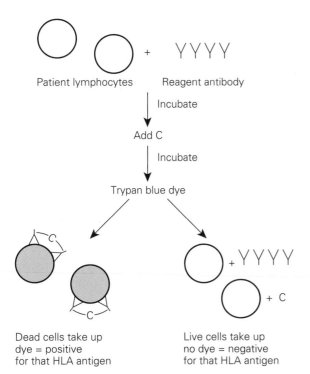

FIG. 17–4. Complement-dependent cytotoxicity testing. Patient lymphocytes are isolated from whole blood by Ficoll-Hypaque density gradient centrifugation and placed in 96 well microtiter plates. The wells contain a panel of antibodies recognizing different HLA antigens. The plate is incubated for 30 minutes, complement is added, the plate is reincubated for 60 minutes, and then trypan blue dye is added. Cells recognized by the antibody will undergo complement-mediated cell membrane damage and become permeable to the dye.

the scoring is performed manually by microscopic assessment. Test sensitivity can be enhanced by the addition of an antihuman IgG (AHG) antibody step (AHG-CDC assay). The readout can be manual microscopic scoring of cell death based on vital staining; alternatively, the readout can be automated using microscopes equipped with mechanical stages. Because patient sera often may contain low levels of HLA antibodies, AHG-CDC assays are used for pretransplant crossmatching and for antibody specificity analysis. Lymphocytes express multiple HLA class I and II antigens encoded by distinct HLA loci, and moreover, individual HLA molecules have multiple epitopes, some of which are shared with other allele products encoded by the same or a different locus. For HLA class I typing or anti–class I antibody identification, a purified T cell population is preferred because human T lymphocytes express class I molecules but not class II molecules. Conversely, B cells are required for class II typing or antibody identification because human B cells express class II as well as class I HLA molecules.

Solid-phase enzyme-linked immunosorbent assays (ELISA) are available for panel-reactive antibody (PRA) determination and antibody-specificity analysis. ELISA-based assays are reproducible, objective, and sensitive. Some ELISA-based HLA tests use HLA antigens solubilized from continuous cell lines and purified by immunoprecipitation with anti–class I or anti–class II antibodies. In this format, antibody specificity analysis can be problematic because of partially overlapping HLA specificities in the cell panel. Newer assays use pure HLA antigens produced by recombinant technology to simplify specificity analysis.

Single-cell analysis by flow cytometry is the most sensitive method for crossmatching and antibody identification. As with the AHG-CDC method, tagged T or B lymphocytes are incubated with the blood serum to permit formation of antigen–antibody complexes on the cell surface. After washing to remove unbound proteins, the bound antibodies are detected with a second antibody (i.e., antihuman IgG labeled with a chromophore, such as fluorescein). In an alternative flow cytometric assay format, lymphocytes are replaced by microparticles coated with HLA antigens of known specificity obtained through a recombinant technique. One advantage of flow cytometry is the ability to identify the lymphocyte population without the need for physical purification. Widely used histocompatibility tests and their indications are briefly described in the following sections.

Donor-Recipient Crossmatch Test

Purpose: Detect clinically significant cytotoxic antibodies in a recipient against alloantigens on cells from a prospective transplant donor.

Test specimen: Pretransplant serum sample(s) from the transplant candidate.

Reagents: Purified T and B lymphocytes from the potential donor and recipient (autologous control); rabbit serum complement.

Utility: A positive T cell test due to donor-reactive IgG alloantibodies is a contraindication for kidney and some other organ transplants because of the high risk for early graft failure. In hematopoietic stem cell (bone marrow) transplantation, a positive crossmatch test is a predictor of engraftment failure.

HLA Antigen Phenotype

Purpose: Identify HLA class I and class II proteins expressed on cells of candidate transplant donors and recipients.

Reagents: Panel of polyclonal/monoclonal antibodies of known HLA specificities; rabbit serum complement.

Test Specimen: Purified T and B lymphocytes from the prospective donor(s) and the recipient.

Utility: Cost-effective low-resolution HLA phenotype method based on serologically defined public, broad, and private epitopes for solid organ transplants, platelet transfusion, or disease association. May be used to determine the epitope relationships of newly described alleles identified by DNA-based methods.

Panel-Reactive Antibody and HLA Specificity Analysis

Purpose: Determine the cell panel percent reactivity and define the specificity of anti-HLA class I and/or class II antibodies.

Test Specimen: Pretransplant or post-transplant recipient serum.

Reagents: Purified T or B lymphocytes from a panel of HLA-typed individuals; rabbit serum complement.

Utility: Detects HLA-specific antibodies induced by pregnancy, transfusion with blood products, or previous transplantation to aid in donor selection for transplantation and platelet transfusion. T cells detect anti–class I Abs; B cells detect anti–class I and II antibodies.

DNA-Based HLA Genotyping

Purpose: Low-resolution (serologic equivalent) or high-resolution HLA allele definition for organ or hematopoietic stem cell transplantation.

Test Specimen: DNA extracted from nucleated cells of blood or tissue cells.

Reagents: DNA primers or probes of specific HLA sequences of selected loci or alleles for use with polymerase-chain reaction (PCR)-based HLA typing or sequencing.

Immunosuppression for Prevention and Treatment of Rejection

Immunosuppression following organ transplantation is necessary to (1) induce the initial acceptance of the graft, (2) prevent rejection while preserving host defenses, and (3) reverse rejection episodes when they occur. Immunosuppression can be associated with an increased risk of infections, especially opportunistic viruses such as cytomegalovirus (CMV). An increased incidence of B cell lymphomas and squamous carcinomas of the skin are associated with chronic herpesvirus and papillomavirus infection, respectively.

Combination immunosuppressive therapy uses drugs that act at different stages of the activation pathway and cell cycle to target critical steps of the allograft response (Table 17–2). The goal is to increase effectiveness while reducing toxicity. All agents interfere with T cell function, but only some suppress B cells directly.

Corticosteroids are potent anti-inflammatory and immunosuppressive agents used for treatment of acute rejection and, in lower doses, for maintenance immunosuppression. Steroids nonspecifically block the production of HLA molecules, adhesion molecules and proinflammatory cytokines (IL-1, TNF-α, IL-6), and chemoattractants that decrease macrophage function and alter leukocyte traffic patterns.[29] Long-term use of corticosteroids is associated with complications, including hypertension and post-transplant diabetes mellitus.

Cyclosporine and tacrolimus block signal transduction pathways in T cells to inhibit cytokine synthesis (especially IL-2, IL-3, IL-4 and INF-γ).[30] These products of microbe fermentation inhibit calcineurin phosphatases and have their effect early in the proliferative cycle ($G_0 > G_1$). MMF is a chemically modified natural product that selectively inhibits inosine monophosphatase dehydrogenase.[31] Unlike other cell types, T and

---

TABLE 17–2. Some Immunosuppressive Agents and their Inhibitory Action

Action Site	Cell Cycle Stage	Drug or Therapeutic Monoclonal Antibody
Immune cell activation	G_0	Corticosteroids Anti-CD3, -CD4, -CD8, -CD40 monoclonal antibodies
Gene transduction in activated T cells	G_0	Cyclosporine (Neoral) Tacrolimus
IL-2 response	G_1	Rapamycin Daclizumab
DNA synthesis	S	Azathioprine (Imuran)
Cell division (mitosis)	G_2	Cyclophosphamide X-rays

IL = Interleukin; DNA = deoxyribonucleic acid.

B lymphocytes are dependent for their proliferation on de novo synthesis of purines. MMF is used in combinations with other agents, such as cyclosporine and corticosteroids. The active metabolite of MMF inhibits T and B cell proliferation and suppresses antibody formation. MMF reduces the incidence of acute rejection and reduces expression of adhesion molecules important in the rejection process.

Monoclonal antibodies specific for T cell surface molecules are available for the treatment of severe acute rejection episodes and GvH reactions. Mouse anti-CD3 monoclonal antibody (OKT3) transiently modulates T cell receptors from the cell membrane, rendering these cells temporarily nonfunctional. At high doses, OKT3 depletes circulating T cells by complement-mediated cytolysis or opsonization for phagocytosis. OKT3 and other mouse monoclonal antibodies are immunogenic in humans, which limits their use to a single course of treatment. Daclizumab is a humanized monoclonal antibody produced by recombinant DNA technology that binds specifically to the alpha subunit of the high-affinity human IL-2 receptor (IL-2R). IL-2R is expressed on activated lymphocytes, but not on resting lymphocytes.[32] It has a serum half-life of 20 days and reduces the frequency of acute rejection in kidney transplant patients.[32] Sirolimus is a microbe product that shares with tacrolimus a common intracellular binding protein. Sirolimus is antiproliferative for B and T cells and inhibits growth factor-induced proliferation. Sirolimus can prevent acute, accelerated, and chronic rejection and may permit withdrawal of steroids as well as reduction of cyclosporine exposure. The effect of these newer prophylactic and maintenance regimens is to reduce the incidence of severe rejection, delay the time to first rejection, and decrease the incidence of severe rejections without side effects or increased adverse events.

SUMMARY

Transplantation of organs and tissues between members of a species engages the immune system in a way that does not occur in nature. The immune system evolved against the threat of infectious agent and not for the purpose of graft rejection. Consequently, the extraordinary diversity of the MHC in the species developed in response to non-MHC antigens and not to alloantigens. During the development of each individual, the T lymphocyte system is selected to recognize nonself peptides bound to a self-MHC molecules. T cells can distinguish between peptides that differ by a single amino acid. Transplant antigens will usually differ from self not only by the peptides they are presenting but also by amino acid differences in the donor MHC molecules. Allogeneic responses are unique in that they are unusually vigorous, and they can be stimulated by two different sets of APCs (i.e., from both donor and recipient). Thus, it is difficult to understand transplant immunology by applying classical immunologic reasoning. Graft rejection can involve unusual types of immune responses. The goal of transplantation biology has been to devise strategies to induce graft tolerance. Although allograft tolerance in adult humans has not been achieved, intense investigation into the problem has contributed to understanding the fundamental mechanisms of immunology. The survival of the fetus as physiologic allograft is attributed in part to the absence of classical HLA-A, -B, -C expression on most trophoblasts that would serve as targets of cytotoxic T cells, as well as protection from viral attack by NK cells, which normally are inhibited by HLA-A, -B, -C, and HLA-G determinants.

The major role of histocompatibility laboratories is to support clinical transplant programs by helping to prevent hyperacute or acute rejection, improving overall graft survival rates, and monitoring HLA sensitization status. Computerized data systems are essential for efficient and equitable organ allocation that takes into account such factors as medical urgency, HLA matching, donor-recipient crossmatching, and individual patient risk factors. A major challenge to histocompatibility laboratories is to provide the laboratory data that will maximize the benefits from the scarce supply of organs and tissues.

Exercise: HLA Haplotype Segregation Analysis

PRINCIPLE

Serologic HLA typing provides information about the HLA protein polymorphisms expressed on the cell surface of an individual. **HLA phenotype** information is limited to the alloantigens that are recognized by the reagent panel selected for a particular indication. Each reagent panel consists of polyclonal antisera or monoclonal antibodies selected to recognize private or shared HLA specificities and HLA antigens. An HLA class I panel might detect the products of HLA-A, -B, -C loci; a class II panel might recognize the products of the DR and DQ loci. Donor-recipient matching for renal (kidney) transplantation is usually based on the HLA-A, -B, -DR, because these antigens seem to be the most immunogenic. By convention, HLA phenotypes are written as a string of antigens (e.g., HLA-A1, 3; B7, 8; DR7, 17). If only one HLA antigen is identified for a locus, then an X or blank is inserted. To help distinguish these possibilities, retyping with a different panel might be needed or the entire family might be typed. Family typing is essential if the goal is to find a genotypic HLA-identical donor (i.e., a sibling that shares two haplotypes with a patient). Each parent–child combination will share only one haplotype. Segregation analysis involves inspection of phenotype data from parental and offspring generations of a nuclear family so that the four haplotypes can be inferred from the HLA phenotype data. Haplotype segregation analysis is based on the principle that HLA genes are transmitted en bloc and yields the **HLA genotype** of the individual.

Sequence-based HLA typing is a method of direct allele typing. Segregation analysis using the HLA allele assignments of family members is still needed to define the segregating haplotypes. Predicted haplotypes of some individuals can be deduced without family studies if the particular HLA alleles at closely linked exhibit linkage disequilibrium. By referring to published allele frequency tables for the appropriate ethnic group, the two haplotypes of many individuals can be assigned.

PROCEDURE

1. Arrange the HLA phenotypes in the order in which the corresponding genes are arranged on chromosome 6, from centromeric (left) to telomeric (right) to recognize and interpret rare intra-HLA recombination events that occur in approximately 1 to 2 percent of families.
2. Identify the antigens at each locus from one parent that could only have come from the father and designate these as haplotypes (a) and (b), or could only have been inherited from the mother (haplotypes [c] and [d], where [a, b, c, d] is a shorthand representation of the inferred haplo-

types). For each child, list the two haplotypes that can account for the phenotype of the child (i.e., ac, ad, bc, bd).
3. Write out each of the four haplotypes (i.e., HLA-DQ_, DR_, B_, C_, A_) where the underline would be replaced with the number corresponding to the particular antigen assigned to each locus in the string.
4. If there is no antigen available to assign a given locus, insert X after the locus designation. A blank X may reflect homozygosity at the locus.
5. Each child will inherit one paternal haplotype and one maternal haplotype. If an extra haplotype is required to explain the data, then consider the following possibilities: (a) incomplete typing or missed antigen, (b) incorrect typing, (c) nonpaternity, or (d) interlocus crossover during meiosis in one of the parents.

JONES FAMILY GENOTYPE ANALYSIS WORKSHEET

1. Using the following worksheet, deduce the haplotypes that segregate in the Jones family. The HLA phenotypes of the Jones Family are listed in the centromeric → telomeric order.

Father:		DQ2,X	DR13,17	B8,X	Cw7,X	A1,24
	(a)	DQ___	DR___	B___	Cw___	A___
	(b)	DQ___	DR___	B___	Cw___	A___
Mother:		DQ1,X	DR1,13	B35,60	Cw3,w4	A2,3
	(c)	DQ___	DR___	B___	Cw___	A___
	(d)	DQ___	DR___	B___	Cw___	A___
Child 1:						
(patient)		DQ1,2	DR1,17	B8,35	Cw4,w7	A3,24
	( )	DQ___	DR___	B___	Cw___	A___
	( )	DQ___	DR___	B___	Cw___	A___
Child 2:		DQ1,2	DR13,17	B8,60	Cw3,w7	A2,24
	( )	DQ___	DR___	B___	Cw___	A___
	( )	DQ___	DR___	B___	Cw___	A___
Child 3:		DQ1,2	DR13,17	B8,60	Cw3,w7	A1,2
	( )	DQ___	DR___	B___	Cw___	A___
	( )	DQ___	DR___	B___	Cw___	A___
Child 4:		DQ1,2	DR13,X	B8,60	Cw3,w7	A1,2
	( )	DQ___	DR___	B___	Cw___	A___
	( )	DQ___	DR___	B___	Cw___	A___
Child 5:		DQ1,2	DR1,13	B8,35	Cw4,w7	A1,3
	( )	DQ___	DR___	B___	Cw___	A___
	( )	DQ___	DR___	B___	Cw___	A___

2. Using the (a, b, c, d) as an abbreviations for the four haplotypes, which paternal and maternal haplotypes were present in each of the five children?
3. Which sibling is the best match for Child 1, who is in need of an organ transplant, and why?

INTERPRETATION OF RESULTS

HLA genotyping is important in histocompatibility testing, especially when serotyping data is incomplete and the possibility of a related donor is under consideration. The chance that two siblings will be HLA-identical by sharing a paternal and a maternal haplotype is 1:4, or 25 percent. The chance that two siblings share one haplotype is 1:2 or 50 percent. The chance that two siblings share zero haplotypes is 1:4 or 25 percent, following the Mendelian principle. If a child needing a renal transplant shares two haplotypes with a sibling (e.g., patient: a, c/sibling: a, c), then it follows that they probably share the same HLA antigens at closely linked loci that may not have been typed, such as −DP, or at a locus where the phenotype assignment is problematic. Allele typing by DNA-based methods yields the genotype directly at the coding level. However, DNA typing results, taken alone, provide no information about whether the allele is expressed. Although HLA expression is codominant, certain virus infections and cancers interfere with HLA gene expression and thus alter the phenotype.

1. The type of allograft rejection associated with vascular and parenchymal injury with lymphocyte infiltrates is which of the following?
   a. Hyperacute rejection
   b. Acute cellular rejection
   c. Acute humoral rejection
   d. Chronic rejection

2. Antigen receptors on T lymphocytes bind HLA class II molecules with the help of which accessory molecule?
   a. CD2
   b. CD3
   c. CD4
   d. CD8

3. Patients at risk for graft-versus-host disease (GvHD) include each of the following except recipients of:
   a. Bone marrow transplants
   b. Lung transplants
   c. Liver transplants
   d. Irradiated leucocytes

4. HLA molecules exhibit all of the following properties except that they:
   a. Belong to the immunoglobulin superfamily
   b. Are heterodimeric
   c. Are integral cell membrane glycoproteins
   d. Are monomorphic

5. Kidney allograft loss from intravascular thrombosis without cellular infiltration 5 days post-transplant raises the suspicion level about which primary rejection mechanism?
   a. Hyperacute rejection
   b. Accelerated humoral rejection
   c. Acute humoral rejection
   d. Acute cellular rejection
   e. Chronic rejection

6. Which reagents would be used in a direct (forward) donor-recipient crossmatch test?
   a. Donor serum and recipient lymphocytes + rabbit serum complement
   b. Recipient serum and donor lymphocytes + rabbit serum complement
   c. Donor stimulator cells + recipient responder cells + complete culture medium
   d. Recipient stimulator cells + donor responder cells + complete culture medium

7. The indirect allorecognition pathway involves which one of the following mechanisms?
   a. Processed peptides from polymorphic donor proteins restricted by recipient HLA class II molecules
   b. Processed peptides from polymorphic recipient proteins restricted by donor HLA class I molecules
   c. Intact polymorphic donor protein molecules recognized by recipient HLA class I molecules
   d. Intact polymorphic donor protein molecules recognized by recipient HLA class II molecules

8. Which immunosuppressive agent selectively inhibits IL-2 receptor-mediated activation of T cells and causes clearance of activated T cells from the circulation?
   a. Mycophenylate mofetil
   b. Cyclosporine mofetil
   c. Corticosteroids
   d. Sirolimus
   e. Daclizumab

References

1. Urban, RG, and Chicz, RM: MHC Molecules. RG Landes Company, Austin, 1996.
2. Gould, DS, and Auchincloss, Jr, H: Direct and indirect recognition: The role of MHC antigens in graft rejection. Immunol Today 20:77–82, 1999.
3. Rossini, AA, Greiner, DL, and Mordes, JP: Induction of immunologic tolerance for transplantation. Physiol Rev 79:141, 1999.
4. Bodmer, JG, Marsh, SGE, et al: Nomenclature for factors of the HLA system. Tissue Antigens 53:407–446, 1999.
5. Loveland, B, and Simpson E: The non-MHC transplantation antigens: Neither weak nor minor. Immunol Today 7:223–229, 1986.
6. Roopenian, DC, Davis, AP, et al: The functional basis of minor histo-compatibility loci. J Immunol 151:4595–4605, 1993.
7. Nelson, PW, Helling, TS, et al: Current experience with renal transplantation across the ABO barrier. Am J Surg 164:541–545, 1992.
8. Galili, U: Interaction of the natural anti-Gal antibody with a-galactosyl epitopes: A major obstacle for xenotransplantation in humans. Immunol Today 14:480–482,1993.
9. Sherman, LA, and Chattopadhyay, C. The molecular basis of allorecognition. Ann Rev Immunol 11:385–402, 1993.
10. Steinman, RM, Gutchinov, B, et al: Dendritic cells are the principal stimulators of the primary mixed leukocyte reaction in mice. J Exp Med 157:613–627, 1983.
11. Bociek, AG, Stewart, DA, et al: Bone marrow transplantation—current concepts. J Invest Med 43:127–135, 1995.

12. Paul, WE: Fundamental Immunology, ed. 4. Lippincott-Raven, Philadelphia, 1999, pp 1175–1235.

13. Ferrara, JLM: Pathogenesis of acute graft-versus-host disease: Cytokines and cellular effectors. J Hematother Stem Cell Res 9:299–306, 2000.

14. Bryson, JS, and Flanagan, DL: Role of natural killer cells in the development of graft-versus-host disease. J Hematother Stem Cell Res 9:307–316, 2000.

15. Kamada, N: Transplantation Biology: Cellular and Molecular Aspects. Lippincott-Raven, Philadelphia, 1996, pp 531–539.

16. Williams, K, et al: Factors predictive of corneal graft survival: Report from the Australian Corneal Graft Registry. Ophthalmology 99:403–414, 1992.

17. Ayliffe, W: Changing assumptions about the mechanism of corneal transplant rejection. Eye 14:121–122, 2000.

18. Hubscher, SG: Histological finding in liver allograft rejection—new insights into the pathogenesis of hepatocellular damage in liver allografts. Histopathology 18:377–383, 1991.

19. Dawson, S, Imagawa, DK, et al: UCLA Liver Transplantation: Analysis of the first 1,000 patients. Clinical Transplants 1994. UCLA Tissue Typing Laboratory, Los Angeles, 1994, pp 189–195.

20. Harihan, S, Johnson, CP, et al: Improved graft survival after renal transplantation in the United States, 1988 to 1996. New Engl J Med 342:605–612, 2000.

21. Ojo, AO, Meier-Kriesche, HU, Hansen, JA, et al: MMF reduces late renal allograft loss independent of acute rejection. Transplantation 69:2405–2409, 2000.

22. Opelz, G, Wujciak, T, et al: HLA compatibility and organ transplant survival. Rev Immunogenet 1:334–342, 1999.

23. Stevenson, S, and Arnoczky, SP: Transplantation of musculoskeletal tissues: Biology and biomechanics of the musculoskeletal system. In Buckwalter, JA, Einhorn, TA, and Simon, SR (eds): Orthopaedic Basic Science, ed. 2. Am Acad Orthopaedic Surgeons, Rosemont, Ill., 2000, pp 568–579.

24. Sykes, M, Sachs, DH, and Strober, S: Mechanisms of tolerance. In Forman, SJ, Blume, KG, and Thomas, ED (eds): Bone Marrow Transplantation. Blackwell Scientific, Boston, 1994, pp 204–219.

25. Petersdorf, EW, Longton, GM, et al: Definition of HLA-DQ as a transplantation antigen. Proc Nat Acad Sc 93:15358–15363, 1996.

26. Armitage, J: Bone marrow transplantation. N Engl J Med 330:827, 1994.

27. Brown, C, and Navarrete, C: Screening for HLA-specific antibodies. In Bidwell, JL, and Navarrete, C (eds): Histocompatibility Testing. Imperial College Press, London, 2000, 65–98.

28. Terasaki, P, and McClelland, JD: Microdroplet assay of human serum cytotoxins. Nature 204:998–1000, 1964.

29. Rock, CS, Coyle, SM, et al: Influence of hypercortisolemia on the acute-phase protein response to endotoxin in humans. Surgery 112:467–474, 1992.

30. Liu, J, Farmer, JDJ, et al: Calcineurin is a common target of cyclophilin-cyclosporin A and FKBP-FK506 complexes. Cell 66:807–815, 1991.

31. Allison, AC, and Eugi, EM: Purine metabolism and immunosuppressive effects of mycophenolate mofetil (MMF). Clin Transplantation 10:74–84, 1996.

32. Vincenti, F, Kirkman, R, et al: Interleukin-2-receptor blockade with daclizumab to prevent acute rejection in renal transplantation. N Engl J Med 338:161–165, 1998.

Tumor Immunology

Kate Rittenhouse-Olson, PhD, SI(ASCP)

Learning Objectives

After completing this chapter, the reader will be able to:
1. Compare and contrast the normal cell and the tumor cell.
2. Discuss evidence to support and to refute the theory of immunosurveillance.
3. Define tumor-associated antigen (TAA) and give examples.
4. Describe the following tumor markers used in immunologic screening: Bence Jones protein, monoclonal immunoglobulins, alpha-fetoprotein (AFP), human chorionic gonadotropin (hCG), calcitonin, and prostate specific antigen (PSA).
5. Discuss use of the following tumor markers in monitoring disease: AFP, calcitonin, carcinoembryonic antigen (CEA), CA-125, PSA, CA-19.9, CA-15.3, and interleukin-1 (IL-2) receptor.
6. List the necessary criteria for a tumor marker to be used for screening.
7. Explain how tumor markers are used for monitoring the course of disease.
8. Describe how tumor markers are used in pathologic diagnosis.
9. Cite examples of how tumor markers are used in immunolocalization and immunotherapy.
10. Compare and contrast passive versus active immunotherapy.

Key Terms

Ab-toxin
Alpha-fetoprotein
Bence Jones protein
CA-125
Calcitonin
Human choronic
  gonadotropin (hCG)

Immunosurveillance
Metastatic growth
Monoclonal immunoglobulin
Neoplastic cells
Oncofetal antigen
Prostate specific antigen
  (PSA)

Tumor-associated antigen
Tumor infiltrating
  lymphocyte (TIL)

Tumor immunology is the study of the antigens associated with tumors, the immune response to tumors, the effect of the tumor on the host's immune status, and the use of the immune system to help eradicate the tumor.[1]

To treat bacterial, viral, and parasitic infections or the uncontrolled growth of a tumor, we must first look for the differences between the organism causing the disease and the normal tissue of the host. This knowledge is critical for any therapeutic effort. For bacterial infections, scientists have targeted the differences between the bacterial cell wall, the bacterial cell membrane and the bacterial ribosomes from related human structures and this has led to successful antibiotics. Similarly, antigenic differences between bacteria and host tissues have led to the development of a myriad of successful vaccines. Correlates of this exist for viruses, parasites, and tumors. Therefore, to under-

stand clinical efforts in tumor immunology, we must begin with a background concerning the differences between tumor cells and normal cells.

Cancer begins with changes in one normal cell. These changes permit the cell to grow and proliferate without regard to normal growth signals or controls. These changes are called malignant transformation, and the resulting cells are called tumor cells or **neoplastic cells.** The tumor cell and its progeny have gained the ability to grow beyond normal tissue boundaries. This is called invasive growth, and the tumor cells often are capable of growing in distant organs after dissociating from the primary site. They are further able to travel through the bloodstream or the lymphatics to accomplish **metastatic growth.** The progeny of the cell that undergoes transformation are monoclonal in origin, meaning they are initially identical phenotypically and genotypically. As rapid uncontrolled proliferation continues, mistakes occur in deoxyribonucleic acid (DNA) replication causing cellular phenotypic and genotypic heterogeneity to develop.[1,2]

Malignant cells are different in appearance from normal cells from the same organ. Cancer is the replacement of normal tissue by the uncontrolled growth of these transformed cells of one lineage. The loss of normal cell and organ function through the growth of cancer cells leads to many of the symptoms of cancer. The malignant cells also differ on a molecular level from normal cells of the same organ. Malignant cells show an increased metabolic rate that causes a need for more oxygen and also can cause increased production of lactic acid. Cancer cells have a higher than normal average DNA content because of their uncontrolled proliferation with a high percentage of cells undergoing mitosis. Cancer cells also may show differences in surface antigens.[3]

Immunosurveillance

Paul Ehrlich formulated a theory stating that the immune system functions as a surveillance mechanism in the prevention of the successful growth and spread of neoplastic cells. Ehrlich postulated that because enormous numbers of cell divisions are required in a normal life, then the potential for development of neoplastic cells is very high. He surmised that malignant transformation is accompanied by a change in cell surface antigens causing them to appear foreign, thereby causing recognition and destruction of the neoplastic cell by cells of the host immune system. Thomas and Burnet modified Ehrlich's theory by stating that the primary reason for development of T cell–mediated immunity was for defense against neoplastic cells. Burnet coined the term **immunosurveillance.** Cell-mediated immunity also has a primary role in antiviral activity, but there is much evidence that the immune system is involved in an antineoplastic response as well.[1,2]

Support for the theory of immunosurveillance has been gathered from observing trends in human cancer incidence and through use of animal experimentation. Observations in humans that lend credence to the theory of immunosurveillance include the fact that there is increased incidence of tumors in the elderly and that these individuals have a less efficient immune system. However, this observation doesn't provide conclusive evidence because the elderly also have a greater cumulative effect of lifelong exposure to carcinogens that may lead to a higher incidence of tumors. Observation of an increased incidence (several thousandfold) of tumors in individuals whose cell-mediated immunity is suppressed also supports the theory of immunosurveillance. However, because the increased tumor incidence in these individuals is of lymphoreticular origin, this may reflect a defect in the lymphoreticular system rather than a defect in immunosurveillance. Patients with acquired immunodeficiency disease (AIDS) also have an increased incidence of tumors, but these are of viral etiology. Patients that are immunosuppressed because of drug treatment for allografts or autoimmune diseases have an increased incidence of tumors of viral or ultraviolet light etiology, so the theory of immunosurveillance is supported for at least these types of tumors.[1,2,4,5]

Observations of occasional spontaneous regression of tumors in choriocarcinomas, lymphomas, and malignant melanomas also lend support to the theory of immunosurveillance by suggesting the possibility that these regressions are caused by a successful immune response against the tumor. Additional support for the immune system battle against malignancy is the regression of metastasis after removal of tumor from the primary site. These occurrences suggest that although the immune system is unable to control a large number of tumor cells, it may be able to respond successfully when that number is reduced.

Support for the theory of immunosurveillance also comes from histologic analysis of tumor tissue. Infiltration of immune cells can be seen within the tumor mass. These cells are lymphocytes called **tumor infiltrating lymphocytes (TIL).** This population of lymphocytes consists of T cells able to react with the antigens on the tumor, indicating the presence of a cellular immune response to the tumor *in situ.* The usefulness of human monoclonal antibodies developed to tumor antigens using B cells from the draining (sentinel) lymph nodes indicates a possible role for a humoral response to tumor antigens as well. Other proof in humans include the fact that delayed type skin tests to some tumor antigens are positive in some cancer patients and that immune complexes containing cancer antigens and antibody are found circulating in some cancer patients.[4,5]

There are some facts that refute the theory of immunosurveillance. Patients have decreased T cell responses in certain diseases such as leprosy and sarcoidosis, but these diseases are not associated with increased tumor incidence. Additionally, immunologically privileged sites such as the brain and the lens of the eye do not have an increased incidence of tumors. However, the consensus is that the immune system does play a role in the prevention of metastasis. Antibody, T cells, natural killer cells, lymphokine-activated killer (LAK) cells, and macrophages all have been found to kill tumor cells. The patient's T cell response to tumor is thought to be the most important of these, although it is believed that this cell does not act alone.[4,5] It is generally accepted that the immune system prevents the occurrence of an even greater number of cancers.

If immunosurveillance is indeed occurring, the question to consider is the reason why tumors are able to form at all. There are tumor-related reasons and patient-related reasons. The tumors may not be targeted through surveillance because the immune stimulus is too weak or because a strong antigenic epitope is absent. The tumor cell may lack class I or II molecule expression, making antigen presentation to T cells impossible. The tumor antigens might not be on all of the tumor cells. The tumor may be resistant to the immune response, and the growth rate of the tumor may exceed the ability of the immune response to destroy it. Soluble antigen released by the tumor may also prevent cellular interaction by binding to the T cell receptor and thereby preventing interaction with the tumor cell. In addition, some tumors secrete factors that are immunosuppressive, including prostaglandins and tumor growth factor–β, and these may facilitate their escape from immunosurveillance. The patient may be tolerant to the tumor antigen, recognizing it as a self-antigen and thus being incapable of generating an effective immune response. Finally, the patient may be immunosuppressed as a result of a carcinogen, tumor burden, infection, or age and incapable of mounting an immune response to the tumor.[1,2,4,5]

Tumor-Associated Antigens

Tumor-associated antigens are antigens present in the tumor tissue in higher amounts than in normal tissue.[1] These are not tumor-specific antigens because they also have been found on some normal human tissue. It is the hope of many scientists to find the perfect tumor-associated antigen that is unique to a particular tumor and will aid in the screening diagnosis, histopathologic evaluation, staging, monitoring, localization, and immunotherapy of various malignancies.

There are thousands of references to antigens associated with neoplasms in the literature. Why are more of these antigens not clinically useful? Why are the approximately 50 antigens currently used clinically better than the others? This chapter attempts to answer these questions and to provide information concerning the currently used markers and the protocols used to find them. The worldwide market for cancer markers is projected to be over 500 million dollars, and the clinical use of these markers is increasing.[6]

Screening and Diagnosis

The criteria for use of a screening test for diagnosis of cancer are quite stringent. The following five criteria must be met for a test to have clinical use:

- The tumor must be an important health problem for the population.
- There must be a recognizable early symptom or marker that can be used for screening.
- It must be a tumor for which treatment at an early stage is more successful than at a later stage.
- The screening test must be acceptable to the population.
- The costs and benefits of the screening test must be acceptable to the population.

The benefits include improved survival time, less radical treatment needed for tumors detected earlier, and reassurance for those with negative results. The costs include longer morbidity in cases whose prognosis is not changed, overtreatment of questionable diagnoses, misleading reassurance for those with false-negative results, anxiety and possible morbidity from more invasive testing for those with false-positive results, the actual physical hazards of the screening tests, and the actual dollar costs of the screening test.[7] To improve the cost-to-benefit ratio, selected subgroups should be screened when possible instead of the entire population.

People are screened for the presence of malignancies by a variety of different methods. Commonly used methods include stool occult blood for colorectal carcinoma, Papanicolaou smear for cervical cancer, self exams for breast and testicular cancer, x-ray mammography for breast cancer, and digital rectal exam for prostate cancer. The two types of laboratory screening methods for malignancies include immunologic screening and genetic screening. Genetic screening usually is performed to find conditions indicating increased risk for cancer. The genetic screening test having received the most use is analysis for the BRCA-1 and BRCA-2 mutations, two susceptibility genes for breast cancer also associated with increased risk of ovarian cancers. Further discussion of genetic screening is outside the scope of this chapter; hence the focus will be on immunologic screening for tumors.

Immunologic Screening

Immunologic screening is used to detect the presence of antigens associated with a particular tumor. An antigen must meet very stringent requirements to be useful for screening the general population:

- It must be produced by the tumor and secreted into some biologic fluid that can be analyzed easily for antigen levels.
- Its circulating half-life must be long enough to permit its concentration to increase with increasing tumor load.
- It must increase to clinically significant levels (above background control levels) while the disease is still treatable.
- The antigen must be absent from or at background levels in all individuals without the malignant disease in question to minimize false-positive test results.
- It must not yield too many false-negative results.[8]

If a particular cancer develops in 1 out of every 10,000 individuals, then a 3-percent false-positive rate will yield 300 false-positive results for every one true cancer detected (Fig. 18–1). Conversely, a false-negative rate of 3 percent will miss 3 out of every 100 true cancers. This underscores the importance of select-

ing highly sensitive and specific tests for screening. Antigens meeting these criteria include Bence Jones protein for multiple myeloma, monoclonal immunoglobulin for multiple myeloma and macroglobulinemia, Alpha-fetoprotein (AFP) and human chorionic gonadotropin (hCG) for nonseminomatous testicular cancer and primary hepatoma, calcitonin for familial medullary thyroid carcinoma and multiple endocrine neoplasia type 2A, and prostate specific antigen (PSA) for prostate cancer.[9,10]

Bence Jones protein consists of immunoglobulin light chains found in urine that are a diagnostic criterion for multiple myeloma. First described in 1846, Bence Jones protein was one of the first tumor-associated antigens described. Bence Jones protein is elevated in 50 to 75 percent of multiple myeloma cases. This is because immunoglobulin chain production can be unbalanced in this disease with production of more light chains than heavy chains. The excess light chains are released into the circulation, and because they are

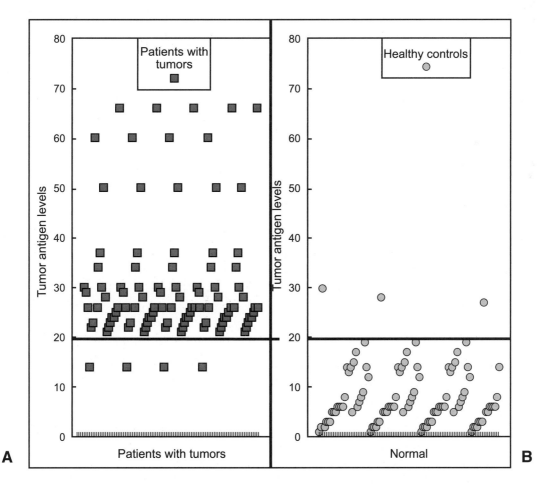

FIG. 18–1. Measurement of a tumor-associated antigen in patients with tumors *(A)* and in a normal population *(B)*. Note that in B, there is a 3-percent false-positive rate using this antigen as an indicator of a tumor.

small molecules, they pass through the glomeruli and are excreted into the urine. They can be detected using immunoelectrophoresis with anti-κ or anti-λ light chain antibody.[10]

Monoclonal immunoglobulin in the serum of patients with multiple myeloma, macroglobulinemia, and heavy chain disease is a diagnostic aid for patients presenting with symptoms of these diseases. These tumor types result from overproduction of B cells or plasma cells and originate from one aberrant cell. Because the progeny of these cells are clones, the products are the result of a monoclonal production of antibody. Both monoclonal immunoglobulins and Bence Jones protein are discussed further in the chapter on immunoproliferative diseases.

Alpha-fetoprotein (AFP) is a glycoprotein structurally related to albumin that is present in extremely low amounts in normal adult human sera. It is in the group of tumor-associated antigens called **oncofetal antigens,** indicating its presence in both tumor tissue and in tissues of fetal origin. Serum levels of AFP aid in the diagnosis of nonseminomatous testicular cancer and primary hepatoma. This marker should be used in conjunction with hCG for testicular tumors to decrease the number of false-negative results. AFP and hCG are never elevated in patients whose scrotal masses are benign. AFP also is elevated in most cases of hepatocellular carcinoma, hereditary tyrosinemia, and ataxia telangiectasia, and in 20 percent or less of patients with pancreatic adenocarcinoma, gastric carcinoma, and colonic carcinoma. Serum AFP is measured using capture or sandwich enzyme immunoassay.[10,11]

Human chorionic gonadotropin (hCG), which is used in conjunction with AFP for testicular tumors, is a heterodimeric glycoprotein hormone with a degree of homology to luteinizing hormone (LH). It also is elevated in gestational tumors including hydatiform mole and choriocarcinoma. Antisera used for the detection of this hormone must react with the C terminus of the β peptide of hCG to prevent cross-reactivity with human LH. A sandwich enzyme immunoassay method is generally used in the clinical laboratory. hCG has long been recognized as a marker present in normal pregnancy. hCG enzyme immunoassays for pregnancy testing are available for both clinical laboratory and home use.[10,11]

Calcitonin is used as a diagnostic marker for evaluation of patients with familial medullary thyroid carcinoma and multiple endocrine neoplasia type 2A. Multiple endocrine neoplasia type 2A is a syndrome that includes the occurrence of medullary thyroid carcinoma, pheochromocytoma, and hyperparathyroidism. Calcitonin is a small polypeptide hormone produced by C cells in the thyroid gland. It is involved in calcium metabolism, and it is secreted in response to elevated calcium levels to prevent bone resorption. Calcitonin levels provide a valuable screening test for family members of medullary thyroid carcinoma patients because 10 to 20 percent of these patients carry a genetically dominant trait related to tumor occurrence. The assay for this marker involves provocation of its release by intravenous administration of calcium and pentagastrin after which levels are measured by direct radioimmunoassay using the sandwich or capture antibody technique with the second antibody labeled with ^{125}I.[13] Detection of the gene involved is also a screening method for family members of patients diagnosed with this type of cancer.[13]

Prostate specific antigen (PSA) serum levels are used to confirm a diagnosis of prostate cancer. Prostate cancer is the most common cause of cancer mortality in men. It occurs mainly in men over 60, with a median age for occurrence of 75 and a median age for death of 79. PSA is a prostate tissue–specific antigen found in epithelial cells lining the prostate gland and ducts in normal, benign hypertrophic and in malignant prostatic tissues. It is not found in any other human tissues. PSA is secreted by the prostate, and it acts as a protease to dissolve the seminal gel formed after ejaculation. It is not present in the serum of females and is present only in very low amounts in the sera of normal male subjects. Serum levels are elevated in most patients with prostatic tumors, although levels are also mildly elevated in patients with benign prostatic hypertrophy. The American Cancer Society suggests that annual PSA screening begin at age 50 for normal white males and at age 45 for black males and for individuals with first-degree relatives with prostate cancer.

PSA is present in the serum either complexed to a protease inhibitor or as free PSA (minor amount). PSA levels are measured by a sandwich radioimmunoassay (RIA) or enzyme immunoassay (EIA) method. The fact that PSA is organ-specific but not disease-specific renders the test somewhat problematic because of false-positive results with benign prostatic hypertrophy. However, measures can be taken to decrease the number of false-positive results. Because PSA levels increase with age, baseline levels can be age-adjusted to decrease false-positive diagnoses. Additionally, the PSA velocity, defined as the annual increase of PSA, can be determined. A rise in the PSA value greater than 0.7 ng/mL per year or 20 percent per year is suggestive of cancer. The free-to-total ratio is an expression of the percent of PSA that is free in the serum compared to the percent that is bound to protease inhibitors. The lower this percent, the more a tumor is indicated. Controversy has surrounded the use of PSA as a screening molecule because many men have slow growing prostatic adenocarcinoma that might not cause any clinical morbidity or mortality if left undetected. There is some concern such individuals would be more harmed if the tumor were detected by PSA determinations because of the potential for unnecessary surgery or radiation therapy. However, PSA is a widely used marker that leads to earlier diagnosis in many patients.[14]

CA-125 is an additional antigen that is sometimes screened for as a marker in ovarian cancer. It is an ovarian carcinoma cell surface glycoprotein that was discovered by Bast. Ovarian cancer is the fifth most common cancer in women, and it has a poor prognosis. There are no early symptoms for this disease, so 65 to 75 percent of patients present with advanced disease. The 5-year survival rate for early stage disease is greater than 90 percent, while late stage disease has a 5-year survival rate of about 10 percent. This suggests that detection of an early marker would improve prognosis. Attempts to use CA-125 as a screening marker have been attempted, but elevations of CA-125 levels in benign conditions (e.g., endometriosis, pelvic inflammatory disease, uterine fibroids, and pregnancy) created many false-positive results. A false positive would result in surgery, and 50 false-positive results were obtained for each one cancer found in screening postmenopausal women alone. CA-125 is used but is not approved by the U.S. Food and Drug Administration (FDA) as a screening marker. CA-125 is measured using a capture EIA with a single bead as the solid support for capture antibody.[6,10,11]

Pathologic Diagnosis

The pathologist may use tumor-associated antigens from tumor tissue for differential diagnosis of tumor type. The technique involves incubation of tumor tissue with antibody to the tumor-associated antigen, then with a secondary antibody enzyme conjugate, and finally with substrate. Color development indicates presence of the tumor-associated antigen. The requirements for clinical use of an antigen to facilitate differential diagnosis by the pathologist are less stringent than the requirements for an antigen to be used for widespread screening. To be useful in pathologic diagnosis, the marker must be differentially expressed in the tumor of origin and other tumors, which may have a similar appearance histologically. It is important to note that the use of these markers must be combined with other clinical results because the differentiation that

occurs with transformation sometimes can result in loss of the marker. This false-negative situation is relatively common. In addition, the DNA changes that occur with malignant transformation sometimes can cause expression of a marker that is not normally associated with the tumor type in question, although this occurrence is relatively uncommon.

Monitoring the Course of Disease

Cancer management with tumor-associated antigens involves performing serial determinations of the antigen in previously diagnosed patients to establish prognosis, detect recurrence, and monitor the results of therapy. This is an area in which many tumor-associated antigens are used clinically. The information provided by these data helps the clinician make important decisions concerning the therapeutic regimen for each patient. The requirements for an antigen to be clinically useful in this way are: (1) The antigen must be released from the tumor into a fluid where it can be measured, (2) the half-life of the antigen must be long enough for concentrations to become measurable, and (3) the half-life must be short enough to correlate decrease in tumor burden with timely decrease in antigen levels. See Figure 18–2 for an idealized curve for a hypothetical tumor marker.

Some of the hallmarks of an ideal antigen for clinical monitoring are shown in the Figure 18–1. At diagnosis, the marker is elevated significantly above normal levels. After surgical removal of the tumor, serum levels of antigen quickly return to normal levels, and this drop correlates with the clinical picture of no evidence of disease. The speed at which levels of the marker drop is equal to the biologic half-life of the marker if there is no residual tumor. The slope of the decrease can be used to indicate whether or not tumor is still present. If marker concentration decreases at a slower rate than its biologic half-life, then a portion of the serum concentration of this marker must be caused by residual tumor. With time, the serum levels of antigen begin increasing in this patient, and this foretells the appearance of clinically evident disease. As the first chemotherapeutic regimen is begun, there is no drop in antigen level. As time goes on and no drop in antigen levels is seen, there is also no clinical improvement. A second chemotherapeutic regimen is tried, and this time antigen levels slowly drop to normal levels. Normal levels of antigen occur when there is no clinical evidence of disease. Certainly, this is an idealized model, but it is representative of a typical situation.

Markers currently being used for this clinical

TABLE 18–1. Summary of Tumor-Associated Antigens and Their Areas of Clinical Use and the Associated Tumors

Antigen	Uses*	Associated Tumor(s)
Bence Jones protein	1	Multiple myeloma
AFP	1, 2, 3	Nonseminomatous testicular cancer, primary hepatoma
hCG	1, 2, 3, 4	Nonseminomatous testicular cancer, choriocarcinoma
Calcitonin	1, 2, 3	Familial medullary thyroid carcinoma
PSA	1–4	Prostate cancer
CA-125	1–4	Ovarian adenocarcinoma, 1 not approved
Cytokeratins	2	Sarcomata, hematopoietic origin
HMB-45	2	Malignant melanoma
Neuron-specific enolase	2	Small cell cancers of the lung, endocrine tumors
S-100	2	Neuroendocrine tumors, melanoma
Beta 2 microglobulin	3	Lymphoma
Lactate dehydrogenase	3	Lymphoma
CEA	2, 3, 4, 5	Tumors of gastrointestinal tract, breast
Estrogen receptor	3	Breast adenocarcinoma
CD45*	2	Hematopoietic malignances
IL-2 receptor (CD25)	4	T cell leukemia
Monoclonal immunoglobulin	1, 2, 3, 4	Clonality indicates B cell malignancy
CA-19.9	4	Colonic AND pancreatic adenocarcinoma
CA-15.3	4	Breast adenocarcinoma
Prostate specific membrane antigen	5	Prostatic adenocarcinoma, Prostascint
NRLU-10 (Ab name)	5	Small cell lung cancer, Verluma
B-1	5	Lymphoma
CD20	6	Lymphoma
MAGE	6	Melanoma

*See discussion for descriptions and limitations.
1 = Screening
2 = Pathologic diagnosis
3 = Staging
4 = Monitoring
5 = Localization of metastasis
6 = Therapy
AFP = Alpha-fetoprotein; hCG = human chorionic gonadotropin; PSA = prostate specific antigen; CEA = carcinoembryonic antigen.

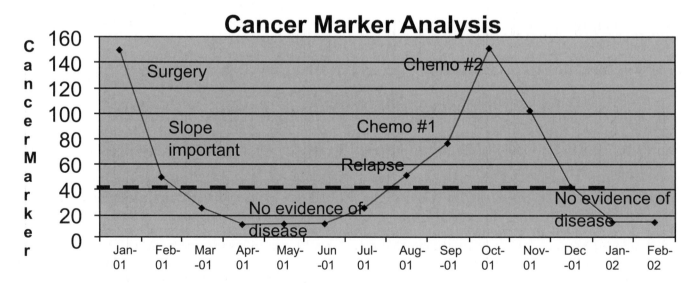

FIG. 18–2. Cancer marker analysis. A curve showing the results of monitoring the cancer patient for tumor recurrence and for therapy efficacy using levels of a tumor-associated antigen.

purpose are AFP, hCG, calcitonin, carcinoembryonic antigen (CEA), CA-125, PSA, CA-19.9, CA-15.3, and interleukin (IL)-2 receptor. Serial AFP levels are used clinically after surgical resection of hepatomas.[10] AFP can be used along with hCG for serial monitoring of nonseminomatous testicular tumors.[11] Calcitonin levels are used to monitor medullary thyroid carcinoma.[13] CEA is predictive of the success or failure of treatment in colon and breast cancer.[15] This marker also has been used for monitoring pancreatic adenocarcinoma, and neuroblastoma.[15] Prostatic acid phosphatase (PAP) was the first serum marker for prostate cancer, but assays for this marker are less than ideal as a result of problems with false negatives and false positives. PAP has been largely replaced by PSA analysis. PSA is so specific to the prostate that any antigen circulating after prostatectomy is indicative of residual disease. The success of antiandrogen therapy for prostate cancer is remarkable, but resistant tumor usually does develop eventually. These facts compel the clinician to postpone hormonal therapy until a certain clinical picture is apparent, and PSA levels can help determine this time.[14]

CA-125 levels are measured serially in the therapy of ovarian adenocarcinoma. CA-125 was found when monoclonal antibodies were produced to a serous cystadenocarcinoma cell line. It is not a tissue-specific antigen, nor a tumor-specific antigen because it is present on a number of normal tissues. However, it is still valuable for detection of residual tumor prior to second-look surgery because serum levels of this marker increase as the tumor grows. Monitoring with this antigen, or any other, is only attempted when the primary tumor is known to produce it. There is an 85-percent sensitivity for detection of the recurrence of ovarian cancer with cutoff levels over 35u/mL.[10]

CA-19.9 is an antigen discovered through immunization of mice with a human colorectal cancer cell line. CA-19.9 is used conditionally in monitoring of colon carcinoma and pancreatic adenocarcinoma.[12] Another marker, CA-15.3, is used conditionally in monitoring breast adenocarcinoma. Most patients with progressive disease show increasing CA-15.3 levels, but it usually is not elevated in early stage disease.[10,12] A change in antigen level by more than 25 percent correlates with disease progression or regression. When one or two measurements show an increase, with subsequent measurements showing a decrease, this may be the result of antigen release caused by tumor cell death.

The IL-2 receptor (CD25) is a protein that is unregulated on T cells when they are exposed to antigen or mitogens. Serum levels of shed CD25 are elevated in patients with adult T cell leukemia and some other tumors. Measurement of CD25 levels can aid in monitoring therapy. This test is approved in the United States for monitoring the response to therapy in patients with hairy cell leukemia.[16]

Immunotherapy

Immunotherapy is the final use of tumor-associated antigens to be discussed. The possibility of stimulating the patient's own immune system to respond to tumor-associated antigens has intrigued scientists for over a century. All the different protocols cannot be discussed here; however, increasing knowledge concerning tumors and the immune system have led to new protocols and recent optimism in this area. The methods used can be separated into two different types of therapy: passive immunotherapy or active immunotherapy. Passive immunotherapy involves transfer of antibody or cells to patients who are not expected to make immune responses of their own. With active immunotherapy, patients are immunized in a manner that stimulates them to mount immune responses to their own tumors.

Passive Immunotherapy

The first use of passive administration of antiserum developed via tumor inoculations to treat cancer patients was by Hericourt and Richet in 1895.[17] More recent attempts at passive transfer of antibody involve treatment with monoclonal antibody. This work has had sporadic success and has led to subsequent research using antibody to tumor-associated antigens covalently linked to a toxic moiety **(Ab-toxins)**. The clinical requirements for an antigen to be used in Ab-toxin conjugate therapy are the following:

- It must be a cell surface antigen with high antigenic density.
- It must be present on the primary tumor and on all metastatic foci.
- Normal tissues must be free from the antigen or not susceptible to the toxin.

The toxins generally chosen are plant and fungal toxins that block ribosomal protein synthesis. Such toxins are abrin, ricin, and saporin. The part of the toxin molecule that normally binds to cells must be removed before attaching it to the antibody (Ab). Drugs used in cancer chemotherapy and radionuclides have also been linked to antibody molecules for this type of immunotherapy. Because the major obstacle in cancer chemotherapy is the toxicity of the drugs to normal host tissue, targeting the chemotherapeutic agent to the tumor cells can avoid this complication.

Antigens for which Ab-toxin conjugate administration has been attempted are CEA and anti-idiotypic antibodies to leukemias. The obstacles involved in Ab-toxin conjugates are:

1. Tumor heterogeneity with regard to antigenic expression
2. Antigenic modulation or the loss of antigen from the tumor cells
3. Failure of conjugate to penetrate tumor tissue
4. Failure to internalize into the cell after binding
5. Toxic effects on other tissues, particularly the hematopoietic organs
6. The limited amount of toxin that can be linked to the antibody without destruction of binding activity
7. Host antibody response to the injected antibody
8. Circulating antigen forming immune complexes with the Ab-toxin conjugate, removing them from circulation
9. Failure to release intact toxin

Success has been achieved with a few antibody conjugates. Anti-p185$^{Her2/neu}$ has received FDA approval for use in patients with metastatic breast cancer. It is used in conjunction with cisplatin. The Her2/neu gene is found to be amplified in about 25 percent of breast tumors. The gene codes for a transmembrane protein, and the anti-p185$^{Her2/neu}$ monoclonal antibody is made against this protein. This gene also is expressed in certain patients with ovarian, gastric, endometrial, and salivary gland tumors. It is associated with poor prognosis in breast cancer and also is associated with familial disease linkage. There is a definite synergistic effect when the antibody is used along with cisplatin because the response to both used together is much greater than the sum of the responses to these treatments used independently.[18]

The recent approval by the FDA of rituximab (Rituxan), an unconjugated chimeric antibody against the CD20 antigen for the treatment of relapsed low-grade or follicular B cell non-Hodgkin's lymphoma (NHL), marked a milestone in the development of these antibody-based treatments.[19] Rituximab (Rituxan; IDEC Pharmaceuticals, San Diego, CA) is a genetically engineered chimeric (murine-human) monoclonal antibody (mAb) directed against the CD20 antigen found on the surface of normal and malignant B cells. Multicenter studies have demonstrated its efficacy against relapsed low-grade and follicular NHL. Because of its human component, rituximab has low immunogenicity and should not significantly hinder future retreatment. Future studies will evaluate the anti-

tumor activity of rituximab combined with various chemotherapeutic or biologic agents in the treatment of B cell lymphoma and other CD20-positive lymphoid neoplasms. Other new drug therapies using both unconjugated and radiolabeled monoclonal antibodies are pending FDA approval. It is anticipated that further new treatment options based on mAb technology will be available soon for the treatment of patients with NHL.

Active Immunotherapy

The goal of active immunotherapy is to develop an immune response by the patient that will help eliminate the tumor. Intralesional injections of Bacillus Calmette Guerin (BCG) or other bacterial components,[8,20] have been attempted to enhance patient immune response to tumor antigens. Superficial bladder cancer is still treated with BCG. BCG is instilled in the bladder and causes an inflammatory response by recruiting lymphocytes, macrophages, and neutrophils to the area. This represents a local nonspecific stimulation of the immune response, which reduces the risk of recurrence in patients after surgery for bladder cancer.[21]

Other attempts at stimulating host immune systems with their own tumor antigens have involved transfection of isolated tumor cells with genes for cytokine production and reinjection of the irradiated modified tumor cells. This has been done with many cytokines, especially IL-2 and granulocyte monocyte-colony stimulating factor (GM-CSF). This procedure is an attempt to cause modified tumor cells to act as antigen presenting cells for the tumor antigens.[22]

Active immunotherapy with anti-idiotypic antibodies (Ab$_2$) has been attempted on colon cancer patients with an Ab$_2$ bearing the internal image of a colon carcinoma-associated antigen.[23] These studies resulted in the production of antibodies to the tumor-associated antigen and some clinical response. The lymphokine-mediated expansion of TILs is a relatively new avenue that is being explored to obtain clinically relevant immune activity directed at tumor-associated antigens. TILs have been reported to be 50 to 100 times more potent than LAK cells.[24]

Irradiated or chemically mutated tumor cells from a patient may stimulate T cell activity against a tumor. Studies conducted by Boone found that the mutation caused the expression of antigens able to stimulate T cell activity on both altered cells and original tumor cells. He was able to clone the genes for these antigens using molecular biology techniques and found several antigens, which he named MAGE 1, MAGE 2, MAGE 3, BAGE and GAGE. These were all melanoma-associated antigens. Importantly, he has since discovered that MAGE 1 can only be presented by human leukocyte antigen (HLA) type A1, an HLA type present on 26 percent of Caucasians. MAGE 1 is on 30 percent of melanoma patients cells; therefore, about 8 percent of these patients can be helped by immunization with MAGE-1. MAGE 3 appears on 70 percent of the tumors and can be presented by both HLA A1 and HLA A2.[25,26] Through new understanding about limitations in antigen presentation of tumor-associated antigens, it now can be predetermined who will benefit from these vaccinations. This is an exciting new area of research that has expanded to other tumor types.

Vaccine trials are currently underway to promote an immune response to tumor antigens. Tumor antigens have been inserted into viral expression vectors such as adenovirus and vaccinia virus, and these have been administered with or without IL-2. Tumor peptides are used as immunogens with incomplete Freund's adjuvant and IL-2.[27] Tumor antigens have been mixed with purified preparations of the patient's dendritic cells to have very effective antigen presentation.[28] It remains to be seen which, if any, of these immunization protocols will work, but after many discouraging years the excitement created by real potential has returned to this field.

SUMMARY

Tumor immunology is the study of the antigens associated with tumors, the immune response to tumors, the effect of the tumor on the host's immune status, and the use of the immune system to help eradicate the tumor. Cancer begins with changes in one normal cell, and these changes allow the cell to grow and proliferate without regard to normal growth signals or controls. As these abnormal cells grow, they may show differences in surface antigens. Such antigens are called tumor-associated antigens.

It is hypothesized that a mechanism called immunosurveillance exists, which protects us against growth of tumors. This involves the ability of the immune system to recognize the tumor cells as foreign and to promptly destroy them. T cells play a major role in this process. Only when the immune system is suppressed or overwhelmed do tumors presumably have the ability to grow. The clinical laboratory's role in detection and monitoring of cancer is based on the presence of specific tumor-associated antigens.

The identification and use of tumor-associated antigens has had an effect in the areas of screening, diagnosis, histopathologic evaluation, staging, monitoring the course of the disease, localization of metastasis, and immunotherapy.

Detection and measurement of these antigens have led to earlier diagnosis, easier monitoring, increased specificity in pathology determinations, successes in determining location of metastatic sites, and some clinical successes in eliminating the tumor with immunotherapeutic protocols. Examples of some of these antigens include Bence Jones protein associated with multiple myeloma, AFP and hCG in testicular cancer and primary hepatoma, calcitonin in familial thyroid carcinoma, and PSA for prostate cancer. Many problems have been encountered in attempts to develop clinical uses for tumor-associated antigens, but each year we see new and productive efforts in surmounting these problems, and new markers are constantly added to our list of clinically relevant ones.

Case Studies

1. A 45-year-old woman came to her physician's office after noticing a lump during her breast self-exam. She had a strong family history of breast cancer. The lump was detected on mammography and found to be a 0.5-cm mass that was adherent to her skin. Analysis found her CA-15.3 levels to be 60 IU/mL, which is significantly above background, with the normal upper range being 30 IU/mL. After surgery the levels of CA-15.3 dropped but at a rate that was slower than the biologic half life, and they remained above 30 IU/mL.

Questions

   a. What should be done? Do you think that there is residual tumor?
   b. During chemotherapy for this tumor the CA-15.3 levels continued to rise. What should be done? Is there any immunotherapy that can be added?

2. A 25-year-old man was admitted to the hospital with fatigue, weakness, weight loss, shortness of breath, and chest and back pain. His previous medical history was unremarkable except for an undescended testis, which wasn't corrected until he was 9 years old. An abnormal chest x-ray showed a large (9- X 3-cm) mass on the chest wall and multiple abnormal areas on his right lung. The surgeon's diagnosis was that the patient had a nonoperable sarcoma and palliative treatment only was suggested. However, the following laboratory values were obtained in clinical chemistry and clinical immunology.

	Patient Results	Reference Range
AFP	150 ng/mL (133 IU)	0–8.5 ng/mL (0–7.55 IU)
hCG	63 mIU/mL	<2mIU/mL

Questions

   a. What are possible tumor types?
   b. What can be done to determine if the tumor in the chest wall had its origin in the testis?

c. For what else will these markers be used in the treatment course of this young man?

3. A 56-year-old black male was seen by a urologist, complaining of frequent urination and with only small volumes of urine creating great urgency. During the digital rectal exam, the urologist felt a hard prostatic nodule approximately 0.5 cm in diameter rather than a normal smooth uniform surface of the prostate. The patient's blood was drawn, and his serum level of PSA was determined and compared to the level from the previous year. The patient's physician also asked that the bound-to-total PSA ratio be determined.

The test results are shown below.

Laboratory Results

Test	Patient's Results	Reference Range
PSA October 1999	6.5 ng/mL	0–3.5 ng/mL
PSA October 1998	3.5 ng/mL	0–3.5 ng/mL
Bound/free PSA	15%	≥23.4%

Questions

a. What do these results indicate?
b. What is the PSA velocity?
c. What will we look for after surgery?

Exercise: Semi-Quantitative PSA Membrane Test for the Detection of Serum Levels of PSA

PRINCIPLE★

This is a solid phase one step capture membrane enzyme immunoassay for the measurement of PSA in patient serum. Elevated PSA is found in men with prostate cancer and in men with benign prostatic hypertrophy. An age-adjusted cut-off should generally be used. This assay uses two controls: 4 ng/mL and 10 ng/mL. Patients without tumors rarely have levels above 10 ng/mL, but many patients with tumors will be in the 4- to 10-ng/mL range. Patients with benign prostatic hypertrophy may be in this range also. A positive above 4 will warrant further investigation with a quantitative test and a digital rectal examination. The membrane is cellulose-based and contains antihuman PSA as the immobilized antibody, and antihuman PSA monoclonal conjugate with red-colored gold as the labeled antibody. Serum is applied, the device is incubated at room temperature for 10 minutes, and a visual interpretation is performed.

This rapid test for PSA performs according to the following principle: The membrane of the test cassette is impregnated with antihuman PSA as the immobilized antibody in the test region and with different antimouse immunoglobulin in the control regions. During the test, the PSA in the patient's serum reacts with the red-colored monoclonal mouse anti-PSA IgG's, in which the pad on the bottom of the cassette is immersed. Through the capillary effect in the membrane of the test cassette, the reaction mixture is carried to each of the impregnated areas. The color-marked mouse mAb regions are bound in the control regions by the mouse antiglobulin, independent of the existence of PSA. Upon positive findings, the colored PSA antibody complex is maintained in the test region: A third red band is created. R2 is an internal standard that will yield a color equivalent to 10-ng/mL PSA; line 2 or T is the test result. R1 is the internal standard that will yield a color equivalent to 4-ng/mL PSA. No line or a line lighter in color than the 4-ng/mL line is a negative result, and a line darker than the 4-ng/mL standard is a positive result.

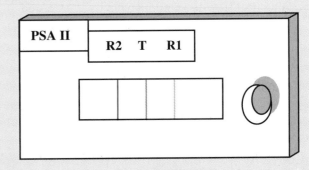

FIG. 18–3. A schematic showing the Seratec rapid PSA test cassette. In this example the patient line T has more PSA than R1 the 4-ng/mL control and less than R2 the 10-ng/mL control.

★ This test is available from Seratec (Telephone: +49 551 50480-0, Fax: +49 551 50480-80, e-mail: seratec@t-online.de).

1. How do tumors differ from normal cells?
   a. Polyclonal in origin
   b. Dependent on normal growth signals and restraints
   c. Lower in DNA content than normal tissue
   d. Produce increased amounts of lactic acid

2. Each of the following supports the theory of immunosurveillance *except:*
   a. There is an increased number of tumors in elderly persons.
   b. There is an increased number of tumors in individuals who are immunosuppressed.
   c. Immunologically privileged sites such as the brain and the lens of the eye do not have increased cancer incidences.
   d. There is evidence of *in situ* tumors in many individuals upon autopsy after death by other causes.

3. Which of the following patients have increased tumor rates?
   a. Transplant patients on cyclosporine
   b. AIDS patients
   c. Thymic aplasia patients
   d. All of the above

4. If a disease is present in one in every 10,000 individuals, and a marker can detect this disease with 100-percent sensitivity and 95-percent specificity, what would be the number of false positives for each cancer found?
   a. 5000
   b. 5
   c. 50
   d. 500

5. Which best describes Bence Jones protein?
   a. Monoclonal intact immunoglobulin molecules
   b. Light chains from the immunoglobulin molecule
   c. Structurally related to albumin
   d. Used to detect spina bifida

6. AFP can be used for the diagnosis of:
   a. Pregnancy
   b. Nonseminomatous germ cell tumors
   c. Myelomas
   d. Thyroid carcinoma

7. HCG is used for cancer screening in conjunction with which molecule?
   a. Calcitonin
   b. CEA
   c. Immunoglobulin
   d. AFP

8. Which best characterizes measurement of calcitonin?
   a. Screened in the general population
   b. Performed by a serum assay after stimulus
   c. Performed by a urine assay after a provoking stimulus
   d. Tested in conjunction with Bence Jones protein

9. Which is true of PSA?
   a. Useful for screening the under 50 population
   b. A tissue specific antigen
   c. Used for screening black males over 60
   d. Suggested for use for black males over 40 and white males over 50

10. A tumor found in the prostate does not stain with antibody to PSA. Is this proof that the tumor came from a different organ?
    a. Yes
    b. No

11. In monitoring the course of the disease, which of the following is true?
    a. The antigen must be released from the tumor into the serum.
    b. The half life of the protein must be long enough so that concentrations become measurable.
    c. The half life of the protein must be short enough that along with a decrease in tumor burden there is a timely decrease in antigen levels.
    d. All of the above.
    e. None of the above.

12. All of the following are markers used for monitoring disease *except:*
    a. Calcitonin
    b. Carcinoembryonic antigen
    c. CA-125
    d. Cytokeratin
    e. PSA

13. IL-2 is used in monitoring which of the following?
    a. Pancreatic adenocarcinoma
    b. Colonic adenocarcinoma
    c. Breast adenocarcinoma
    d. Hairy cell leukemia

14. CA-15.3 is used conditionally in the monitoring of:
    a. Pancreatic adenocarcinoma
    b. Colonic adenocarcinoma
    c. Breast adenocarcinoma
    d. Hairy cell leukemia

15. CA-19.9 is used conditionally in the monitoring of:
   a. Pancreatic adenocarcinoma
   b. Colonic adenocarcinoma
   c. Breast adenocarcinoma
   d. Hairy cell leukemia

References

1. Greenberg, PD: Mechanisms of tumor immunology. In Stites, DP, Terr, AI, and Parslow, TG (eds): Medical Immunology, ed. 9. Appleton & Lange, Stamford, Conn.,1997.
2. Goldsby, RA, Kindt, TJ, and Osborne, BA: Kuby Immunology, ed. 4. WH Freeman, New York, 2000.
3. Robbins, SL, and Cotran, RS: Pathologic Basis of Disease, ed. 1. WB Saunders, Philadelphia, 1979.
4. Abbas, AK, Lichtman, AH, and Pober, JS: Cellular and Molecular Immunology, ed. 4. WB Saunders, Philadelphia, 2000.
5. Screiber, H: Tumor immunology. In Paul, WE (ed): Fundamental Immunology, ed. 4. Lippincott Williams & Wilkins, Philadelphia, 1999.
6. Owen, NC: New cancer products. Predicting market outcome. In Sell, S (ed): Serological Cancer Markers (Contemporary Biomedicine). Humana Press, Totowa, NJ, 1992.
7. Austoker, J: Screening for ovarian, prostatic, and testicular cancers. BMJ 309:315–20. 1994.
8. Diakun, KR: Tumor-associated antigens. In Van Oss, CJ, and Van Regenmortel, MHV (eds): Immunochemistry. Marcel Dekker, New York, 1994.
9. Tumor immunology. Beers, MH, Berkow, R, and Burs, M (eds): Merck Manual Diagnosis & Therapy, ed. 17. Merck & Co, Whitehouse Station, NJ, 1999.
10. Pandha, HS, and Waxman, J: Tumour markers. QJM 88:233, 1995.
11. Horwich, A, Huddart, R, and Dearnaley, D: Markers and management of germ-cell tumours of the testes. Lancet 352:1535, 1998.
12. Ahern, H: Tumor marker measurement aids in cancer diagnosis, therapy. Advance for Medical Laboratory Professionals, 1995.
13. Lips, CJ, Landsvater, RM, and Hoppener, JW, et al: Clinical screening as compared with DNA analysis in families with multiple endocrine neoplasia type 2A. N Engl J Med 331:828, 1994.
14. Plaut, D: Testing for prostate cancer—A numbers game and then some. Advance for Medical Laboratory Professionals 10:9, 1998.
15. Gold, P, and Goldenberg, NA: The carcinoembryonic antigen (CEA): Past, present and future. MJM 3:46, 1997.
16. Arun, B, Curti, BD, and Longo, DL, et al: Elevations in serum soluble interleukin-2 receptor levels predict relapse in patients with hairy cell leukemia. Cancer J Sci Am 6:21, 2000.
17. Hericourt, J, and Richet: Traaitment dd'un cas de sarcome par iaa, Serotheraapie, Compt. Rendd. Acad. D. sc. 948–950. 1895.
18. Dillman, RO: Perceptions of Herceptin: A monoclonal antibody for the treatment of breast cancer. Cancer Biother Radiopharm 14:5, 1999.
19. Press, OW: Radiolabeled antibody therapy of B-cell lymphomas. Semin Oncol 26(5 Suppl 14):58, 1999.
20. Eilber, FR, Morton, DL, and Holmes EC, et al: Adjuvant immunotherapy with BCG in treatment of regional-lymph node metastases from malignant melanoma. N Engl J Med 294:237, 1976.
21. Melekos, MD, and Moutzouris, GD: Intravesical therapy of superficial bladder cancer. Curr Pharm Des 6:345, 2000.
22. Nawrocki, S, and Mackiewicz, A: Genetically modified tumour vaccines—where we are today. Cancer Treat Rev 25:29, 1999.
23. Basak, S, Eck, S, and Gutzmer, R, et al: Colorectal cancer vaccines: Antiidiotypic antibody, recombinant protein, and viral vector. Ann NY Acad of Sci 910:237, 2000.
24. Wang, RF, and Rosenberg, SA: Human tumor antigens for cancer vaccine development. Immunol Rev 170:85, 1999.
25. Van den Eynde, BJ, and Boon, T: Tumor antigens recognized by T lymphocytes. Int J Clin Lab Res 27:81, 1997.
26. Visseren, MJ, van der Burg, SH, and van der Voort, EI, et al: Identification of HLA-A*0201-restricted CTL epitopes encoded by the tumor-specific MAGE-2 gene product. Int J Cancer 73:125, 1997.
27. Hadzantonis, M, and O'Neill, H: Review: Dendritic cell immunotherapy for melanoma. Cancer Biother Radiopharm 14:11, 1999.
28. Fox, C: Andy's last shot. Life May:82–94, 1998.

Part IV

Serologic Diagnosis of Infectious Diseases

chapter 19

Spirochete Diseases

Learning Objectives

After finishing this chapter, the reader will be able to:

1. Describe identifying characteristics of *Treponema pallidum* and *Borrelia burgdorferi*.
2. Explain how syphilis and Lyme disease are transmitted.
3. Discuss the different stages of syphilis.
4. Discuss the advantages of direct fluorescent staining for *T. pallidum* over darkfield examination without staining.
5. Define reagin.
6. Distinguish treponemal from nontreponemal tests for syphilis.
7. Describe the principle of the following tests for syphilis: Venereal Disease Research Laboratory (VDRL), rapid plasma reagin (RPR), fluorescent treponemal antibody absorption (FTA-ABS), and agglutination assays.
8. Give reasons for false-positive reagin test results.
9. Compare and contrast sensitivity and specificity of treponemal and nontreponemal testing for the various stages of syphilis.
10. Discuss the advantages and disadvantages of polymerase chain reaction (PCR) and enzyme immunoassay (EIA) testing.
11. Discuss limitations of cerebrospinal fluid (CSF) testing and testing for congenital syphilis.
12. Describe early and late manifestations of Lyme disease.
13. Relate various aspects of the immune response to Lyme disease to disease stages.
14. Compare immunofluorescence assay (IFA), EIA, and immunoblot testing for Lyme disease as to sensitivity and ease of performance.
15. Discuss causes of false positives and false negatives in serologic testing for Lyme disease.

Key Terms

Borrelia burgdorferi	FTA-ABS test	RPR test
Chancre	Immunoblotting	Tabes dorsalis
Congenital syphilis	Polymerase chain reaction (PCR)	Tertiary syphilis
Erythema chronicum migrans		*Treponema pallidum*
Flocculation	Reagin	VDRL test

Spirochetes are long, slender, helically coiled bacteria containing *axial filaments,* or periplasmic flagella, that wind around the bacterial cell wall and are enclosed by an outer sheath.[1] These gram-negative, microaerophilic bacteria exhibit a characteristic corkscrew flexion or motility. Diseases caused by these organisms have many similarities, including a localized skin infection that becomes disseminated to numerous organs as the disease progresses, a latent stage, and cardiac and neurologic involvement if the disease remains untreated. This chapter discusses disease manifestations and testing for the two major spirochete diseases, syphilis and Lyme disease. Serologic testing plays a key role in diagnosis of these diseases because isolation of the organism itself is difficult to accomplish in the laboratory, and clinical symptoms are not always apparent.

Syphilis

Syphilis remains the most commonly acquired spirochete disease in the United States today.[2] It is typically spread through sexual transmission. Although the incidence of cases in the United States is at a low of 2.2 cases per 100,000 individuals,[3] it is most often seen in localized outbreaks among certain high-risk populations. Homosexual transmission between men is responsible for a number of these outbreaks.[4,5] In countries such as the United Kingdom in Western Europe, the incidence appears to be on the rise again.[6,7,8] Thus, despite the current emphasis on safe sexual practices, syphilis remains a major health problem in many areas of the world. Early detection of the disease is of major importance. Characteristics of the organism and the disease are presented, as well as a discussion of the most frequently used serologic methods of identification.

Characteristics of the Organism

The causative agent of syphilis is *Treponema pallidum,* subspecies *pallidum,* a member of the family Spirochaetaceae. Organisms in this family have no natural reservoir in the environment and must multiply within a living host. Three other pathogens in this group have been found to be so morphologically and antigenically similar to *T. pallidum* that all but one are now classified as subspecies.[9] These other organisms are *T. pallidum* subspecies *pertenue,* the agent of yaws; *T. pallidum* subspecies *endemicum,* the cause of nonvenereal endemic syphilis; and *T. carateum,* the agent of pinta. Yaws is found in the tropics, pinta is found in Central and South America, and endemic syphilis is found in desert regions.

T. pallidum (which will hereafter be used to refer to subspecies pallidum) varies in length from 6 to 20 μm and in width from 0.1 to 0.2 μm, with 6 to 14 coils (Fig. 19–1).[1,10] The outer membrane of *T. pallidum* is a phospholipid bilayer with very few exposed proteins. Several newly identified membrane proteins, called treponemal rare outer membrane proteins (TROMPs) have been characterized.[11] It appears that the scarcity of such proteins delays the host immune response.

Mode of Transmission

Pathogenic treponemes are rapidly destroyed by heat, cold, and drying out, so they are almost always spread by direct contact. Sexual transmission is the primary mode of dissemination, and this occurs through abraded skin or mucous membranes coming in contact with an open lesion. Approximately one-third to 50 percent of the individuals who are exposed to a sexual partner with active lesions will acquire the disease.[10] Congenital infections can also occur during pregnancy. Transmission to the fetus is possible in mothers with clinically latent disease.

Other potential means of transmission include parenteral exposure through contaminated needles or blood, but this is extremely rare. The lack of transfusion-transmitted syphilis in the United States for the past 30 years has actually called into question the

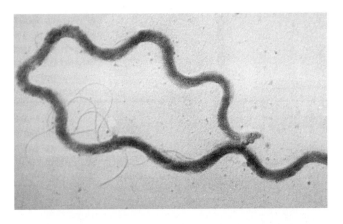

FIG. 19–1. *Treponema pallidum.* Electron micrograph showing the colis and periplasmic flagella. (Courtesy of CDC Archives, Atlanta, GA.)

necessity of testing potential donors for presence of the disease.[12] Because syphilis can only be transmitted by means of fresh blood products, the use of stored blood components has virtually eliminated the possibility of transfusion-associated syphilis.[10]

Stages of the Disease

Once contact has been made with a susceptible skin site, endothelial cell thickening occurs with aggregation of lymphocytes, plasma cells, and macrophages.[13] The initial lesion, called a **chancre,** develops between 10 and 90 days after infection, with about 21 days being the average.[6] A chancre is a painless, solitary lesion characterized by raised and well-defined borders (Fig. 19–2). These usually occur on the external genitalia such as the penis in males, but in women they may appear in the vagina or cervix, and thus may go undetected. This primary stage lasts from 1 to 6 weeks, during which time the lesion heals spontaneously.

If the initial chancre is untreated, about 25 percent of such cases progress to the *secondary stage,* in which systemic dissemination of the organism occurs. This stage is usually observed about 1 to 2 months after the primary chancre disappears, but in up to 15 percent of reported cases, the primary lesion may still be present.[14] Symptoms of the secondary stage include generalized lymphadenopathy, or enlargement of the lymph nodes, malaise, fever, pharyngitis, and a rash on the skin and mucous membranes.[7,10,14] The rash may appear on the palms of the hands and the soles of the feet.[10] Involvement of the central nervous system may occur earlier than previously suspected because viable organisms have been found in the cerebrospinal fluid (CSF) of a number of patients with primary or secondary syphilis.[9] Approximately 40 percent of patients with

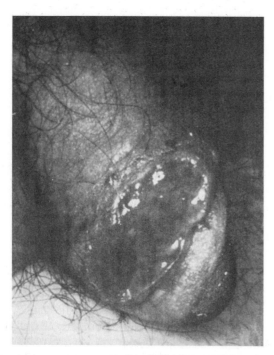

FIG. 19–2. Primary chancre in the early stage of syphilis. (From Bryant, NJ: Laboratory Immunology and Serology. WB Saunders, Philadelphia, 1992, p 115, with permission.)

secondary syphilis may exhibit neurologic signs such as visual disturbances, hearing loss, tinnitus, and facial weakness.[6] Lesions persist from a few days up to 8 weeks. After this time, spontaneous healing occurs, as in the primary stage. The latent stage follows the disappearance of secondary syphilis.

The *latent stage* is characterized by a lack of clinical symptoms. It is arbitrarily divided into early latent, less than 1 year's duration, and late latent, in which the primary infection has occurred more than 1 year previously. Patients are noninfectious at this time, with the exception of pregnant women, who can pass the disease on to the fetus even if they exhibit no symptoms.

About one-third of the individuals who remain untreated develop **tertiary syphilis.**[6,10] This stage appears anywhere from months to years after secondary infection. Typically, this occurs most often between 10 and 30 years following the secondary stage.[6,10] Tertiary syphilis has three major manifestations: gummatous syphilis, cardiovascular disease, and neurosyphilis.

Gummas are localized areas of granulomatous inflammation that are most often found on bones, skin, or subcutaneous tissue. Such lesions can reach up to several centimeters in diameter, and they contain lymphocytes, epithelioid cells, and fibroblastic cells.[14] They may heal spontaneously with scarring, or they may remain destructive areas of chronic inflammation. It is likely that they represent the host response to infection.

Cardiovascular complications usually involve the ascending aorta, and symptoms are due to destruction of elastic tissue, especially in the ascending and transverse segments of the aortic arch.[14] This may result in aortic aneurysm, thickening of the valve leaflets causing aortic regurgitation, or narrowing of the ostia, producing angina pectoris.[10]

Neurosyphilis is the complication most often associated with the tertiary stage, but as previously discussed, it actually can occur anytime after the primary stage and can span all stages of the disease. During the first 2 years following infection, however, central nervous system involvement often takes the form of acute meningitis.

Late manifestations of neurosyphilis include **tabes dorsalis,** a degeneration of the lower spinal cord, and general paresis, or chronic progressive dementia. It usually takes more than 10 years for these to occur, but both are the result of structural central nervous system damage and cannot be reversed. Fortunately, these symptoms are now very rare because of early detection and treatment with penicillin.[6,10]

Congenital Syphilis

Congenital syphilis occurs when a woman who has early syphilis or early latent syphilis transmits treponemes to the fetus. Due in large measure to a national plan launched by the Centers for Disease Control and Prevention, the occurrence of congenital syphilis dropped to an all time low of 529 cases in the year 2000.[15] Although the disease can be transmitted at any stage of pregnancy, typically the fetus is most affected during the second or third trimester of pregnancy, and fetal or perinatal death occurs in approximately 10 percent of the cases.[14]

Infants who are liveborn often have no clinical signs of disease during the first few weeks of life. Some may remain asymptomatic, but between 60 and 90 percent of such infants develop later symptoms if not treated at birth.[16] Inflammation of the umbilical cord, called necrotizing funisitis, may be the first indication of the disease.[10,17] The infant may exhibit clear or hemorrhagic rhinitis, or runny nose. Skin eruptions, in the form of a macropapular rash that is especially prominent around the mouth, the palms of the hands, and soles of the feet, are also common.[9] Other telltale symptoms include generalized lymphadenopathy, hepatosplenomegaly, jaundice, anemia, painful limbs, and bone abnormalities such as saddle nose or saber shins.[9,10,15] Neurosyphilis may occur in up to 60 percent of infants with congenital disease.[18]

Nature of the Immune Response

The primary body defenses against treponemal invasion are intact skin and mucous membranes. Once skin is penetrated, T cells and macrophages play a key role in the immune response. Primary lesions show the presence of both CD4+ and CD8+ T cells. Cytokines produced activate macrophages, and it is ultimately phagocytosis by macrophages that causes healing of the primary chancre.[14] The protective role of antibody is uncertain, however, as coating of treponemes with antibody does not necessarily bring about their destruction.[11] In fact, circulating immune complexes may actually prevent the host from synthesizing further specific treponemal antibody.[19] *T. pallidum* is also capable of coating itself with host proteins, which delays the recognition of the pathogen by the immune system.[10] Newly discovered proteins, the TROMPS, appear to be important in bringing about complement activation that ultimately kills the organism.[11] However, the chronic nature of the disease is an indicator that the organisms are able to evade the immune response. Treponemes may persist in the host for years if antibiotic therapy is not obtained.

Laboratory Diagnosis

Laboratory diagnosis of syphilis can be divided into three sections: direct detection of spirochetes, nontreponemal serologic tests, and treponemal serologic tests.

These vary in sensitivity and ease of performance. Principles and procedures of each type of testing are discussed and are compared and summarized in Table 19–1.

Direct Detection of Spirochetes

Dark-Field Microscopy. Primary and secondary syphilis can be diagnosed by demonstrating the presence of *T. pallidum* in exudates from skin lesions.[2,9] In *dark-field microscopy*, a dark-field condenser is used to keep all incident light out of the field except for that captured by the organisms themselves. It is essential to have a good specimen in the form of serous fluid from a lesion. This is usually obtained by cleaning the lesion with sterile saline and rubbing with clean gauze. Pathogenic treponemes are identified on the basis of characteristic corkscrew morphology and flexing motility.[10]

Because observation of motility is the key to identification, specimens need to be examined as quickly as possible, before they become dried out. False results are possible because of delay in evaluation of the slides, obtaining an insufficient specimen, or pretreatment with antibiotics.[10] Thus, a negative test does not exclude a diagnosis of syphilis. In addition, an experienced microscopist is needed to perform testing. If a specimen is obtained from the mouth or the rectal area where morphologically identical nonpathogens can be found, these must be differentiated from the true pathogens.

TABLE 19–1. Comparison of Tests Used for the Diagnosis of Syphilis

Test	Antigen	Antibody	Comments
Direct Microscopic			
Darkfield	*T. pallidum* from patient	None	Must have good specimen, experienced technologist; inexpensive
Fluorescent antibody	*T. pallidum* from patient	Antitreponemal antibody with fluorescent tag	More specific than darkfield; specimen does not have to be live
Nontreponemal			
VDRL RPR TRUST	Cardiolipin	Reagin	Flocculation; good for screening tests, treatment monitoring; false positives
Treponemal			
FTA-ABS	Nichols strain of *T. pallidum*	Antitreponemal	Confirmatory; specific, sensitive; may be negative in primary stage
EIA	Treponemal or recombinant	Antitreponemal	Simple to perform; can be automated; not as sensitive as FTA-ABS
	Enzyme-labeled treponemal antigen	Anti-IgG or anti-IgM, antitreponemal antibody from patient	Simple to perform; sensitive in primary syphilis, but sensitivity decreases in later stages
DNA probe	Patient DNA matched to treponemal DNA	None	Technically demanding; very specific; lacks sensitivity

VDRL = Venereal disease research laboratory; RPR = rapid plasma reagin; TRUST = toluidine red unheated serum test; FTA-ABS = fluorescent treponemal antibody absorption; EIA = enzyme immunoassay; DNA = deoxyribonucleic acid.

Fluorescent Antibody Testing of a Specimen. The use of a fluorescent-labeled antibody is a sensitive and highly specific alternative to dark-field microscopy. This can be performed by either a direct method, which uses a fluorescent-labeled antibody conjugate to *T. pallidum*, or an indirect method using antibody specific for *T. pallidum* and a second labeled anti-immunoglobulin antibody.[9] An advantage of this method is the fact that live specimens are not required. A specimen can be brought to the laboratory in a capillary tube, or fixed slides can be prepared for later viewing. Slides are fixed by air drying, followed by either heat fixing, placing in acetone for 10 minutes, or by dipping in 10-percent methanol for 20 minutes. Even after fixing, treponemes can be washed off the slide, so each slide must be handled individually, and rinsing must be carefully done.[9] Development of monoclonal antibodies has made this method very sensitive and specific.[9] However, monoclonal antibodies do react with other subspecies of *T. pallidum*, and this must be taken into account when making a diagnosis.

Nontreponemal Serologic Tests

If a patient does not have active lesions, as may be the case in secondary or tertiary syphilis, then serologic testing is the key to diagnosis. Serologic tests can be classified as nontreponemal or treponemal, depending on the type of antibody that is detected. Nontreponemal tests determine the presence of **reagin,** an antibody that is formed against lipid material from damaged cells. This is found in the sera of patients with syphilis as well as in several other disease states. An antigen that is a combination of cholesterol, lecithin, and cardiolipin is used in the reaction. The term *reagin* should not be confused with the same word that was originally used to describe IgE. They are not related at all because reaginic antibodies are either IgG or IgM.

All of the nontreponemal tests are based on flocculation reactions in which patient antibody complexes with the cardiolipin antigen. **Flocculation** is a specific type of precipitation that occurs over a narrow range of antigen concentration. The antigen consists of very fine particles.

In general, nontreponemal tests are positive within 1 to 4 weeks after the appearance of the primary chancre.[2,9] Titers usually peak during the secondary or early latent stages. In primary disease, between 13 and 41 percent of individuals appear nonreactive, but by the secondary stage, almost all patients have reactive test results.[2,9] Testing of sera from patients in the secondary stage, however, is subject to false negatives because of

the prozone phenomenon. Typically this creates a nonreactive pattern that is granular or rough in appearance.[9] If a prozone is suspected, serial twofold dilutions should be made to obtain a titer.

Reagin titers tend to decline in later stages of the disease, even if the patient remains untreated. After a number of years, about 25 percent of untreated syphilis cases were shown to become nonreactive for reagin.[10] This decline occurs more rapidly in individuals who have received treatment. A first-time infection, if in the primary or secondary stage, should show a fourfold decrease in titer by the third month following treatment, and an eightfold decrease by 6 to 8 months.[14] Following successful treatment, tests typically become completely nonreactive within 1 to 2 years.

Examples of nontreponemal tests include Venereal Disease Research Laboratory (VDRL), rapid plasma reagin (RPR), toluidine red unheated serum test (TRUST), unheated serum reagin (USR), and reagin screen test (RST). RPR and the VDRL are the most widely used of these tests.

Venereal Disease Research Laboratories Test. The **VDRL test,** which was designed by the Venereal Disease Research Laboratories, is both a qualitative and quantitative slide flocculation test for serum, and there is a modification for use on spinal fluid.[20] Antigen for all tests must be prepared fresh daily. It consists of an alcoholic solution of 0.03 percent cardiolipin, 0.9 percent cholesterol, and 0.21 percent lecithin. A 1-percent buffered saline solution with a pH of 6.0 is used to mix with the antigen. The antigen suspension is prepared by pipetting 0.4 mL of the buffered saline solution onto the bottom of a 30-mL bottle. The VDRL antigen (0.5 mL) is added directly to the saline solution, using the lower half of a 1.0-mL pipette graduated to the tip. The antigen is added drop by drop while the bottle is continuously rotated on a flat surface. The pipette tip should remain in the upper third of the bottle, and rotation should not be vigorous enough to splash saline onto the pipette. The last drop of antigen should be expelled out of the pipette without touching the saline solution. Rotation of the bottle should continue for another 10 seconds. Lastly, 4.1 mL of the buffered saline solution is added, using a 5-mL pipette, and the bottle is shaken about 30 times in 10 seconds.

A Hamilton syringe is used to deliver one drop of antigen for the slide test. This must be calibrated before use by filling the syringe with the antigen mix. The syringe is fitted with an 18-gauge needle without bevel that will deliver 60 drops (± 2 drops) of antigen suspension per mL when the syringe and needle are held vertically. If the delivery is off by more than 2 drops, the system must be cleaned with alcohol and recalibrated.

Serum is heated at 56°C for 30 minutes to inactivate complement, and 0.05 mL is pipetted into a ceramic ring of a glass slide. Three control sera—nonreactive, minimally reactive, and reactive—are pipetted into rings on the glass slide in the same manner. Sera and patient samples are spread out to fill the entire ring. One drop (1/60 mL) of the VDRL antigen is then added to each ring. The slide is rotated for 4 minutes on a rotator at 180 rpm. It is read microscopically to determine the presence of flocculation, or small clumps. The results are recorded as reactive, moderately reactive, weakly reactive, or nonreactive.[20] Tests must be performed at room temperature within the range of 23°C to 29°C (73°F to 85°F) because results may be affected by temperature changes. All sera with reactive or weakly reactive results must be tested using the quantitative slide test, in which dilutions of serum up to 1:32 are used.

The VDRL test is the only one routinely used for the testing of spinal fluid.[9,10] For spinal fluid testing, the antigen is prepared by diluting the VDRL serum slide test antigen on a 1:1 basis with a 10-percent saline solution. This is mixed by inversion and allowed to stand for at least 5 minutes but not more than 2 hours before use. A Boerner agglutination slide, which has concave wells 16 mm in diameter and 1.75 mm deep, is used for this test. For each spinal fluid sample, 0.05 mL is pipetted into a well, and the sample is spread to fill the entire surface. One drop of antigen is added to each well, using a 1/100 mL syringe that has been calibrated to deliver 100 drops/mL with a 21- or 22-gauge needle. The slide is rotated on a mechanical rotator for 8 minutes at 180 rpm. The test is read microscopically, as in the VDRL serum test. If a test is reactive, twofold dilutions are made and retested following the same protocol. A positive VDRL test on spinal fluid is diagnostic of neurosyphilis because false positives are extremely rare.[10]

Rapid plasma reagin (RPR) test is a modified VDRL test. The antigen suspension contains charcoal particles, which make the test easier to read. The suspension is contained in small glass vials, which are stable for up to 3 months after opening. The antigen is similar to the VDRL antigen with the addition of ethylenediaminetetra-acetic acid (EDTA), thimerosal, and choline chloride, which stabilize the antigen and inactivate complement so that serum does not have to be heat inactivated before use. Patient serum (approximately 0.05 mL) is placed in an 18-mm circle on a plastic-coated disposable card using a capillary tube or

Dispenstir device. Antigen is dispensed from a small plastic dispensing bottle with a 20-gauge needle, according to test kit instructions. The needle is calibrated to deliver 60 drops/mL. One free-falling drop is placed onto each test area, and the card is mechanically rotated under humid conditions at 100 rpm for 8 minutes.[2] Cards are read under a high-intensity light source, and if flocculation is evident, the test is positive. All reactive tests should be confirmed by retesting using doubling dilutions in a quantitative procedure. The RPR test appears to be more sensitive than the VDRL in primary syphilis.[10]

Standard Treponemal Serologic Tests

Treponemal tests use specific treponemal antigens and detect antibody directed against the organism itself. The two main types include the fluorescent treponemal antibody absorbed (FTA-ABS) test and agglutination tests. Typically, these tests are more difficult to perform and more time consuming, so they are used for confirmation rather than screening.

Fluorescent Treponemal Antibody Absorption Test. One of the most used confirmatory tests is the **FTA-ABS,** an indirect fluorescent antibody test. A 1:5 dilution of heat-inactivated patient serum is made with a sorbent consisting of an extract of nonpathogenic treponemes (Reiter Strain). This removes cross-reactivity with treponemes other than *T. pallidum*. Slides used for this test have the Nichols strain of *T. pallidum* fixed to them. They are kept frozen until use and then are equilibrated at room temperature for 30 minutes.

Diluted patient samples and controls are measured (0.01 mL) and applied to individual wells on the test slide. Slides are then incubated in a covered moist chamber at 37°C for 30 minutes. They are rinsed with deionized water and placed in a Coplin jar with phosphate-buffered saline for 5 minutes. After a second rinsing, the slides are air dried, and 0.01 mL of antibody conjugate that has been appropriately standardized is added to each well. Slides are reincubated as before for 30 minutes, and a similar washing procedure is followed. Mounting medium is applied, and coverslips are placed on the slides. They are examined under a fluorescence microscope as soon as possible.

If specific patient antibody is present, it will bind to the *T. pallidum* antigens. The antibody conjugate, consisting of anti-immunoglobulin with a fluorescein isothiocyanate label, will only bind where immunoglobulin is present and bound. When slides are read under a fluorescence microscope, the intensity of the green color is reported on a scale of 0 to 4+. No fluorescence indicates a negative test, and a 2+ or above is considered reactive.[9] A result of 1+ means that the specimen was minimally reactive, and the test must be repeated with a second specimen drawn in 1 to 2 weeks.[9] Experienced personnel are required to read and interpret fluorescent test results.

The FTA-ABS is highly sensitive and specific, but it is time consuming to perform. This test is usually positive before reagin tests, although 20 percent of primary syphilis cases are nonreactive.[19] In secondary and latent syphilis, tests are usually 100 percent reactive. Once a patient is reactive, that individual remains so for life. Although there are fewer false positives compared to reagin tests, reactivity is seen with other treponemal diseases, notably yaws and pinta.[10]

Agglutination Tests. Several varieties of passive hemagglutination tests have been used to detect specific treponemal antibody. These are no longer available in the United States, and microhemagglutination tests have largely been replaced by particle agglutination tests such as the Serodia TP-PA test.[21] Particle agglutination tests use gel particles coated with treponemal antigens and are more sensitive in detecting primary syphilis.[14]

Comparison of Nontreponemal and Treponemal Serologic Tests

Nontreponemal tests are inexpensive, simple to perform, and can yield quantitative results. Thus, they are extremely useful as a screening tool, in monitoring the progress of the disease, and in determining the outcome of treatment. The main disadvantage is that they are subject to false positives. Transient false positives occur in diseases such as hepatitis, infectious mononucleosis, varicella, herpes, measles, malaria, and tuberculosis, and during pregnancy.[9] Chronic conditions causing sustained false-positive results include systemic lupus erythematosus, leprosy, intravenous drug use, autoimmune arthritis, advanced age, and advanced malignancy.[2,14]

A reactive nontreponemal test should be confirmed by a more specific treponemal test. In pregnancy, this is especially important because nontreponemal titers from a previous syphilis infection may increase nonspecifically.[2,14] Under the following conditions, titers can be considered to be a nonspecific increase: lesions are absent, the increase in titer is less than fourfold, and documentation of previous treatment is available.[2]

Although treponemal tests are usually reactive before reagin tests in primary syphilis, they suffer from a lack of sensitivity in congenital syphilis and neurosyphilis. Nontreponemal tests should be used for these purposes.[2,10] Treponemal tests, however, are not subject to as many false positives as the nontreponemal tests, but because they are more difficult to perform, they are best used as confirmatory tests to distinguish false-positive from true-positive reagin results. They also help establish a diagnosis in late latent syphilis or late syphilis because they are more sensitive than nontreponemal tests in these stages.[2] See Table 19–2 for a comparison of sensitivities of some of the most widely used serologic tests.

Newer Technologies in Syphilis Testing

Enzyme Immunoassay. Several enzyme immunoassay (EIA) tests have been developed for serodiagnosis of syphilis. One of these, Reagin II, uses a cardiolipin antigen similar to that used in the VDRL test. Screening of a large number of samples can be easily accomplished by this method, and it is reported to have a sensitivity of 93 percent in primary syphilis.[21] However, it also has a slightly higher rate of false positives than RPR tests.

Other EIA tests have been developed to capture a specific class of antibody, either IgM or IgG. Microtiter wells are coated with antibody to IgM or IgG and reacted with patient serum. Then treponemal antigens that are labeled with an enzyme are added (Fig. 19–3). These have a fairly high sensitivity in primary syphilis, but the sensitivity decreases as the disease progresses.[22] Specificity is similar to other treponemal tests. EIA tests are especially useful in diagnosis of congenital syphilis in infants to look for presence of IgM, which cannot cross the placenta.

TABLE 19–2. Sensitivity of Commonly Used Serologic Tests for Syphilis				
Stage Test	**Primary (%)**	**Secondary (%)**	**Latent (%)**	**Late (%)**
Nontreponemal (Reagin) Tests				
Venereal Disease Research Laboratory Test (VDRL)	78	100	95	71(37–94)
Rapid plasma reagin card test (RPR)	86	100	98	73
Specific Treponemal Tests				
Fluorescent treponemal antibody absorption (FTA-ABS) test	84	100	100	96
T. pallidum microhemagglutination assay (MHA-TP)	76	100	97	94

Adapted from Smith, MB et al: Spirochete Infections. In Henry, JB (ed): Clinical Diagnosis and Management by Laboratory Methods, ed. 20, Philadelphia, WB Saunders, 2001, p 1134.

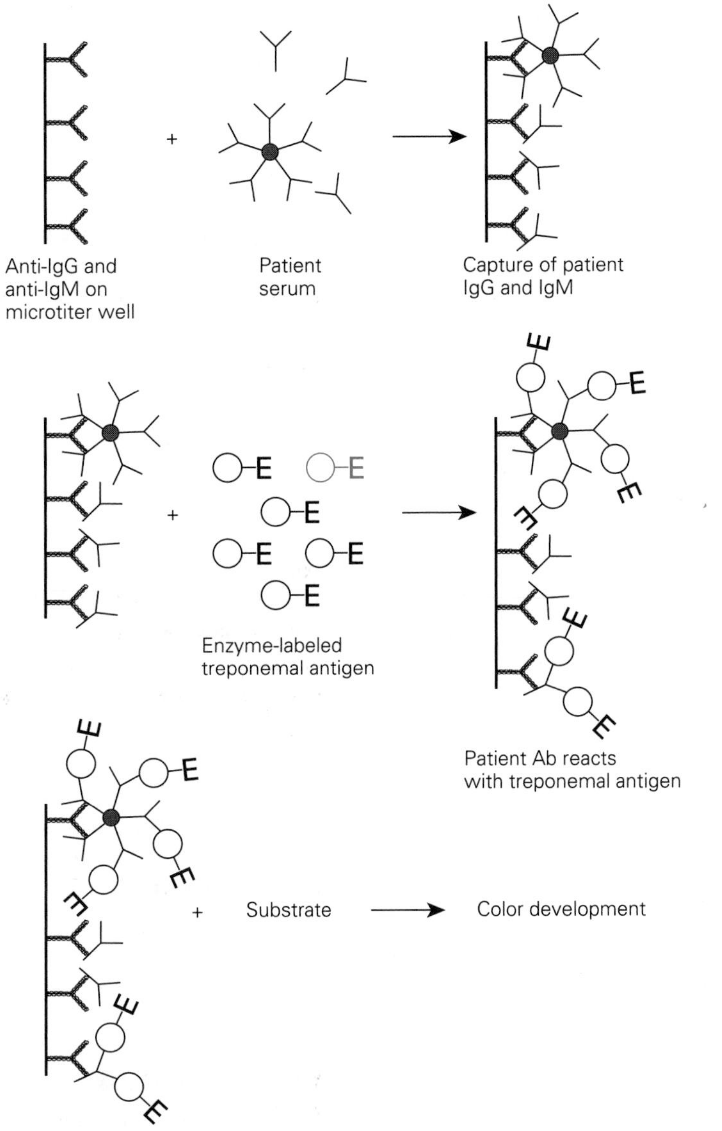

FIG. 19–3. Antibody capture enzyme-linked immunosorbent assay (ELISA) test. Only specific antitreponemal antibody will react with enzyme-labeled antigen.

Polymerase Chain Reaction Technique. Polymerase chain reaction (PCR) technology, which involves separation and isolation of a sequence of deoxyribonucleic acid (DNA) that is unique to a particular antigen, has been applied to testing of spinal fluid for the presence of treponemes. DNA is extracted from the sample and then amplified or increased using a polymerase enzyme and a primer that starts the reaction. The newly made DNA is then subjected to agarose gel electrophoresis using a technique known as *Southern blotting.* Nitrocellulose paper is used to make a copy or blot of the gel. A labeled probe, which is a sequence of DNA specific to the antigen being tested for, is added to the nitrocellulose paper. The probe will adhere only to a complementary strand of DNA. Presence of the radiolabel on the nitrocellulose paper confirms the presence of treponemal antigen (Fig. 19–4).

Preliminary findings indicate that PCR is an extremely sensitive technique, capable of detecting as little as one treponeme in a CSF sample.[23] For other fluids, especially serum, although the specificity appears to be 100 percent, sensitivity is closer to 70 percent.[24] Once sensitivity problems are solved for serum samples, this technique will have wide applicability for the future. PCR has been used in conjunction with fine-needle aspiration of material from the inguinal

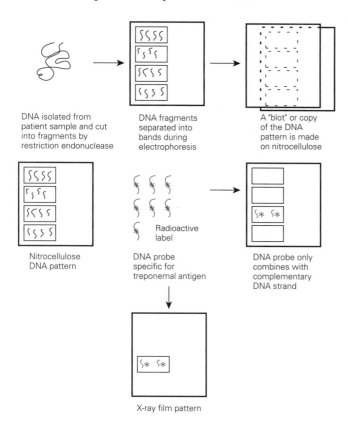

DNA isolated from patient sample and cut into fragments by restriction endonuclease

DNA fragments separated into bands during electrophoresis

A "blot" or copy of the DNA pattern is made on nitrocellulose

Nitrocellulose DNA pattern

DNA probe specific for treponemal antigen

Radioactive label

DNA probe only combines with complementary DNA strand

X-ray film pattern

FIG. 19–4. Southern blotting technique for determining the presence of treponemal DNA.

lymph nodes. Preliminary results indicate that this could be a useful new tool for diagnosis where serologic testing is not conclusive.[25]

Diagnostic Problem Areas

Congenital Syphilis. Nontreponemal tests for congenital syphilis performed on cord blood or neonatal serum detect the IgG class of antibody.[26] It is difficult to differentiate passively transferred maternal antibodies from those produced by the neonate, so that there are problems in establishing a definitive diagnosis. Late maternal infection may result in a nonreactive test because of low levels of fetal antibody. Additionally, testing of spinal fluid for presence of treponemes often lacks sensitivity.[27] Nontreponemal titers in the infant that are higher than the mother may be a good indicator of congenital disease, but this does not always occur.[9]

Several approaches have focused on the detection of IgM in the infant. An FTA-ABS test for IgM alone has been found to lack sensitivity, and the test is subject to interference because of the presence of rheumatoid factor.[27] However, an IgM capture assay is more sensi-

tive, and a Western blot assay (see Chapter 9 for details) using four major treponemal antigens has demonstrated a high sensitivity and specificity.[9]

Currently it is recommended that in high-risk areas, nontreponemal tests be performed on both mother and infant at birth, regardless of previous negative maternal tests. Since symptoms are not always present at birth, if congenital syphilis is suspected because of maternal history, tests should be repeated on infant serum within a few weeks.[16] If infection is present in the infant, the titer will remain the same or increase. The Western blot test is recommended for congenital syphilis.[10]

Cerebrospinal Fluid Tests. CSF is typically tested to determine whether treponemes have invaded the central nervous system. Such testing is usually more reliable if central nervous system symptoms are present. The traditional test performed on spinal fluid is the VDRL, which is a highly specific indicator of neurosyphilis.[10] If blood contamination of the specimen is not present, a positive VDRL confirms neurosyphilis.[13] However, sensitivity is lacking because samples from fewer than 70 percent of patients with active neurosyphilis have been found to give positive tests.[10,14] If a negative test is obtained, other indicators, such as increased lymphocyte and elevated total protein (>45 mg/dL) count, are used as signs of active disease.[14] PCR has been advocated in diagnosis of neurosyphilis and may play an important future role.[10]

Treatment

Penicillin is still the drug of choice for treatment of primary or secondary syphilis. A single intramuscular injection is usually effective.[28] Doxycycline can be used as an alternative if the patient is allergic to penicillin. Neurosyphilis is treated with crystalline penicillin or procaine penicillin to achieve a high enough concentration in the central nervous system. Probenecid is recommended for use along with penicillin in neurosyphilis patients.[28] For congenital syphilis, crystalline penicillin is administered for 10 days.

Lyme Disease

When an unusually large number of cases of juvenile arthritis appeared in a rural setting in southern Connecticut, local mothers became suspicious and persisted until there was a response from health officials. Because most cases developed in the summer, it was postulated that an infectious agent transmitted by an arthropod bite might be the cause. In 1982 the agent was isolated and identified as a new spirochete and named ***Borrelia burgdorferi***.[29]

Lyme disease, named after the little town in Connecticut where cases were first reported, was soon recognized as a multisystem illness involving the skin, the nervous system, the heart, and the joints. This syndrome is the most common vector-borne infection in the United States today, as more than 17,000 cases were reported in the year 2000.[30]

Characteristics of the Organism

Three closely related species, referred to as the *Borrelia burgdorferi sensu lato* complex, are now recognized as causative agents of Lyme disease. They are *B. burgdorferi sensu stricto,* responsible for cases in the United States, and *B. afzelii* and *B. garinii,* which are found in Europe.[31] All share the same characteristics and for simplicity will be referred to as *B. burgdorferi.* The organism is a loosely coiled spirochete, 5 to 25 μm long and 0.2 to 0.5 μm in diameter.[1,31] The outer membrane, which consists of glycolipid and protein, is extremely fluid and only loosely associated with the organism. Several important lipoprotein antigens, labeled OSP-A through OSP-F, are located within this structure and are actually encoded by plasmids.[32] There are also surface proteins that allow the spirochetes to attach to mammalian cells.

Just underneath the outer envelope are *endoflagellae* or *periplasmic flagellae.* These run parallel to the long axis of the organism and are made up of 41-kd subunits that elicit a strong antibody response. The flagellin subunit is homologous to that of other spirochetes, notably *B. recurrentis* and *T. pallidum,* thus causing cross-reactivity in serologic testing.[1] The organism divides by binary fission approximately every 12 hours. It can be cultured in the laboratory in a complex liquid medium (Barbour-Stoenner-Kelly) at 33°C, but it is extremely difficult to isolate from patients and is found only early on in illness.[31] Cultures often must be incubated for 6 weeks or longer to detect growth.[1]

The main reservoir in nature is *Peromyscus leucopus,* the white-footed mouse, although in California and Oregon the spirochete is harbored by the dusky-footed woodrat.[32] Vectors are several types of *Ixodes* ticks: *I. scapularis* in the Northeast and Midwest United States, *I. pacificus* in the West, *I. ricinus* in Europe, and *I. persulcatus* in Asia. White-tailed deer are the main host for the tick's adult stage (Fig. 19–5) and seem to be critical for survival of the tick. All stages of the tick can transmit the disease, but the most likely one is the nymph stage, which is most active in the summertime.[1] The tick must take a blood meal and be attached for 24 hours for infection to occur.

Stages of the Disease

Lyme disease resembles syphilis in that manifestations occur in several stages. These have been characterized as (1) localized rash, (2) dissemination to multiple organ systems, and (3) a chronic disseminated stage often including arthritic symptoms.[33] Because these stages are not always sharply delineated, however, it may be easier to view Lyme disease as a progressive, chronic infectious disease that involves diverse organ systems.

The first distinguishing feature is often the rash known as **erythema chronicum migrans,** which appears between 2 days and 2 weeks after a tick bite; the average is about 7 days.[34] The rash is usually found on the lower extremities. A small red papule where the bite occurred expands to form a large ringlike erythema with a central area that exhibits partial clearing (Fig. 19–6). This expansion occurs over a week or more, and even if untreated, the lesion gradually fades within 3 to 4 weeks. At this point, there may be accompanying nonspecific flulike symptoms such as

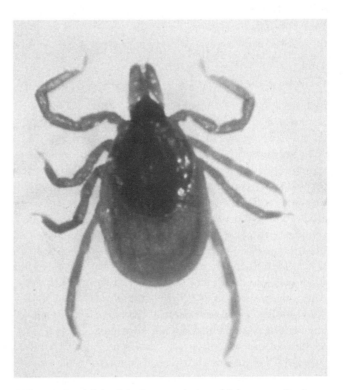

FIG. 19–5. Adult tick *I. scapularis,* which transmits Lyme disease. (Courtesy of Steven M. Opal, MD, Assistant Professor of Medicine, Brown University, Providence, RI.)

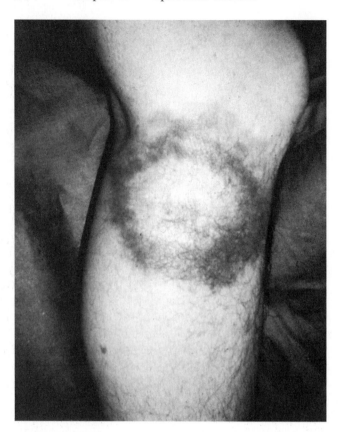

FIG. 19–6. Erythema chronicum migrans rash, which appears after a tick bite in Lyme disease. (Courtesy of Steven M. Opal, MD, Associate Professor of Medicine, Brown University, Providence, RI.)

malaise, headache, fever, and fatigue.[10,35,36] Approximately 80 percent of patients develop the rash.[33,35,36] At this early stage, antibody response is minimal.

Dissemination occurs by way of the bloodstream, and once this takes place, the disease can take many forms. Approximately 10 to 15 percent of patients will display multiple lesions.[32] Various systems may be affected, and there is often migratory pain in the joints, tendons, muscle, and bones. If treatment is not obtained, neurologic or cardiac involvement is seen in about 15 percent of patients within 4 to 6 weeks after the onset of infection.[32,37] Cardiac involvement typically manifests itself as varying degrees of atrioventricular block. Occasionally, acute myopericarditis or mild left ventricular dysfunction are also seen.[33]

The most prevalent neurologic sign is facial palsy.[32,38] This is a peripheral neuritis that usually involves one side of the face. Other peripheral nerve manifestations include pain and weakness in the limb that has been bitten. The central nervous system may be involved as well, and this is termed *neuroborreliosis*.

Some patients develop sleep disturbances, mild chronic confusional states, or difficulty with memory and intellectual functioning.[33] An aseptic meningitis, characterized by severe headache, photophobia, and mild elevation of spinal fluid protein, can also be seen.[10]

A late disseminated stage occurs months after the onset of disease in untreated patients. Between 50 and 60 percent of these individuals will develop brief attacks of arthritis.[32,38] This usually affects the large joints, especially the knee, and is episodic in nature. Many of these patients had earlier signs of dissemination of the organism, including secondary skin lesions and neurologic signs such as stiffness of the neck. Only about 10 percent of patients experience a continued chronic course, as spontaneous remission usually occurs. A link may exist between individuals who are susceptible to these chronic manifestations and the human leukocyte antigen (HLA) gene DRB1★0401, as a higher than normal percentage of those so affected have this phenotype.[32]

Nature of the Immune Response

The first detectable antibody in Lyme disease is of the IgM class. It does not peak until between the third and fourth weeks of infection.[35] If patients with symptoms are tested in less than 7 days, seropositivity is only about 30 percent.[35,39] IgG synthesis lags behind that of IgM, and it is often not detectable until approximately 4 to 6 weeks after the onset of erythema migrans.[34] It is not known why the antibody response is delayed, nor why once antibody is formed, it is not necessarily protective because secondary and tertiary stages occur despite high levels of circulating antibody. Spirochete lipoproteins do also trigger production of macrophage-derived cytokines, which enhance the immune response.[32]

Laboratory Diagnosis

Diagnosis of Lyme disease is not an easy task. If the characteristic rash is present, this can be used as a presumptive finding, but in as many as 20 percent of patients, the rash is not apparent. Direct isolation of the organism from skin scrapings, spinal fluid, or blood is possible, but the yield of positive cultures is extremely low. IgM response often does not appear until 3 to 6 weeks after the tick bite, and IgG is further delayed. Antibiotic therapy begun shortly after the appearance of erythema migrans may further delay or eliminate an antibody response. Therefore, diagnosis needs to be based on several criteria that include a history of a tick bite, the clinical symptoms, and a confirmation of the presence of *B. burgdorferi* through either direct or indirect methods.[35,39] Some of the current testing procedures are discussed and compared in Table 19–3.

Immunofluorescence Assay

Immunofluorescence assay (IFA) was the first test used to evaluate antibody response. Microscope slides are coated with antigen from whole or processed spirochetes, and then patient serum is added and allowed to react. An antihuman globulin with a fluorescent tag attached is added next and reacts with any specific antibody present. Typically a test result is only considered positive if a titer of 1:256 is obtained.[39] Specimens obtained in the first few weeks may be falsely negative.[39] In addition, there are problems with false positivity. Other diseases such as syphilis and relapsing fever can give positive results. Chronic diseases such as rheumatoid arthritis can also produce false positives, and this is indicated by a beaded fluorescent pattern. Reading of fluorescent patterns tends to be highly subjective, and the procedure is extremely labor intensive. Positive results need to be confirmed by the Western blot.[39,40]

Enzyme Immunoassay

EIA testing is a good primary screening method that is quick, reproducible, relatively inexpensive, and lends itself well to automation.[39] EIA methods involve antigen preparation by means of sonication of *B. burgdorferi* and concentration of the resulting protein fractions. This material is then coated onto 96-well microtiter plates. Patient sera is added and allowed to incubate with the antigen. After a washing step, antihuman globulin conjugated with an enzyme tag such as alkaline phosphatase is added to each well. Adding specific substrate produces a color change. Plates are

read in a spectrophotometer, and quantitation of antibody is possible, so that the test is more precise than IFA.[39]

Drawbacks of EIA include a lack of sensitivity during the early stages of Lyme disease. The sensitivity for early serum specimens has been reported to be anywhere from 58 to 92 percent.[41] Specificity has also been a problem with EIA testing. False positives occur with syphilis and other treponemal diseases such as yaws, relapsing fever, and leptospirosis.[1,41] If serum is absorbed to decrease cross-reactivity, this also decreases specific Lyme antibody titers. Additionally, patients with infectious mononucleosis, Rocky Mountain spotted fever, and other autoimmune diseases have been known to be positive with EIA.[39] Lyme disease patients do not test positive with RPR, so this can be run concurrently to rule out syphilis.[39]

Western Blot

Immunoblotting, or Western blotting, has been used in reference laboratories and is the technique against which most others are compared. It is recommended as a confirmatory test.[40,42] The technique consists of electrophoresis of antigens in an acrylamide gel and then transfer of this pattern to nitrocellulose paper. The nitrocellulose is reacted with patient serum and developed with an antihuman globulin to which an enzyme or a radioactive label is attached. Bands are then analyzed and interpreted.

Ten proteins are used in the interpretation of this test. They are designated by their molecular weight 18, 23, 28, 30, 39, 41, 45, 58, 66, and 93 kD.[10] For a result to be considered positive for presence of specific IgM antibody, two of the following bands must be present: 23(Osp C), 39, and 41 (flagellin) kD.[43,44] An IgG immunoblot is considered positive if 5 of the

TABLE 19–3. Comparison of Tests for the Diagnosis of Lyme Disease

Test	Antigen	Antibody	Comments
IFA	Whole or processed *B. burgdorferi*	Anti-Borrelia antibody from patient, antihuman globulin with fluorescent tag	Difficult to perform; false positives; lack of sensitivity
EIA	Sonicated *B. burgdorferi*	Anti-Borrelia antibody from patient, antihuman globulin with enzyme tag	Easy to perform; false positives; more sensitive than IFA
	Purified flagellin protein	Antiflagellin antibody from patient, antihuman globulin with enzyme tag	Easy to perform; highly specific; sensitive in early Lyme disease
DNA probe	Patient DNA matched to Borrelial DNA	None	Technically demanding, very specific; lacks sensitivity

IFA = Immunofluorescence assay; EIA = enzyme immunoassay; DNA = deoxyribonucleic acid.

10 listed bands are positive.[43,44] However, immunoblotting is technically involved and requires special equipment. The currently accepted testing protocol calls for a two-step approach with the use of EIA or IFA as initial screening tools. Then if a test is equivocal or positive, it should be confirmed by Western blot.[40]

Polymerase Chain Reaction

In testing for Lyme disease, the best hope for both sensitivity and specificity may be PCR. A piece of target DNA that is only present in strains of *B. burgdorferi* has been located and identified.[45] Only a few organisms need be present for detection. DNA from the patient sample is extracted and amplified by adding DNA polymerase and nucleotides.

Once a sufficient amount of the unknown DNA is made, this is combined with the known DNA probe to see if binding takes place. The single-stranded Borrelia DNA will only bind to an exact complementary strand, thus positively identifying the presence of the organism in the patient sample. This is much more specific than testing for antibody because there is no cross-reactivity with other spirochete antigens. Recent studies indicate that quantitative PRC performed on material from a skin biopsy right after the onset of the erythema migrans rash is the most sensitive method of detecting Lyme disease.[46] However, the sensitivity is lacking with other specimens such as blood, CSF, and synovial fluid, and the testing remains to be standardized.[10,35]

Treatment

Borrelia is sensitive to a number of orally administered antibiotics including penicillins, cephalosporins, tetracyclines, and macrolides. For early Lyme disease, doxycycline is the drug of choice, followed by amoxicillin.[33] A single dose of doxycycline has been found to be effective in prevention of Lyme disease if administered shortly after a tick bite occurs.[47] Neuroborreliosis requires the use of intravenous therapy. Ceftriaxone, cefotaxime, or penicillin G are the antibiotics used for this purpose.[35] A vaccine made with the Osp-A surface antigen has had limited usefulness and has been recalled from the market.[48]

SUMMARY

Syphilis and Lyme disease are the two major diseases caused by spirochetes. Spirochetes are distinguished by the presence of axial filaments that wrap around the cell wall inside a sheath and give the organisms their characteristic motility.

Syphilis is caused by the organism *Treponema pallidum,* subspecies *pallidum*. The disease is acquired by direct contact, usually through sexual transmission. Transmission to the fetus occurs in an infected mother after the 18th week of pregnancy.

The disease can be separated into four main clinical stages. In the primary stage, a chancre, or lesion, develops on the genitalia at the site of contact. Typically, this heals spontaneously, but untreated patients often progress to the secondary stage, in which systemic dissemination of the organism occurs. The secondary stage is characterized by fever, malaise, swollen lymph nodes, and a rash that involves skin and mucous membranes.

The latent stage follows the disappearance of the secondary stage. Patients are usually free of clinical symptoms, but serologic tests are still positive, and transmission to the fetus can occur at this stage. About one-third of the individuals who remain untreated develop tertiary syphilis, which can manifest itself as cardiovascular disease, gummatous syphilis with areas of granulomatous lesions, or neurosyphilis with damage to the central nervous system. Early diagnosis and treatment help to prevent later complications.

Direct laboratory diagnosis involves detection of the organism itself from a lesion, using either dark-field or fluorescence microscopy. If an active lesion is not present, diagnosis must be made on the basis of serologic tests. These can be classified as either nontreponemal or treponemal, depending on the type of antibody that is detected. Nontreponemal tests determine the presence of reagin, and the VDRL, RPR, and RST tests are examples of such tests. These are good screening tests because they are fairly sensitive and simple to perform, but they lack specificity.

Treponemal antibody tests include the FTA-ABS, hemagglutination, and particle agglutination. These detect antibody formed against the organism itself. For the FTA-ABS test, specially prepared slides containing treponemal antigens are used. Patient antibody is allowed to react with the fixed antigen, and then an anti-immunoglobulin, which has a fluorescent tag, is added to determine specific antigen–antibody combination. In passive agglutination tests, specially treated particles coated with treponemal antigens are used as indicators. Hemagglutination tests have largely been replaced by particle agglutination tests that use antigen-coated gel particles. If patient antibody is present, agglutination occurs.

Treponemal tests are more specific and sensitive in early stages of the disease, but they are expensive and more difficult to perform. Titers of these antibodies remain for life, while nontreponemal titers drop after successful treatment. New developments in testing include EIA technology and PCR. EIAs test for antibody to specific treponemal antigens, and class separation of antibodies is possible. PCR detects specific treponemal DNA.

Lyme disease represents the most common vector-borne infection in the United States today. The organism responsible is a spirochete named *Borrelia burgdorferi,* which is transmitted by the bite of a deer tick. Although an expanding red rash is often the first symptom noted, the disease can be characterized as a progressive, chronic infectious syndrome involving diverse organ systems.

The presence of IgM and IgG cannot usually be detected until 3 to 6 weeks after symptoms initially appear. The appearance of antibody is actually preceded by a T cell response that seems to suppress immunoglobulin production within the first few weeks of the disease. Because of this phenomenon of suppression, serologic tests for Lyme disease are often falsely negative during the early weeks.

The most sensitive test developed to date is immunoblotting, which involves electrophoresis of *Borrelia* antigens followed by reaction with patient serum to detect antibody to specific fractions. In more common use are IFA and EIA tests. These are easier to perform but are subject to false positives because of cross-reactivity with other spirochete diseases, such as syphilis and relapsing fever, and with certain autoimmune diseases. Current testing protocol involves screening with IFA or EIA and follow-up of equivocal or positive tests with immunoblotting. All serologic findings must be interpreted carefully and in conjunction with clinical diagnosis.

Case Studies

1. A 30-year-old woman saw her physician, complaining of repeated episodes of arthritis-like pain in the knees and hip joints. She recalled having seen a very small tick on her arm about 6 months prior to the development of symptoms. No rash was ever seen, however. A blood specimen was obtained with the following results: rheumatoid arthritis—negative; lupus—negative; RPR—negative; EIA test for Lyme disease—indeterminate.

Questions

   a. Does the absence of a rash rule out the possibility of Lyme disease?
   b. What might cause an indeterminate EIA test?
   c. What confirmatory testing would help in determining the cause of the patient's condition?

2. A mother who had no prenatal care appeared at the emergency room in labor. A baby boy was safely delivered, and he appeared to be normal. A blood sample was obtained from the mother for routine screening. An RPR test performed on the mother's serum was positive. The mother had no obvious signs of syphilis and denied any past history of the disease. She indicated that she had never received any treatment for a possible syphilis infection. Cord blood from the baby also exhibited a positive RPR result.

Questions

   a. Is the baby at risk for congenital syphilis?
   b. What is the significance of a positive RPR on a cord blood?
   c. How should these results be handled?

Exercise: RPR Card Test for Serologic Detection of Syphilis

PRINCIPLE

The RPR (rapid plasma reagin) 18-mm Circle Card Test is a nontreponemal serologic test for syphilis that detects reagin, an antibody formed against cardiolipin during the progress of the disease. The antigen consists of cardiolipin mixed with carbon particles, cholesterol, and lecithin. If antibody is present in the patient specimen, flocculation occurs with coagglutination of the carbon particles, resulting in black clumps against the white background of the plastic-coated card. Nonreactive specimens appear to have an even, light-gray color.

SAMPLE PREPARATION

Either plasma or serum can be used for this procedure. Collect blood by venipuncture using aseptic technique. Centrifuge the specimen at a force sufficient to sediment cellular elements. Keep the plasma or serum in the original collecting tube. Heat inactivation is not necessary for this procedure.

REAGENTS, MATERIALS, AND EQUIPMENT

1. Macro-Vue 18-mm Circle Card Test Kit, which contains the following:
   a. Antigen suspension: 0.003-percent cardiolipin, 0.020- to 0.022-percent lecithin, 0.09-percent cholesterol, EDTA (0.0125 mol/L), Na2HPO4 (0.01 mol/L), 0.1-percent thimerosal (preservative), 0.02-percent charcoal, 10-percent choline chloride (w/v), and distilled water. Refrigerate to store. Unopened ampules have a shelf life of 12 months from date of manufacture. Once opened, antigen in the dispensing bottle may be used for approximately 3 months or until the expiration date.
   b. Brewer diagnostic cards, which are specially prepared plastic-coated cards designed for use with the RPR card antigen.
   c. Dispenstirs
   d. Needles, 20 gauge
   e. Stirrers
   f. Dispensing bottle
2. Serologic pipette, 1 mL
3. Controls: known reactive and weakly reactive sera prepared from pooled rabbit sera and nonreactive pooled human sera. These need to be stored at 4°C and may be used until the expiration date on the label.
   WARNING: Because no test method can offer complete assurance that human immunodeficiency virus, hepatitis B virus, or other infectious agents are absent, specimens and these reagents should be handled as though capable of transmitting an infectious disease. The Food and Drug Administration recommends such material be handled at a Biosafety Level 2.
4. A rotator, 100 rpm, circumscribing a circle 2 cm in diameter with an automated timer and a cover containing a moistened sponge or blotter.

PROCEDURE★

1. Controls, RPR card antigen suspension, and test specimens should be at room temperature for use. The antigen suspension should be checked with controls using the regular test procedure. Only those suspensions that give the prescribed reactions should be used.
2. Attach the needle to the tapered fitting on the dispensing bottle.
3. To prepare the antigen suspension, vigorously shake the ampule for 10 to 15 seconds to resuspend the antigen and disperse any carbon particles lodged in the neck of the ampule. Overagitating will produce a coarse antigen, so disregard any particles left in the neck of the ampule after this time.
4. Snap the ampule neck, making sure that all the antigen is below the break line. Withdraw all the antigen into the dispensing bottle by collapsing the bottle and using it as a suction device.
5. To check the delivery of the needle, place it firmly on a 1-mL pipette. Fill the pipette with antigen suspension. Holding the pipette in a vertical position, count the number of drops delivered in 0.5 mL. This should be 30 ± 1 drops for a yellow 20-gauge needle.
6. Hold a Dispenstir device between the thumb and forefinger near the sealed end. Squeeze and do not release until open end is below surface of the specimen. Hold specimen tube vertically to minimize stirring up of cellular elements when using original blood tube. Release finger pressure to draw up the sample.
7. Hold Dispenstir in a vertical position over the card test area. Do not touch the surface of the card. Squeeze, allowing one drop to fall onto card.
8. Measure out controls in the same manner.
9. Gently shake antigen dispensing bottle before use. Hold in a vertical position, and dispense several drops into bottle cap to make sure the needle passage is clear. Place 1 free-falling drop onto each test or control area. Return

---

★ Adapted from the package insert for the Macro-Vue RPR 18-mm Circle Card Test (Brewer Diagnostic Kit), manufactured by Becton Dickinson and Company, Cockneysville, MD.

test droplets from the bottle cap to the dispensing bottle. Do not mix antigen and specimen. Mixing is accomplished during rotation.

10. Rotate for 8 minutes, under humidifying cover, on a mechanical rotator at 100 rpm.

11. Immediately following mechanical rotation, briefly rotate by hand with tilting of the card (three to four to-and-fro motions). Read macroscopically in the "wet" state under a high-intensity incandescent lamp or strong daylight.

12. Report as reactive any specimen showing characteristic clumping, ranging from slight but definite to marked and intense, and as nonreactive any specimen showing slight roughness or no clumping.

NOTE: There are only two possible reports with the card test: reactive or nonreactive, regardless of degree of activity. Any specimen demonstrating slight but definite clumping is always reported as reactive.

13. Upon completion of tests, remove the needle from the dispensing bottle and rinse with distilled or deionized water. Do not wipe the needle because this may remove the silicon coating and affect accuracy of delivery.

INTERPRETATION

The diagnosis of syphilis should not be made on a single reactive result without the support of a positive history or clinical evidence. As with all cardiolipin antigen tests, biologic false positives are possible with a number of diseases and conditions mentioned elsewhere. Therefore, reactive specimens should be subjected to further serologic study, including confirmatory testing.

RPR card tests should not be used for spinal fluids, however. Additionally, the Public Health Service has indicated that little reliance may be placed on cord blood serologic tests for syphilis.

Lipemia will not interfere with the card tests. However, if the degree of lipemia is so great that antigen particles are obscured, the specimen should be considered unsatisfactory. Hemolyzed specimens are acceptable unless they are so hemolyzed that printed material cannot be read through them.

1. *Treponema pallidum* and *Borrelia burgdorferi* can be distinguished from one another on the basis of which of the following?
   a. Only *T. pallidum* has axial filaments.
   b. Only *B. burgdorferi* has an outer sheath.
   c. Only *B. burgdorferi* can be grown in the laboratory on artificial media.
   d. Only *T. pallidum* stimulates IgM production to the membrane proteins.

2. False-positive nontreponemal tests for syphilis may be due to which of the following?
   a. Infectious mononucleosis
   b. Systemic lupus
   c. Pregnancy
   d. All of the above

3. In the fluorescent treponemal antibody absorption (FTA-ABS) test, what is the purpose of absorption with Reiter treponemes?
   a. It removes reactivity with lupus antibody.
   b. It prevents cross-reactivity with antibody to other *T. pallidum* subspecies.
   c. It prevents cross-reactivity with antibody to nonpathogenic treponemes.
   d. All of the above.

4. Which test is recommended for testing cerebrospinal fluid for detection of neurosyphilis?
   a. RPR
   b. VDRL
   c. FTA-ABS
   d. Enzyme immunoassay

5. Advantages of direct fluorescent antibody testing to *T. pallidum* include all of the following except:
   a. Reading is less subjective than with dark-field testing.
   b. Monoclonal antibody makes the reaction very specific.
   c. Slides can be prepared for later reading.
   d. Careful specimen collection is less important than in dark-field testing.

6. Which of the following is true of reagin?
   a. It can be detected in all patients with primary syphilis.
   b. It is antibody directed against cardiolipin.
   c. Reagin tests remain positive after successful treatment.
   d. It is only found in patients with syphilis.

7. Which syphilis test detects specific treponemal antibodies?
   a. RPR
   b. VDRL
   c. FTA-ABS
   d. Agglutination

8. Which of the following is true of treponemal tests for syphilis?
   a. They are usually negative in the primary stage.
   b. Titers decrease with successful treatment.
   c. They should be used as confirmatory tests rather than for screening.
   d. They are subject to a greater number of false positives than reagin tests.

9. An RPR test done on a 19-year-old woman as part of a prenatal workup was negative but exhibited a rough appearance. What should the technologist do next?
   a. Report the result out as negative.
   b. Do a VDRL test.
   c. Send off for confirmatory testing.
   d. Make serial dilutions and do a titer.

10. Treponemal EIA tests for syphilis are characterized by all of the following *except:*
    a. They are adaptable to automation.
    b. They are useful in diagnosing secondary or tertiary syphilis.
    c. Subjectivity in reading is eliminated.
    d. They can be used to distinguish between IgG and IgM antibodies.

11. Which of the following tests is the most sensitive during the early phase of Lyme disease?
    a. IFA
    b. EIA
    c. Immunoblotting
    d. Isolation of the spirochete

12. False-positive serologic tests for Lyme disease may be due to all of the following *except:*
    a. Shared antigens between *Borrelia* groups
    b. Cross-reactivity of antibodies
    c. Resemblance of flagellar antigen to that of *Treponema* organisms
    d. Patient in the early stage of the disease

13. Advantages of polymerase chain reaction PCR testing for syphilis include all of the following *except:*
    a. It is extremely specific.
    b. Many false positives are eliminated.
    c. Testing of serum is extremely sensitive.
    d. It can be used on CSF.

14. A 24-year-old man who had just recovered from infectious mononucleosis had evidence of a genital lesion. His RPR test was positive. What should the technologist do next?
    a. Report out as false positive.
    b. Do a confirmatory treponemal test.
    c. Do a VDRL.
    d. Have the patient return in 2 weeks for a repeat test.

15. A 15-year-old girl returned from a camping trip. Approximately a week after her return, she discovered a small red area on her leg that had a larger red ring around it. Her physician had her tested for Lyme disease, but the serologic test was negative. What is the best explanation for these results?
    a. She definitely does not have Lyme disease.
    b. The test was not performed correctly.
    c. Antibody response is often suppressed in early stages.
    d. Too much antibody was present, causing a false negative.

16. Which of the following is a true statement about late manifestations of Lyme disease?
    a. Treatment cannot reverse complications.
    b. Both central and peripheral nervous systems may be affected.
    c. Cardiac or neurologic damage occurs in all cases.
    d. Arthritis only appears in elderly patients.

17. Problems encountered in IFA testing for Lyme disease include all of the following *except:*
    a. Cross-reactivity with antibodies to syphilis
    b. False negatives in the later stages of disease
    c. False positives with rheumatoid factor
    d. Subjectivity in the reading of fluorescent patterns

References

1. The spirochetes. In Forbes, BA, Sahm, DF, and Weissfeld, AS: Bailey and Scott's Diagnostic Microbiology, ed. 11. Mosby, St. Louis, MO, 2002, pp 595–602.
2. Pope, V, Larsen, SA, and Schriefer, M: Immunological methods for the diagnosis of spirochetal diseases. In Rose, NR, et al: Manual of Clinical Laboratory Immunology, ed. 5. American Society for Microbiology, Washington, DC, 1997, pp 510–525.
3. Centers for Disease Control and Prevention: Primary and secondary syphilis—United States, 2000–2001. MMWR 51(43):971–973, 2002.
4. Centers for Disease Control and Prevention: Primary and secondary syphilis among men who have sex with men—New York City, 2001: MMWR 51(38):853–856, 2002.
5. Centers for Disease Control and Prevention: Outbreak of syphilis among men who have sex with men—Southern California, 2000: MMWR 50(38):117–120, 2001.
6. Schiff, E, and Lindberg, M: Neurosyphilis. South Med J 95:1083–1087, 2002.
7. Doherty, L, et al: Syphilis: Old problem, new strategy. BMJ 325:153–165, 2002.
8. Nicholl, A, and Hamers, FF: Are trends in HIV, gonorrhoea, and syphilis worsening in western Europe? BMJ 324:1324–1327, 2002.
9. Larsen, SA, Norris, SJ, and Pope, V: Treponema and other host-associated spirochetes. In Murray, PR, et al (eds): Manual of Clinical Microbiology, ed. 7. American Society for Microbiology, Washington, DC, 1999, pp 759–776.
10. Smith, MB et al: Spirochete infections. In Henry, JB (ed): Clinical Diagnosis and Management by Laboratory Methods, ed. 20. WB Saunders, Philadelphia, 2001, pp 1131–1143.
11. Blanco, DR, Miller, JN, and Lovett, MA: Surface antigens of the syphilis spirochete and their potential as virulence determinants. Emerg Infect Dis 3:11–20, 1997.

12. Orton, S: Syphilis and blood donors: What we know and, what we do not know, and what we need to know. Transfus Med Rev 15:282–291, 2001.

13. Goldmeier, D, and Hay, P: A review and update on adult syphilis, with particular reference to its treatment. Int J STD AIDS 4:70–82, 1993.

14. Lukehart, SA: Syphilis. In Braunwald, E., et al (eds): Harrison's Principles of Internal Medicine, ed. 15, New York, McGraw-Hill, 2001, pp 1044–1052.

15. Congenital syphilis—United States, 2000. MMWR 50:573–577, 2001.

16. Chhabra, RS, et al: Comparison of maternal sera, cord blood, and neonatal sera for detecting presumptive congenital syphilis: Relationship with maternal treatment. Pediatrics 91:88–91, 1993.

17. Guarner, J, et al: Testing umbilical cords for funisitis due to Treponema pallidum infection, Bolivia. Emerg Infect Dis 6:487–492, 2000.

18. Michelow, IC, et al: Central nervous system infection in congenital syphilis. N Engl J Med 346:1792–1798, 2002.

19. Pavia, CS, and Drutz, DJ: Spirochetal diseases. In Stites, DP, Terr, AI, and Parslow, TG (eds): Medical Immunology, ed. 9, 1997, pp 739–747.

20. Larsen, SA, et al (eds): A Manual of Tests for Syphilis. American Public Health Association, Washington, DC, 1998.

21. Pope, V, et al: Comparison of the Serodia Treponema pallidum Particle Agglutination, Captia Syphilis-G, and SpiroTek Reagin II tests with standard test techniques for diagnosis of syphilis: J Clin Micro 38:2543–2545, 2000.

22. Van der Sluis, JJ: Laboratory techniques in the diagnosis of syphilis: A review. Genitourin Med 68:413–419, 1992.

23. Noordhoek, G, et al: Detection by polymerase chain reaction of Treponema pallidum DNA in cerebrospinal fluid from neurosyphilis patients before and after antibiotic treatment. J Clin Microbiol 29:1976–1984, 1991.

24. Grimprel, E, et al: Use of polymerase chain reaction and rabbit infectivity testing to detect Treponema pallidum in amniotic fluid, fetal and neonatal sera, and cerebrospinal fluid. J Clin Microbiol 29:1711–1718, 1991.

25. Kouznetsov, AV, and Prinz, JC: Molecular diagnosis of syphilis: The Schaudinn-Hoffmann lymph-node biopsy. Lancet 360:388–389, 2002.

26. Patel, JA, and Chonmaitree, T: Syphilis screen at delivery: a need for uniform guidelines. Am J Dis Child 147:256–258, 1993.

27. Sanchez, PJ, et al: Evaluation of molecular methodologies and rabbit infectivity testing for the diagnosis of congenital syphilis and neonatal central nervous system invasion by Treponema pallidum. J Infect Dis 167:148–157, 1993.

28. Workowski, KA, and Levine, WC: Sexually transmitted diseases treatment guidelines—2002. MMWR 51(RR06):1–80, 2002.

29. Burgdorfer, W, et al: Lyme disease—A tick-borne spirochetosis? Science 216:1317, 1982.

30. Centers for Disease Control and Prevention: Lyme disease—United States, 2000. MMWR 51:29–31, 2002.

31. Schwan, TG, Burgdorfer, W, and Rosa, PA: Borrelia. In Murray, PR, et al (eds): Manual of Clinical Microbiology, ed. 7. American Society for Microbiology, Washington, DC, 1999, pp 746–758.

32. Steere, AC: Lyme disease. N Engl J Med 345:115–124, 2001.

33. Steere, AC: Lyme borreliosis. In Braunwald, E, et al (eds): Harrison's Principles of Internal Medicine, ed. 15, New York, McGraw-Hill, 2001, pp 1061–1065.

34. Centers for Disease Control Division of Vector-Borne Infectious Diseases: Lyme disease: Diagnosis. www.cdc.gov/ncidod/dvbid/lyme/diagnosis.htm, accessed November 3, 2002.

35. Smith, RP, et al.: Clinical characteristics and treatment outcome of early Lyme disease in patients with microbiclogically confirmed erythema migrans. Ann Intern Med 136:421–428, 2002.

36. Hercogova, J: Review: Lyme borreliosis. Int J Dermatol 40:547–550, 2001.

37. Nadelman, RB, et al: Praphylaxis with single-dose dowycycline for the prevention of Lyme disease after an Ixodes scapularis tick bite. N Engl J Med 345:79–84, 2001.

38. Kalish, RA, et al: Evaluation of study patients with Lyme disease, 10–20 year follow-up. J Infect Dis 183:453–460, 2001.

39. Johnson, RC, and Johnson, BJB: Lyme disease: Serodiagnosis of Borrelia burgdorferi sensu lato infection. In Rose, NR, et al: Manual of Clinical Laboratory Immunology, ed. 5. American Society for Microbiology, Washington, DC, 1997, pp 526–533.

40. Centers for Disease Control and Prevention: Recommendations for test performance and interpretation from the Second National Conference on Serological Diagnosis of Lyme Disease. MMWR 44:590, 1995.

41. Brown, SL, Hansen, SL, and Langone, JJ: Role of serology in diagnosis of Lyme disease. JAMA 282:62–66, 1999.

42. Pfister, HW, Wilske, B, and Weber, K: Lyme borreliosis: Basic science and clinical aspects. Lancet 343:1013–1016, 1994.

43. Engstrom, SM, Shoop, E, and Johnson, RC: Immunoblot interpretation criteria for serodiagnosis of early Lyme disease. J Clin Microbiol 33:419–427, 1995.

44. Dressler, F, et al: Western blotting in the serodiagnosis of Lyme disease. J Infect Dis 167:392–400, 1993.

45. Rosa, PA, and Schwan, TG: A specific and sensitive assay for the Lyme disease spirochete Borrelia burgdorferi using the polymerase chain reaction. J Infect Dis 160:1018–1029, 1989.

46. Nowakowski, J, et al: Laboratory diagnostic techniques for patients with early Lyme disease associated with erythema migrans: A comparison of different techniques. Clin Infect Dis 33:2023–2027, 2001.

47. Nadelman, RB, et al: Prophylaxis with single-dose doxycycline for the prevention of Lyme disease after an Ixodes scapularis tick bite. N Engl J Med 345:79–84, 2001.

48. Centers for Disease Control Division of Vector-Borne Infectious Diseases: Lyme disease: Vaccine recommendations. www.cdc.gov/ncidod/dvbid/lyme/vaccine.htm, accessed November 2, 2002.

chapter 20

Streptococcal Serology

Christine Stevens and Diane Wyatt, MS, MT(ASCP)

Learning Objectives

After completion of this chapter, the reader will be able to:

1. Describe how the M protein contributes to the virulence of *Streptococcus pyogenes.*
2. Distinguish suppurative from nonsuppurative complications of streptococcal infections.
3. Describe symptoms of acute rheumatic fever.
4. Discuss how pathogenesis occurs in glomerulonephritis.
5. List and describe five exoantigens produced by group A streptococci.
6. Discuss reasons for performing antibody rather than antigen testing for sequelae of streptococcal infections.
7. State the principle of the antistreptolysin O (ASO) titer.
8. List causes for false-negative results in an ASO titer.
9. Explain how the presence of antideoxyribonuclease B (anti-DNase B) is detected.
10. Compare the sensitivity of the Streptozyme test to other tests for streptococcal antibodies.
11. State advantages and disadvantages for each antibody detection method.
12. Interpret laboratory data to diagnose sequelae of streptococcal infections.

Key Terms

Acute rheumatic fever	Hyaluronidase	Pyrogenic exotoxins
Anti-DNase B	Lancefield group	Serotype
ASO titer	Nephritogenic strain	Streptolysin O
Exoantigen	Nonsuppurative	Suppurative complications
Glomerulonephritis	complications	

Streptococci are gram-positive spherical, ovoid, or lancet-shaped organisms that are catalase negative and often seen in pairs or chains.[1] They are divided into groups or **serotypes** on the basis of certain cell wall components. The outermost cell wall component contains two major proteins know as M and T, and these determine the serogroup or serotype. The serotype is based on minor variations in the proteins that can be identified serologically. Interior to the protein layer is the group specific carbohydrate which divides streptococci into 20 defined groups, designated A-H and K-V[2] (Fig. 20–1). These are known as the **Lancefield groups,** based on the pioneering work of Dr. Rebecca Lancefield. Some strains possess, outside the cell wall, a hyaluronic acid capsule that contributes to the bacterium's antiphagocytic properties.

Streptococcus pyogenes, which belongs to Lancefield group A, is one of the most common and ubiquitous pathogenic bacteria and causes a variety of infections.

The M protein is the major virulence factor of the group. M protein is a filamentous molecule consisting of two α-helical chains twisted into a ropelike structure that extends out from the cell surface. There is a net negative charge at the amino-terminal end that helps to inhibit phagocytosis. In addition, presence of the M protein limits deposition of C3 on the bacterial surface, thereby diminishing complement activation.[3,4]

Immunity to group A streptococci appears to be associated with antibodies to the M protein. There are more than 100 serotypes of this protein, and immunity is serotype specific.[4,5] Therefore, infection with one strain will not provide protection against another strain.

The genome of an M1 strain of *Streptococcus pyogenes* has just been sequenced, and of the 1752 genes, it is estimated that more than 40 code for various virulence factors.[6] Thirteen different surface proteins have been identified. In addition, numerous **exoantigens,** proteins excreted by the bacterial cell as it metabolizes,

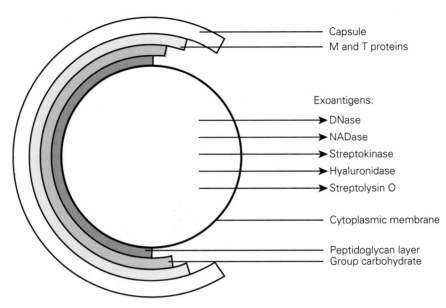

FIG. 20–1. Diagram of antigenic components of *Streptococcus pyogenes.*

are also produced. One of these is called streptococcal inhibitor of complement, which interferes with the membrane attack complex of complement.[7] **Pyrogenic exotoxins** A, B, and C are responsible for the rash seen in scarlet fever and also appear to contribute to pathogenicity.[5,8,9]

Antibodies to several of the exoantigens are produced during the course of streptococcal infections. Such exoantigens include the enzymes streptolysin O, deoxyribonuclease B (DNase), hyaluronidase, nicotinamide adenine dinucleotidase (NADase), and streptokinase. Characteristics of these enzymes are discussed, along with methods for detection of antibodies to these streptococcal products. Culture and rapid screening methods can be used for diagnostic testing early in infection. However, diagnosis of the sequelae to infection such as glomerulonephritis and acute rheumatic fever is best achieved by detection of antibodies. The advantages and disadvantages of each type of testing are presented.

Characteristics of Group A Streptococcal Infection

The two major sites of infection in humans are the upper respiratory tract and the skin with pharyngitis and impetigo being the most common.[2,10] Symptoms of pharyngitis include fever, chills, severe sore throat, headache, tonsillar exudates, petechiae on the soft palate, and anterior cervical lymphadenopathy.[10] About 20 percent of school children are asymptomatic carriers of group A streptococci.[5] The most common skin infection is streptococcal pyoderma or impetigo, characterized by vesicular lesions on the extremities that become pustular and crusted. Such infections tend to occur in young children.[5]

Other acute or **suppurative complications** include otitis media, scarlet fever, erysipelas, cellulitis, puerperal sepsis, and sinusitis. Septic arthritis, acute bacterial endocarditis, and meningitis also can result from a pharyngeal infection.[2,11] In recent history, increases have been noted in severe invasive infections associated with group A streptococci, notably toxic shock syndrome and necrotizing fasciitis.[8,12,13] Toxic shock syndrome is a life-threatening multisystem disease that initiates as a skin or soft tissue infection and may proceed to abdominal pain or pain in the extremities, shock, and renal failure.[14,15] Necrotizing fasciitis results from a skin infection that invades the muscles of the extremities or the trunk and causes fever and severe pain. The onset is quite acute and can be considered a medical emergency. Previously, the disease was associated with predisposing conditions, such as chronic illness in the elderly or varicella in children, but recent data indicate that young healthy persons are affected as well.[13,16] Reporting of necrotizing fasciitis and toxic shock syndrome is part of a Centers for Disease Control and Prevention surveillance program designed to follow emerging pathogens. It is projected that more than 10,000 such cases occur per year in the United States alone.[17]

In cases of **nonsuppurative complications,** the inflammatory response is not present in the infected organs, but elsewhere in the body. This may result in acute rheumatic fever or poststreptococcal glomerulonephritis that are damaging sequelae to streptococcal infections resulting from the host response to infections with *Streptococcus pyogenes.*[1] Serologic testing plays a major role in the diagnosis of these two diseases.

Acute Rheumatic Fever

Acute rheumatic fever was the leading cause of death in individuals between the ages of 5 and 20 years in the 1920s.[18] The incidence of the disease has generally declined in North America and Western Europe since that time. This may be the result of improved living conditions, such as better nutrition and hygiene, and less crowding. The advent of antibiotics has also had a significant effect.[11,19] Since the mid-1980s, however, there has been a resurgence of rheumatic fever in isolated epidemics with involvement of only certain serotypes.[11,20] These scattered outbreaks occurred among both adults and children. Isolates from these infections were found to be rich in M protein and heavily encapsulated, perhaps representing more invasive strains.[21,22] Worldwide, rheumatic fever remains a major determinant of heart disease and causes approximately 400,00 deaths annually, mainly in children and young adults.[23]

Acute rheumatic fever develops as a sequel to pharyngitis or tonsillitis in 2 to 3 percent of infected individuals. It does not occur as a result of skin infection. It appears that a limited number of rheumatogenic serotypes are associated with the disease.[2] The latency period is 20 days after onset of the sore throat. Characteristic features of acute rheumatic fever include pain caused by inflammation in the joints, along with inflammation of the heart and Sydenham's chorea in some patients.[2,19] Sydenham's chorea is characterized by involuntary jerking movements of the arms, legs, and face caused by inflammation of brain tissue, and it may appear as late as 6 months after the initial infection.

Acute rheumatic fever is most likely caused by the host response to the infection manifested as autoimmunity with either antibodies or cell-mediated immunity produced against streptococcal antigens cross-reacting with human heart tissue.[6,24] Chief among the antibodies are those directed toward the M proteins. M proteins appear to have at least three epitopes that resemble antigens in heart tissue, permitting cross-reactivity to occur. Titers of some antibodies may remain high for several years following infection.

Poststreptococcal Glomerulonephritis

The second main complication following a streptococcal infection is **glomerulonephritis,** a condition characterized by damage to the glomeruli in the kidney. This complication may follow infection of either the skin or the pharynx, while rheumatic fever follows only upper respiratory infections. Glomerulonephritis is associated with certain **nephritogenic strains** of streptococci.[1,2] It is most common in children between the ages of 2 and 12, and is especially prevalent in the winter months.[25]

A latent period averaging 10 days follows the initial infection.[2] Symptoms of glomerulonephritis may include hematuria, proteinuria, edema and hypertension. Patients may also experience malaise, backache, and abdominal discomfort.[26] Renal function is usually impaired because of reduction of the glomerular filtration rate, but renal failure is not typical.

The most widely accepted theory for the pathogenesis of poststreptococcal glomerulonephritis is that it results from deposition of antibody–streptococcal antigen immune complexes in the glomeruli. These immune complexes stimulate an inflammatory response causing damage and impaired function of the kidney due to release of the lysosomal contents of leukocytes and activation of complement.[1,2,25]

Rapid Streptococcal Screening Methods

Diagnosis of acute streptococcal infections typically is made by culture of the organism from the infected site. As an alternative to culture, approximately 30 commercial kits have been developed for the detection of group A streptococcal antigen from throat swabs. Antigen is extracted by either enzymatic or chemical means, and the process takes anywhere from 2 to 30 minutes depending on the particular technique. Either enzyme immunoassay (EIA) or latex agglutination is then used to identify the antigen. Many of these tests require no more than 2 to 5 minutes of hands-on time providing a distinct advantage over culture. However, while the specificity is high, the sensitivity is much lower, ranging anywhere from 60 to 95 percent. For this reason, it is recommended that cultures be performed when rapid test results are negative.[1,2,5]

Detection of Streptococcal Antibodies

Culture or rapid screening methods are extremely useful for diagnosis of acute pharyngitis. However, serologic diagnosis must be relied on for rheumatic fever and glomerulonephritis because the organism is unlikely to be present in the pharynx or on the skin at that time.[24] This is caused by either administration of antibiotics or the latent period of the disease itself.

Group A streptococci elaborate more than 20 exotoxins, and it is the antibody response to one or more of these that is used as documentation of non-suppurative disease. Some of these products include streptolysins O and S; deoxyribonucleases A, B, C, and D; streptokinase; NADase; hyaluronidase; diphosphopyridine nucleotidase; and pyrogenic exotoxins.[1,2] Streptolysins O and S are hemolysins that destroy both red and white blood cells.[25] Streptolysin O is oxygen and heat labile while streptolysin S is stable; however, it is to the former that antibodies are formed. **Hyaluronidase** also is known as spreading factor, and it breaks down hyaluronic acid, which acts as a binding substance for connective tissue. Pyrogenic exotoxins cause fever, changes in the blood-brain barrier, organ damage, and alterations in T cell function.[27] Diphosphopyridine nucleotidase is cardiotoxic.[11]

Antibody response to these streptococcal products is variable. The most diagnostically important antibodies are the following: ASO, anti-DNase B, anti-NADase and antihyaluronidase. Assays for detection of these antibodies can be performed individually or through use of the Streptozyme kit (Wampole Laboratories, Cranbury, NJ), which detects antibodies to all these products.[28]

Serologic evidence of disease is based on an elevated or rising titer of streptococcal antibodies. The onset of clinical manifestations of rheumatic fever or glomerulonephritis typically coincides with the peak of antibody response, so a serum specimen tested at that time should demonstrate an elevation in these antibodies. If acute and convalescent phase sera are tested in parallel, a fourfold rise in titer (a two-tube difference in doubling serial dilutions) is considered significant. The use of at least two tests for different exotoxins is recommended because production of detectable ASO does not occur in all patients. The most commonly used tests are those for ASO and anti-DNase B.[2]

Antistreptolysin O Titer

The **ASO titer** was the first test developed to measure streptococcal antibodies. This test is based on neutralization of the hemolytic activity of streptolysin O. **Streptolysin O** is one of the exoantigens released by streptococcal bacteria as they grow. ASO titers increase within 1 to 2 weeks after infection and peak between 3 to 6 weeks following the initial symptoms.[24] However, an antibody response only occurs in about 85 percent of acute rheumatic fever patients within this period. If chorea is the only symptom, ASO titers may be borderline or low. Additionally, ASO titers usually do not increase in individuals with skin infections.[2]

The range of expected normal values is variable and depends on the patient's age, the geographic location, and the season of the year. Thus the upper limits of normal must be established for specific populations.[21] Typically, however, a single ASO titer is considered to be moderately elevated if the titer is at least 240 Todd units in an adult and 320 in a child.[24,29] A titer that is two dilutions above the upper limit is considered to be significant.[2] ASO titers tend to be highest in school-age children and young adults.

The traditional ASO titer involves dilution of patient serum, to which a measured amount of streptolysin O reagent is added. These are allowed to combine during an incubation period after which reagent red blood cells are added as an indicator. If enough antibody is present, the streptolysin O is neutralized and no hemolysis occurs. The titer is reported as the reciprocal of the highest dilution demonstrating no hemolysis. This may be expressed in either Todd or International Units depending upon the standard used.[2] Reagent ASO is diluted for use as a standard. For the test to be valid, the ASO standard must demonstrate a titer that does not differ by more than one dilution from the manufacturer's stated value.

Several commercial slide agglutination tests are available for ASO that can be used for screening purposes. If such a test is negative but a streptococcal sequela is suspected, then a titration should be performed.[29] The possibility of false-negative results is reduced if two or more antibody tests are performed.[2]

Other standard tests include titration of anti-DNase B, antistreptokinase and antihyaluronidase. It has been reported that use of two different antibody tests results in findings of an elevated titer for at least one antibody in 95 percent of patients with acute rheumatic fever, with the exception of those patients whose only symptom is Sydenham's chorea.[20,29] In this case, positive antibody tests are found in about 80 percent of cases.

Anti-DNase B Testing

Testing for the presence of **anti-DNase B** is gaining popularity because these antibodies sometimes appear earlier than antistreptolysin O in streptococcal pharyngitis. Sensitivity is increased for the detection of glomerulonephritis preceded by streptococcal skin infections as ASO antibodies often are not stimulated by this type of disease. DNase B is mainly produced by group A streptococci, so testing for anti-DNase B is highly specific for group A streptococcal sequelae.[2] Macrotiter, microtiter, and EIA methods now are available for anti-DNase B testing.

Measurement of anti-DNase activity is based on a neutralization methodology. If anti-DNase B antibodies are present, they will neutralize reagent DNase B, preventing it from depolymerizing deoxyribonucleic acid (DNA). Presence of DNase is measured by its effect on a DNA-methyl green conjugate. This complex is green in its intact form, but when hydrolyzed by DNase, the methyl green is reduced and becomes colorless. An overnight incubation at 37°C is required to permit antibodies to inactivate the enzyme. Tubes are graded for color, with a 4+ indicating that the intensity of color is unchanged, and a 0 indicating a total loss of color. The result is reported as the reciprocal of the highest dilution demonstrating a color intensity of between 2+ and 4+. Normal titers for children from 2 to 12 years of age have been reported to range from 240 to 640 units.[24]

The test should be performed on paired acute and convalescent sera. A fourfold rise in titer (a difference of two tubes in a doubling serial dilution) is indicative of a recent streptococcal infection. An advantage of this method over the ASO titer is the stability of reagents. DNase B enzyme can be stored for two to three months at 2°C to 8°C without loss of activity, while ASO reagents must be used almost immediately after reconstitution.[2]

Streptozyme Testing

The Streptozyme test is a slide agglutination screening test for the detection of antibodies to several streptococcal antigens. Sheep red blood cells are coated with streptolysin, streptokinase, hyaluronidase, DNase, and NADase so that antibodies to any of the streptococcal antigens can be detected. Reagent red blood cells are mixed with a 1:100 dilution of patient serum. Hemagglutination represents a positive test, indicating that antibodies to one or more of these antigens are present.

The test is rapid and simple to perform, but it appears to be less reproducible than other antibody tests. More false positives and false negatives have been reported for this test than for the ASO and anti-DNase assays.[2] Because a larger variety of antibodies are included in this test, the potential is higher for detection of streptococcal antibodies. However, single determinations are not as significant as several titrations performed at weekly or biweekly intervals following the onset of symptoms.[26] The Streptozyme test is an excellent screening tool but should not be used for definitive testing.[2]

SUMMARY

Group A streptococci are widely distributed pathogens that are responsible for a variety of diseases ranging from pharyngitis and skin infections to rheumatic fever and acute glomerulonephritis. It is in diagnosis of the latter two diseases that serologic testing plays a major role. Rheumatic fever develops in a small percentage of the population as a sequel to throat infection, and damage to the smooth muscle of the heart may result. Glomerulonephritis may follow either a throat or a skin infection. The glomerular membrane is affected, resulting in impaired renal function.

The pathogenesis of these diseases is believed to be caused by cross-reactive antibodies reacting with cardiac tissue and immune complex deposition in the kidney. These activate complement to initiate an inflammatory response causing tissue damage. Antibody titers to streptococcal antigens typically remain high in both of these diseases.

Group A streptococci produce more than 20 exotoxins, and it is the antibody response to several of these products that can be measured in the laboratory. The most important of the products are streptolysin O, DNase B, streptokinase, NADase, and hyaluronidase. Evidence of nonsuppurative sequelae is based on a rise in titer in antibodies to one or more of these antigens because it usually is not possible to detect the organism itself at this time.

The ASO titer is based on the principle of neutralization of the action of streptolysin O on indicator red blood cells. If patient antibody is present, no lysis of red blood cells occurs. This test is somewhat time-consuming to perform, and antibody response only occurs in about 85 percent of individuals with clinical symptoms of disease. Agglutination tests using latex particles coated with streptolysin O are available, but the sensitivity of these is not as high as that of a traditional titration.

Anti-DNase B testing, a second method of detecting streptococcal antibodies, is gaining more extensive use. It, too, is based on neutralization of an enzyme by patient antibody. DNA is conjugated to an indicator that changes color when the DNA is depolymerized by enzyme action. Anti-DNase B antibodies may be detected earlier than ASO antibodies, and these are triggered by both throat and skin infections.

The Streptozyme test is a slide agglutination test that can detect antibodies to five streptococcal exoantigens. These antigens are coated on sheep red blood cells and mixed with patient antibody. If any of the five antibodies is present, a positive test will result. However, results are less reproducible than with other testing, so this should be used as a screening tool only.

In general, a negative antibody test does not rule out the presence of disease. Different patients will exhibit varying responses to streptococcal antigens, so it is recommended that more than one type of test be performed. In addition, titers should be performed in parallel on acute and convalescent sera to document ongoing infection. A fourfold rise in titer is considered significant for disease.

Case Study

1. A 6-year-old boy was brought to the pediatric clinic. His mother indicated he had been ill for several days with fever and general lethargy. The morning of the visit he had told his mother that his back hurt and she had observed what appeared to be blood in his urine. History and physical examination indicated a well-nourished child with an unremarkable health history other than a severe sore throat with fever three weeks ago that was medicated with aspirin and throat lozenges. This child's temperature was 101.5°F, and the physician noted edema in his hands and feet. Blood and urine specimens were collected for a Streptozyme test, complete blood cell count, and urinalysis. Laboratory test results were as follows:

White blood cell count:	12.7×10^9/L
Hematocrit:	36%
Hemoglobin:	12.1 gm/dL
White cell differential:	
N. neutrophils	73%
N. bands	4%
Lymphocytes	16%
Monocytes	5%
Eosinophils	2%
Basophils	0%
Red cell count:	normal
Urinalysis:	
Color:	red
Clarity:	cloudy
SG:	1.025
pH:	6.0
Protein:	2+
Glucose:	neg
Ketones:	neg
Blood:	large
Bilirubin:	neg
Urobilinogen:	neg
Nitrite:	neg
Leukocytes:	trace
Sediment:	3–5 white cells/hpf
	100 red cells/hpf
	0–1 granular cast/lpf
	0–1 red cell cast/lpf
Streptozyme:	positive

Questions

a. What disorder is indicated by this child's history, physical, and laboratory test results?

b. What was the most likely causative agent of the sore throat preceding the current symptoms?

c. Discuss the most widely accepted theory explaining the physiologic basis for this disease.

Exercise: Antistreptolysin O Titer

PRINCIPLE

The ASO titer is performed to detect antibodies to streptolysin O, an exotoxin produced by group A streptococci that has the biologic property of hemolyzing red blood cells. The ASO titer is a neutralization assay in which dilutions of patient serum are incubated with a standardized preparation of streptolysin O. If specific antibody is present, it will neutralize the reagent streptolysin O, thereby preventing the hemolysis of reagent group O human red blood cells added after the incubation period. The ASO titer is used in diagnosis of nonsuppurative sequelae of streptococcal infection, which include glomerulonephritis and rheumatic fever.

SAMPLE PREPARATION

Blood is collected aseptically, avoiding hemolysis, and permitted to clot. Serum should be removed and refrigerated or frozen if not tested immediately. One test requires 0.5 mL of serum.

REAGENTS, MATERIALS, AND EQUIPMENT

Test tubes, glass, 12 × 75 mm
Test tubes, glass, 16 × 110 mm
Water bath, 37°C
Serologic pipettes, disposable
Streptolysin O buffer (Difco Laboratories Inc., Detroit, MI)
Streptolysin O reagent (Difco Laboratories Inc., Detroit, MI)
ASO standard (Difco Laboratories Inc., Detroit, MI)
5-percent human group O red blood cell suspension

PROCEDURE★

1. Prepare streptolysin O buffer as follows: Pour one vial of buffer concentrate into a 100-mL volumetric flask. Bring the volume up to the mark with distilled water. Working buffer should have a pH of 6.6 ±0.1. Prepared buffer should be stored at 2°C to 8°C and may be used as long as there is no visible contamination. Undiluted buffer is stored at room temperature.

2. Reconstitute the streptolysin O reagent by adding distilled water in the amount stated on the vial. Mixing must be performed gently to avoid oxidation. Unopened vials may be stored at 2°C to 8°C, but once it is recon-

stituted, the reagent is labile and must be used within 15 minutes.

3. The ASO standard consists of lyophilized human gamma globulin, which is stored at 2°C to 8°C until ready for use. Reconstitute with the stated amount of distilled water. It should be used within 8 hours or frozen at −10°C or below.

4. A 5-percent suspension of human group O red blood cells is prepared by obtaining anticoagulated blood and washing cells three to four times in saline. By the fourth washing, the supernatant should be clear. If a reddish tinge is still evident at this point, the cells should not be used. Suspend 5 mL of the washed and packed cells in 95 mL of the working buffer.

5. Prepare dilutions of patient serum as follows:
   1:10 dilution: 0.5 mL of serum and 4.5 mL of working buffer
   1:100 dilution: 1.0 mL of 1:10 dilution and 9.0 mL of working buffer
   1:500 dilution: 2.0 mL of 1:100 dilution and 8.0 mL of working buffer.

6. Ten 12- × 75-mm test tubes are labeled for each patient sample using the numbers from the following chart. In addition, label one tube for the red blood cell control and one for the streptolysin O control (numbers 13 and 14). Five more tubes (numbered 3 through 7) are labeled to use for the ASO standard.

7. To each labeled patient tube, add the volumes of working buffer and serum predilutions as indicated in the chart, using disposable serologic pipettes.

8. For the ASO standard tubes, add the standard to tubes 3 to 7 in the same amounts as those given for patient serum. Add the corresponding amount of buffer to each tube.

9. Tubes 13 and 14 receive a measured amount of buffer only in the amounts noted in the chart below.

10. Add 0.5 mL of reconstituted streptolysin O reagent to all tubes except number 13.

11. Shake gently to mix and cover with plastic wrap. Incubate for 15 minutes at 37°C.

12. Add 0.5 mL of 5-percent red blood cell suspension to all tubes. Shake gently to mix, and incubate at 37°C for 30 minutes. Shake tubes gently after the first 15 minutes of incubation.

13. Centrifuge the tubes for 3 minutes at 1500 rpm.

14. Read for the highest dilution showing no hemolysis.

15. Tube 13 (red blood cell control) should show no hemolysis, and tube 14 (ASO control) should show complete hemolysis.

16. The ASO standard should have a titer of 166 Todd units (tube 5) ± 1 tube.

★ Adapted from the package insert for Antistreptolysin O Titer, Difco Laboratories Inc., Detroit, MI, 1999.

Serum Dilution														
	1:10		**1:100**					**1:500**					**Controls**	
Tube	1	2	3	4	5	6	7	8	9	10	11	12	13	14
Serum (mL)	0.8	0.2	1.0	0.8	0.6	0.4	0.3	1.0	0.8	0.6	0.4	0.2	—	—
Buffer (mL)	0.2	0.8	0.0	0.2	0.4	0.6	0.7	0.0	0.2	0.4	0.6	0.8	1.5	1.0
Todd units	12	50	100	125	166	250	333	500	625	833	1250	2500		

INTERPRETATION

The serum titer is reported as the reciprocal of the highest dilution showing no hemolysis. Generally, a titer of 166 Todd units or below is considered normal. For this reason, tubes 1 and 2 typically are not performed, and the titer begins with tube 3. All controls and the ASO standard must be within range for the test to be considered valid.

A single ASO titer does not have a great deal of diagnostic significance because normal values may vary for a given individual or population. Therefore, it is recommended that a repeat titer be performed within 2 weeks and that paired testing of the two sera be performed. A fourfold rise in titer is considered to be significant.

The streptolysin O reagent is not stable. If not handled according to directions, the reagent may become inactive, resulting in no hemolysis and yielding a false-positive result. This source of error is controlled by observation of the streptolysin O control.

The ASO titer is a useful tool in the diagnosis of acute rheumatic fever or glomerulonephritis, but interpretation of the results must be done cautiously. Only 75 to 80 percent of patients with rheumatic fever develop antibodies to streptolysin O. Those patients who had a skin infection prior to the development of acute glomerulonephritis do not develop ASO antibodies at all. Thus, a negative test does not rule out presence of the disease. Final diagnosis should take into account both laboratory and clinical findings.

Exercise: Streptozyme Test

PRINCIPLE

The Streptozyme Rapid Slide Test is an agglutination test that detects antibodies to five group A streptococcal exoantigens, including streptolysin O, streptokinase, hyaluronidase, DNase B, and NADase. These antigens are attached to aldehyde-fixed sheep red blood cells. When patient serum is added to these reagent red blood cells, agglutination of the red blood cells occurs if the patient has antibodies to one or more of these antigens.

SAMPLE PREPARATION

Blood is collected aseptically. Either serum or plasma may be used, as well as peripheral blood from a finger-tip or earlobe. If blood is collected from a finger or ear puncture, a heparinized capillary tube or the tube supplied with the Streptozyme kit may be used. If serum or plasma cannot be tested with 24 hours of collection, it should be stored frozen.

REAGENTS, MATERIALS, AND EQUIPMENT

Streptozyme Rapid Slide Test Kit (Wampole Laboratories, Cranbury, NJ), which contains the following:

Streptozyme reagent
Positive control serum
Negative control serum

Calibrated capillary tubes and bulbs
Mirrored glass slide

Additional materials needed:

Stirrers
Test tubes
Isotonic saline (0.85 percent)
Pipettes

WARNING

Because no test method can offer complete assurance that human immunodeficiency virus, hepatitis B virus, or other infectious agents are absent, controls should be handled as though capable of transmitting an infectious disease. The Food and Drug Administration recommends such material be handled at a Biosafety Level 2.

CAUTION

The reagents in this kit contain sodium azide. Sodium azide may react with lead and copper plumbing to form highly explosive metal azides. Upon disposal, flush with a large volume of water to prevent azide buildup.

PROCEDURE*

1. Dilute serum or plasma sample 1:100 with isotonic saline.
2. If the sample is peripheral blood from the earlobe or fingertip, fill the capillary tube (supplied with the kit) to the line. Without allowing the blood to clot, and using the bulb supplied, expel the sample into a tube containing 2.5 mL of isotonic saline. This technique yields an approximate 1:100 dilution.
3. Fill the capillary tube to the mark (0.05 mL) with the diluted specimen. Using the bulb supplied, expel the specimen onto a section of the glass slide provided with the kit.

4. Repeat step 3 for the positive and negative controls, placing each on a section of the slide that borders the patient specimen.
5. Add 1 drop of reagent to each section. Be sure the reagent is mixed well before it is used.
6. Thoroughly mix all samples using a disposable stirrer. Use a clean stirrer for each sample.
7. Rock the mirrored slide back and forth gently for 2 minutes at the rate of 8 to 10 times per minute.
8. At the end of 2 minutes, place the slide on a flat surface and observe for agglutination.
9. Agglutination must be read within 10 seconds. Reading is facilitated by a direct light source above the slide.
   NOTE: If the test is positive, a titer can be obtained by preparing the following dilutions and testing each by the above method.

Preparation of Sample		Resulting Dilution
1.0 mL of primary dilution (1:100)	+ 1.0 mL saline	1:200
0.5 mL of primary dilution	+ 1.5 mL saline	1:400
0.5 mL of primary dilution	+ 2.5 mL saline	1:600
0.5 mL of primary dilution	+ 3.5 mL saline	1:800

INTERPRETATION

A single Streptozyme determination is not as significant as serial titrations performed on a weekly or biweekly basis for up to 6 weeks following a streptococcal infection. Any positive serum should be further diluted to determine the titer. Positive results with Streptozyme are often obtained when the ASO titer is negative because of the fact that multiple antibodies can be detected. Titers considered to be within normal limits may vary with the season of the year, geographic location, and the age group of the patients.

* Adapted from the package insert for the Streptozyme Rapid Slide Test by Wampole Laboratories, Division of Carter-Wallace, Inc, Cranbury, NJ 08512.

1. All of the following are characteristics of streptococcal M protein *except:*
   a. It is the chief virulence factor of group A streptococci.
   b. It provokes an immune response.
   c. Antibodies to one serotype protect against other serotypes.
   d. It limits phagocytosis of the organism.

2. A technologist is performing an ASO titer. The streptolysin O reagent was reconstituted with distilled water, after which it was shaken vigorously and placed in the refrigerator overnight before use. Assuming all other testing procedures were performed correctly, what do you expect results to show?
   a. An accurate titer
   b. A mucin clot in all patient tubes
   c. A falsely decreased titer
   d. A falsely increased titer

3. Which of the following would invalidate an ASO titer?
   a. Lack of hemolysis in the red blood cell control
   b. A titer of 250 Todd units for the ASO standard
   c. Partial hemolysis in the streptolysin O control
   d. A titer of 166 Todd units for patient serum

4. An ASO titer and a Streptozyme test are performed on a patient's serum. The ASO titer demonstrates hemolysis in all patient tubes with controls and the standard showing expected results. The Streptozyme test is positive, and both positive and negative controls react appropriately. What can you conclude from these test results?
   a. The patient has a high titer of ASO.
   b. The patient has an antibody to a streptococcal exoenzyme other than streptolysin O.
   c. The patient has not had a previous streptococcal infection.
   d. The patient has scarlet fever.

5. Which of the following applies to acute rheumatic fever?
   a. Symptoms begin after either a throat or a skin infection.
   b. Antibodies to group A streptococci cross-react with heart tissue.
   c. Diagnosis is usually made by culture of the organism.
   d. All patients suffer permanent disability.

6. Antibodies are formed to all of the following streptococcal exotoxins *except:*
   a. Streptolysin O
   b. Streptolysin S
   c. DNase B
   d. Hyaluronidase

7. Which of the following indicates the presence of anti-DNase B activity in serum?
   a. Reduction of methyl green to colorless
   b. Clot formation when acetic acid is added
   c. Inhibition of red blood cell hemolysis
   d. Lack of change in the color indicator

8. Which of the following is considered to be a nonsuppurative complication of streptococcal infection?
   a. Acute rheumatic fever
   b. Scarlet fever
   c. Impetigo
   d. Pharyngitis

9. All of the following are reasons for false-negative results in an ASO titer *except:*
   a. Skin infection preceding glomerulonephritis
   b. Presence of Sydenham's chorea as the only symptom of rheumatic fever
   c. Failure to add the streptolysin O reagent to all tubes
   d. Serum obtained very early in infection

10. In an ASO titer, the red blood cell control tube should show which of the following?
    a. No hemolysis
    b. Red cell agglutination
    c. Complete hemolysis
    d. Partial hemolysis

References

1. Forbes, BA, Sahm, DF, and Weissfeld, AS: Bailey and Scott's Diagnostic Microbiology, ed. 11. Mosby, St. Louis, 2002, pp 298–315.

2. Ayoub, EM, and Hardin, E: Immune response to streptococcal antigens: Diagnostic methods. In Rose, NR, De MacArio, EC, and Folds, JD, et al (eds): Manual of Clinical Laboratory Immunology, ed. 5. American Society for Microbiology, Washington, D.C., 1997.

3. Fischetti, VA: Streptococcal M protein. Sci Am 264:58, 1991.

4. Larsen, HS: Streptococcaceae. In Mahon, CR, and Manuselis, G (eds): Textbook of Diagnostic Microbiology, ed. 2. WB Saunders, Philadelphia, 2000, pp 345–371.

5. Wessels, MR: Streptococcal and enterococcal infections. In Braunwald, E, Fauci, AS, and Kasper, DL, et al (eds): Harrison's Principles of Internal Medicine, ed. 15. McGraw-Hill, New York, 2001, pp 901–909.

6. Ferretti, JJ, McShan, WM, and Ajdic, D, et al: Complete genome sequence of an M1 strain of Streptococcus pyogenes. Proc Natl Acad Sci USA 98:4658–4663, 2001.

7. Akesson, P, Sjoholm, AG, and Bjorck, L: Protein SIC, a novel extracellular protein of Streptococcus pyogenes interfering with complement function. J Biol Chem 271:1081–1088, 1996.

8. Kiska, DL, Thiede, B, and Caracciolo, J, et al: Invasive group A streptococcal infections in North Carolina: Epidemiology, clinical features, and genetic and serotype analysis of causative organisms. J Infect Dis 176:992–1000, 1997.

9. Saouda, M, Wu, W, and Conran, P, et al: Streptococcal pyrogenic exotoxin B enhances tissue damage initiated by other Streptococcus pyogenes products. J Infect Dis 184:723–731, 2001.

10. Ruoff, KL, Whiley, RA, and Beighton, D: Streptococcus. In Murray, PR, Baron, EJ, and Pfaller, MA, et al (eds): Manual of Clinical Microbiology, ed. 7. American Society for Microbiology, Washington, D.C., 1999.

11. Bisno, AL: Group A streptococcal infections and acute rheumatic fever. N Engl J Med 325:783, 1991.

12. Cockerill, FR III, MacDonald, KL, and Thompson, RL, et al: An outbreak of invasive group A streptococcal disease associated with high carriage rates of the invasive clone among school-aged children. JAMA 277:38–43, 1997.

13. Moses, AE, Goldberg, S, and Korenman, Z, et al: Invasive group A streptococcal infections, Israel. Emerg Infect Dis 8:421–426, 2002.

14. Hoge, CW, Schwartz, B, and Talkington, DF, et al: The changing epidemiology of invasive group A streptococcal infections and the emergence of streptococcal toxic shock-like syndrome. A retrospective population-based study. JAMA 269:384, 1993.

15. Wolf, JE, and Rabinowitz, LG: Streptococcal toxic shock-like syndrome. Arch Dermatol 131:73–77, 1995.

16. Davies, HD, McGeer, A, and Schwartz, B, et al: Invasive group A streptococcal infections in Ontario, Canada. Ontario Group A Streptococcal Study Group. N Engl J Med 335:547–554, 1996.

17. Schuchat, A, Hilger, T, and Zell, E, et al: Active bacterial core surveillance of the emerging infections program network. Emerg Infect Dis 7:92–99, 2001.

18. Bland, EF: Rheumatic fever: The way it was. Circulation 76:1190, 1987.

19. Sell, S: Immunology, Immunopathology and Immunity, ed. 6. American Society for Microbiology, Washington, D.C., 2001, pp 313–325.

20. Williamson, L, Bowness, P, and Mowat, A, et al: Lesson of the week: Difficulties in diagnosing acute rheumatic fever-arthritis may be short lived and carditis silent. BMJ 320:362–365, 2000.

21. Bisno, AL, Shulman, ST, and Dajani, AS: The rise and fall (and rise?) of rheumatic fever. JAMA 259:728, 1988.

22. Veasy, LG, Wiedmeier, SE, and Orsmond, GS, et al: Resurgence of acute rheumatic fever in the intermountain area of the United States. N Engl J Med 316:421, 1987.

23. Attacking the attacker: WHO steps up its fight against rheumatic fever. http://www.who.int/inf-pr-1999/en/pr99-73.html. Accessed June 5, 2002.

24. Kaplan, EL, Rothermel, CD, and Johnson, DR: Antistreptolysin O and anti-deoxyribonuclease B titers: Normal values for children ages 2 to 12 in the United States. Pediatrics 101:86–88, 1998.

25. Brady, HR, and Brenner, BM: Pathogenesis of glomerular injury. In Braunwald, E, Fauci, AS, and Kasper, DL, et al (eds): Harrison's Principles of Internal Medicine, ed. 15. McGraw-Hill, New York, 2001, pp 1572–1580.

26. Lang, MM, and Towers, C: Identifying poststreptococcal glomerulonephritis. Nurse Pract 26:34, 2001.

27. Defining the group A streptococcal toxic shock syndrome. Rationale and consensus definition. The Working Group on Severe Streptococcal Infections. JAMA 269:390, 1993.

28. Wampole Laboratories: Package Insert for Streptozyme Rapid Slide Test Kit. Cranbury, NJ, 1990.

29. Guidelines for the diagnosis of rheumatic fever. Jones Criteria, 1992 update. Special Writing Group of the Committee on Rheumatic Fever, Endocarditis, and Kawasaki Disease of the Council on Cardiovascular Disease in the Young of the American Heart Association. JAMA 268:2069, 1992.

Serology of Viral Infections

Linda E. Miller, PhD, SI(ASCP)

Learning Objectives

After finishing this chapter, the reader will be able to:

1. Differentiate between the different hepatitis viruses and their modes of transmission.
2. Correlate the various serologic markers of hepatitis with their diagnostic significance.
3. Indicate the laboratory methods that are most commonly used to screen for or confirm hepatitis virus infections.
4. Associate the Epstein–Barr virus (EBV) with the specific diseases it causes.
5. Correlate the heterophile antibody and antibodies to the EBV with their clinical significance.
6. Indicate the laboratory methods used to test for heterophile antibodies and EBV antibodies.
7. List the diseases associated with varicella zoster virus, rubella virus, rubeola virus, and mumps virus.
8. State the most common serology method used to detect antibodies to these viruses.
9. Indicate how serology is used to detect current infection with or immunity to each of the preceding viruses.
10. Discuss the clinical significance of cytomegalovirus, human T lymphotropic virus type I, and human T lymphotropic virus type I.
11. Discuss the laboratory methods used to detect exposure to the preceding viruses.
12. Correlate viral IgM and IgG antibodies with their clinical significance in terms of detecting current infections, congenital infections, or immunity to infections.

Key Terms

Anti-Hbe	HBeAg	IgM anti-HBc
Anti-HBs	HbsAg	Rubella virus
Cytomegalovirus	Hepatitis	Shell vial
Epstein-Barr virus	Herpes simplex virus	Varicella-zoster virus
HBcAg		

As our knowledge of viruses has increased, so has the development of serologic assays to detect viral infections. These assays have become some of the most important and frequently performed tests in clinical immunology. Because viral culture is typically a difficult and lengthy process, while serologic tests for viral infections can be easily and rapidly performed by the clinical laboratory, the latter play an essential role in helping physicians establish a presumptive diagnosis so that treatment may be initiated promptly. In addition, serologic tests are important in monitoring the course of infection, detecting past infections, and assessing immune status.

In general, presence of virus-specific IgM antibodies in a sample of patient serum indicates a current or recent viral infection, while IgG antibodies to the virus signify either a current or a past infection and, in most cases, immunity. Specific IgM antibodies in the newborn's serum indicate congenital infections with viruses; on the other hand, IgG antibodies in the infant's serum are mainly maternal antibodies that have crossed the placenta. Current infections in the adult or newborn may also be indicated by immunoassays for viral antigens in serum or other clinical samples from the patient or by viral nucleic acids that can be detected by molecular methods.

Some of the most important viral infections detected by serology, which will be discussed in this chapter, are those caused by the hepatitis viruses, viruses of the herpes group, measles, mumps, rubella, and the human T cell leukemia viruses. Serology of the human immunodeficiency virus is discussed in Chapter 22.

Hepatitis

Hepatitis is a general term that means inflammation of the liver. It can be caused by a number of viruses as well as noninfectious agents, including ionizing radiation, chemicals, and autoimmune processes. The primary hepatitis viruses, which are listed in Table 21–1, are viruses whose main clinical effects are on the liver. Other viruses, such as cytomegalovirus, Epstein-Barr virus (EBV), and herpes simplex virus, can also produce liver inflammation, but it is secondary to other disease processes. This section will focus on the primary hepatitis viruses. Two of these viruses, the hepatitis A virus (HAV) and the hepatitis E virus (HEV) are transmitted primarily by the fecal-oral route, while the hepatitis B virus (HBV), the hepatitis D virus (HDV), the hepatitis C virus (HCV), and the hepatitis G virus (HGV) are transmitted mainly by the parenteral route (i.e., through contact with blood and other body fluids). All may produce similar clinical manifestations. The early, or acute, stages of hepatitis are characterized by general flulike symptoms such as fatigue, fever, myalgia, loss of appetite, nausea, vomiting, diarrhea or constipation, and mild to moderate pain in the right upper quadrant of the abdomen.[1] Progression of the disease can lead to liver enlargement (hepatomegaly) and tenderness, jaun-

TABLE 21–1. Summary of Hepatitis Viruses

Hepatitis Virus	Type/Family	Transmission	Acute	Chronic	Complications
Hepatitis A (HAV)	RNA picornaviridae	Fecal, oral	Yes	No	Low risk of fulminant liver disease
Hepatitis B (HBV)	DNA hepadnaviridae	Parenteral, sexual, perinatal	Yes	Yes	33% of chronic cases may progress to chronic active hepatitis, liver cirrhosis, and hepatocellular carcinoma
Hepatitis C (HCV)	RNA flaviviridae	Parenteral, sexual, perinatal	Yes	Yes	Cirrhosis (10%–20%); hepatocellular carcinoma (15%); autoimmune-type chronic active hepatitis and cryoglobulinemia
Hepatitis D (HDV)	RNA	Mostly parenteral, but also sexual, perinatal; HBV infection required	Yes	Yes	Fulminant hepatitis, cirrhosis
Hepatitis E (HEV)	RNA calciviridae	Fecal, oral	Yes	No	Fulminant liver failure in pregnant women

RNA = Ribonucleic acid; DNA = deoxyribonucleic acid.

dice, dark urine, and light feces. Initial laboratory findings typically include elevations in bilirubin (~25-fold), and 10- to 100-fold elevations in the liver enzymes, alanine aminotransferase (ALT), and aspartate aminotransferase (AST).[1,2] These findings are nonspecific indicators of liver inflammation and must be followed by specific serologic tests to identify the cause of hepatitis more definitively.

Hepatitis A

HAV is a single-stranded ribonucleic acid (RNA) virus that belongs to the *Picornaviridae* family. It is the most common cause of acute viral hepatitis throughout much of the world.[3] HAV is transmitted primarily through the fecal-oral route, by close person-to-person contact or ingestion of contaminated food or water.[1-4] Conditions of poor personal hygiene, poor sanitation, and overcrowding facilitate transmission. Occasional transmission through contact with contaminated blood has been reported and may occur during a short period within the acute stage of infection when a high number of viral particles can be found in the source blood.[3,5]

Following an average incubation period of 28 days, the virus produces symptoms of acute hepatitis in the majority of infected adults; most infections in children are asymptomatic.[1,2,4] Symptoms typically have an abrupt onset, continue for 1 to 8 weeks, and then resolve. Massive hepatic necrosis resulting in fulminant hepatitis and death are rare, and are usually associated with underlying liver disease. The infection does not progress to a chronic state, and liver enzymes usually drop to normal levels within 6 months.[5]

HAV antigens are shed in the feces of infected individuals during the incubation period and early acute stage of infection, but decline to low levels by the time symptoms appear and are thus not a clinically useful indicator of disease.[2,4] Serologic tests for antibody are therefore critical in establishing diagnosis of the infection, and acute hepatitis A is indicated by the presence of IgM antibodies to HAV. These antibodies are routinely detected by a solid-phase antibody-capture enzyme-linked immunosorbent assay (ELISA) test; they typically peak during the first month of illness and decline to undetectable levels within 6 to 12 months.[1,4,5]

Competitive inhibition ELISA tests are available to detect total HAV antibodies, which consist predominantly of IgG.[5] These antibodies indicate immunity to HAV and are produced as a result of natural infection or immunization. Vaccination against HAV by administration of formalin-killed whole virus is recommended for travelers to endemic areas of the world and for other high-risk individuals.[3,6] Infection with HAV may be prevented in nonimmunized individuals who have been exposed to the virus by intramuscular injection of gamma globulin that contains antibodies to HAV.

Hepatitis E

Like HAV, HEV is an RNA virus that is transmitted by the fecal-oral route. The most common mode of transmission is through fecally contaminated drinking water in developing nations of the world; occurrence in the United States is mainly associated with travel to endemic regions.[1,7,8]

Hepatitis E usually presents as an acute, self-limiting hepatitis without progression to a chronic carrier state.[1,8] However, it is associated with a high rate of mortality in pregnant women.[1,7]

Serologic tests for HEV have been developed but are not commercially available in the United States.[4,7,8] Diagnostic tests available in research laboratories include ELISA, Western blot, and fluorescent antibody blocking assay to detect antibodies to HEV, as well as polymerase chain reaction (PCR) to detect HEV RNA. Studies have shown that IgM anti-HEV is typically present during the acute infection but declines rapidly in the early recovery period; while IgG anti-HEV persists, it may provide some immunity to the host.[4,8] HEV RNA can be detected in the feces of most patients for about 2 weeks after the onset of illness, but may persist longer in some cases.[7]

Hepatitis B

HBV is transmitted through the parenteral route by intimate contact with HBV-contaminated blood or other body fluids, especially semen, vaginal secretions, saliva, and breast milk.[1,2,8,9] Transmission has thus been associated with sexual contact, blood transfusions, sharing of needles and syringes by intravenous drug users, tattooing, and occupational needle-stick injury. Unapparent transmission of HBV may occur through close personal contact of broken skin or mucous membranes with the virus. Studies of health-care workers have estimated that the risk for a nonimmune person to acquire the infection ranges from 6 to 30 percent following a single percutaneous exposure to HBV.[10] Infection with HBV may be prevented through immunization or through intramuscular injection of gamma globulin containing antibodies to HBV given soon after exposure to the virus. Transmission of HBV may also occur via the perinatal route, from infected mother to infant, most likely during the time of delivery or through breast milk feedings.

After transmission to the host, HBV undergoes an average incubation period of 60 to 90 days, followed by a highly variable clinical course.[1,9,11,12] Many individuals may remain asymptomatic. About 30 to 50 percent of older children and adults, and less than 10 percent of children younger than 5 years of age, develop clinical symptoms of acute hepatitis, which typically last 1 to 4 weeks. Most HBV-infected adults recover within 6 months and develop immunity to the virus, but 1 to 2 percent develop fulminant liver disease with hepatic necrosis, which has a high rate of fatality. Chronic HBV infection develops in 5 to 10 percent of infected adults, 30 to 60 percent of infected children less than 4 years old, and 90 percent of infected infants. About 25 percent of these persons become chronic carriers of the virus, with increased risk of developing cirrhosis and hepatocellular carcinoma. Worldwide, about 300 million people are thought to be chronic carriers of HBV, and about 1 million deaths per year have been attributed to this virus.[12,13]

HBV is a deoxyribonucleic acid (DNA) virus belonging to the *Hepadnaviridae* family.[14,15] The virion is a 42-nm sphere consisting of a nucleocapsid core surrounded by an outer envelope of lipoprotein. The core of the virus contains circular partially double-stranded DNA, a DNA-dependent DNA polymerase enzyme, and two proteins: the hepatitis B core antigen **(HBcAg)** and the hepatitis Be antigen (HBeAg). A protein called the hepatitis B surface antigen (HBsAg) can be found in the outer envelope of the virus as well as in particles circulating freely in the blood.

These antigens, or antibodies to them, serve as serologic markers for hepatitis B and have been used in differential diagnosis of HBV infection, monitoring the course of infection in patients, assessing immunity to the virus, and screening blood products for infectivity. The levels of these markers vary with the amount of viral replication and the host's immune response and are useful in establishing the initial diagnosis and in monitoring the course of infection. Typical patterns of these markers during acute and chronic hepatitis B are shown in Figure 21–1 and are described following.[1,2,9,11,16]

The hepatitis B surface antigen, or **HBsAg,** is the first marker to appear, becoming detectable 2 to 12 weeks after exposure to HBV. Its levels peak during the acute stages of infection, then gradually decline as the patient develops antibodies to the antigen and recovers. Serum HBsAg usually becomes undetectable by 12 to 20 weeks after the onset of symptoms in patients with acute hepatitis B. In patients with chronic HBV infection, HBsAg remains elevated. HBsAg is thus an indicator of active infection and is an important marker in detecting initial infection, monitoring the course of infection and progression to chronic disease, and in the screening of donor blood.

The hepatitis Be antigen, or **HBeAg,** appears shortly after HBsAg and disappears shortly before HBsAg in recovering patients. It may be elevated during chronic infection. This marker is present during periods of active replication of the virus and thus indicates a high degree of infectivity when present. The HBcAg is not detectable in serum because the viral envelope masks it.

As the host develops an immune response to the virus, antibodies appear. First to appear is IgM antibody to the core antigen, or **IgM anti-HBc.** This antibody is an indicator of current or recent acute infection. It

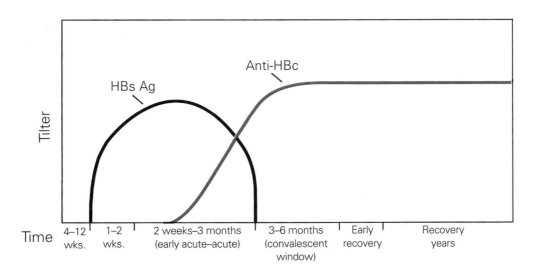

FIG. 21–1. HbsAG and anti-HBc as markers of acute hepatitis B.

typically appears 2 weeks after HBsAg during acute infection and can be detected up to 6 months later. This marker is useful in detecting infection during the "core window," or the time between the disappearance of HBsAg and the appearance of antibodies to HBsAg, and is therefore used in addition to HBsAg for the screening of donor blood. IgG antibodies to the core antigen are produced before IgM anti-HBc disappears, and then persist for the lifetime of the individual. They are the predominant antibodies detected in the test for total anti-HBc, and they can be used to indicate a past HBV infection.

The appearance of antibodies to the HBe antigen, or **anti-HBe,** occurs shortly after the disappearance of HBeAg and indicates that the patient is recovering from HBV infection.

Antibodies to HBsAg, or **anti-HBs,** also appear during the recovery period of acute hepatitis B, weeks to months after HBsAg disappears. These antibodies persist for years and provide protective immunity. Anti-HBs are also produced after immunization with the hepatitis B vaccine, which consists of recombinant HBsAg produced from genetically engineered yeast. Protective titers of the antibody are considered to be 10 mIU/mL of serum or higher.[9,17] Anti-HBs are not produced during chronic HBV infection in which immunity fails to develop.

The most widely used method for detecting serologic markers for hepatitis B has been the ELISA because of its high level of sensitivity and ease of use for batch testing in the clinical laboratory.[2,16] A prototype of this assay for detection of HBsAg is shown in Figure 21–2. Any positive results should be verified by repeated testing of the same specimen in duplicate, followed by a confirmatory ELISA test, which uses anti-HBs to neutralize HBsAg in the patient sample. A competitive assay for anti-HBc is shown in Figure 21–3.

Newer, fully automated assays that use microparticles and computerized instrumentation have also been manufactured.[16,18] Molecular methods have been developed to detect HBV DNA and are used primarily to evaluate the effectiveness of antiviral therapy in patients with chronic hepatitis B or to diagnose atypical cases of hepatitis B originating from mutations in the HBV genome.[11,19]

Hepatitis D

Hepatitis D is a parenterally transmitted infection that can only occur in the presence of hepatitis B. This is because the HDV virion incorporates the HBsAg of HBV into its outer protein coat, which it requires to replicate and infect host cells.[1,2,11] Infection with the two viruses occurs either simultaneously, as a coinfection, or sequentially as a superinfection in chronic HBV carriers. Presence of HDV in a patient with hepatitis B results in a greater risk of developing fulminant hepatitis or chronic liver disease.[1,2,8] Hepatitis D infection is routinely indicated by the presence of anti-HDV in the patient's serum,[2,8,11,16] which is most often detected by ELISA. IgM anti-HDV typically appears 6 to 7 weeks after exposure, remains elevated during the acute phase of the illness, and then declines. IgG anti-HDV is produced during convalescence and then declines to subdetectable levels if the infection resolves. Both IgM and IgG antibodies tend to remain elevated during chronic infection.

Hepatitis C

Hepatitis C is a major public health problem, causing

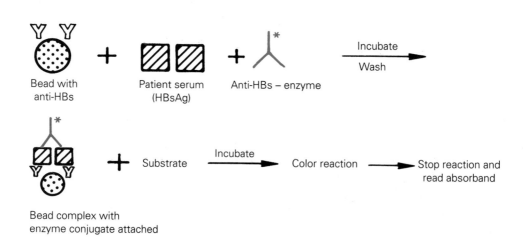

FIG. 21–2. Detection of HbsAg by ELISA. (From Miller, LE: Testing for viral hepatitis. The Learning Laboratorian Series 3:5, 1991, with permission.)

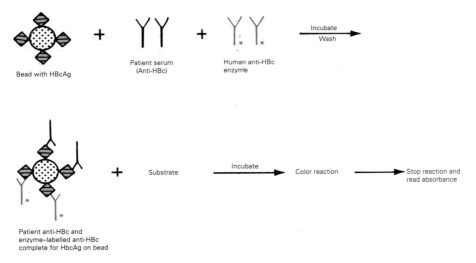

FIG. 21–3. Competitive enzyme immunoassay (EIA) for detection of anti-HBc. (From Miller, LE: Testing for viral hepatitis. The Learning Laboratorian Series 3:5, 1991, with permission.)

chronic infection in about 1.8 percent of individuals in the United States and 3 percent of the world's population.[1,20–23] It is the cause of the majority of infections previously classified as "nonA-nonB" prior to the discovery of HCV in 1989.[24]

Hepatitis C is transmitted mainly by exposure to contaminated blood, with intravenous drug use being the main source of infection.[1,20,22] Blood transfusion was also a major source of infection before 1992, when routine screening of blood donors for HCV antibody was implemented, but testing has reduced this risk to about 0.001 to 0.01 percent per unit of blood transfused.[23] Other risk factors for acquiring hepatitis C include organ transplantation before 1992, occupational exposures to contaminated blood, chronic hemodialysis, and possibly intranasal cocaine use, body piercing, and tattooing. Sexual transmission of HCV is thought to be less common, but is higher in those who have had multiple sex partners or a history of sexually transmitted diseases.[20,22,23] Perinatal transmission has been estimated to occur at a rate of about 6 percent.

Following an average incubation period of 7 to 8 weeks, HCV produces symptoms of acute hepatitis in only about 20 percent of cases.[1,21–23] Although the majority of infections are asymptomatic, about 85 percent of persons are thought to develop chronic infection, with cirrhosis developing slowly over 20 to 25 years in about 20 percent of these individuals.[1,21–23] Those with cirrhosis are at an increased risk of developing hepatocellular carcinoma. End-stage liver disease related to HCV accounts for one-third of the liver transplantations performed in industrialized nations.[20] HCV is also the most common cause of mixed essential cryoglobulinemia, which is characterized by production of immune complexes containing HCV

particles, anti-HCV, immunoglobulins, rheumatoid factor, and complement.[21] These complexes deposit themselves in various locations in the body, causing glomerulonephritis, vasculitis, and neuropathy.

HCV is a single-stranded RNA virus belonging to the *Flaviviridae* family. Its genome contains an open reading frame that codes for three structural proteins (C, E1, and E2) and six nonstructural proteins (NS1, NS2, NS3, NS4a, NS4b, and NS5). Six different genotypes and more than 50 subtypes of the virus have been discovered.[23] The high mutation rate of the virus allows it to escape the immune response and persist in the host. This has created difficulty in developing an effective vaccine.

A number of laboratory tests have been developed to diagnose and monitor persons with HCV infection. Screening assays are based on ELISA methods in which antibodies to HCV are captured onto microtiter plates or plastic beads coated with antigens from the virus. These assays are used in the screening of blood and organ donors and in the initial diagnosis of symptomatic patients; they are also recommended in the screening of individuals with high risk factors.[20,22,25]

The first ELISAs developed, or first-generation ELISAs, used a recombinant HCV antigen called c100 from the NS4 protein. This test was limited in that its sensitivity was only 81 to 89 percent, and antibodies usually did not become detectable until 15 to 20 weeks after exposure.[24,26] Second- and third-generation ELISA tests use a larger number of antigens from the NS3, NS4, and NS5 proteins of HCV, thus increasing sensitivity and specificity. With the current third-generation assays, antibodies can usually be detected at the time symptoms appear, or 7 to 8 weeks after exposure.[26]

Although third-generation ELISAs have a specificity greater than 99 percent, false-positive results can occur due to cross-reactivity present in persons with other viral infections or autoimmune disorders.[26] Recombinant immunoblot assays (RIBAs) have been developed to confirm positive ELISA results to reduce the number of false-positives.[22,25] In the RIBA, antibodies in the patient serum bind to different HCV antigens that have been immobilized onto a nitrocellulose strip. Bound antibodies are detected after adding a peroxidase-labeled goat-antihuman IgG conjugate, and the appropriate substrate. A colorimetric reaction follows, producing visible bands in the locations of the specific HCV antigens to which antibodies are present in the test sample. The result is considered positive if a specific pattern of bands is produced.

Molecular assays have also been developed to detect HCV RNA in a patient's serum or plasma and may replace the RIBA in confirmation of positive ELISA results.[20,25,26] A reverse transcriptase polymerase chain reaction (RT-PCR), which is based on amplification of DNA that is produced from HCV RNA in the test sample, is available as a qualitative or quantitative assay. A branched DNA amplification (bDNA), which is a branched-chain signal amplification assay, is available as a quantitative test that involves amplification of the assay's detection signal following binding of HCV RNA in the sample to specific molecular probes.

In addition to confirming positive results, the molecular assays can be used in the following ways: (1) to make an earlier diagnosis because HCV RNA appears as early as 1 week after exposure,[21] (2) to detect infection in babies born to HCV-positive mothers, and (3) to detect exposure in immunosuppressed individuals who are unable to mount an adequate antibody response to the virus.[26] Quantitative assays have been useful in monitoring the amount of virus, or "viral load," carried by patients before, during, and after antiviral therapy in chronically infected individuals.[22,23,25,26] HCV genotyping by molecular or serologic methods is also available but is mainly considered a research tool.[23,26]

Current laboratory tests for HCV are not able to distinguish between acute and chronic infection or definitively predict resolution of the infection.[21,26] Research is underway to try to identify additional markers that could be used for this purpose.

Hepatitis G

In 1995 and 1996, another virus associated with hepatitis was discovered independently by two research groups. They named the infectious agent GB virus-C (GBV-C) and HGV, respectively.[15,27,28] This RNA virus is transmissible by the bloodborne route and has been found in serum from patients with acute or chronic liver diseases as well as in 1 to 2 percent of blood donors.[15,28] Its exact clinical significance needs to be defined more clearly by further studies. Detection of the virus has been based primarily on RT-PCR methods, which amplify HGV RNA.[27,28] Serology tests based on ELISA and Western blot methods have also been developed.[27,29] Studies indicate that antibodies to the HGV envelope protein E2 may be associated with recovery from hepatitis G infection.[27,29]

Herpes Virus Infections

The Herpes viruses are DNA viruses that are surrounded by a protein capsid, an amorphous tegument, and outer envelope.[30] These viruses are all capable of establishing a latent infection with lifelong persistence in the host. The *Herpesviridae* family includes the Epstein-Barr virus, cytomegalovirus, varicella-zoster, the **herpes simplex viruses** (HSV-1 and HSV-2), and the human herpes viruses (HHV-6, HHV-7, and HHV-8). The serology of some of these viruses will be discussed following.

Epstein-Barr Virus

The **Epstein-Barr virus** (EBV), also known as human herpes virus-4, or HHV-4, causes a wide spectrum of diseases, including infectious mononucleosis, lymphoproliferative disease, and a number of malignancies.[31-33] Most EBV infections result from oral contact with infected saliva; transmission through bloodborne and perinatal routes is much less frequent.[31,34-36]

The virus infects epithelial cells in the oropharynx, where it enters a lytic cycle, characterized by viral replication, lysis of host cells, and release of infectious virions until the acute infection is resolved. Another major target of EBV is the B lymphocyte, which the virus enters by binding to CD21 (a receptor for both EBV and the C3d protein of complement) on the surface of the B cell membrane.[31] Infected B cells spread the virus throughout the lymphoreticular system and become polyclonally activated, proliferating and secreting a number of antibodies, including EBV-specific antibodies, heterophile antibodies, and autoantibodies.[35,36] In healthy individuals, this process is kept in check by the immune response of natural killer cells and specific cytotoxic T cells. However, EBV can persist in the body indefinitely in a small percentage of B cells in which it establishes a latent infection.[31]

Several antigens have been identified in EBV-infected cells that are associated with different phases of the viral infection, and antibodies to these antigens have become an important diagnostic tool.[33,37,38] Antigens produced during the initial stages of viral replication in the lytic cycle are known as the early antigens (EA). These antigens can be further classified into two groups based on their location within the cells: EA-D, which has a diffuse distribution in the nucleus and cytoplasm, and EA-R, which is restricted to the cytoplasm only. The late antigens of EBV are those that appear during the period of the lytic cycle following viral DNA synthesis. They include the viral capsid antigen (VCAs) in the protein capsid and the membrane antigens in the viral envelope. Antigens appearing during the latent phase include the EBV nuclear antigen (*EBNA*) proteins, EBNA-1, EBNA-2, EBNA-3A, EBNA-3B, EBNA-3C, and EBNA-LP, and the latent membrane proteins (LMPs), LMP-1, LMP-2A, and LMP-2B (Table 21–2).

The clinical manifestations of EBV vary with the age and immune status of the host. Infections in infants and young children are generally asymptomatic or mild, while primary infections in healthy adolescents or adults commonly result in infectious mononucleosis (IM).[31-36] More than half of patients with IM present with three classic symptoms: fever, lymphadenopathy, and sore throat. Other symptoms, including splenomegaly, hepatomegaly, and periorbital edema, may also be seen. Although these symptoms are essential in diagnosing IM, they can also be caused by a number of other infectious agents, and laboratory testing plays an important role in differentiating IM from other infections.

Characteristic laboratory findings in patients with IM include an absolute lymphocytosis (>50 percent of the total leukocytes, with a count >4500/μL) and at least 10-percent atypical lymphocytes (thought to be activated cytotoxic T cells).[34,35] Serologic findings include presence of a heterophile antibody and antibodies to certain EBV antigens.

Heterophile antibodies, by definition, are antibodies that are capable of reacting with similar antigens from two or more unrelated species. The heterophile antibodies associated with IM are IgM antibodies produced as a result of polyclonal B cell activation and are capable of reacting with horse red blood cells, sheep red blood cells, and beef red blood cells. These antibodies are produced by 60 to 70 percent of patients with IM during the first week of clinical illness and by up to 90 percent of patients by the fourth week.[34,35] They disappear in most patients by 3 months after the onset of symptoms, but can be detected in some patients for up to 1 year.[34,35] For many years, these heterophile antibodies were detected by a rapid slide agglutination method, the Monospot, which tested the ability of serum absorbed with guinea pig kidney or beef erythrocyte antigens to agglutinate horse red blood cells. The antibody could then be titered by incubating serial dilutions of the patient's serum with sheep red blood cells in the Paul-Bunnell test. These methods have been replaced today by rapid latex agglutination tests or solid phase immunoassays using purified bovine red blood cell extract as the antigen. Studies have shown the sensitivity of these kits varies from 63 to 84 percent, and the specificity ranges from 84 to 100 percent.[35,36,39] False-positive results, although uncommon, can occur in patients with lymphoma, viral hepatitis, and autoimmune disease.[36]

Negative heterophile antibody results occur in about 20 percent of patients with IM overall and 50 percent of children less than 4 years old.[35,36] In these patients, who demonstrate symptoms of IM but are negative for the heterophile antibody, further testing for EBV-specific antibodies is indicated.[36,38] These antibodies can be detected by indirect immunofluorescence, ELISA, or immunoblot techniques.[35,38] IgM antibody to the VCA is the most useful marker for acute IM because it usually appears at the onset of clinical symptoms and disappears by 3 months.[34-36,38] IgG anti-VCA is also present at the onset of IM but persists for life and can thus indicate a past infection. Antibodies to EA-D are seen during acute IM, and anti-EBNA appears during convalescence. A summary of serologic responses during acute, convalescent, and post-IM is shown in Table 21–3.

Some individuals develop chronic active EBV infection, with severe illness for more than 6 months.[31,32] In addition, EBV has been associated with a number of malignancies, both hematologic (e.g., Burkitt's

TABLE 21–2. Epstein-Barr Virus Antigens

Early Acute Phase	Late Phase	Latent Phase
EA-R (early antigen restricted)	VCA (viral capsid antigen)	EBNA (EBV nuclear antigen)
EA-D (early antigen diffuse)	MA (membrane antigen)	EBNA-1
		LYDMA (lymphocyte-detected membrane antigen)

lymphoma and Hodgkin's disease) and nonhematologic (e.g., nasopharyngeal carcinoma and gastric carcinoma).[31–33] EBV can also cause a lymphoproliferative disorder in immunocompromised patients, including those with primary immunodeficiencies, acquired immunodeficiency syndrome (AIDS), or organ transplantation.[31,33] Serology tests for EBV antibodies, tests to detect EBV antigens in tissue biopsies, and molecular methods to detect EBV DNA have been useful in the diagnosis of these disorders.[32,33,38] The typical patterns of EBV antibodies seen in some of these disorders is shown in Table 21–3.

Cytomegalovirus

Cytomegalovirus (CMV), also known as human herpes virus-5 (HHV-5) is a widespread virus that has infected significant numbers of individuals, up to 100 percent of those in some populations studied.[40,41] It is spread by close, prolonged contact with infected body secretions, by intimate sexual contact, and perinatally, from infected mother to infant.[40–42] The virus has been isolated in saliva, urine, stool, vaginal and cervical secretions, semen, breast milk, and blood.

Primary, or initial, infections in healthy individuals are usually asymptomatic, but may occasionally produce an IM-like illness with fever and hepatitis.[41–43] An immune response against the virus is stimulated, but the virus persists in a latent state in myeloid cells and may be reactivated at a later time in the life of the individual.

The clinical consequences of CMV infection are much more serious in the immunocompromised host, most notably organ transplant recipients and patients with AIDS. Infection associated with organ transplant may result from reactivation of CMV in the recipient or transmission of CMV from the donor. It can manifest as a CMV mononucleosis-like syndrome with or without localized infection of selected organs and is associated with an increased risk for allograft failure when a previously unexposed recipient becomes infected with CMV from the donor organ.[41,43] In patients with AIDS, dissemination of the virus most commonly occurs to the retina, lungs, gastrointestinal tract, or central nervous system and may produce serious consquences.[42,43]

CMV is also the most common cause of congenital infections, occurring in 0.3 to 2 percent of all live births throughout the world.[44,45] About 10 to 15 percent of infected infants exhibit symptoms of central nervous system and multiple organ involvement at birth, and 20 to 30 percent of these will die from the infection.[44–47] Ninety percent of the surviving infants will develop clinical sequelae, such as hearing loss, visual impairment, and mental retardation, in their early childhood years. Mothers who acquire primary CMV infection during their pregnancy have a greater risk of giving birth to an infected infant with severe clinical consequences than do women in whom CMV was reactivated during the pregnancy.

A number of laboratory methods have been developed to detect CMV infection, including serology, viral culture, viral antigen assays, and molecular assays. The serology methods performed most commonly are ELISA and latex agglutination.[48] These assays are most useful in documenting a past CMV infection in healthy individuals such as blood and organ donors.[49] A fourfold rise in antibody titers of serial serum specimens in persons older than 6 months of age suggests a recent infection,[47,48] but rapid detection of infection is not possible by this process. Assays for IgM CMV antibodies have been developed but are limited in value

TABLE 21–3. Serologic Responses of Patients with Epstein-Barr Virus–Associated Diseases

Condition	Heterophile Anti-VCA			Anti-EA		Anti-EBNA	Heterophile (IgM)
	IgM	IgG	IgA	Diffuse EA	Restricted EA		
Uninfected	−	−	−	−	−	−	−
IM	+	++	±	+	−	−	+
Convalescent IM	−	+	−	−	±	+	±
Past infection IM	−	+	−	−	−	+	−
Chronic active infection IM	−	+++	±	+	++	±	−
Posttransplant lymphoproliferative disease	−	++	±	+	+	±	−
Burkitt's lymphoma	−	+++	−	±	++	+	−
Nasopharyngeal carcinoma	−	+++	+	++	±	+	−

Adapted from Straus, SE, et al: Epstein-Barr virus infections: Biology, pathogenesis, and management. Ann Intern Med 118:45, 1993, with permission.
VCA = Viral capsid antigen; EA = early antigen; EBNA = EBV nuclear antigen; IM = infectious mononucleosis.

because of the potential for false-negative results in newborns and immunocompromised patients and for false-positive results due to other infections or the presence of rheumatoid factor.[47–49] In addition, IgM antibodies may not necessarily indicate primary CMV infection because they can be produced as a result of CMV reactivation as well and may persist for up to 18 months.[44,47] Serologic methods that use recombinant antigens to detect CMV antibodies of different avidities are being developed in an attempt to increase the sensitivity and specificity of tests for CMV disease.[44,48] Because of the limitations of serology testing, direct methods of detecting CMV infection are essential.

The traditional method of viral culture involves observation of characteristic cytopathic effects in cell lines inoculated with CMV-infected specimens. This method is limited, however, because results do not appear until several days to weeks after inoculation. Implementation of the **shell vial** assay has reduced the time of detection to 24 to 48 hours after inoculation.[49,50] This assay is an immunofluorescence method that uses monoclonal antibodies to detect immediate early CMV antigens in infected cells grown on coverslips in shell vials. More rapid detection has been made possible by the introduction of a CMV antigenemia assay, which detects the CMV lower matrix protein, pp65, in CMV-infected peripheral blood leukocytes by immunocytochemical or immunofluorescent staining.[50,51] This method, which is commercially available and can be performed in 2 hours, has become a valuable tool in decisions to initiate early antiviral therapy in infected patients.[49] Molecular assays to detect CMV DNA have also been developed. Studies indicate that results from quantitative PCR for CMV viral load are helpful in distinguishing active CMV disease from latent infection in immunocompromised hosts,[52–54] monitoring the effectiveness of antiviral treatment,[49] and predicting symptomatic congenital CMV infections.[44,45]

Varicella-Zoster Virus

The **varicella-zoster virus** (VZV), also known as human herpes virus 3 (HHV-3), is the cause of two distinct diseases: varicella, more commonly known as chickenpox, and herpes zoster, or shingles. The virus is transmitted by inhalation of infected respiratory secretions or contact with infectious skin lesions.[55,56]

Primary infection with VZV results in chickenpox, which is characterized by a blister-like rash with intense itching and fever.[55,57] In a typical infection, these vesicular lesions first appear on the face and scalp, then spread to the trunk and extremities, and break down to form a crust over the next 12 to 14 hours. The

illness is usually mild and self-limiting in healthy children, but may in some cases produce complications, the most common of which are secondary bacterial skin infections.[56] Primary infections in adults, neonates, or pregnant women tend to be more severe, with a larger number of lesions and a greater chance of developing complications such as pneumonia. Varicella infection in pregnant women may also cause premature labor or congenital malformations if the infection is acquired during the first 20 weeks of pregnancy.[55–57] Infections in immunocompromised patients are more likely to result in disseminated disease, with extensive skin rash, neurologic conditions (e.g., encephalitis), pneumonia, or hepatitis.[57,58]

During the course of primary infection, VZV is thought to travel from the skin to the sensory nerve endings to the dorsal ganglion cells, where it establishes a latent state.[55] Reactivation of the virus occurs in 20 percent of persons with a history of varicella infection, probably as a result of a decrease in cell-mediated immunity.[55] Reactivation results in movement of the virus down the sensory nerve to the dermatome supplied by that nerve, resulting in eruption of the painful vesicular rash known as shingles in the affected area.[55,57] The rash may persist for weeks to months and is more severe in immunocompromised and elderly individuals.

In most cases, diagnosis of primary varicella or herpes zoster is based on clinical findings, and confirmation by laboratory testing is not necessary.[57,58] Laboratory tests are of benefit the following circumstances: (1) Differential diagnosis of skin lesions in immunocompromised patients and neonates who would benefit from prompt initiation of antiviral therapy, (2) diagnosis confirmation in certain cases so that prophylactic administration of varicella immune globulin can be given to high risk contacts, and (3) determination of immune status.[58,59]

Rapid identification of the virus can be performed by microscopic examination of smears made from the base of the vesicles and stained with hematoxylin-eosin, Wright Giemsa, toluidine blue, or Papanicolaou's stain to reveal multinucleated giant cells called Tzanck cells; however, this procedure cannot distinguish between VZV and HSV.[58,59] Traditional viral culture is a time-consuming, intensive method; however, detection of VZV antigens by direct immunofluorescence in shell vial cultures may be made 24 to 48 hours after inoculation.[58,59] VZV DNA in skin lesions, peripheral blood mononuclear cells, cerebrospinal fluid, and tissues can be detected by PCR with a high degree of sensitivity and specificity. This method is being used increasingly in clinical settings.[55,58]

A number of serologic methods have been developed

to detect antibodies to VZV; of these, the ELISA is most commonly used.[58,59] Serology is of limited use in detecting current infections because accurate detection requires demonstration of a fourfold rise in antibody titer between acute and convalescent samples, a process that takes 2 to 4 weeks to perform.[58,60] IgM antibodies to VZV may not be detectable until the convalescent stage of illness; furthermore, they cannot distinguish between primary and reactivated infection.[59] Although IgM tests may have some use in the diagnosis of congenital infections,[59,60] they are difficult to perform and interpret and are available only in highly specialized laboratories.[61]

Serology is most useful in determining immunity to VZV or in confirming a history of VZV infection. More than 90 percent of the population has detectable antibody titers, mostly as a result of natural infection, but more recently resulting from immunization with the live attenuated varicella vaccine.[58] As a result of natural illness, varicella antibodies are produced within 2 weeks after appearance of the rash and persist for years.[60]

Viral Infections of Childhood

Rubella

The **rubella virus** is a single-stranded, enveloped RNA virus belonging to the family *Togaviridae*.[62,63] It is transmitted through respiratory droplets or through transplacental infection of the fetus during pregnancy.

This virus is the cause of the typically benign, self-limited disease known as German measles. Prior to widespread use of the rubella vaccine, this was mainly a disease of young children. However, it occurs most often now in young, unvaccinated adults.[62,64] Following an incubation period of 12 to 23 days, the virus replicates in the upper respiratory tract and cervical lymph nodes. It produces a characteristic erythematous, maculopapular rash, which appears first on the face, then spreads to the trunk and extremities, and usually resolves in 3 days.[63,65] In adolescents and adults, this is usually preceded by a prodrome of low-grade fever, malaise, swollen glands, and upper respiratory infection lasting 1 to 5 days.[64,65] However, 25 to 50 percent of rubella infections are asymptomatic.[64,65] The infection usually resolves without complications. A significant number of infected adult women experience arthralgias and arthritis, but chronic arthritis is rare.[63,65,66] Other clinical manifestations, including encephalitis, thrombocytopenia, and myocarditis, are infrequent.[63,66]

If rubella infection occurs during pregnancy, espe-cially the first trimester, severe consequences are likely to follow, including miscarriage, stillbirth, or the congenital rubella syndrome (CRS).[64–66] Infants born with CRS may present with a number of abnormalities, the most common of which are deafness, eye defects including cataracts and glaucoma, cardiac abnormalities, mental retardation, and motor disabilities. In mild cases, symptoms may not be recognized until months to years after birth.

A vaccine consisting of live, attenuated rubella virus was developed with the primary goal of preventing infection of pregnant women by preventing dissemination of the virus in the population as a whole.[64,66] The vaccine is part of the routine immunization schedule in infants and children and is usually given in combination with vaccines for measles and mumps (measles/mumps/rubella [MMR] vaccine). Following licensure of the vaccine in 1969, the number of rubella infections and cases of CRS in the United States has dropped dramatically, although outbreaks have occurred, particularly among unvaccinated adults or immigrants to this country.

Laboratory testing is helpful in confirming suspected cases of German measles, whose symptoms may mimic those of other viral infections. It is essential in the diagnosis of CRS and in the determination of immune status in other individuals. Rubella virus can be grown in cultures inoculated with respiratory secretions or other clinical specimens; however, growth is slow and does not produce characteristic cytopathic effect. Demonstration of the virus must therefore be accomplished by its ability to interfere with the growth of another virus added to the culture and by neutralization of this effect with specific rubella antibody.[67,68] For these reasons, viral culture is not routinely used to diagnose rubella infections, and serology testing is the method of choice.[62]

A number of methods have been developed to detect rubella antibodies, including hemagglutination inhibition (HI), complement fixation, radial hemolysis, latex agglutination, and ELISA.[67] Although HI was once the standard technique for measuring rubella antibodies, the most commonly used method today is the ELISA because of its sensitivity, specificity, ease of performance, and adaptability to automation.[64,66,68] Solid-phase capture ELISAs can be used to detect rubella-specific IgM antibodies.

Serology tests can be used in both the diagnosis of rubella infections and in screening for rubella immunity. IgM and IgG antibodies to rubella appear as the rash of German measles begins to fade.[62,67] IgM antibodies generally decline by 4 or 5 weeks but may persist in low levels for 6 months to a year in some cases. IgG antibodies provide immunity and persist for life. Primary rubella infection is indicated by the presence of rubella-specific IgM antibodies or by a fourfold rise in rubella-specific IgG antibody titers between acute- and convalescent-phase samples.[62,63,66,67] False-positive IgM test results have occurred in individuals with other viral infections, heterophile antibody, or rheumatoid factor;[66] the latter may be reduced by using IgM capture ELISAs. Presence of IgG antibodies indicates immunity to rubella as a result of natural infection or immunization.[62]

Laboratory confirmation of congenital rubella infection is indicated by presence of rubella-specific IgM antibodies in cord blood or serum from the infant.[67,68] To eliminate false-positive results, this can be confirmed by viral culture or by demonstration of persistently high titers of rubella IgG antibodies.[63,67] RT-PCR can be used to detect rubella RNA in samples of chorionic villi, placenta, amniotic fluid, fetal blood, lens tissue, or products of conception as an aid in prenatal or postnatal diagnosis.[62,67,68]

Rubeola

The rubeola virus is a single-stranded RNA virus belonging to the *Paramyxoviridae* family.[62,63] It is spread by direct contact with aerosolized droplets from the respiratory secretions of infected individuals.

Rubeola virus is the cause of the disease commonly known as measles. Following an incubation period of about 10 to 12 days, the virus produces prodromal symptoms of fever, cough, coryza (runny nose), and conjunctivitis, which last 2 to 4 days.[62,63,69] During the prodromal period, characteristic areas known as Koplik spots appear on the mucous membranes of the inner cheeks or lips; these appear as gray-to-white lesions against a bright red background and persist for several days. The typical rash of measles appears about 14 days after exposure to the virus and is characterized by an erythematous maculopapular eruption that begins on the face and head, spreads to the trunk and extremities, and lasts 5 to 6 days.

Measles is a systemic infection that can result in complications. These are most common in adults, children less than 5 years of age, and immunocompromised persons, and include otitis media, croup, bronchitis, pneumonia, and encephalitis.[62,69] Rarely, a fatal degenerative neurologic disease called subacute sclerosing panencephalitis (SSPE) can result from persistent replication of measles virus in the brain years after primary measles infection. Measles infection during pregnancy results in a higher risk of premature labor and spontaneous abortion, but unlike rubella, it is not associated with a defined pattern of congenital malformations in the newborn.[63,69]

The incidence of measles has been greatly reduced in developed nations of the world since the introduction of a live, attenuated measles virus vaccine. The vaccine was originally licensed in 1963; a more effective vaccine was licensed in 1968 and is used in the routine immunization schedule of infants and children, most commonly in combination with rubella and mumps (MMR).[64,69] Recommended administration of the vaccine is in two doses, the first between the ages of 12 and 15 months, and the second between ages 4 to 6; administration of the first dose prior to the age of 12 months may result in vaccine failure because of interference of the immune response by the presence of maternal antibodies.

The diagnosis of measles has typically been based on clinical presentation of the patient. However, this basis for diagnosis has been complicated by decreased ability of physicians to recognize the clinical features of measles because of a reduction in the number of cases as a result of the effectiveness of our immunization program.[62,70] In addition, atypical presentations of measles can occur in individuals who received the earlier form of measles vaccine, who have low antibody titers, or who are immunocompromised.[62,70] Laboratory tests are therefore of value in ensuring rapid, accurate diagnosis of sporadic cases; in addition, they are important for epidemiological surveillance and control of community outbreaks.[62]

Isolation of rubeola virus in conventional cell cultures is technically difficult and slow and is not generally performed in the routine diagnosis of measles but may be useful in epidemiologic surveillance of measles virus strains.[62,69] The optimal time to recover measles virus from nasopharyngeal secretions or blood is from the prodrome period up to 2 days after rash onset. From urine, it is 1 week after appearance of the rash.[62]

Serology testing provides the most practical means of confirming a measles diagnosis.[62] A variety of methods have been developed to detect rubeola antibodies, including hemagglutination inhibition, endpoint neutralization, complement fixation, indirect fluorescent antibody tests, and ELISA. The most commonly used is ELISA.[69,70] In conjunction with clinical symptoms, a diagnosis of measles is indicated by the presence of rubeola-specific IgM antibodies or by a fourfold rise in the rubeola-specific IgG antibody titer between serum samples collected soon after the onset of rash, and 10 to 30 days later.[69] The sensitivity of the IgM tests is highly dependent on the time of sample collection, with 3 to 11 days after the onset of rash being optimal.[62,71] Samples collected before 72 hours may yield false-negative results. The incidence of false-positive results because of rheumatoid factor can be reduced by the use of an IgM capture ELISA. Presence of rubeola-specific IgG antibodies indicates past infection or immunization, with subsequent immunity to measles.[62]

Other tests that have been developed to detect measles infection include fluorescent antibody staining of urine or nasopharyngeal specimens to identify measles antigen and RT-PCR to detect rubeola RNA in a variety of clinical specimens.[62]

Mumps

The mumps virus, like rubeola, is a single-stranded RNA virus that belongs to the *Paramyxoviridae* family. It is transmitted by infected respiratory droplets.[62,72] Following an incubation period of 12 to 25 days, the virus spreads to various tissues, including the meninges of the brain, and salivary glands, pancreas, testes, and ovaries and produces inflammation at those sites.[73] Inflammation of the parotid glands, or parotitis, is the most common clinical manifestation of mumps, occurring in 30 to 40 percent of cases.[64,73] The swelling of parotitis results in earache and tenderness of the jaw, which can be bilateral or unilateral; it resolves in 7 to 10 days. Although parotitis is the classic symptom of mumps, 15 to 20 percent of infections are asymptomatic, and another 40 to 50 percent have nonspecific or respiratory symptoms with no parotitis.[64,73]

Complications of mumps infections include asymptomatic meningitis (50 to 60 percent of cases), symptomatic meningitis (15 percent of patients), testicular inflammation (in up to 50 percent of postpubertal males), ovarian inflammation (in about 5 percent of postpubertal females), and deafness (in about 1 case per 20,000).[73] Pancreatitis, encephalitis, and polyarthritis occur infrequently but are important complications of mumps.[62] Mumps infection in pregnant women results in increased risk for fetal death when it occurs in the first trimester of pregnancy, but it is not associated with congenital abnormalities.[64] The number of mumps cases in the United States has declined steadily since the introduction of a live attenuated mumps virus vaccine in 1967 and its routine use in childhood immunization schedules in 1977.[64]

The diagnosis of mumps is usually made on the basis of clinical symptoms, especially parotitis and does not require laboratory confirmation.[62,73] However, laboratory testing is very useful in cases in which parotitis is absent or when differentiation from other causes of parotitis is required. Mumps virus can be isolated within the first few days of illness from saliva, urine, cerebrospinal fluid, or swabs from the area around the excretory duct of the parotid gland, but growth of the virus may be slow and difficult and is not performed on a routine basis.[62,72,73]

Serologic tests are the method of choice in confirmation of a mumps diagnosis, when indicated.[62,72,73] Although a variety of methods have been developed to detect mumps antibodies, including complement fixation, hemagglutination inhibition, hemolysis-in-gel, neutralization assays, immunofluorescence assay, and ELISA, the latter two methods are used most commonly because they are sensitive, specific, cost effective, and readily performed by the routine clinical laboratory. Use of solid-phase IgM capture assays reduces the incidence of false-positive results because of rheumatoid factor. Current or recent infection is indicated by the presence of mumps-specific IgM antibody in a single serum sample or by at least a fourfold rise in specific IgG antibody between two specimens collected during the acute and convalescent phases of illness. Cross-reactivity between antibodies to mumps and parainfluenza viruses has been reported in tests for IgG, but is usually not a problem because of differentiation in clinical symptoms.[62,72] IgM antibodies can be detected within the first 5 days of illness. They peak at 1 week, and persist for at least 6 weeks.[72] IgG antibodies persist for a long period of time and indicate immunity to mumps.

Fluorescence antibody staining for mumps antigens and RT-PCR to detect mumps virus RNA in clinical specimens have been developed, but are not widely available at this time.[62]

Human T Cell Lymphotropic Viruses

Human T cell lymphotropic virus type I (HTLV-I) and human T cell lymphotropic virus type II (HTLV-II) are both classified as retroviruses. These viruses have RNA as their nucleic acid and an enzyme called reverse transcriptase, whose function is to transcribe the viral RNA into DNA. The DNA then becomes integrated into the host cell's genome. The viruses can then proceed to complete their replication cycle or remain in a latent state within infected cells for a prolonged period of time. Both viruses infect T lymphocytes, cause T cell proliferation, and they have the potential to establish persistent infection.

Both viruses have three structural genes, called gag, pol, and env, and two major regulatory genes, called tax and rev.[74,75] In HTLV-I, the gag gene codes for the viral core proteins p19, p24, and p15, the pol gene codes for the reverse transcriptase enzyme, and the env gene codes for the envelope glycoproteins gp46 and gp21.

HTLV-I can be transmitted by three major routes: bloodborne (mainly through transfusions containing cellular components or through intravenous drug abuse), sexual, and mother-to-child (mainly through breast feeding).[74,76,77] HTLV-II is thought to be transmitted by the same routes. HTLV-I infection is endemic in southern Japan, the Caribbean, portions of Africa, the Middle East, South America, the Pacific Melanesian Islands, and Papua New Guinea.[74,76] In the United States and Europe, infections result mainly from immigrants from endemic areas. HTLV-II infections are highest in various Native American populations and intravenous drug abusers in North America, certain European nations, and Southeast Asia.[78]

HTLV-I is known to cause two diseases: adult T cell leukemia/lymphoma (ATL), a mature T cell non-Hodgkin's lymphoma with a leukemic phase of circulating, activated CD4+/CD25+ T cells, and HTLV-I-associated myelopathy or tropical spastic paraparesis (HAM or TSP), a slowly progressing neurologic disorder.[74,77] These diseases appear in 2 to 5 percent of individuals infected with HTLV-I,[74] and symptoms do not appear until several years after the initial infection. Evidence suggests that HTLV-I is also associated with a variety of chronic inflammatory or autoimmune disorders such as infective dermatitis, uveitis, and Sjögren's syndrome.[74,77] The role of HTLV-II in causing human disease has not been clearly defined, but evidence suggests that this virus may also be associated with lymphoproliferative, neurologic, and inflammatory disorders.[77,78]

Serologic testing plays an important role in testing for HTLV-I and HTLV-II infections because culture of the viruses requires sophisticated techniques that cannot be performed in routine clinical laboratories.[77] ELISA, particle agglutination assay, and immunofluorescence assay have all been developed to screen for HTLV-I antibodies, with ELISA being the method of choice in the United States.[75,79] This method is used to detect HTLV-I infection in individuals and to screen blood donors. The ELISA method uses HTLV-I–infected cell lysates and recombinant proteins or synthetic peptides as the source of antigen bound to the solid phase.[75,80] This assay is also used to screen for HTLV-II antibodies because there is a significant amount of cross-reactivity between HTLV-I and HTLV-II due to their structural homology. The assay cannot distinguish between HTLV-I and HTLV-II infection. Because false-positive results may also occur, any sample producing a reactive result in the initial ELISA screen is retested by ELISA and subsequently tested by a more specific, confirmatory method.

The confirmatory method of choice is the Western blot, which identifies antibodies to separate HTLV antigens. Specimens are considered positive for HTLV-I or HTLV-II by this test if bands representing antibodies to gag protein p24, and the env glycoprotein gp46 or an envelope precursor, gp61/68 are present.[75,79] Differentiation of HTLV-I from HTLV-II antibodies can then be performed using modified ELISA or Western blot techniques.[75] PCR can be used to detect HTLV-I or HTLV-II RNA in various samples in order to differentiate between the two viruses, to demonstrate presence of virus in different tissues, and to assess patient responses to therapy.[77]

Other Viral Infections

See Table 21–4 for laboratory methods used to detect infections with other viruses and their clinical significance.

SUMMARY

Serologic tests for viral antibodies are among the most important tests performed by the clinical immunology laboratory. These tests can be used to indicate current infections, congenital infections, and previous exposure to viruses or the vaccines used to prevent viral infections with subsequent immunity.

The hepatitis viruses are those whose primary effect is inflammation of the liver. Hepatitis A and hepatitis E are transmitted by the fecal-oral route, while hepatitis B, hepatitis C, hepatitis D, and hepatitis G are transmitted primarily by the parenteral route. Hepatitis B, hepatitis C, and hepatitis D may lead to chronic infections. The method of choice to test for hepatitis infections is the ELISA. IgM anti-HAV antibodies indicate current or recent hepatitis A infection, while IgG antibodies indicate immunity to hepatitis A. Hepatitis B infection is indicated by the presence of the antigen HBsAg; HBe Ag indicates high infectivity. IgM antibodies to hepatitis B core antigen are present in acute hepatitis B, while IgG anti-HBc is present during past or chronic hepatitis B infection. Antibodies to HBsAg can be present as a result of past hepatitis B infection or immunization with the hepatitis B vaccine and indicate immunity. Exposure to hepatitis C virus is detected by ELISA measuring anti-HCV, and HCV infection is confirmed by RIBA testing or RT-PCR. Hepatitis D occurs as super- or coinfection with hepatitis B and is indicated by antibodies to hepatitis D. Serologic tests for hepatitis E and hepatitis G have been developed but are not widely available.

There are eight human herpes viruses, including the Epstein-Barr virus, cytomegalovirus, and varicella-zoster virus. The Epstein-Barr virus is the cause of

TABLE 21–4. Other Important Viruses Detected by Viral and Serologic Tests

Virus	Route of Infection; Latent Site	Clinical Manifestations	Susceptible Individual	Viral Tests	Serologic Tests
Adenovirus	Respiratory; latent in adenoidal and tonsillar tissues	Acute respiratory disease, keratoconjunctivitis, pharyngoconjunctival fever, hemorrhagic cystitis, gastroenteritis	Swimmers in improperly chlorinated pools; industrial workers exposed to eye trauma; individuals in crowded conditions; school children; immunocom-promised patients	Culture; electron microscopy DNA probes	EIA, IFA, RIA, HI
Arbovirus	Skin by biting mosquitoes, ticks, flies, or other arthropods	Fever encephalitis, aseptic meningitis, hemorrhagic fever, rash, acute arthritis, hepatitis, retinitis	Seasonal exposure in specific ecologic habitats and geographic locations	EIA antigen capture assay; PCR; RNA probes	EIA, IFA, HI
Influenza	Respiratory; airborne	Fever, chills, fatigue, headache, myalgia, cough; pulmonary complications of viral or bacterial origin	Seasonal in winter, spring; all individuals susceptible	Fluorescent antibody staining of nasal secretions; EIA antigen capture assay; culture, rapid culture shell vials	EIA, HI
Rotavirus	Fecal-oral route	Infectious gastroenteritis	Seasonal in winter, spring; infants and young children	Direct or indirect EIA; electron microscopy	EIA
Mumps	Respiratory; airborne	Bilateral or unilateral parotitis; more serious manifestations: meningitis, encephalitis, epididymoorchitis, oophoritis, polyarthritis, pancreatitis	Young children	Culture, CF, HI, neutralization	EIA, HI, CF, neutraliza-tion, IF
Measles	Respiratory; airborne; latent CNS involvement	Sneezing, cough, fever, redness of eyes and photophobia, Koplik's spots on mouth epithelium, macular or maculopapular rash; more serious complications include acute encephalitis, postinfectious encephalomyelitis	Young children	Electron microscopy, IF, culture	HI, CF, EIA

DNA = Deoxyribonucleic acid; EIA = enzyme immunoassay; IFA = immunofluorescence assay; RIA = radioimmunoassay; HI = hemagglutination inhibition; PCR = polymerase chain reaction; RNA = ribonucleic acid; CF = complement fixation; IF = immunofluorescence; CNS = central nervous system.

infectious mononucleosis, a number of hematologic and nonhematologic malignancies, and lymphoproliferative disorders in immunosuppressed individuals. Most patients with infectious mononucleosis produce heterophile antibodies, which can react with antigens from beef, horse, or sheep red blood cells. Although these antibodies were once routinely screened for by the Monospot test, they are now commonly detected by rapid immunochromatographic or agglutination methods used to detect antibodies to bovine antigens. ELISA or immunofluorescence assay (IFA) tests for EBV-specific antigens are used to detect heterophile-negative cases of infectious mononucleosis and to diagnose other EBV-associated diseases.

CMV infection is asymptomatic in most healthy individuals, but may produce a mononucleosis-like syndrome in some. The virus can remain latent for years and become reactivated later in life. CMV infection can have more serious consequences in immunocompromised individuals or congenitally infected infants. Active CMV infection is best detected by shell vial assays to identify CMV antigens by immunofluorescence, CMV antigenemia assays for pp65 antigen, or molecular assays to detect CMV viral load. Serologic assays for CMV antibody are most helpful in documenting a past infection in potential blood and organ donors.

The primary infection with varicella virus causes chickenpox, while reactivation of the virus in nerve cells supplying the skin causes shingles. Diagnosis of current varicella virus infection is usually based on clinical findings, but detection of varicella virus antigens by shell vial assay and immunofluorescence or of varicella DNA by PCR may be helpful in some clinical settings. Serologic methods, most commonly ELISA, are used mainly to document immunity to varicella virus.

Immunization programs have greatly reduced the incidence of three childhood infections: rubella, rubeola, and mumps. Rubella infection is the cause of German measles, but can result in severe congenital abnormalities if it occurs during pregnancy. Rubeola viruses cause measles, a systemic infection that can cause complications in some individuals. Mumps virus is the cause of mumps, whose classic feature is swelling of the parotid glands; complications may occur. Although the diagnosis of these three infections is usually based on clinical findings, laboratory testing may be helpful in confirmation. Because culture of these viruses is slow and difficult, serology is most often used for this purpose. Current infections are indicated by the presence of IgM antibodies specific for the appropriate virus or by a fourfold rise in virus-specific IgG antibodies in two separate specimens collected during the acute and convalescent phases of disease.

Testing for IgG antibodies is most commonly performed, however, to screen for immunity to these viruses.

The human T cell lymphotropic viruses, HTLV-I and HTLV-II are retroviruses that infect T lymphocytes. HTLV-I is the cause of adult T cell leukemia/lymphoma, and HTLV-I-associated myelopathy, also known as tropical spastic paraparesis, while the disease associations of HTLV-II are not completely understood. ELISA tests are used routinely to screen blood donors for antibodies to the cross-reacting HTLV-I and HTLV-II viruses and to detect exposure to HTLV in other individuals. Positive results are confirmed by Western blot. Specialized serologic or molecular tests can be performed to differentiate between HTLV-I and HTLV-II infection.

Serology tests have also been developed to detect exposure to other viruses, including adenoviruses, arbovirus, herpes simplex-1 and -2, parainfluenza, parvovirus B19, respiratory syncytial virus, and rotavirus.

Case Studies

1. A 25-year-old male had been experiencing flulike symptoms, loss of appetite, nausea, and constipation for 2 weeks. His abdomen was tender, and his urine was dark in color. Initial testing revealed elevations in his serum alanine aminotransferase (ALT) and aspartate aminotransferase (AST) levels.

Questions

   a. What laboratory tests should be used to screen this patient for viral hepatitis?
   b. If the patient tested positive for hepatitis B, which tests should be used to monitor his condition?
   c. If the patient developed chronic hepatitis B, which markers would be present in his serum?

2. An 5-lb infant was born with microcephaly, purpuric rash, low platelet count, cardiovascular defects, and a cataract in the left eye. The infant's mother recalled experiencing flulike symptoms and a mild skin rash early in her pregnancy. She had not sought medical attention at the time. The infant's physician ordered tests to investigate the cause of the newborn's symptoms.

Questions

   a. What virus is the most likely cause of the infant's symptoms?
   b. What serology test would you suggest that the doctor order on the mother to support your suggested diagnosis?
   c. What serology test should be performed on the infant's serum to support this diagnosis?

Exercise: Testing for the Heterophile Antibody of Infectious Mononucleosis by the MONO-plus® Test

PRINCIPLE

The MONO-plus® test uses direct solid-phase immunoassay technology for the qualitative detection of infectious mononucleosis (IM) heterophile antibodies in human serum, plasma, or whole blood. In the test procedure, 10 μL of serum or plasma is added to the sample well (S) located directly below the test region (T). For the fingertip or whole blood, 25 μL of blood is collected in a capillary tube and added to the sample well (S). If IM-specific heterophile antibody is present in the sample, it will be captured in the antigen band (bovine erythrocyte extracts) impregnated in the test membrane. The developer solution is then added to the sample well (S). As the specimen and the developer solution move by capillary action to the antigen band, the solution mobilizes the dye conjugated to the anti-human IgM antibodies. Visualization of the antigen band in the test region (T) will occur only when the antibody-dye conjugate binds to the IM-specific heterophile antibody, which has been bound to the extracted antigen obtained from bovine erythrocytes. As the antibody-dye conjugate continues to move along the test membrane, it will bind to another band located in the control region (C) to generate a colored band regardless of the presence of IM heterophile antibodies in the sample. Therefore, the presence of two colored bands, one in the test region (T) and the other in the control region (C), indicates a positive result, while the presence of a colored band in the control region (C) only indicates a negative result.

REAGENTS, MATERIALS, AND EQUIPMENT

MONO-plus® test kit (Wampole Laboratories, Princeton, N.J. 08540), containing:

> MONO-plus® test devices
> MONO-plus® Developer Solution
> MONO-plus® Negative Control serum
> MONO-plus® Positive Control serum
> Capillary tubes
> Micropipettes (optional)
> Patient serum, plasma, or whole blood to be tested

PROCEDURE*

Capillary tube directions:

a. Insert the unmarked end of the capillary tube into the rubber bulb far enough to penetrate the thin membrane within the bulb.

b. Fill the tube with sample by capillary action to the appropriate line (black line for whole blood = 25 μL, or red line for serum/plasma = 10 μL). Do not draw specimen into bulb. If specimen is drawn into bulb, discard the bulb and use a new one.

c. Place finger on hole in bulb.

d. Squeeze bulb to empty blood into the upper end of the sample well (S) of the test device.

e. Save the bulb and discard the used capillary into the biohazard waste.

1. Step 1. Remove 3 test devices from their packaging and label "Positive Control," "Negative Control," or "Patient Specimen." Using the capillary tubes provided in the kit or separate micropipettes, place the positive control, negative control, and patient specimen into the upper end of the sample well of the appropriately labeled test device. For each control, serum, or plasma specimen, pipette 10 μL; for each sample of whole blood, pipette 25 μL.

2. Step 2. Add 2 to 3 drops of developer solution into the lower end of the sample well (S).

3. Step 3. Read test results at 8 minutes. A strong positive result may appear in less than 3 minutes. Waiting 8 minutes is required to report a negative result. Results are stable up to 15 minutes after the addition of the developer solution.

INTERPRETATION OF RESULTS

Positive

One pink-purple colored horizontal band each in the test region (T) and the control region (C) indicate that IM-specific heterophile antibodies have been detected. **NOTE:** A positive result may be read as soon as a distinct pink-purple colored band appears in the test region (T) and in the control region (C). Any shade of pink-purple colored horizontal band in the test region (T) should be reported as a positive result. The intensity of the colored band in the test region (T) may be different than the intensity of the band in the control region (C).

---

*MONO-plus® kit package insert, Wampole Laboratories, Princeton, N.J. 08540, ©2000. MONO-plus® is manufactured by Princeton Biomeditech, Monmouth Junction, N.J. 08852.

Negative

One pink-purple colored band in the control region (C), with no distinct colored horizontal band in the test region (T) other than faint background color, indicates the IM-specific heterophile antibodies have not been detected.

Invalid

A distinct colored horizontal band in the control region (C) should always appear. The test is invalid if no such band forms in the control region (C).

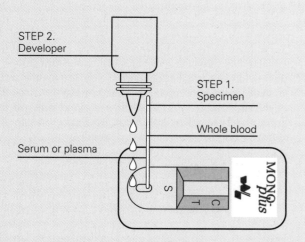

FIG. 21-4. MONO-plus® test device. For each control, serum, or plasma specimen, 10 μL is pipetted into well. If whole blood is used, 25 μL is added. Then 2 to 3 drops of developer is placed into sample well.

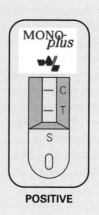

FIG. 21-5. Positive.

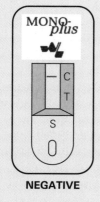

FIG. 21-6. Negative.

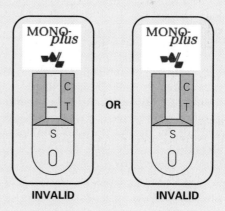

FIG. 21-7. Invalid or invalid.

Exercise: Testing for the Heterophile Antibody of Infectious Mononucleosis by the Paul-Bunnell Test

PRINCIPLE

This test is used to determine the titer of the heterophile antibody in patients with infectious mononucleosis. Serial dilutions of patient serum are prepared and incubated with sheep red blood cells. The titer of the antibody is the reciprocal of the last dilution to show agglutination of the red blood cells.

REAGENTS, MATERIALS, AND EQUIPMENT

0.9-percent saline solution

Sheep erythrocytes stored in Alsever's solution Refrigerate until use

Positive control serum containing heterophile antibody of infectious mononucleosis

Patient serum to be tested

13- × 100-mm glass test tubes

0.1-mL and 1.0-mL pipettes

PROCEDURE[81]

1. Inactivate complement in sera to be tested by heating in a 56°C water bath for 30 minutes.
2. Place sheep red blood cells into a tube and wash the cells three times in saline.
3. Prepare 5 mL of a 2-percent sheep red blood cell suspension by pipetting 0.1 mL of washed, packed red blood cells into 4.9 mL of saline.
4. Set up and label 2 rows of 10 test tubes in a rack. One row is for a positive-control serum and the other for the patient serum to be tested. Label the control tubes C1-C10, and the patient tubes, P1-P10.
5. Pipette 0.4 mL of saline in the first tube of each row and 0.25 mL of saline in each remaining tube.
6. Pipette 0.1 mL of positive control serum into tube #1 of the control row.
7. Mix and serially transfer 0.25 mL through tube #9, discarding 0.25 mL from tube #9. *Tube #10 of this row contains no serum and serves as a negative control.*

8. Obtain a sample of patient serum to be tested. Pipette 0.1 mL of patient serum into tube #1 of the patient row.
9. Mix and serially transfer 0.25 mL through tube #10, discarding 0.25 mL from tube #10.
10. Add 0.1 mL of the 2-percent sheep red blood cell suspension (prepared in step #3 above) to each tube in the control and patient rows.
11. Shake the tubes to obtain an even mixture. Cover the tubes with parafilm and incubate at room temperature for at least 15 minutes. A more accurate reading may be obtained by allowing the tubes to incubate for 2 hours.
12. Following the incubation period, read each tube individually for macroscopic agglutination, as follows: gently shake the tube to resuspend the red blood cells, tilt the tube, and hold up to light. Compare each tube to the negative control tube and record results.

INTERPRETATION OF RESULTS

The antibody titer is reported as the reciprocal of the dilution in the last tube, which shows visible agglutination (Fig. 21–8). Titers less than or equal to 56 are considered normal.

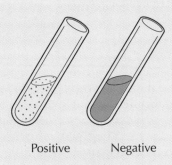

FIG. 21–8. Interpretation of Paul-Bunnell test results.

Review Questions

1. An individual with hepatomegaly, jaundice, and elevated liver enzymes has the following laboratory results: IgM anti-HAV (negative), HBsAg (positive), IgM anti-HBc (positive), and anti-HCV (negative). These findings support a diagnosis of:
   a. Hepatitis A
   b. Acute hepatitis B
   c. Chronic hepatitis B
   d. Hepatitis C

2. Which of the following hepatitis viruses is transmitted by the fecal-oral route?
   a. Hepatitis B
   b. Hepatitis C
   c. Hepatitis D
   d. Hepatitis E

3. The most useful application of testing for HCV RNA is to:
   a. Screen for hepatitis C
   b. Differentiate hepatitis C from hepatitis B infection
   c. Differentiate acute HCV infection from chronic HCV infection
   d. Monitor hepatitis C patients on antiviral therapy

4. The serum of an individual who received all doses of the hepatitis B vaccine should contain
   a. Anti-HBs
   b. Anti-HBe
   c. Anti-HBc
   d. All of the above

5. A 12-year-old girl presented to her physician with a sore throat, lymphadenopathy, and fatigue. Her laboratory results were: 5000 lymphocytes/μL with 10-percent atypical lymphocytes, CMV antibody negative, and heterophile antibody screen negative. These laboratory results
   a. Confirm a diagnosis of infectious mononucleosis
   b. Indicate that the diagnosis is not infectious mononucleosis because the heterophile antibody screen is negative
   c. Suggest a diagnosis of infectious mononucleosis, but should be followed by a heterophile antibody titer to strengthen the diagnosis
   d. Suggest a diagnosis of infectious mononucleosis, but should be followed by a test for IgM anti-VCA to strengthen the diagnosis

6. In the laboratory, heterophile antibodies are routinely detected by their reaction with:
   a. B lymphocytes
   b. Bovine erythrocyte antigens
   c. Sheep erythrocyte antigens
   d. Epstein-Barr virus antigens

7. Presence of IgM antirubella antibodies in the serum from an infant born with a rash suggests:
   a. A diagnosis of measles
   b. A diagnosis of German measles
   c. Congenital infection with the rubella virus
   d. Passive transfer of maternal antibodies to the infant's serum

8. A pregnant woman is exposed to a child with a rubella infection. She had no clinical symptoms, but had a rubella titer performed. The titer was 1:8. Three weeks later, she had a repeat test, and the titer was 1:128. She still had no clinical symptoms. Was the laboratory finding indicative of rubella infection?
   a. No, the titer must be greater than 256 to be significant.
   b. No, the change in titer is not significant if no clinical signs are present.
   c. Yes, a greater than fourfold rise in titer indicates early infection.
   d. Yes, but clinical symptoms must also correlate with laboratory findings.

9. The most common cause of congenital infections is:
   a. CMV
   b. Rubella
   c. VZV
   d. HTLV-I

10. A positive result on a screening test for HTLV-I antibody:
   a. Is highly specific for HTLV-I infection
   b. Cannot distinguish between HTLV-I and HTLV-II infection
   c. Must be confirmed by PCR
   d. Must be confirmed by viral culture

References

1. Abbott Diagnostics Educational Services: Hepatitis Learning Guide. Abbott Diagnostics, Abbott Park, Ill., 1998, pp 1–68.
2. Miller, LE, Ludke, HR, Peacock, JE, and Tomar, RH: Manual of Laboratory Immunology, ed. 2. Lea & Febiger, Philadelphia, 1991, pp 242–244, 248–253.
3. Koff, RS: Hepatitis A. Lancet 351:1643–1649, 1998.
4. Winn, WC: Enterically transmitted hepatitis. Clin Lab Med 19(3): 661–673, 1999.
5. Lemon, SM: Type A viral hepatitis: Epidemiology, diagnosis, and prevention. Clin Chem 43(8B):1494–1499, 1997.
6. Moyer, L, Warwick, M, and Mahoney, FJ: Prevention of hepatitis A virus infection. Am Fam Physician 54(1):107–114, 1996.
7. Krawczynski, K, Aggarwal, R, and Kamili, S: Hepatitis E. Infect Dis Clin North Am 14(3):669–687, 2000.
8. Centers for Disease Control and Prevention: Viral Hepatitis. Available from: http://www.cdc.gov/ncidod/diseases/hepatitis [Accessed October 12, 2000].
9. Zimmerman, RK, Ruben, FL, and Ahwesh, ER: Hepatitis B virus infection, hepatitis B vaccine, and hepatitis B immune globulin. J Fam Pract 45(4):295–315, 1997.
10. Cardo, DM, and Bell, DM: Bloodborne pathogen transmission in health care workers. Infect Dis Clin North Am 11(2):331–346, 1997.
11. Gitlin, N: Hepatitis B: Diagnosis, prevention, and treatment. Clin Chem 43:8(B):1500–1506, 1997.
12. Shapiro, CN, Mahoney, FJ, and Mast, EE: Hepatitis B. Available from: http://www.cdc.gov/nip/publications/manual/wpd/hepb.wpd [Accessed May 17, 1999].
13. Evans, AA, and London, WT: Epidemiology of hepatitis B. In Zuckerman, AJ, and Thomas, HC (eds): Viral Hepatitis, ed. 2. Churchill Livingstone, London, 1998, pp 107–114.
14. Kann, M, and Gerlich, W: Hepadnaviridae: Structure and molecular virology. In Zuckerman, AJ, and Thomas, HC (eds): Viral Hepatitis, ed. 2. Churchill Livingstone, London, 1998, pp 77–105.
15. Dienstag, JL, and Isselbacher, KJ: Acute viral hepatitis. In Fauci, AS, Braunwald, E, Isselbacher, KJ, et al (eds): Harrison's Principles of Internal Medicine, ed. 14. McGraw-Hill, New York, 1998, pp 1677–1692.
16. Decker, RH: Diagnosis of acute and chronic hepatitis B. In Zuckerman, AJ, and Thomas, HC (eds): Viral Hepatitis, ed. 2. Churchill Livingstone, London, 1998, pp 201–215.
17. Centers for Disease Control and Prevention: Recommendations of the Advisory Committee on Immunization Practices (ACIP) and the Hospital Infection Control Practices Advisory Committee (HICPAC). MMWR 46 (RR-18):1, 1997.
18. Weber, B, et al: Improved detection of hepatitis B surface antigen by a new rapid automated assay. J Clin Microbiology 37(8):2639–2647, 1999.
19. Pawlotsky, JM, et al: Routine detection and quantification of hepatitis B virus DNA in clinical laboratories: Performance of three commercial assays. J Virological Methods 85 (1–2):11–21, 2000.
20. EASL Consensus Panel: EASL International consensus conference on Hepatitis C: Consensus statement. J Hepatol 31(suppl 1):3–8, 1999.
21. Marcellin, P: Hepatitis C: The clinical spectrum of disease. J Hepatol 31(suppl 1):9–16, 1999.
22. Catalina, G, and Navarro, V: Hepatitis C: A challenge for the generalist. Hosp Prac 35(1):97–98, 101–104, 107–108, 2000.
23. Lam, NP: Hepatitis C: Natural history, diagnosis, and management. Am J Health-Syst Pharm 56:961–973, 1999.
24. Morton, TA, and Kelen, GD: Hepatitis C. Ann Emerg Med 31:381–390, 1998.
25. Urdea, MS, et al: Hepatitis C—diagnosis and monitoring. Clin Chem 43 (8B):1507–1511, 1997.
26. Pawlotsky, JM: Diagnostic tests for Hepatitis C. J Hepatol 31(suppl 1):71–79, 1999.
27. Simons, JN, Desai, SM, and Mushahwar, IK: The GB viruses. Curr Top Microbiol Immunol 242:341–375, 2000.
28. Tanaka, T, Hess, G, Tanaka, S, and Kohara, M: The significance of hepatitis G virus infection in patients with non-A to C hepatic diseases. Hepatogastroenterology 46:1870–1873, 1999.
29. Tacke, M, et al: Detection of antibodies to a putative hepatitis G virus envelope protein. Lancet 349:318–320, 1997.
30. Nauschuetz, WF: Clinical Virology. In Mahon, CR, and Manuselis, G (eds): Textbook of Diagnostic Virology, ed. 2. WB Sanders, Philadelphia, 2000, pp 866–870.
31. Cohen, JI: Epstein-Barr virus infection. N Eng J Med 343(7):481–492, 2000.
32. Kawa, K: Epstein-Barr Virus-associated diseases in humans. Int J Hematol 71:108–117, 2000.
33. Okano, M: Epstein-Barr virus infection and its role in the expanding spectrum of human diseases. Acta Paediatr 87:11–18, 1998.
34. Peter, J, and Ray, CG: Infectious mononucleosis. Pediatr Rev 19(8):276–279, 1998.
35. Hickey, SM, and Strasburger, VC: What every pediatrician should know about infectious mononucleosis in adolescents. Pediatr Clin North Am 44(6):1541–1556, 1997.
36. Godshall, SE, and Kirchner, JT: Infectious mononucleosis: Complexities of a common syndrome. Postgrad Med 107(7):175–179, 183–184, 186, 2000.
37. Okano, M, Gross, TG: A review of Epstein-Barr virus infection in patients with immunodeficiency disorders. Am J Med Sci 319(6): 392–396, 2000.
38. Jenson, HB, Ench, Y, and Sumaya, CV: Epstein-Barr virus. In Rose, NR, et al (eds): Manual of Clinical Laboratory Immunology, ed. 5. ASM Press, Washington, D.C., 1997, pp 634–643.
39. Linderholm M, et al: Comparative evaluation of nine kits for rapid diagnosis of infectious mononucleosis and Epstein-Barr virus-specific serology. J Clin Microbiol 32(1):259–261, 1994.
40. Smith, MA, and Brennessel, DJ: Cytomegalovirus. Infect Dis Clin North Am 8(2):427–438, 1994.
41. Gershon, AA, Gold, E, and Nankervis, GA: Cytomegalovirus. In Evans, AS, and Kaslow, RA (eds): Viral Infections of Humans, ed. 4. Plenum Medical Book Co, New York, 1997, pp 229–251.
42. Nauschuetz, WF: Clinical Virology. In Mahon, CR, and Manuselis, G: Textbook of Diagnostic Microbiology, ed. 2. WB Saunders, Philadelphia, 2000, pp 833–874.
43. Yanowitz, J, and Grose, C: Congenital Infections. In Storch, GA: Essentials of Diagnostic Virology. Churchill Livingstone, New York, 2000, pp 187–201.
44. Lazzarotto, T, et al: Prenatal indicators of congenital cytomegalovirus infection. J Pediatr 137(1):90–95, 2000.
45. Guerra, B, et al: Prenatal diagnosis of symptomatic congenital cytomegalovirus infection. Am J Obstet Gynecol 183(2):476–482, 2000.
46. Halwachs-Baumann, G, et al: Screening and diagnosis of congenital cytomegalovirus infection: A 5-y study. Scan J Infect Dis 32:137–142, 2000.
47. Scott, LL, Hollier, LM, and Dias, K: Perinatal herpesvirus infections: Herpes simplex, varicella, and cytomegalovirus. Infect Dis Clin North Am 11(1):27–53, 1997.
48. Waner, JL, and Stewart, JA: Cytomegalovirus. In Rose, NR et al (eds): Manual of Clinical Laboratory Immunology, ed. 5. ASM Press, Washington, D.C., 1997, pp 644–648.
49. Zaia, JA: Diagnosis of CMV. Pediatr Infect Dis J 18(2):153–154, 1999.
50. Smith, TS, et al: New developments in the diagnosis of viral diseases. Infect Dis Clin North Am 7(2):183, 1993.
51. Landry, ML, and Ferguson, D: 2-Hour cytomegalovirus pp65 antigenemia assay for rapid quantitation of cytomegalovirus in blood samples. J Clin Microbiol 38(1):427–428, 2000.

52. Caliendo, AM, et al: Comparison of quantitative cytomegalovirus (CMV) PCR in plasma and CMV antigenemia assay: Clinical utility of the prototype AMPLICOR CMV MONITOR test in transplant recipients. J Clin Microbiol 38(6):2122–2127, 2000.

53. Rao, M, et al: Cytomegalovirus infection in a seroendemic renal transplant population: A longitudinal study of virological markers. Nephron 84:367–373, 2000.

54. Blank, BS, et al: Value of different assays for detection of human cytomegalovirus (HCMV) in predicting the development of HCMV disease in human immunodeficiency virus-infected patients. J Clin Microbiol 38(2):563–569, 2000.

55. McCrary, ML, Severson, J, and Trying, SK: Varicella zoster virus. J Am Acad Dermatol 41:1–14, 1999.

56. Stover, BH, and Bratcher, DF: Varicella-zoster virus: Infection, control, and prevention. Am J Infect Control 26(3):369–381, 1998.

57. Cohen, JI, et. al: Recent advances in varicella-zoster virus infection. Ann Intern Med 130 (11):922–932, 1999.

58. Liesegang, TJ: Varicella zoster viral disease. Mayo Clin Proc 74:983–398, 1999.

59. Breuer, J, Harper, DR, and Kangro, HO: Varicella zoster. In Zuckerman, AJ, Banatvala, JE, and Pattison, JR: Principles and Practice of Clinical Virology, ed. 4. John Wiley & Sons, Ltd, Chichester, England, 2000, pp 47–77.

60. Chapman, SJ: Varicella in pregnancy. Seminars in Perinatology 22(4):339–346, 1998.

61. Brunell, PA: Varicella zoster virus. In Rose, NR, et al (eds): Manual of Clinical Laboratory Immunology, ed. 5. ASM Press, Washington, D.C., 1997, pp 339–346.

62. Hodinka, RL, and Moshal, KL: Childhood infections. In Storch, GA: Essentials of Diagnostic Virology. Churchill Livingstone, New York, 2000, pp 167–186.

63. Rosa, C: Rubella and rubeola. Semin Perinatol 22(4):318–322, 1998.

64. Centers for Disease Control and Prevention: Measles, mumps, and rubella—vaccine use and strategies for elimination of measles, rubella, and congenital rubella syndrome and control of mumps: recommendations of the advisory committee on immunization practices (ACIP). MMWR 47(RR-8):1, 1998.

65. Kimberlin, DW: Rubella immunization. Pediatr Ann 26(6):366–370, 1997.

66. Centers for Disease Control and Prevention: Rubella. Available from: http://www.cdc.gov/nip/publications/pink/rubella.pdf [Accessed November 7, 2000].

67. Mahony, JB, and Chernesky, MA: Rubella virus. In Rose, NR, et al (eds): Manual of Clinical Laboratory Immunology, ed. 5. ASM Press, Washington, D.C., 1997, pp 693–698.

68. Best, JM, and Banatvala, JE: Rubella. In Zuckerman, AJ, Banatvala, JE, and Pattison, JR: Principles and Practice of Clinical Virology, ed. 4. John Wiley & Sons, Ltd, Chichester, England, 2000, pp 387–418.

69. Centers for Disease Control and Prevention: Measles. Available from: http://www.cdc.gov/nip/publications/pink/meas.pdf [Accessed November 7, 2000].

70. Black, FL: Measles and mumps. In Rose, NR, et al (eds): Manual of Clinical Laboratory Immunology, ed. 5. ASM Press, Washington, D.C., 1997, pp 688–692.

71. Helfand, RF, et al: Diagnosis of measles with an IgM capture EIA: The optimal timing of specimen collection after rash onset. J Infect Dis 175:195–199, 1997.

72. Holmes, SJ: Mumps. In Evans, AS, and Kaslow, RA (eds): Viral Infections of Humans: Epidemiology and Control, ed. 4. Plenum Medical Book Co, New York, 1997, pp 531–550.

73. Centers for Disease Control and Prevention: Measles. Available from: http://www.cdc.gov/nip/publications/pink/mumps.pdf [Accessed November 7, 2000].

74. Manns, A, Hisada, M, and Grenade, LL: Human T-lymphotropic virus type I infection. Lancet 353 (9168):1951–1958, 1999.

75. Lal, RB: Delineation of immunodominant epitopes of human T-lymphotropic viruses types I and II and their usefulness in developing serologic assays for detection of antibodies to HTLV-I and HTLV-II. J AIDS Hum Retro 13(suppl 1):S170–S178, 1996.

76. Larson, CJ, and Taswell, HF: Human T-cell leukemia virus type I (HTLV-I) and blood transfusion. Mayo Clin Proc 63:869–875, 1988.

77. Mueller, NE, and Blattner, WA: Retroviruses—Human T-cell lymphotropic virus. In Evans, AS, and Kaslow, RA (eds): Viral Infections of Humans: Epidemiology and Control, ed. 4. Plenum Medical Book Co, New York, 1997, pp 785–813.

78. Hall, WW, et al: Human T lymphotropic virus type II (HTLV-II): Epidemiology, molecular properties, and clinical features of infection. J AIDS Hum Retro 13 (suppl 1):S204–S214, 1996.

79. Centers for Disease Control and Prevention: Current Trends Licensure of Screening Tests for Antibody to Human T-Lymphotropic Virus Type I. MMWR 37(8):736, 1988.

80. Sabino, EC, et al: Evaluation of the INNO-LIA HTLV I/II assay for confirmation of human T-cell leukemia virus-reactive sera in blood bank donations. J Clin Micro 37:1324–1328, 1999.

81. Paul, JR, and Bunnell, WW: The presence of heterophile antibodies in infectious mononucleosis. Am J Med Sci 183:90, 1932.

HIV Serology

Linda E. Miller, PhD, (SI)ASCP

Learning Objectives

After finishing this chapter, the reader will be able to:

1. Explain conditions under which transmission of human immunodeficiency virus (HIV) can occur.
2. Describe the makeup of the HIV particle.
3. Differentiate the three main structural genes of HIV and their products.
4. Describe replication of the HIV virus.
5. Describe the effects of HIV on the immune system.
6. Describe retroviral treatments and the impact they have had on HIV infection.
7. Discuss flow cytometric methods for CD4 T cell enumeration.
8. Compare first generation, second generation, and third generation enzyme-linked immunosorbent assay (ELISA) tests for HIV antibody.
9. Give reasons for false positives and false negatives in HIV antibody testing.
10. Define positive predictive value and relate this to HIV antibody testing.
11. Describe the Western blot test.
12. Interpret a Western blot test, given the types of reactive bands.
13. Discuss advantages and disadvantages of p24 antigen testing.
14. Differentiate between reverse transcriptase polymerase chain reaction (RT-PCR), branched DNA (bDNA) amplification, and nucleic acid sequence-based amplification (NASBA) testing for HIV nucleic acid.
15. Discuss the clinical utility of HIV viral load testing and drug-resistance testing.
16. Select the appropriate HIV test for a particular situation.

Key Terms

AIDS	Gag	Polymerase chain reaction
Amplicon	HAART	Positive predictive value
Branched chain DNA	HIV	Reverse transcriptase
CD4 T cell	Hybridization	Seroconversion
ELISA	NASBA	Viral load tests
Env	p24 antigen	Western blot test
Flow cytometry	Pol	

Human immunodeficiency virus **(HIV)** is the etiologic agent of the Acquired Immunodeficiency Syndrome, or **AIDS,** a disease that has reached epidemic proportions in many areas of the world and for which there is no cure. In 2001, AIDS was reported to be the fourth leading cause of death worldwide and the leading cause of death in Africa.[1] Although the majority of infected persons reside in developing countries, HIV infection has also created a significant problem in developed nations. In the United States alone, for example, over 774,000 cases of AIDS and close to 450,000 AIDS-related deaths were reported from 1981, when the first cases of AIDS were identified, through the year 2000.[2] Accurate diagnosis is essential for early intervention and halting the spread of the disease. This chapter emphasizes techniques for laboratory diagnosis of HIV infection, while presenting some characteristics of the virus itself and outlining immunologic manifestations of the disease.

The virus that is responsible for causing AIDS, HIV-

1, was identified independently by the laboratories of Luc Montagnier of France and Robert Gallo and Jay Levy of the United States in 1983 and 1984.[3,4,5] It was formerly called human T cell lymphotrophic virus-type III (HTLV-III), lymphadenopathy-associated virus (LAV), and AIDS-associated retrovirus (ARV). Isolates of HIV-1 have been classified into three groups, Group M (the main group), Group N (the new group), and Group O (the outlier group).[6,7] Group M viruses are responsible for the majority of HIV-1 infections world-wide, while Groups N and O are largely confined to part of West Central Africa.

A related but genetically distinct virus, HIV-2, was discovered in 1986.[8] This virus is endemic in West Africa, although it has also been identified in patients in other parts of the world.[6,7] HIV-2 appears to be transmitted in the same manner as HIV-1 and may also cause AIDS, but is less pathogenic and has a lower rate of transmission.[6] Although differences in the viruses are discussed in this chapter, the focus is on HIV-1 because it is much more prevalent throughout the world. Throughout this chapter, the term *HIV* is used to refer to HIV-1, and HIV-2 is so named.

HIV Transmission

Transmission of HIV occurs by one of three major routes: (1) through intimate sexual contact, (2) through contact with blood or other body fluids, or (3) by the perinatal route, from infected mother to infant.[3,9–11] The majority of cases of HIV infection have occurred by sexual transmission, through either vaginal or anal intercourse; transmission by oral sex has been reported in some cases.[11,12] Worldwide, about 75 percent of cases of HIV infection can be attributed to heterosexual contact, while in the United States, the largest number of cases has resulted from anal intercourse in homosexual males.[12] The presence of other sexually transmitted diseases such as syphilis, gonorrhea, or genital herpes appears to increase the likelihood of transmission, probably because of disruption of protective mucous membranes and increased immune activation in the genital areas.[11,12]

The second route of transmission is by parenteral exposure to infected blood or body fluids. This has occurred through the sharing of contaminated needles by intravenous drug users, through blood transfusions or the use of clotting factors by hemophiliacs, through occupational injuries with needle sticks or other sharp objects, or by mucous membrane contacts in health-care workers exposed to infectious fluids.[9,12–14] The virus has also been acquired by transplantation of infected tissue. Screening of blood and organ donors for HIV has dramatically decreased the incidence of infection in recipients of blood transfusions, clotting factors, and organ transplants.[2] Studies by the Centers for Disease Control and Prevention (CDC) have estimated the risk of transmission to health-care workers to be approximately 0.3 percent after a percutaneous exposure to HIV-infected blood and about 0.09 percent after a mucous membrane exposure, although other factors may increase or decrease the risk in individual situations.[14] Body fluids considered to be potentially infectious include blood, semen, vaginal secretions, cerebral spinal fluid, synovial fluid, pleural fluid, peritoneal fluid, pericardial fluid, amniotic fluid, and other fluids containing visible blood.[13–15] Saliva, sputum, tears, sweat, urine, vomitus, and feces are not considered to be infectious unless they contain visible blood.[13]

The third route of transmission is perinatal, from infected mother to her fetus or infant. Transmission by this route can occur during pregnancy, by transfer of blood during delivery, or through breast-milk feedings.[15] Vertical transmission from an infected mother to her infant has been reported in 15 to 35 percent of HIV-positive mothers who have not been treated with antiviral agents during their pregnancies.[15]

Characteristics of HIV

Composition of the Virus

HIV belongs to the genus *Lentivirinae* of the virus family *Retroviridae*.[11] It is classified as a retrovirus because it contains ribonucleic acid (RNA) as its nucleic acid and a unique enzyme, called **reverse transcriptase,** that transcribes the viral RNA into deoxyribonucleic acid (DNA), a necessary step in the virus' life cycle.[16] HIV is a spherical particle, ~100 nm in diameter, which contains an inner core with two identical strands of RNA, surrounded by a protein coat or capsid, and an outer envelope of glycoproteins embedded in a lipid matrix.[17] These knoblike structures are involved in binding the virus to host cells during infection. Figure 22–1 shows the structure of the HIV virion.

Structural Genes

The genome of HIV includes three main structural genes, *gag, env,* and *pol,* as well as a number of regulatory genes. Figure 22–2 shows the relative locations of the major HIV genes and indicates their gene products. The **gag** gene codes for *p55,* a precursor protein with a molecular weight of 55 kd (kilodaltons), from which three core structural proteins are formed, *p15, p17,* and

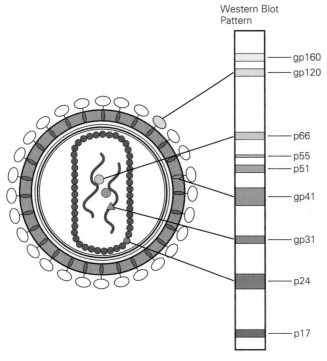

Western Blot
Pattern

— gp160
— gp120

— p66
— p55
— p51

— gp41

— gp31

— p24

— p17

FIG. 22–1. Structure of HIV, showing corresponding Western blot pattern. The viral antigens, including core (p17, p24, and p55), envelope (gp 160, gp 120, and gp 41), and polymerase (p66, p51, and gp 31), are shown as they appear on a Western blot. Location of these antigens in the particle itself is indicated. Those antigens not indicated in the particle itself are precursors, which are cleaved to form smaller viral proteins that are incorporated into the particle. (From Sloand, E, et al: HIV testing: State of the Art. JAMA 266: p 2862, 1991, with permission.)

p24.[7,12,16,18] All three are located in the nucleocapsid of the virus. The capsid that surrounds the internal nucleic acids is made up of *p24* and *p15*, while *p17* lies between the protein core and the envelope and is actually embedded in the internal portion of the envelope.[19]

The **env** gene codes for the glycoproteins *gp160*, *gp120*, and *gp41*, which are found in the viral envelope. Gp160 is a precursor protein that is cleaved to form *gp120* and *gp41*. It is *gp120* that forms the 72 knobs or spikes found protruding from the outer envelope, while *gp41* is a transmembrane glycoprotein that spans the inner and outer membrane and attaches to *gp120*. Both *gp120* and *gp41* are involved with fusion and attachment of HIV to receptors on host cells.[20]

The third structural gene, **pol,** codes for enzymes necessary for HIV replication,[12,16,19] namely *p66* and *p51*, which are subunits of reverse transcriptase, *p31*, or integrase, which mediates integration of the viral DNA into the genome of infected host cells, and *p10*, a protease that cleaves protein precursors into smaller

active units. The *p66* protein is also involved in degradation of the original HIV RNA. These proteins are located in the core, close to the nucleic acids.

Several other genes in the HIV genome code for products that have a regulatory function.[7,12,16] Although these products are not an integral part of the viral particle itself, they serve important functions in viral synthesis: *vpu* codes for *p16*, which is required for efficient assembly and budding of the virions off infected host cells, while *nef* codes for *p27*, which may modify the host cell to enhance later viral replication; *tat* codes for *p14*, which increases viral gene expression by acting as a transactivator, or long-distance activator, for several genes; *rev* codes for *p19*, which transports viral RNA out of the nucleus; and *vif* codes for *p23*, which acts as a viral infectivity factor. Table 22–1 summarizes the major HIV-1 genes, their products, and their functions.

HIV-2 also has *gag, env,* and *pol* genes that serve a similar function. The homology between the genomes of the two viruses is approximately 50 percent.[21] The *gag* and *pol* regions are most similar, while the *env* region differs greatly. Thus, the viruses can most easily be distinguished on the basis of antigenic differences in their *env* proteins.

Viral Replication

The first step in the reproductive cycle of HIV is attachment of the virus to a susceptible host cell. This interaction is mediated through the host-cell CD4 antigen, which serves as a receptor for the virus by binding the *gp120* glycoprotein on the outer envelope of HIV. T helper cells are the main target for HIV infection because they express high numbers of CD4 molecules on their cell surface and bind the virus with high affinity.[12] Other cells, such as macrophages, monocytes, dendritic cells, Langerhans cells, and microglial brain cells can also be infected with HIV, because they have some surface CD4.

Entry of HIV into the host cells to which it has attached requires an additional binding step involving coreceptors that promote fusion of the HIV envelope with the plasma cell membrane. These coreceptors belong to a family of proteins known as chemokine receptors, whose main function is to direct white blood cells to sites of inflammation. The chemokine receptor CXCR4 is required for entry of HIV into T lymphocytes, while the chemokine receptors CCR5 and CCR2 are required for entry into macrophages.[20] Binding of the coreceptors allows for entry of HIV by inducing a conformational change in the gp41 glycoprotein, which mediates fusion of the virus to the cell membrane.

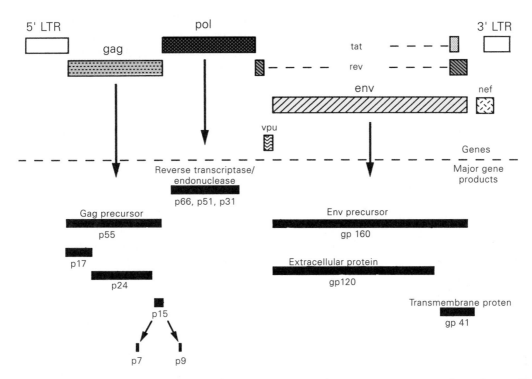

FIG. 22–2. The HIV-1 genome. The relative locations of the major genes in the HIV-1 genome are indicated, as well as their gene products. (Constantine, NT, Callahan, JD, and Watts, DM: Retroviral Testing: Essentials for Quality Control and Laboratory Diagnosis. CRC Press, Boca Raton, Fla., 1992, p 13, with permission.)

TABLE 22–1. Major HIV Genes and Their Products

Gene	Protein Product	Function
gag	p17	Inner surface of envelope
	p24	Core coat for nucleic acids
	p9	Core-binding protein
	p7	Binds to genomic RNA
env	gp120	Binds to CD4 on T cells
	gp41	Transmembrane protein
pol	p66	Subunit of reverse transcriptase
	p51	Subunit of reverse transcriptase
	p31	Integrase
tat	p14	Transactivates transcription
rev	p19	Production of viral mRNA
vif	p23	Infectivity factor
nef	p27	Unknown regulatory function
vpu	p16	Maturation of viral particles

RNA = Ribonucleic acid; mRNA = messenger RNA.

After fusion occurs, the viral particle is taken into the cell, and uncoating of the particle exposes the viral genome. Action of the enzyme reverse transcriptase produces complementary DNA from the viral RNA. This so-called provirus becomes integrated into the host's genome and is copied along with the cell's DNA (Fig. 22–3). The provirus may direct the production of new HIV virions or may remain in a latent state until viral expression is induced by environmental stimuli such as infections with cytomegalovirus (CMV) or herpes simplex.[22] When viral production occurs, viral DNA within the cell nucleus is transcribed into genomic RNA and messenger RNA (mRNA), which are transported to the cytoplasm. Translation of mRNA occurs, with production of viral proteins and assembly of viral particles. As the virions bud from the cell membrane, host cells may be destroyed by lysis.[12] Viral replication occurs to the greatest extent in antigen-activated T helper cells.[22]

Immunologic Manifestations

Immune Responses to HIV

In healthy individuals, an initial burst of HIV replication is followed by a slowing down of virus production as the host's immune response develops and keeps the virus in check.[12,23] This initial viral replication can be detected in the laboratory by the presence of increased levels of **p24 antigen** and viral RNA in the host's bloodstream (see discussion later). As the virus replicates, some of the viral proteins produced form complexes with major histocompatibility complex (MHC) class I antigens and are transported to the

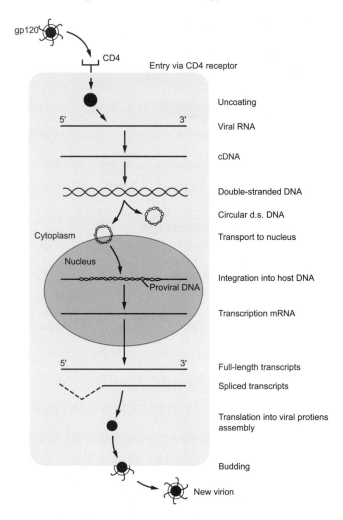

gp120

CD4

Entry via CD4 receptor

Uncoating

5'   3'   Viral RNA

cDNA

Double-stranded DNA

Circular d.s. DNA

Cytoplasm   Transport to nucleus

Nucleus

Integration into host DNA

Proviral DNA

Transcription mRNA

5'   3'   Full-length transcripts

Spliced transcripts

Translation into viral protiens assembly

Budding

New virion

FIG. 22–3. Replication cycle of HIV. (From Crowe, S, and Mills, J: Virus infections of the immune system, In Parslow, TG et al: Medical Immunology. Lange Medical Books, McGraw-Hill, New York, NY, 2001, p 646, with permission.)

host-cell surface, where they stimulate lymphocyte responses.

B lymphocytes are stimulated to produce antibodies to HIV, which can usually be detected in the serum of the host by 6 weeks after primary infection.[23,24] Antibodies may be produced to all the major HIV antigens, including p15, p17, p24, p31, gp41, p51, p55, p66, gp120, and gp160.[19] The first ones to appear are usually those directed against the gag proteins p24 and p55. This is followed by antibody to p51, gp120, and gp41. Most patients have antibody to the precursor gp160 as well.

Immune complexes are formed between the antibodies, circulating HIV virions, and complement. These complexes bind to receptors on follicular dendritic cells and cells of the reticuloendothelial system and are cleared from the circulation, resulting in a decrease in the level of virus in the blood. For reasons

to be discussed later, the virus cannot be completely eliminated by this and other immune mechanisms, and a chronic, persistent infection develops in the host, which ultimately leads to profound immunosuppression. After chronic infection has been established, neutralizing antibodies are produced that bind to HIV and inhibit its infection of new target cells.[23,25] Antibody titers drop significantly, however, during the advanced stages of HIV infection, as the level of immunosuppression increases.[23]

HIV infection also results in the stimulation of T lymphocytes. The most protective immune responses against HIV are thought to be mediated by the cytotoxic T lymphocytes, also known as CD8 T cells or cytolytic T cells (CTLs), which have been observed to increase up to 20 times more than normal during the initial weeks of HIV infection.[26] Although antibodies can only attach to virions circulating freely outside of host cells, CTLs are able to attack host cells harboring viruses internally. This process involves the binding of CTL with HIV-specific antigen receptors to HIV proteins in association with MHC class I molecules on the surface of infected host cells.[27] HIV-specific CTL are stimulated to develop into mature, activated clones through the effects of cytokines released by activated **CD4 T** helper **cells,** a process that is common to immune responses against other viruses (see Chapter 6 for details). After the CTLs bind to HIV-infected host cells, proteolytic enzymes are released from their granules and lyse the target cells. Free virions are released from the lysed cells and can be bound by antibodies. CTL can also suppress replication and spreading of HIV by producing cytokines that have antiviral activity.[23,27]

Effects of HIV Infection on the Immune System

Although the humoral and cell-mediated immune responses of the host usually reduce the level of HIV replication, they are generally not sufficient to completely eliminate the virus. This is because HIV has developed several mechanisms by which it can escape immune responses. First of all, HIV can be harbored in a silent state for long periods by numerous cells in the body, including resting CD4 T cells, dendritic cells, cells of the monocyte/macrophage lineage, and cells at sites such as the brain, retina, and testes, which are protected by blood-tissue barriers. Secondly, immune complexes containing HIV may become trapped by follicular dendritic cells in the lymph nodes, which can chronically present antigen and activate CD4 T cells, increasing the susceptibility of these cells to viral replication.[22,23,26,28,29] Third, genetic mutations occurring in HIV over time can result in the production of altered viral antigens to which prior immune responses are ineffective.[30]

The ability of HIV to evade the immune response results in a persistent infection that is capable of destroying the immune system. Because the prime targets of the virus are the CD4 T helper cells, these cells are most severely affected, and a decrease in this cell population has been long recognized as the hallmark feature of HIV infection.[31] CD4 T helper cells are killed or rendered nonfunctional as a result of infection with HIV, and these effects appear to result from a variety of mechanisms.[12,22,25,32]

Because T helper cells play a central role in the immune system by regulating the activities of B and T lymphocytes (see Chapter 6), destruction of the T helper cells by HIV results in decreased effectiveness of both antibody- and cell-mediated immune responses. For example, a decreased ability of B cells to respond to an immunologic challenge with specific antigens has been observed in HIV-infected individuals.

Cell-mediated immunity is also affected, as seen by an overall reduction in CTL activity and a decrease in delayed-type hypersensitivity responses in advanced disease.[23] Altered production of cytokines and chemokines have been seen in HIV-infected individuals, including decreases in the levels of interleukin (IL)-2, IL-4, and IL-6, and increased levels of the proinflammatory cytokines interferon-γ, IL-10, and tumor necrosis factor-α.[23]

Other immunologic abnormalities, including decreased monocyte/macrophage chemotaxis and decreased natural killer (NK) cell activity, have also been observed in AIDS patients.[31]

Clinical Symptoms

Although the course of disease can vary in individual patients, HIV infection has been observed to progress through three clinical stages, which coincide with the level of viral replication and the amount of immune destruction: (1) primary infection, (2) clinical latency, and (3) AIDS.[11,22] The primary stage, which soon follows infection, is characterized by a rapid burst of viral replication prior to the development of HIV-specific immune responses. In this stage, high levels of circulating virus, or viremia, can be seen in the blood of infected individuals, and HIV begins to disseminate to the lymphoid organs. As the immune system becomes activated, an acute retroviral syndrome may develop. This syndrome, which has been noted in 50 to 70 percent of patients with primary HIV infection, is characterized by flulike or infectious mononucleosis-like symptoms, such as fever, lymphadenopathy, sore throat, arthralgia, myalgia, fatigue, rash, and weight loss.[11,22]

Symptoms of the primary stage usually appear 3 to 6 weeks after initial infection and resolve within a few days to a few weeks. Some patients are asymptomatic during this stage.

As HIV-specific immune responses develop, they begin to curtail replication of the virus, and patients enter a period of clinical latency. This stage is characterized by a decrease in viremia as the virus is cleared from the circulation, and the absence of clinical symptoms.[11,22] Studies have demonstrated, however, that the virus is still present in the plasma, albeit at lower levels, and more so in the lymphoid tissues, where it causes a gradual deterioration of the immune system. The length of clinical latency can vary widely in individual patients, but typically lasts for several years.

Untreated individuals will ultimately progress to the final stage of HIV infection, the acquired immunodeficiency syndrome or AIDS, which is characterized by profound immunosuppression, along with a resurgence of viremia and the appearance of life-threatening infections and malignancies. The rate at which individuals progress to the development of AIDS varies, but progression typically occurs within a median time of 10 years after initial infection.[23,25] The rate of progression has been dramatically decreased with the use of antiretroviral therapies (see following discussion).

The CDC first defined AIDS as "a disease, at least moderately predictive of a defect in cell mediated immunity, occurring in a person with no known cause for diminished resistance to that disease."[33] The definition has been revised several times over the years as more information has been acquired about HIV and additional laboratory tests for HIV have been developed. In the 1993 case definition, the CDC classified HIV-infected adults and adolescents into nine categories (A1-C3), based on CD4 T cell counts, in association with clinical conditions found in HIV infection (Table 22–2).[34] According to this definition, HIV-infected individuals have been classified as having AIDS if they have an absolute CD4 T lymphocyte count of less than 200/μL and/or certain opportunistic infections or malignancies indicative of AIDS (Table 22–3). Individuals with AIDS are classified in categories A3, B3, C1, C2, or C3.

In addition to opportunistic infections and malignancies, HIV-infected individuals often demonstrate neurologic symptoms resulting from the ability of HIV to infect cells in the brain. In early HIV infection, these symptoms may manifest as forgetfulness, poor concentration, apathy, psychomotor retardation, and withdrawal, while progression to late disease may result in confusion, disorientation, seizures, dementia, gait disturbances, ataxia, or paraparesis.[35]

A separate case definition for AIDS in children has also been published by the CDC.[36] Symptoms of AIDS in infants include failure to thrive, persistent oral candidiasis, hepatosplenomegaly, lymphadenopathy, recurrent diarrhea, or recurrent bacterial infections.[15,37] In addition, abnormal neurologic findings may be present. The rate by which HIV infection progresses in children varies and may be influenced by factors such as maturity of the immune system at the time of infection, the dose of virus to which the child was exposed, and the route of infection.[15]

Since the advent of new antiretroviral therapies that have delayed progression to AIDS (see discussion in Treatment section), the CDC has found it necessary to track individuals who are HIV-positive but who have not developed AIDS, in addition to tracking people with AIDS. As a result, they published a revised surveillance case definition for HIV infection in 1999.[38] According to this definition, adults, adolescents, and children aged 18 months or older are considered to be HIV-infected if they meet the previously published clinical criteria[34] *or* if they demonstrate positive test results on screening and confirmatory tests for HIV antibody or a positive test result for an HIV virologic test (i.e., HIV nucleic acid detection, HIV p24 antigen test, or HIV isolation in culture). The principles of these tests will be discussed in the section on Laboratory Testing.

Treatment

Treatment of HIV infection involves supportive care of individual infections and malignancies seen in patients, and administration of antiretroviral drugs. Three different classes of antiretroviral drugs are available for treatment of HIV infection: nucleoside analogue reverse transcriptase inhibitors, nonnucleoside reverse transcriptase inhibitors, and protease inhibitors.[13,14,39] The nucleoside analogue reverse transcriptase inhibitors are similar in structure to nucleosides and inhibit further action of the reverse transcriptase enzyme when they incorporate themselves into the viral DNA being generated. This class of drugs includes zidovudine (also known as ZDV or azidothymidine [AZT]), lamivudine (deoxythiacytidine or 3TC), didanosine (dideoxyinosine or ddI), abacavir (ABC), and stavudine (dideoxydidehyrothymidine or d4T). The second class of drugs, the nonnucleoside reverse transcriptase inhibitors, stops reverse transcriptase from transcribing RNA into DNA by binding directly to the enzyme. This class of drugs includes nevirapine (NVP), delavirdine (DLV), and efavirenz (EFV). The third class of drugs, the protease inhibitors, prevents HIV from being assembled and released during the last stage of the viral reproductive cycle. These drugs include saquinavir (SQV), indinavir (IDV), ritonavir (RTV), nelfinavir (NFV), amprenavir (AMP), and lopinavir. New drugs continue to be developed as advances in this area are made.

Studies have shown that treatment with multiple drugs is more effective than treatment with a single drug in killing the virus and avoiding viral resistance. Potent multidrug regimens involving drugs from two or three of the classes mentioned previously are now the standard of treatment and are referred to as **HAART,** or highly active antiretroviral therapy.[40] Consequently, HAART has had a dramatic effect on the clinical course of HIV infection, as evidenced by a significant decline in the incidence of opportunistic infections, a delay in progression to AIDS, and decreased mortality in patients who have received this multidrug treatment.[41] Retroviral drugs have also had a significant impact in reducing perinatal transmission of HIV. In 1994, investigators from the United States and

TABLE 22–2. 1993 Revised Classification System for HIV Infection and Expanded AIDS Surveillance Case Definition for Adolescents and Adults

Clinical Categories			
	(A)	(B)	(C)
CD41 T cell Categories	Asymptomatic, Acute (Primary) HIV or PGL*	Symptomatic, Not (A) or (C) Conditions†	AIDS-Indicator Conditions
(1) = 500/mL	A1	B1	C1§
(2) 200–499/mL	A2	B2	C2§
(3) < 200/mL AIDS-indicator T cell count	A3§	B3§	C3§

*PGL 5 persistent generalized lymphadenopathy. Clinical Category A includes acute (primary) HIV infection.
†See text for discussion.
§These cells illustrate the expanded AIDS surveillance case definition. Persons with AIDS-indicator conditions (Category C) as well as those with CD41 T lymphocyte counts <200/mL (Categories A3 or B3) are reportable as AIDS cases in the United States and Territories, effective January 1, 1993.
For more information visit the Centers for Disease Control website: http://www.cdc.gov/mmwr/preview/mmwrhtml/00033545.htm

TABLE 22–3. Clinical Categories of HIV Infection Category A

One or more of the conditions listed following in an adolescent (=13 years) or adult with documented HIV infection. Conditions listed in Categories B and C must not have occurred.
- Asymptomatic HIV infection
- Persistent generalized lymphadenopathy
- Acute (primary) HIV infection with accompanying illness or history of acute HIV infection

Category B

Symptomatic conditions in an HIV-infected adolescent or adult that are not included among conditions listed in Category C and that meet at least one of the following criteria: (a) conditions are attributed to HIV infection or are indicative of a defect in cell-mediated immunity or (b) conditions considered by physicians to have a clinical course or require management that is complicated by HIV infection. Examples include:
- Bacillary angiomatosis
- Candidiasis, oropharyngeal (thrush)
- Candidiasis, vulvovaginal; persistent, frequent, or poorly responsive to therapy
- Cervix dysplasia (moderate or severe)/cervix carcinoma in situ
- Constitutional symptoms, such as fever (38.5°C) or diarrhea lasting >1 month
- Hairy leukoplakia, oral
- Herpes zoster (shingles), involving at least two distinct episodes or more than one dermatome
- Idiopathic thrombocytopenic purpura
- Pelvic inflammatory disease
- Peripheral neuropathy

Category C

- Candidiasis of bronchi, trachea, or lungs
- Candidiasis, esophageal
- Cervical cancer, invasive
- Coccidiomycosis, disseminated or extrapulmonary
- Cryptococcosis, extrapulmonary
- Cryptosporidiosis, chronic intestinal (>1 month's duration)
- Cytomegalovirus (other than liver, spleen, or nodes)
- Cytomegalovirus retinitis (with loss of vision)
- Encephalopathy, HIV-related
- Herpes simplex: chronic ulcer(s) (>1 month's duration); or bronchitis, pneumonitis, or esophagitis
- Histoplasmosis, disseminated or extrapulmonary
- Isosporiasis, chronic intestinal (>1 month's duration)
- Kaposi's sarcoma
- Lymphoma, Burkitt's
- Lymphoma, immunoblastic
- Lymphoma, primary, of brain
- *Mycobacterium avium* complex or *M. kansasii,* disseminated or extrapulmonary
- *Mycobacterium tuberculosis*, any site
- *Mycobacterium*, other species or unidentified species, disseminated or extrapulmonary
- *Pneumocystis carinii* pneumonia
- Pneumonia, recurrent
- Progressive multifocal leukoencephalopathy
- Salmonella septicemia, recurrent
- Toxoplasmosis of brain
- Wasting syndrome due to HIV

For more information visit the Centers for Disease Control website: http://www.cdc.gov/mmwr/preview/mmwrhtml/00018871.htm

France published the results of a large clinical trial demonstrating that ZDV administered to HIV-positive women during pregnancy and labor and to the newborn during its first few weeks of life reduced transmission of HIV to the infant by two-thirds.[42] As a result of this study, ZDV treatment, along with advice to avoid breastfeeding, are recommended routinely for pregnant women who are HIV positive.[15]

Although antiretroviral drugs and HAART have significantly improved morbidity and mortality in HIV-infected patients, they cannot be considered a cure for AIDS because restoration of the immune system in patients receiving these treatments is incomplete.[41] Viral resistance to the drugs may also develop, albeit at a slower rate than when single-drug therapy was used, and some patients may not be able to take the drugs because they cannot tolerate their side effects. Many approaches toward dealing with this virus have therefore been directed toward measures to prevent initial infection from occurring. Community-based education aimed at high-risk groups such as homosexual males and intravenous drug users has provided beneficial information on reducing transmission of the virus, and precautions to prevent transmission of HIV and other bloodborne pathogens in health-care workers have been published by the CDC and the Occupational Safety and Health Administration.[9,43] Prophylactic therapy with antiretroviral drugs is also offered to health-care workers who may have been exposed to HIV through percutaneous or mucous membrane contact with potentially infected blood or body fluids, in hopes that early treatment will prevent infection.[13,14] The specific treatment protocols recommended in these situations vary according to level of risk.[13,14]

The ultimate means of preventing infection with HIV would be the development of an effective vaccine. Much research has been directed in this area, but the task has been a very difficult one because of a number of reasons, including the ability of HIV to rapidly mutate and escape immune recognition, the capability of HIV to persist despite vigorous immune responses of the host, genetic variability in HIV clades, the need to induce mucosal immunity because HIV is usually transmitted through mucosal surfaces, and the lack of an ideal animal model.[44,45] Some of the strategies used in development of an HIV vaccine include subunit vaccines, which consist of recombinant HIV envelope glycoproteins, live vector-based vaccines, which use other viruses that have been genetically altered to carry HIV genes, and DNA vaccines involving injections with DNA that codes for HIV proteins.[44–47] It is hoped that research currently underway will hold promise of a breakthrough for the future.

Laboratory Testing for HIV Infection

Four types of laboratory tests have been used in the diagnosis and monitoring of HIV infection: CD4 T cell enumeration, antibody detection, antigen detection, and testing for viral nucleic acid. Culturing for the virus, although a definitive method of demonstrating HIV infection, has been used primarily in research settings. Principles of each of these methods are discussed along with their particular applicability to diagnosis at various stages of the disease.

CD4 T Cell Enumeration

As discussed earlier, destruction of the CD4 T lymphocytes is central to the immunopathogenesis of HIV infection, and CD4 lymphopenia has long been recog-

nized as the hallmark feature of AIDS. Therefore, enumeration of CD4 T cells in the peripheral blood has played a central role in evaluating the degree of immune suppression in HIV-infected patients for a number of years. In untreated patients, there is a progressive decline in the number of CD4 T cells during the course of infection (Fig. 22-4), and as discussed earlier, CD4 T cell counts have been used by the CDC to classify patients into various stages of HIV infection, with those whose counts fall below 200/μL being classified as having AIDS.[34] Since the advent of HAART, CD4 T cell numbers may fluctuate more, with rebounds in counts indicating success of therapy, and declining counts indicating failure.[42,48,49] Therefore, CD4 T cell counts are routinely determined every 3 to 6 months in HIV-infected patients and provide important information to the clinician in documenting the effects of therapy, determining whether a change in therapy should be made, assessing the likelihood for opportunistic infections to develop, and determining when to administer medications aimed at preventing such infections.[50–52]

CD4 T cell counts may be reported as absolute cell counts, percents of total lymphocytes, or the ratio of CD4:CD8 cells. Although a number of methods have been developed to enumerate CD4 T cells, including manual bead assays, enzyme immunoassays, and ELISA,[53] the classic method for enumeration has been immunophenotyping by **flow cytometry.** The basic principle of this method involves incubation of whole peripheral blood with a panel of fluorescent-labeled monoclonal antibodies, removal of the erythrocytes by lysis, and stabilization of the leukocytes by fixation with paraformaldehyde. The results are analyzed through the use of histograms that display the patterns of light scatter and fluorescence emitted by individual cell populations. Guidelines to standardize the performance of CD4 T cell determinations by flow cytometry have been published by the CDC.[54]

Data for CD4 T cell enumeration are reported both as percentages and absolute numbers.[54] To determine the percentage of CD4 T cells in a sample, the number of lymphocytes positive for the CD4 marker is divided by the total number of lymphocytes counted by the flow cytometer:

$$\% \text{ CD4 T cells} = \frac{\# \text{ CD4 lymphocytes} \times 100}{\text{total } \# \text{ lymphocytes}}$$

The percentage obtained is compared to a reference range established by the laboratory performing the test. Patients with HIV infection are classified as having AIDS if this number is decreased below 14 percent.[34]

Absolute numbers of CD4 T cells are calculated by

multiplying the absolute number of lymphocytes (calculated either by the flow cytometer or by the whole blood cell [WBC] count and differential from a hematology analyzer) by the percentage of CD4 T cells in the sample:

$$\text{Absolute \# CD4 T cells} = \text{WBC count} \times \% \text{ Lymphocytes} \times \% \text{ CD4 T cells}$$

The normal number of CD4 T cells ranges from 500 to 1300 cells/μL peripheral blood.[55] When the CD4 T cell number falls below 200/μL, the patient is classified as having AIDS.[34]

Finally, the ratio of CD4 T cells to CD8 T cells may be reported to assess the dynamics between the two T cell populations. In patients with AIDS, the large decrease in the number of CD4 T cells results in an inverted ratio, or a ratio that is less than 1:1.

Detection of HIV Antibody

Blood tests for HIV antibody are generally the first laboratory assays performed in the initial detection of HIV infection because most individuals will develop antibody to the virus within a few weeks to a few months after exposure.[56] The standard screening method for HIV antibody is the ELISA, and the standard confirmatory test is the Western blot. In addition to these, other methods such as rapid test kits, home test kits, and tests using urine and saliva have been developed. The principles of these methods are discussed later.

Screening Tests Using ELISA Testing

Principles of ELISA   ELISAs, or enzyme-linked immunosorbent assays, for the detection of HIV antibody were first implemented in the United States in 1985 in response to the need to screen donated blood to curtail spread of the infection. ELISAs remain the cornerstone of screening procedures for HIV because they are easy to perform, can be adapted to test a large number of samples, and are highly sensitive and specific.[11,19,56] Commercial kits have been developed by a number of manufacturers and are useful in screening blood products and in diagnosing and monitoring patients.

The first-generation of ELISAs were developed based on a solid–phase, indirect-assay system that detected antibodies to HIV-1 only.[6,19,56] (See Chapter 11 for general principles of ELISA.) These tests used a solid support system such as microtiter plate wells, polystyrene beads, or latex beads, coated with viral lysate antigens prepared from whole disrupted HIV-1 virions cultured in human T cell lines. The solid phase is incubated with patient serum or plasma, allowing HIV antibody in the sample to combine with the antigen. After washing carefully, an antihuman immunoglobulin with an enzyme label such as alkaline phosphatase or horseradish peroxidase is added. Washing is repeated, and then a substrate that forms a colored end product is used. The intensity of color formation, as determined by optical density, is directly proportional to the antibody concentration. Using positive and negative controls, a standard curve can be generated to relate

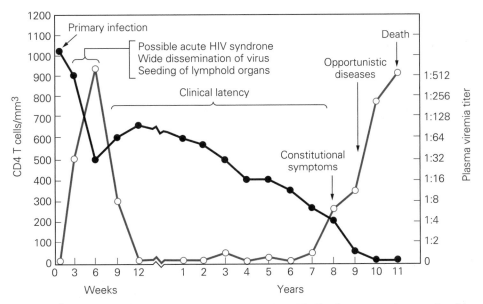

FIG. 22–4. CD4 T cells/mm³ (From Pantaleo, G, Graziosi, C, & Fancim, AS: The immunopathogenesis of human immunodeficiency virus infection. N Engl J Med, 328:327–335, 1993.)

optical density to antibody concentration and to create a cutoff point for negative samples. These first-generation assays had important limitations in that they were more prone to false positives caused by reactions with HLA antigens or other components from the cells used to culture the virus, and they were unable to detect antibodies to HIV-2.[11,56]

The second-generation ELISAs, introduced in the late 1980s, were indirect binding assays that used highly purified recombinant (i.e., genetically engineered) or synthetic antigens from both HIV-1 and HIV-2, rather than crude cell lysates.[11,56] These assays demonstrated improved specificity and sensitivity overall and were able to detect antibodies to both HIV-1 and HIV-2. However, decreased sensitivity resulted when samples containing antibodies to certain subtypes of HIV that lacked the limited antigens used in the assays were tested.

Third-generation assays use the sandwich technique, which is based on the capacity of antibody to bind with more than one antigen.[11,56] In this method, antibodies in patient serum or plasma bind to recombinant HIV-1 and HIV-2 proteins coated onto the solid phase. After washing, enzyme-labeled HIV-1 and HIV-2 antigens are added and bind to the already bound HIV-specific patient antibodies. After substrate is added, color development is proportional to the amount of antibody in the test sample. This format allows for the simultaneous detection of HIV antibodies of different immunoglobulin classes, but may exhibit problems in detecting low affinity antibodies.

Fourth-generation assays have recently been developed.[56] These are enzyme immunoassays or immunofluorescence assays that simultaneously detect HIV-1 antibodies, HIV-2 antibodies, and p24 antigen. These combination assays appear to allow for slightly earlier detection of HIV infection than the third-generation assays because of inclusion of the p24 antigen (see following).

Interpretation of ELISA Results   Studies on large numbers of individuals who are at high risk of acquiring HIV infection have found most of the commercially manufactured tests for HIV antibodies have a sensitivity of at least 99.5 percent and a specificity greater than 99.8 percent.[56] False-negative results occur infrequently but may be due to the collection of the test serum prior to the development of HIV antibodies by the patient (i.e., prior to **seroconversion**), administration of immunosuppressive therapy or replacement transfusion, conditions of defective antibody synthesis such as hypogammaglobulinemia, or technical errors attributed to improper handling of kit reagents.[56] The likelihood of false negatives occurring because the assay was performed prior to seroconversion has been reduced by the technical advances of the second- and third-generation ELISAs, which can detect HIV antibodies an average of 20 days after infection, as compared to the first-generation tests, which had an average window period of 45 days.[11]

False-positive results occur more frequently in the highly sensitive ELISAs and can result because of a number of factors, including heat inactivation of serum prior to testing, repeated freezing/thawing of specimens, presence of autoreactive antibodies, history of multiple pregnancies, severe hepatic disease, passive immunoglobulin administration, recent exposure to certain vaccines, and certain malignancies.[56] The rate of false positives is substantially higher in low-risk populations than in high-risk populations (i.e., the ELISAs have a low **positive predictive value** in low-risk populations). This positive predictive value was been estimated to be only 13 percent in a study done by the American Red Cross on low-risk blood donors, meaning that only 13 percent of all positives were true positives, and 87 percent were false positives in this population.[57] Any positive results obtained by ELISA must therefore be confirmed by additional testing.

According to the testing algorithm established by the CDC, a single sample should be tested first, and if it is positive, then duplicate samples from the original specimen must be retested by ELISA. If two out of the three specimens are reactive, then the results must be confirmed by a more specific method, usually Western blot (see following).[58] Repeatedly reactive units of blood are not used for transfusion, regardless of results of confirmatory testing.

Other Screening Tests

Although ELISAs are ideal screening tests for HIV antibodies in many clinical settings, they may not be suitable for laboratories that have a low volume of testing or in laboratories in developing world countries that have limited financial resources, a lack of complex instrumentation, and a shortage of skilled technicians to perform the tests.[59,60] For these reasons, more rapid and simpler methods to screen for HIV antibody have also been developed. These tests can be performed quickly (typically in 2 to 10 minutes) and have a high level of sensitivity. They are not cost effective for laboratories with a high testing volume, but may be useful in selected situations, such as developing nations of the world that lack sophisticated equipment and clinical settings in which faster notification of test results is desired. Such situations may include publicly funded clinics in which the rate of return visits of clients is low or in cases of potentially hazardous bloodborne exposures by health-care workers who are in the process of deciding whether to begin prophylactic therapy with antiretroviral drugs.[59] The types of rapid methods most commonly used have been microfiltration enzyme immunoassay, agglutination tests, and dot blot tests.[56,60]

Microfiltration Enzyme Immunoassay At the time of this writing, the microfiltration enzyme immunoassay is the only rapid test licensed for use in the United States. In this assay, human serum or plasma is placed in a sample cup, where it is incubated with latex particles that have been coated with purified p24 and gp41 HIV antigens. If the test sample contains antibodies to these antigens, they will bind to the particles. The contents of the cup are then transferred to a test cartridge, washed, incubated with a goat-antihuman immunoglobulin, washed, and then incubated with a substrate. A positive test is indicated by development of a blue color in the center of the test device.

Agglutination Tests Several agglutination tests have been developed using latex particles, gelatin particles, or microbeads. Recombinant HIV antigens have been adsorbed onto these carrier particles, and if antibody is present in the patient sample, clumping occurs. These tests are rapid, are simple to perform, and can be read visually.

Dot-Blot Testing This test is also simple to perform but more expensive than other types of tests.[19] Absorbent nitrocellulose paper serves as the solid support for HIV antigens. Patient specimen is allowed to filter through the paper or membrane, and then an antihuman immunoglobulin with an enzyme label is added. A color reaction is produced in a confined area after addition of substrate.

Home Testing The Food and Drug Administration (FDA) has approved the use of home test kits for individuals who prefer this format to being tested by a clinic or private physician. In this test system, individuals are provided with written information about HIV and AIDS, obtain a small blood sample by performing a fingerstick with a sterile lancet, and apply the sample to a designated area on a test card.[56] The card is then mailed to a certified laboratory, in which traditional ELISA testing for HIV antibody is performed, followed with confirmation by Western blot. The results can be obtained by telephone using a personal identification number. True home test kits, similar to home pregnancy tests, are available for use in other countries.[56]

Urine and Saliva Tests Commercial companies have also developed assays that use urine, saliva, or other body fluids instead of serum or plasma. These tests have the advantage of easier collection of the test sample, with no invasive procedures. Studies are underway to determine if these tests will be able to provide an accurate alternative to blood testing.[56]

Confirmatory Tests

Because of the possibility of obtaining false-positive results, as discussed earlier, all positive samples from HIV screening tests must be referred for testing with a more specific confirmatory method. Confirmatory methods using the principles of Western blotting, immunofluorescence assay, and radioimmunoprecipitation have been developed. The most widely used confirmatory test for HIV antibody, and the standard test in use today, is the Western blot test. This method will be discussed following.

Western Blot Testing

Principles The **Western blot test** for HIV antibodies was introduced in 1984 and has been used for systematic confirmation of positive ELISA results since 1985.[11] This technique is more technically demanding than ELISA, but has the advantage of providing an antibody profile of the patient sample that reveals the specificities to individual HIV antigens present. Several commercial kits are available for this type of testing and can provide results within a few hours.[56]

The first Western blot methods developed used a lysate of HIV antigens that was separated into individual proteins by polyacrylamide gel electrophoresis and blotted onto nitrocellulose paper. Antigens with lower molecular weight migrated faster and were positioned toward the bottom of the test strip, while antigens of higher molecular weight remained toward the top. The newer line immunoassays use recombinant HIV antigens, which are applied as separate bands to the test membranes.[11] These assays have a better sensitivity and specificity than the Western blot tests, which use viral lysate and can discriminate between HIV-1 and HIV-2.[11]

In the Western blot procedure, a nitrocellulose test strip containing HIV antigens is reacted with patient serum.[56] During the incubation period, any HIV antibodies present will bind to their corresponding antigen, and unbound antibody is removed by washing. Next, an antihuman immunoglobulin with an enzyme label (i.e., the conjugate) is added directly to the nitrocellulose paper and binds to specific HIV antibodies from the patient sample. Unbound conjugate is removed by washing, and bound conjugate is detected after addition of the appropriate substrate, which produces a chromogenic reaction. Colored bands will appear in the positions where antigen-specific HIV antibodies are present. Both HIV-1 and HIV-2 specific Western blot tests have been developed.

In HIV-1 infection, antibodies to the p24 and p55 antigens appear relatively early after exposure to the virus, but tend to decrease or become undetectable as clinical symptoms of AIDS appear.[61] Antibodies to gp31, gp41, gp120, and gp160 appear slightly later, but remain throughout all disease stages in an HIV-infected individual, making them a more reliable indicator of the presence of HIV.[62] Other antibodies commonly detected by this method are those directed against p51 and p66, while antibodies against the regulatory gene products are usually not detectable by conventional methods.[56] The bands produced by the test sample are examined visually for the number and types of antibodies present. Densitometry can also be performed to quantitate the intensity of the bands, which would reflect the amount of each antibody produced. Patients can be followed over time to determine whether there is a change in the antibody pattern.

Because Western blot testing is highly dependent on the technical skill and subjective interpretation of the laboratorian, it should only be performed in laboratories that have an adequate proficiency testing program. Including positive and negative control sera in the test run provides quality control for the Western blot. For the test to be valid, the negative control should produce no bands, the positive control should be reactive with p17, p24, p31, gp41, p51, p55, p66, and gp120/160, and the weakly positive control should react with p24 or p31 and gp41 or gp120/160. In addition, a vigorous external proficiency program should be in place.

Interpretation of Western Blot Results A negative test result is reported if either no bands are present or if none of the bands present correspond to the molecular weights of any of the known viral proteins.[56]

Criteria for determination of a positive test result have been published by the Association of State and Territorial Public Health Laboratory Directors and CDC, the Consortium for Retrovirus Serology Standardization, the American Red Cross, and the Food and Drug Aministration.[11,56,61,62] Although some controversy exists as to what banding pattern constitutes a positive result, most laboratories today follow the criteria of the Association of State and Territorial Public Health Laboratory Directors and CDC.[56] According to these criteria, a result should be reported as positive if at least two of the following three bands are present: p24, gp41, and gp120/gp160.[61]

Specimens that have some of the characteristic bands present but do not meet the criteria for a positive test result are considered to be *indeterminate*. This result may be produced if the test serum is collected in the early phase of seroconversion or if the serum contains antibodies that cross-react with some of the immunoblot antigens, producing false-positive results. False positives may be caused by antibodies produced to cellular contaminants if viral lysates were used as antigen,

autoantibodies including those directed against nuclear, mitochondrial, or T cell antigens, antibodies produced after infection with viruses such as CMV or herpes viral-1, or antibodies produced after vaccinations.[11,56] The use of recombinant antigens instead of viral lysates has reduced the incidence of false-positive results. If an indeterminate test result is obtained, it is recommended that the test be repeated with the same or a fresh specimen; if the test is still indeterminate, testing may be performed with a new specimen obtained a few weeks later, and if the pattern converts to positive, it can be concluded that the first specimen was obtained during the early phase of seroconversion. Failure of an indeterminate test pattern to convert to positive after a few months strongly suggests that the pattern is due to a false-positive test rather than HIV infection.[56]

Because of the possibility of false-positive results, the level of technical difficulty, and the time-consuming nature of the Western blot, this test is inappropriate for use as an initial screen for HIV infection. In the standard testing algorithm described earlier, in which samples determined to be repeatedly reactive by ELISA are then tested by Western blot, the Western blot has been determined to have a positive predictive value greater than 99 percent for both low-risk and high-risk populations.[56]

Detection of HIV Antigen

p24 Antigen Testing

Principles This test detects p24 antigen from the core of the HIV-1 virion. Levels of this antigen in the circulation are thought to correlate with the amount of HIV replication because they are high in the initial weeks of infection during the early burst of viral replication, then become undetectable as antibody to p24 develops and rise again during the later stages of infection when impairment of the immune system allows the virus to replicate.

The FDA licensed HIV antigen testing for research purposes in 1988 and for screening of blood donors in the United States in 1996. The rationale behind its use in the latter situation is to shorten the window period during which HIV infection cannot be detected, because p24 antigen production precedes the appearance of antibody by about 6 days.[24]

A solid-phase antigen capture enzyme immunoassay is used to detect p24 antigen[11,56] (see Chapter 11 for details of capture assays). In this method, a solid support coated with monoclonal anti-HIV-1 antibody is incubated with patient serum or plasma. After washing to remove any unbound antigens, a second anti-HIV-1 antibody conjugated with an enzyme label is added to the reaction. When substrate is added, color development indicates the presence of captured antigen. Optical density can be measured against a standard curve to make a quantitative determination of antigen present.

All positive results should be confirmed by a neutralization assay. This is accomplished by preincubating the patient specimen with human anti-HIV-1 antibody prior to performing the antigen assay. If p24 antigen is present, the neutralizing antibody will form immune complexes and prevent binding of the antigen to the HIV antibody on the solid support. In a positive test, absorbance should decrease by at least 50 percent.[56]

Evaluation of p24 Antigen Testing   Because p24 antigen becomes undetectable as antibody is produced by the host and binds the antigen in immune complexes, the p24 antigen test cannot replace the ELISA test for HIV antibody as the primary screening test for HIV-1 infection. The overall sensitivity of the p24 test is less than that of the ELISA for HIV antibody because only 20 to 30 percent of asymptomatic individuals with HIV infection have detectable serum levels of p24 antigen,[56] and only 50 to 60 percent of patients with full-blown AIDS demonstrate p24 antigen.[19]

The lack of sensitivity that is sometimes encountered with p24 antigen testing is thought to be due largely to complexing of free antigen with p24 antibody. Studies have shown that sensitivity may be improved by dissociating these immune complexes with heat, or by lowering the pH, prior to assay.[11,56]

The p24 antigen test has been most useful in situations in which antibody is not detectable or in which antibody test results are confusing, such as the period before seroconversion, infection in the newborn, and testing of cerebrospinal fluid from patients with dementia and encephalopathy.[11,19,56] The test has also been used to monitor disease progression, and to evaluate the efficacy of antiretroviral therapy, although this application has largely been replaced by nucleic acid testing for HIV (see following).

Nucleic Acid Testing

Tests for HIV nucleic acid have been incorporated into routine clinical practice and have had an important impact on the management of HIV-infected patients. These tests are used to determine the amount of virus present in patients and to determine whether and what type of drug resistance has developed. Quantitative tests for HIV nucleic acid are also know as **viral load tests** and are used routinely to help predict disease progression, predict response to antiretroviral therapy, and

monitor effects of the therapy.[52,63] Viral load testing is performed by nucleic acid amplification methods. Tests for drug resistance can be performed by genotypic or phenotypic assays.

Viral Load Assays

Viral load assays are based on amplification methods that increase the number of HIV RNA copies (or their derivatives) in test samples to detectable levels. Three amplification methods have been developed for this purpose: the reverse transcriptase **polymerase chain reaction** (RT-PCR), which amplifies complementary DNA generated from HIV RNA; the **branched chain DNA** assay (bDNA), which amplifies the labeled signal bound to the test plate; and nucleic acid sequence-based amplification **(NASBA),** which amplifies HIV RNA. The basic principles of each of these methods will be discussed briefly following and in more detail in Chapter 12.

Reverse Transcriptase Polymerase Chain Reaction (RT-PCR)   A commercial RT-PCR was the first assay to be licensed by the FDA for quantitative measurement of circulating HIV nucleic acid. The basic principle of this test is amplification of a DNA sequence that is complementary to a portion of the HIV RNA genome.[63,64,65]

In this assay, HIV RNA is isolated from patient plasma by lysis of the virions and precipitation with alcohol. The RNA is treated with a thermostable DNA polymerase enzyme that has both reverse transcriptase activity and the ability to initiate DNA synthesis in the presence of the appropriate reagents; the enzyme is also stable at high temperatures. The reverse transcriptase activity of the enzyme transcribes the HIV RNA into complementary DNA (cDNA). The cDNA is then amplified by standard polymerase chain reaction (PCR) methodology. In this process, double-stranded cDNA molecules are separated into single strands by heating, and each can then serve as a template for synthesis of a new DNA strand. The separated strands are incubated with primers, or short pieces of DNA that are complementary to the ends of a highly conserved region of the HIV-1 gag gene. Cooling of the reaction allows the primers to bind to the cDNA at the appropriate sites. The reaction is heated again, and the region in between the primers is synthesized in the presence of the DNA polymerase enzyme and the four deoxynucleoside triphosphates. This series of steps, referred to as one cycle, generates a copy of the selected portion of the cDNA, called an **amplicon.** This process is repeated for a number of cycles in an automated thermocycler, resulting in exponential growth in the number of amplicons produced. After the amplification process is complete, the amplicons are chemically denatured into single strands, bound to microtiter plates, and quantitated by addition of an enzyme-labeled probe, followed by a substrate. The amount of color change produced in each well (i.e., the optical density of the sample) is proportional to the amount of HIV RNA contained in the specimen.

The standard RT-PCR method can detect 400 to 750,000 copies of HIV-1 RNA per mL of plasma, while an ultrasensitive version of the test quantitates HIV-1 RNA over a range of 50–75,000 copies/mL.[65] Technical care must be taken when performing the RT-PCR because this assay is susceptible to crosscontamination of test samples with amplicon, target DNA, or target RNA.[65] To minimize crosscontamination, physically separate work areas should be designated for reagent preparation, sample preparation, amplification, and detection.

Branched-Chain DNA (bDNA) Assay The bDNA method is based on amplification of the detection signal generated rather than amplification of the HIV target sequence, in contrast to RT-PCR. This is accomplished through use of a solid-phase sandwich **hybridization** assay that incorporates multiple sets of oligonucleotide probes and hybridization steps to create a series of "branched" molecules.[63,64,66] First, RNA isolated from lysed virions in patient plasma is captured on wells of a microtiter plate coated with a number of probes. The captured RNA is then hybridized with branched amplifier probes and incubated with an enzyme-labeled probe that will bind to the DNA branches. Finally, a chemiluminescent substrate is added, and color change is measured with a luminometer. Quantitative results are generated from a standard curve.

The standard bDNA test can detect 500 to 1,000,000 copies of HIV RNA/mL of plasma, while an ultrasensitive version of the method has a detection range of 50 to 500,000 copies/mL.[63] As compared to the RT-PCR, the bDNA has higher upper limits in its detection ranges, does not require separate rooms for its various steps because amplification of the target is not involved, and is better at detecting all known subtypes of HIV; however, it is more conducive for laboratories with higher testing volumes and requires a larger sample volume.[63]

Nucleic Acid Sequence-Based Amplification (NASBA) NASBA is a target amplification assay based on amplification of HIV RNA.[63,64,66] In this complex procedure, HIV viral RNA is isolated from the clinical specimen to be tested and is initially treated with reverse transcriptase to form cDNA. An RNase H enzyme is used to remove RNA from the RNA:cDNA

hybrid formed, and the cDNA generated serves as a template to generate new RNA molecules in the presence of RNA polymerase, primers specific for a region of the gag gene, and the ribonucleotide triphosphates. All steps of the reaction are performed at a constant temperature. The amplicons produced are captured onto probes bound to magnetic beads, which are in turn hybridized with chemiluminescent probes and attached to the surface of an electrode, where an electrochemiluminescent reaction occurs. The amount of light generated is proportional to the amount of amplicon in the sample, and quantitative results are obtained through the use of internal calibrators that are used to produce a standard curve.

The NASBA method has a wide detection range: 80 to 10,000,000 copies of HIV-1 RNA/mL of specimen. It requires a small volume of specimen, making it conducive to testing of neonates and children, and it can be used for a variety of specimens in addition to plasma, including cerebrospinal fluid, whole blood, semen, cervical washings, and sputum.[63] However, NASBA is a more technically complex method to perform than RT-PCR or bDNA and may be best suited for research laboratories.

Clinical Utility of Viral Load Tests The amount of HIV RNA, or the viral load, in a patient's plasma reflects the natural history of HIV infection in that individual.[64,67] HIV RNA levels become detectable about 11 days after infection and rise to very high levels shortly thereafter, during the initial burst of viral replication. Typically, over a period of a few months, the viral load drops as the individual's immune system clears viral particles from the circulation, and a stable level of plasma HIV RNA, known as the "set point" is achieved (see Fig. 18-4). In untreated individuals, this level can persist for a long time and then rise again later as the immune system deteriorates and the patient progresses to develop AIDS. Successful therapy with antiretroviral drugs will result in a drop in the viral load level.

Viral load tests can therefore be used to monitor patients during the course of HIV infection and have played a critical role in the clinical management of these individuals. Studies performed by the Multicenter AIDS Cohort and other groups have demonstrated that information obtained from viral load tests has prognostic value.[49,52,67–69] These studies have shown that baseline plasma viral load values obtained in patients prior to the start of antiretroviral therapy are an important predictor of disease progression, in that a higher number of HIV RNA copies/mL plasma is associated with more rapid development of an AIDS-defining illness or AIDS-related death.

In addition, viral load values have been instrumental in monitoring patients during the course of antiretroviral therapy. Patients who attain a lower number of HIV-RNA copies/mL of plasma are more likely to achieve a longer treatment response.[28,52,64] The optimal goal of therapy is to reach undetectable levels of HIV RNA (i.e., <50 copies/mL).[70] Patients who fail to achieve a significant decrease in viral load after receiving antiretroviral drugs may not be adhering to the appropriate drug administration schedule or may have problems with absorption of the drugs, while patients whose viral loads increase over a period may have developed viral resistance to the drugs.[52]

Viral load testing may also be used to diagnose primary HIV infection, especially in those individuals who are seronegative or who may have equivocal antibody test results (e.g., those tested prior to seroconversion, or infants). The U.S. Department of Health and Human Services recommends that plasma HIV RNA testing be performed at the time of initial patient evaluation to obtain a baseline value and every 3 to 4 months thereafter in untreated individuals.[52,70] Initiation of antiretroviral therapy is recommended for patients whose HIV RNA levels and CD4 T cell counts reach critical values.[67,70] For patients already undergoing antiretroviral treatment, viral load testing is recommended prior to the initiation of therapy, at 8 weeks, and every 3 to 4 months thereafter in patients who have achieved a stable response. Viral load testing is also recommended for individuals who develop symptoms consistent with primary HIV infection, who develop a clinically significant opportunistic infection, or whose CD4 T cell counts drop unexpectedly.

Drug Resistance Testing

Because HIV has high replication and mutation rates and because no treatment completely eradicates the virus, it is possible for drug-resistant subpopulations to emerge during the course of antiretroviral therapy. Two types of laboratory methods can be used to test for drug resistance: genotype resistance assays and phenotype resistance assays.[52,65]

Genotype resistance assays detect mutations in the reverse transcriptase and protease genes of HIV. In these tests, RNA is isolated from patient plasma, the desired genes are amplified by RT-PCR, and the products are analyzed for mutations associated with drug resistance by automated DNA sequencing or hybridization.[52,65] Commercial kits for genotyping assays are widely available.

Phenotype resistance assays determine the ability of clinical isolates of HIV to grow in the presence of anti-

retroviral drugs.[52,65] Varying concentrations of the drugs are used in these tests, and the results are reported in terms of IC_{50} and IC_{90} values, or the drug concentrations needed to suppress the replication for the patient's viral isolate by 50 or 90 percent as compared to wild-type HIV.[52,71]

Genotype resistance assays are performed more frequently than phenotype resistance assays because they are less expensive, are more widely available, and have a shorter turnaround time.[52] Phenotype resistance assays are technically more difficult to perform and have limited commercial availability. Both assays require that a viral load of at least 500 to 1000 copies of HIV RNA/mL be present in the test sample and for the resistant virus to constitute more than 20 percent of the total viral population in the patient to be detected.[52] Despite these limitations, studies have shown that patients undergoing drug-resistance testing, particularly by genotyping methods, have a better chance of receiving antiretroviral therapy regimens that are more likely to result in greater reductions in viral load.[52,72,73] Therefore, the U.S. Department of Health and Human Services recommends that drug-resistance testing be performed in patients in whom HAART has failed or in whom viral load values have not been optimally reduced by antiretroviral therapy.[52,70]

Virus Isolation

Definitive evidence of HIV infection can be provided through the use of cell culture techniques to isolate viral particles from patient cells and tissues. A cocultivation system has been used, in which cells from patients are mixed with phytohemagglutininstimulated peripheral blood mononuclear cells from HIV-seronegative donors.[11,19] The best patient sample is peripheral blood, but virus can be isolated from other body fluids, such as cerebrospinal fluid, saliva, cervical secretions, semen, and tears, and from organ biopsies.[19] Samples other than peripheral blood, however, have varying levels of virus, which makes culture less efficient.

Infection can be confirmed by detection of reverse transcriptase activity or p24 antigen in the culture supernatant, detection of the HIV genome by molecular methods, or observation of characteristic cytopathic effects.[7] Presence of the virus can also be demonstrated by using fluorescent-labeled monoclonal anti-HIV antibody. Typically, culture results become positive within 2 weeks of incubation, but periods of up to 60 days may be required for some samples.[11]

This procedure is laborious, time consuming, and costly and may be hazardous to laboratory personnel involved in the testing process. Additionally, although the overall sensitivity of the test is about 90 percent, it is much lower for those individuals who are asymptomatic.[11,19] Because of these reasons, viral culture is not suitable for implementation in the clinical laboratory, and information regarding HIV infection can be obtained in a more practical manner by performing other tests such as RT-PCR and p24 antigen in most cases.[11]

Testing of Neonates

Diagnosis of HIV infection in infants is difficult because of placental passage of IgG antibodies from an infected mother to her child. More than 15 months may elapse before uninfected infants who harbor maternal HIV IgG test negative for antibody.[11] Thus, screening tests for antibody done on serum samples taken before this time are unreliable as indicators of infection. Serologic testing for IgA or IgM HIV-specific antibodies is not recommended either, despite the fact that they are not transferred through the placenta.[11] This is because IgA antibody testing lacks sensitivity in the first few months of life, and IgM antibodies directed against HIV in the newborn lack specificity.

Because of the difficulties with serologic testing, HIV infection in infants is best diagnosed using tests that measure components of the virus.[11] One method that has been used is measurement of p24 antigen in neonatal plasma. This test has been shown to have an overall diagnostic sensitivity of 96 percent when heat is used to dissociate immune complexes in the samples prior to testing.[11]

RT-PCR testing has been very useful in the early determination of neonatal infection because of its ability to detect very small amounts of viral DNA in a blood sample. Furthermore, the ability to perform this test with a very small volume of blood makes it ideal for the testing of neonates. The sensitivity of this method in detecting HIV infection in infants has been shown to be 96 percent at ages 1 to 6 months and 98 percent in children older than 6 months, and the specificity of the test is greater than 99 percent.[64] However, the sensitivity of the test in infants less than 1 month of age is much lower, necessitating the need to perform follow-up testing in infants who are suspected of being infected, but who demonstrate negative test results. Determination of HIV status should be based on the results of two RT-PCR assays performed at age 1 month or older.[64,74] Infant testing should be performed as soon as possible so that medical intervention can begin early.[74] Increased emphasis on screening pregnant women for HIV infection should also help in earlier identification of HIV-positive infants.[74]

SUMMARY

Human immunodeficiency virus type 1 (HIV-1) is responsible for the majority of AIDS cases throughout the world. A related virus, HIV-2, may also cause AIDS, but is generally less pathogenic. These viruses belong to the retrovirus family, which contains RNA as the genetic material from which DNA is transcribed. Transmission of HIV occurs by three major routes: through intimate sexual contact, through contact with contaminated blood or body fluids, or through vertical transmission from infected mother to her fetus or infant.

The three main structural genes of HIV are *gag, env,* and *pol.* The gag gene codes for the core proteins of the virus, including p24 antigen, the first to appear during infection. Products of the pol gene are the enzymes reverse transcriptase, integrase, and protease. The env gene codes for the envelope proteins gp120 and gp41, which facilitate attachment of the virus to the CD4 receptor and chemokine coreceptors on susceptible host cells. Several other genes are present that function to regulate replication of the virus.

After HIV binds to a host cell, fusion occurs, and the viral particle is taken inside the cell. Reverse transcriptase produces DNA from the viral RNA, and HIV is incorporated into the host-cell DNA as a provirus. A burst of viral replication occurs after initial infection. This is followed by a period of latency that begins as an immune response to the virus develops and can last for 10 years or more as viral replication is held in check. The prime targets of HIV infection are the T helper cells, which have large numbers of CD4 molecules on their cell surface. Untreated HIV infection results in a progressive destruction of these cells, with resumption of high rates of viral replication and development of profound immunosuppression in the host.

Clinical symptoms of HIV infection are associated with the levels of viral replication and helper T cell destruction in the host. The infection progresses through three stages: primary infection, clinical latency, and AIDS. During the latent period, the virus is harbored in the lymphoid tissues, where it causes gradual destruction of the immune system. In untreated patients, this will eventually result in AIDS, which is characterized by an increase in viral reproduction, with profound immunosuppression and host susceptibility to a number of opportunistic infections and malignancies. The use of HAART, a combination of antiretroviral drugs that inhibit HIV replication, has resulted in improved immune function in infected individuals, with a decline in the incidence of opportunistic infection and a delay in progression to AIDS. Antiretroviral drugs have also played an important role in decreasing perinatal transmission.

The main laboratory tests for HIV infection are CD4 T cell enumeration, HIV antibody detection, p24 antigen detection, and testing for HIV nucleic acid. The standard method for CD4 T cell enumeration is three- or four-color immunofluorescence staining, followed by analysis with flow cytometry. CD4 T cell counts are routinely monitored in HIV-infected individuals and provide important information regarding likelihood of disease progression and development of opportunistic infections, and effectiveness of antiretroviral therapy. These counts are also used in the CDC classification system for HIV infection and AIDS.

Detection of HIV antibodies is performed with an initial ELISA screening test. Third-generation ELISAs employ a sandwich technique in which HIV antibodies in patient serum or plasma are sandwiched between two sets of HIV antigens, one bound to a solid phase and a second containing an enzyme label. ELISA testing is sensitive but is subject to false-positive reactions because of a number of disease states and to reactivity with HLA antigens. Therefore, confirmatory testing of positive specimens is necessary. The Western blot is the most commonly used confirmatory test. In this test, patient serum is reacted with a nitrocellulose strip containing separate areas of distinct HIV antigens. HIV antibodies to specific antigens on the strip are detected after addition of an enzyme-labeled antihuman immunoglobulin and substrate. Colored bands develop in the areas on the strip where HIV antibodies have bound. A positive test result is indicated by presence of two of the following three major bands: p24, gp41, or gp120/160.

Detection of p24 antigen was designed to identify HIV infection during the window period before antibody is detectable. This test may be used to detect infection in seronegative patients and is also used in the screening of blood donor units. An antigen capture or sandwich assay is employed, which uses a solid-phase antibody to capture p24 in the patient specimen. A second labeled antibody is added and adheres only to antigen caught on solid phase.

Nucleic acid testing for HIV is used to determine the amount of virus harbored by patients and the development of drug-resistant strains of virus. Quantitative tests for HIV nucleic acid are known as viral load tests.

These tests have had an important impact on the clinical management of HIV-infected patients by allowing physicians to predict disease progression, to predict response to antiretroviral therapy, and to monitor effects of the therapy. Viral load tests are performed by one of three molecular methods: reverse transcriptase polymerase chain reaction (RT-PCR), a method that converts HIV RNA into cDNA and then amplifies the cDNA generated; branched chain DNA assay (bDNA), which amplifies a labeled signal bound to a test plate; and nucleic acid sequence-based amplification (NASBA), which amplifies HIV RNA. Drug-resistance testing can be performed by genotypic assays that use molecular methods or by phenotypic assays in which HIV replication in clinical isolates is assessed in the presence of varying concentrations of antiretroviral drugs.

Isolation of HIV in culture represents another technique for identification of HIV infection. Because of the fact that it is time consuming, costly, and hazardous to workers, it is not used to a great extent.

Diagnosis of HIV in neonates is more complex than testing in adults. The presence of maternally acquired antibody in newborns makes ELISA tests for HIV antibody unreliable until a child is over 18 months old. PCR testing is usually not sensitive enough to identify infection until the infant is at least 1 month old. Careful monitoring of HIV-infected mothers and early testing of infants at risk is being implemented to facilitate prompt medical intervention.

Case Study

1. A young woman recently discovered that her boyfriend tested HIV-positive. She was concerned that she may have also contracted the infection because she had experienced flulike symptoms 1 month ago. She decided to visit her physician for a medical evaluation.

Questions

   a. What initial laboratory tests should be performed on the young woman to determine if she has been exposed to HIV?

   b. If the woman tests positive in the initial evaluation, how can it be determined whether her test results are truly because of HIV infection or if they represent a false-positive result?

   c. If the woman's test results are truly positive, what tests can be done to monitor the woman over time?

Exercise: Simulation of HIV-1 Detection

PRINCIPLE: AN HIV SCREENING SIMULATION

Enzyme-linked immunosorbent assay (ELISA) tests were originally developed for antibody measurement. These immunoassays have also been adapted to successfully detect samples that contain antigens. This ELISA simulation experiment has been designed to detect a hypothetical patient's circulating IgG directed toward the viral (HIV) antigen. First, the antigens are added to the microtiter wells where some remain absorbed by hydrophobic association to the walls after washing away the excess. The antigens can be the whole HIV lysate, specific HIV proteins, or a mixture of the two. There is no specificity involved with the adsorption process although some substances may exhibit low binding to the walls. After washing away unabsorbed material, the unoccupied sites on the walls of the plastic wells are blocked with proteins, typically gelatin or bovine serum albumin.

Infection by HIV-1 causes the individual to mount an antibody response that eventually results in plasma IgG molecules that bind to different HIV proteins (and/or different areas or the same polypeptide). In this experiment, if these antibodies are present in the plasma sample, they will bind to the adsorbed antigens in the well and remain there after washing.

A solution containing the IgG antibody that binds to any kind of human IgG is then added to the wells. If the primary antibody has remained in a well, then the secondary antibody will bind to it and also remain attached after washing. These secondary antibodies are usually raised in rabbits and goats immunized with human IgG fractions. The second IgG antibodies are purified and covalently cross-linked to horseradish peroxidase. This modification does not significantly affect the binding specificity and affinity of the antibody or the enzymatic activity of the peroxidase.

After washing, a solution containing hydrogen peroxide and aminosalicylate is added to each well. Peroxidase possesses a high catalytic activity and can exceed turnover rates of 10^6 per second. Consequently, amplification of a positive sample can occur over several orders of magnitude. Many hydrogen donor cosubstrates can be used by peroxidase. These cosubstrates include o–diansidine, aminoantipyrine, aminosalicylic acid, and numerous phenolic compounds that develop color on oxidation. The substrate solution added is nearly colorless. Peroxidase converts the peroxide to $H_2O + O_2$ using the salicylate as the hydrogen donor.

The oxidized salicylate is brown and can be easily observed in wells containing anti-HIV-1 IgG (positive plasma).

It should be noted that polyclonal antibody preparations to a given antigen can have variable binding affinities because of differences in the immunologic responses between animals. The use of monoclonal antibodies directed against a single epitope eliminates this variability. Western blot analysis of positive samples is used to confirm infection by HIV.

REAGENTS, MATERIALS, AND EQUIPMENT

EDVOTEK Kit #271: AIDS Kit 1: Simulation of HIV-1 Detection, containing:

HIV antigens (simulated)
Positive control (primary antibody)
Donor 1 serum (simulated)
Donor 2 serum (simulated)
Anti-IgG-peroxidase conjugate (secondary antibody)
Hydrogen peroxide, stabilized
Aminosalicylic acid (peroxide cosubstrate)
Phosphate buffered saline concentrate
Microtiter plates
Transfer pipettes
Microtest tubes with attached caps
1 mL pipettes
plastic tubes, 50 mL

This experiment does not contain HIV virus or its components. None of the components have been prepared from human sources.

Additional Materials Required

Distilled or deionized water
Beakers
37°C incubation oven
Disposable lab gloves
Safety goggles
Automatic micropipets and tips recommended

Make sure glassware is clean, dry, and free of soap residue.

LABORATORY SAFETY

Gloves and goggles should be worn routinely as good laboratory practice.

PROCEDURE★

General Instructions and Procedures

1. Equilibrate a 37°C incubation oven before starting the experiment.
2. Label the Microtiter Plate:
   a. Place the microtiter plate vertically. Mark the plate with your initials or lab group number and number the rows 1 to 4 down the side, as follows:

   Row 1
   Row 2
   Row 3
   Row 4

3. Label the Plastic Transfer pipets:
   a. Label 5 transfer pipettes as follows:

   (−)   (negative)
   (+)   (positive)
   DS 1   (Donor Serum 1)
   DS 2   (Donor Serum 2)
   PBS   (Phosphate Buffered Saline)

4. Use the appropriately labeled plastic transfer pipette for liquid removals and washes as outlined in the experimental procedures.

Instructions for Adding Liquids and Washing Wells

Adding reagents to wells: For adding reagents to the wells, use the same 1-mL pipette. RINSE THE PIPETTE THOROUGHLY with distilled water before using the pipette for adding the next reagent.

If available, reagents should be dispensed with an automatic micropipette using disposable tips.

Liquid Removal and Washes

When instructed in the experimental procedures, remove liquids with the appropriately labeled transfer pipette, and then wash the wells as follows.

1. Use the transfer pipette labeled "PBS" to add PBS buffer to the wells in all rows. Add PBS buffer until each well is almost full.

The capacity of each well is approximately 0.2 mL. Do not allow the liquids to spill over into adjacent wells.

2. With the appropriately labeled transfer pipet, remove all the liquid (PBS buffer) from the wells in each row. Dispose the liquid in the beaker labeled "waste."

Experimental Steps for the Enzyme-Linked Immunosorbent Assay

Wear safety goggles and gloves.

1. To all 12 wells, add 0.1 mL of "HIV" (viral antigens)
2. Incubate for 5 minutes at room temperature.

3. Remove all the liquid (viral antigens) with a transfer pipette.
4. Wash each well once with PBS buffer as described earlier ("Liquid Removal and Washes").
5. Add reagents as outlined following:

Remember to rinse the 1-mL pipette thoroughly with distilled water before adding a new reagent. If you are using automatic micropipettes, use a clean micropipette tip for each reagent.

   Add 0.1 mL of PBS Buffer to the three wells in Row 1. (This is the negative control.)

   Add 0.1 mL of "+" (positive) to the three wells in Row 2. (This is the positive control.)

   Add 0.1 mL of Donor Serum "DS1" to the 3 wells in Row 3.

   Add 0.1 mL of Donor Serum "DS2" to the 3 wells in Row 4.

6. Incubate at 37°C for 15 minutes.
7. Remove all the liquid from each well with the appropriately labeled transfer pipette.
8. Wash each well once with PBS buffer (as described under "Liquid Removal and Washes").
9. Add 0.1 mL of the anti-IgG peroxidase conjugate to all 12 wells.
10. Incubate at 37°C for 15 minutes.

At this time you can obtain the substrate to be used in step 13. Because the substrate must be prepared just prior to use, your instructor will prepare it toward the end of the incubation in step 10.

11. Remove all the liquid from each well with the appropriately labeled transfer pipette.
12. Wash each well once with PBS buffer (as described under "Liquid Removal and washes").
13. Add 0.1 mL of the substrate to all 12 wells.
14. Incubate at 37°C for 5 minutes.
15. Remove the plate for analysis.
16. If color is not fully developed after 5 minutes, incubate at 37°C for a longer period of time.

REMINDERS

Adding Reagents

Be sure to rinse the 1 mL pipette thoroughly before adding a new reagent (Steps 1, 5, 9, and 13). Alternatively, if you are using automatic micropipettes, use a fresh tip for each reagent.

Liquid Removals

Use the appropriately labeled transfer pipette to remove all liquid from the wells in each row (steps 3, 7, and 11) and after washes (steps 4, 8, and 12).

| Transfer pipette | (−) | Row 1 |
| Transfer pipette | (+) | Row 2 |

★ Permission granted to reproduce the following information by EDVOTEK®—The Biotechnology Education Company (edvotek@aol.com).

| Transfer pipette | DS 1 | Row 3 |
| Transfer pipette | DS 2 | Row 4 |

Dispose the liquid in the beaker labeled "waste."

Washes

For all rows, use the transfer pipette labeled "PBS" to add PBS until each well is almost full (steps 4, 8, and 12).

INTERPRETATION OF RESULTS

The positive control, which contains IgG directed against HIV antigens, is the primary antibody. Positive serum samples will also contain anti-HIV IgG. Wells containing positive control or positive serum samples will develop a brown color. Negative serum samples will not contain anti-HIV IgG, and will remain colorless.

1. All of the following apply to HIV *except:*
   a. It possesses an outer envelope.
   b. It contains an inner core with p24 antigen.
   c. It contains DNA as its nucleic acid.
   d. It is a member of the retrovirus family.

2. Which of the following genes is responsible for the coding of reverse transcriptase?
   a. Env
   b. Pol
   c. Gag
   d. Tat

3. HIV virions bind to host T cells through which receptor(s)?
   a. CD4 and CD8
   b. CD4 and the IL-2 receptor
   c. CD4 and CXCR4
   d. CD8 and CCR2

4. Antibodies to which of the following viral antigens are usually the first to be detected in HIV infection?
   a. gp120
   b. gp160
   c. gp41
   d. p24

5. Which of the following is typical of the latent stage of HIV infection?
   a. Proviral DNA is attached to cellular DNA.
   b. Large numbers of viral particles are synthesized.
   c. A large amount of viral RNA is synthesized.
   d. Viral particles with no envelope are produced.

6. The decrease in T cell numbers in HIV-infected individuals is due to:
   a. Lysis of host T cells by replicating virus
   b. Fusion of the T cells to form syncytia
   c. Killing of the T cells by HIV-specific cytotoxic T cells
   d. All of the above

7. The most common means of HIV transmission worldwide is through:
   a. Blood transfusions
   b. Intimate sexual contact
   c. Sharing of needles in intravenous drug use
   d. Transplacenta passage of the virus

8. All of the following are likely immunologic manifestations of HIV infection *except:*
   a. Decreased CD4 T cell count
   b. Increased CD8 T cell count
   c. Increased response to vaccine antigens
   d. Increased serum immunoglobulins

9. The drug zidovudine is an example of a:
   a. Nucleoside analogue reverse transcriptase inhibitor
   b. Nonnucleoside reverse transcriptase inhibitor
   c. Protease inhibitor
   d. Immunotherapeutic drug

10. Which of the following methods is used in third-generation ELISA tests for HIV antibody?
    a. Binding of patient antibody to solid-phase recombinant HIV antigens followed by addition of enzyme-labeled antihuman immunoglobulin
    b. Binding of patient antibody to solid-phase recombinant HIV antigens, followed by addition of enzyme-labeled HIV-specific antibodies
    c. Binding of patient antibody to solid-phase recombinant HIV antigens, followed by addition of enzyme-labeled HIV antigens
    d. Binding of patient antibody to a solid-phase coated with antigens purified from HIV viral lysates, followed by addition of enzyme-labeled antihuman immunoglobulin

11. If a test has a high positive predictive value, which of the following is true?
    a. There will be no false negatives.
    b. Most positives are true positives.
    c. It is not a good screening test.
    d. The number of true positives will vary with the population.

12. False-negative test results in the ELISA test for HIV antibody may be because of:
    a. Heat inactivation of the serum prior to testing
    b. Collection of the test sample prior to seroconversion
    c. Interference by autoantibodies
    d. Recent exposure to certain vaccines

13. Which of the following combinations of bands would represent a positive Western blot for HIV antibody?
    a. p24 and p55
    b. p24 and p31
    c. gp41 and gp120
    d. p31 and p55

14. Which of the following tests would give the least reliable results in a 6-month-old infant?
    a. p24 antigen test
    b. ELISA for HIV antibody
    c. RT-PCR for HIV nucleic acid
    d. NASBA for HIV nucleic acid

15. The RT-PCR is a highly sensitive method that involves
    a. Direct amplification of HIV RNA
    b. Amplification of a label attached to HIV RNA
    c. Amplification of a complementary DNA sequence to a portion of the HIV RNA
    d. DNA sequencing of a portion of HIV RNA

References

1. Centers for Disease Control and Prevention: The global HIV and AIDS epidemic, 2001. MMWR 50(21):434–439, 2001.
2. Centers for Disease Control and Prevention: HIV and AIDS—United States, 1981–2000. MMWR 50(21):430–434, 2001.
3. Barre-Sinoussi, F, et al: Isolation of a T-lymphotropic retrovirus from a patient at risk for acquired immunodeficiency syndrome (AIDS). Science 220:868–870, 1983.
4. Gallo, RC, et al: Human T-lymphotropic retrovirus, HTLV-III isolated from AIDS patients and donors at risk for AIDS. Science 224:500–503, 1984.
5. Levy, JA, et al: Isolation of lymphocytopathic retroviruses from San Francisco patients with AIDS. Science 225:840–842, 1984.
6. Schupbach, J, and Gallo, RC: Human retroviruses. In Spector, S, Hodinka, RL, and Young, SA (eds): Clinical Virology Manual, ed. 3. ASM Press, Washington, D.C., 2000, pp 513–560.
7. Weiss, RA, Dalgleish, AG, and Loveday, C: Human immunodeficiency viruses. In Zuckerman, AJ, Banatvala, JE, and Pattison, JR (eds): Principles and Practice of Clinical Virology, ed. 4. John Wiley & Sons Ltd, Chichester, England, 2000, pp 659–693.
8. Clavel, F, et al: Isolation of a new human retrovirus from West African patients. Science 223:343–346, 1986.
9. Centers for Disease Control and Prevention: Recommendations for prevention of HIV transmission in health-care settings. MMWR 36 (suppl no 2S):1S–17S, 1987.
10. Lifson, AR: Do alternate modes for transmission of human immunodeficiency virus exist? JAMA 259:1353–1356, 1988.
11. Schupbach, J: Human immunodeficiency viruses. In Murray, PR, et al (eds): Manual of Clinical Microbiology, ed. 7. American Society for Microbiology, Washington, D.C., 1999, pp 847–870.
12. Goldsby, RA, Kindt, TJ, and Osborne, BA: Kuby Immunology, ed. 4. WH Freeman, New York, 2000, pp 467–496.
13. Centers for Disease Control and Prevention: Updated U.S. public health service guidelines for the management of occupational exposures to HBV, HCV, and HIV and recommendations for postexposure prophylaxis. MMWR 50(RR11):1–42, 2001.
14. Centers for Disease Control and Prevention: Public health service guidelines for the management of health-care worker exposures to HIV and recommendations for postexposure prophylaxis. MMWR 47:211–215, 1998.
15. Peckham, C, and Gibb, D: Mother-to-child transmission of the human immunodeficiency virus. N Engl J Med 333(5):298–302, 1995.
16. Folks, TM, and Hart, CE: The life cycle of Human Immunodeficiency Virus type 1. In Curran, J, Essex, M, and Fauci, AS (eds): AIDS: Etiology, Diagnosis, Treatment, and Prevention, ed. 4. Lippincott-Raven, Philadelphia, 1997, pp 29–43.
17. Gallo, RC, and Montagnier, L: AIDS in 1988. Scientific American 259(4):41–48, 1988.
18. Fauci, AS: The human immunodeficiency virus: Infectivity and mechanisms of pathogenesis. Science 239:617–622, 1988.
19. Constantine, NT, Callahan, JD, and Watts, DM: Retroviral Testing: Essentials for Quality Control and Laboratory Diagnosis. CRC Press, Boca Raton, Fla., 1992.
20. O'Brien, SJ. AIDS: A role for host genes. Hosp Pract 33(7):53–79, 1998.
21. O'Brien, TR, George, JR, and Holmberg, SD: Human immuno-deficiency virus type 2 infection in the United States: epidemiology, diagnosis, and public health implications. JAMA 267:2775–2779, 1992.
22. Pantaleo, G, Graziosi, C, and Fauci, AS: The immunopathogenesis of Human Immunodeficiency Virus infection. N Engl J Med 328(5):327–335, 1993.
23. Pantaleo, G, and Fauci, AS: Immunopathogenesis of HIV infection. Annu Rev Microbiol 50:825–854, 1996.
24. Centers for Disease Control and Prevention: U.S. Public Health Service guidelines for testing and counseling blood and plasma donors for human immunodeficiency virus type-1 antigen. MMWR 45(RR-2):1–9, 1996.
25. Haynes, BF, Pantaleo, G, and Fauci, AS: Toward an understanding of the correlates of protective immunity to HIV infection. Science 271:324–328, 1996.
26. Pantaleo, G, Graziosi, C, and Fauci, AS: Virologic and immunologic events in primary HIV infection. Springer Semin Immunopathol 18:257–266, 1997.
27. Yang, OO: CD8 T cells in HIV infection: Mechanisms of immunity. Hosp Pract 33(11):105–127, 1998.
28. Powderly, WG, et al: Predictors of optimal virological response to potent antiretroviral therapy. AIDS 13:1873–1880, 1999.
29. Weissman, D, and Fauci, AS: Role of dendritic cells in immunopathogenesis of Human Immunodeficiency Virus infection. Clin Microbiol Rev 10(2):358–367, 1997.
30. Nowak, MA, and McMichael, AJ. How HIV defeats the immune system. Scientific American 273(2):58–65, 1995.
31. Lane, HC, and Fauci, AS: Immunologic abnormalities in the Acquired Immunodeficiency Syndrome. Annu Rev Immunol 3:477–500, 1985.
32. Pantaleo, G: Unraveling the strands of HIV's web. Nat Med 5(1):27–28, 1999.
33. Centers for Disease Control and Prevention: Update on acquired immunodeficiency syndrome (AIDS)—United States. MMWR 31:507–514, 1982.
34. Centers for Disease Control and Prevention: 1993 Revised classification system for HIV infection and expanded surveillance case definition for AIDS among adolescents and adults. MMWR 41(RR-17):1–19, 1992.
35. Price, RW, et al: The brain in AIDS: Central nervous system HIV-1 infection and AIDS dementia complex. Science 239:586–592, 1988.
36. Centers for Disease Control and Prevention: 1994 Revised classification system for human immunodeficiency virus infection in children less than 13 years of age. MMWR 43(RR-12):1–19, 1994.
37. European Collaborative Study: Children born to women with HIV-1 infection: Natural history and risk of transmission. Lancet 337:253–260, 1991.

38. Centers for Disease Control and Prevention: Appendix: Revised surveillance case definition for HIV infection. MMWR 48(RR13):29–31, 1999.

39. Deeks, S, and Volberding, P: Combined antiretroviral therapy: The emerging role. Hosp Pract 30 (suppl 1):23–31, 1995.

40. Tashima, KT, and Flanigan TP: Antiretroviral therapy in the year 2000. Infect Dis Clin North Am 14(4):827–849, 2000.

41. Powderly, WG, Landay, A, and Lederman, MM: Recovery of the immune system with antiretroviral therapy. JAMA 280:72–77, 1998.

42. Connor, EM, et al: Reduction of maternal-infant transmission of human immunodeficiency virus type 1 with zidovudine treatment. N Engl J Med 331:1173–1180, 1994.

43. OSHA: The OSHA bloodborne pathogens standard 29 CFR 1910.1030. http://www.afscme.org/health/faq-bbp.htm [Accessed March 25, 2002].

44. Johnston, MI: HIV vaccines: Problems and prospects. Hosp Pract 32(5):125–140, 1997.

45. Letvin, NL: Progress in the development of an HIV-1 vaccine. Science 280:1875–1880, 1998.

46. Dolin, R: HIV vaccines for prevention of infection and disease in humans. Infect Dis Clin North Am 14(4):1001–1006, 2000.

47. Mulligan, MJ, and Weber J: Human trials of HIV-1 vaccines. AIDS 13 (suppl A):S105–S112, 1999.

48. Autran, B, et al: Positive effects of combined antiretroviral therapy on CD4 T cell homeostasis and function in advanced HIV disease. JAMA 277(5322):112–116, 1997.

49. Mellors, JW, et al: Plasma viral load and CD4+ lymphocytes as prognostic markers of HIV-1 infection. Ann Intern Med 126:946–954, 1997.

50. Brando, B, et al: Cytofluorometric methods for assessing absolute numbers of cell subsets in blood. Cytometry 42:327–346, 2000.

51. Hengel, RL, and Nicholson, JKA: An update on the use of flow cytometry in HIV infection and AIDS. Clin Lab Med 21(4):841–856, 2001.

52. Urban, AW, and Graziano, FM: Laboratory monitoring in the management of HIV infection. Lab Med 33(3):193–202, 2002.

53. Kutok, JL, et al: Four-color flow cytometric immunophenotypic determination of peripheral blood CD4+ T-lymphocyte counts. Am J Clin Pathol 110:465–470, 1998.

54. Centers for Disease Control and Prevention: 1997 Revised guidelines for performing CD4+ T-cell determinations in persons infected with human immunodeficiency virus. MMWR 46(RR2):1–29, 1997.

55. Cohen, PT: Understanding HIV disease. In Cohen, PT, Sande, MA, and Volberding, PA (eds): The AIDS Knowledge Base, ed. 3. Lippincott Williams & Wilkins, Philadelphia, 1999, pp 175–194.

56. Vasudevachari, MB, et al: Principles and procedures of human immunodeficiency virus serodiagnosis. In Rose, NR, Hamilton, RG, and Detrick, B (eds): Manual of Clinical Laboratory Immunology, ed. 6. American Society for Microbiology, Washington, D.C., 2002, pp 790–803.

57. Houn, HY, Pappas, AA, and Walker, EM: Status of current clinical tests for human immunodeficiency virus (HIV): Applications and limitations. Ann Clin Lab Sci 17:279–285, 1987.

58. Centers for Disease Control and Prevention: Update: Serologic testing for antibody to Human Immunodeficiency Virus. MMWR 36:833–843, 1988.

59. Centers for Disease Control and Prevention: Update: HIV counseling and testing using rapid tests, United States, 1995. MMWR 47(RR-7):1–33, 1998.

60. World Health Organization: The importance of simple/rapid assays in HIV testing. Wkly Epidemiol Rec 73:321–328, 1998.

61. Centers for Disease Control and Prevention: Interpretation and use of the Western blot assay for serodiagnosis of human immunodeficiency virus type 1 infections. MMWR 38(S-7):1–7, 1989.

62. Consortium for Retrovirus Serology Standardizations: Serological diagnosis of human immunodeficiency virus infection by Western blot testing. JAMA 260:674–679, 1988.

63. Weikersheimer, PB: Viral load testing for HIV: Beyond the CD4 count. Laboratory Medicine 30(2):102–108, 1999.

64. Arens, M: Human Immunodeficiency Virus (HIV) and other retroviruses. In Storch, GA (ed): Essentials of Diagnostic Virology. Churchill Livingstone, New York, 2000, pp 250–267.

65. Elbeik, T, et al: Quantitation of viremia and determination of drug resistance in patients with Human Immunodeficiency Virus infection. In Rose, NR, Hamilton, RG, and Detrick B (eds): Manual of Clinical Laboratory Immunology, ed. 6. American Society for Microbiology, Washington, D.C., 2002, pp 772–789.

66. Nolte, FS: Quantitative molecular techniques. In Spector, S, Hodinka, RL, and Young, SA (eds): Clinical Virology Manual, ed. 3. ASM Press, Washington, D.C., 2000, pp 198–210.

67. Mylonakis, E, et al: Plasma viral load testing in the management of HIV infection. Am Fam Physician 63(3):483–490, 2001.

68. Hughes, M, et al: Monitoring plasma HIV/RNA levels in addition to CD4+ lymphocyte count improves assessment of antiretroviral therapeutic response. Ann Intern Med 126:929–938, 1997.

69. Mellors, JW, et al: Prognosis in HIV-1 infection predicted by the quantity of virus in plasma. Science 272:1167–1170, 1996.

70. U.S. Department of Health and Human Services and the Henry J. Kaiser Family Foundation. Guidelines for the use of antiretroviral agents in HIV-infected adults and adolescents. August 2001. Available at: http://www.hivatis.org/guidelines/adult/May23_02/AAMay23.pdf [Accessed August 9, 2002].

71. Hirsch, M, et al: Antiretroviral drug resistance testing in adult HIV-1 infection. Recommendations of an International AIDS Society—USA panel. JAMA 28:2417–2426, 2000.

72. Baxter, J, et al: A randomized study of antiretroviral management based on plasma genotypic antiretroviral resistance testing in patients failing therapy. AIDS 14:F83–93, 2000.

73. Durant, J, et al: Drug-resistance genotyping in HIV-1 therapy. Lancet 353:2195–2199, 1999.

74. Centers for Disease Control and Prevention: Revised recommendations for HIV screening of pregnant women. MMWR 50(RR-19):63–110, 2001.

chapter 23

Miscellaneous Serology

Russell F. Cheadle, MS, MT(ASCP), Norma Cook, MA, MT(ASCP), and
Diane Wyatt, MS, MT(ASCP)

Learning Objectives

After finishing this chapter, the reader will be able to:
1. Explain reasons why a host has a more difficult problem overcoming parasitic diseases than those caused by bacteria or viruses.
2. State five outcomes that may follow invasion by a parasite and give a reason for each outcome.
3. List five ways parasites evade host defenses.
4. List three examples illustrating how host responses to parasites cause other pathology for the host.
5. Discuss the role of IgE in parasitic infections.
6. State important diagnostic information provided by serologic testing for *Toxoplasma gondii*.
7. Explain how serologic tests for *Entamoeba histolytica*, *E. histolytica/dispar*, *Giardia lamblia*, *Trichomonas vaginalis*, and *Cryptosporidium parvum* differ from serologic tests for other parasites.
8. Name the best immunologic test method for each of the diseases listed in number 7 and give a reason for the choice.
9. List four possible limitations associated with parasitic serology.
10. List factors that have led to a notable increase in fungal infections in the last 25 years.
11. Describe the etiologic and physiologic factors to be examined when a mycosis is suspected.
12. Discuss the importance of serodiagnosis in making a rapid and presumptive diagnosis of fungal infections.
13. List three areas of testing in which immunologic procedures have major application for mycotic diagnosis.
14. Describe how the stage of the mycosis is important in determining the most effective immunodiagnostic test to be used.
15. Discuss how related cross-reacting mycotic antigens are evaluated.
16. Recognize the ecology, epidemiology, and clinical disease of aspergillosis, candidiasis, cryptococcosis, and coccidioidomycosis.
17. List at least three serologic tests currently used for the serodiagnosis of aspergillosis, candidiasis, cryptococcosis, and coccidioidomycosis.

Key Terms

Antigen switching	Cyst	Mycoses
Aspergillosis	Eosinophil chemotactic factor	Spherule
Candidiasis	Fungi	Thermal dimorphism
Coccidioidomycosis	Hyphae	Toxoplasmosis
Conida	Mold	Yeast
Cryptococcosis	Mycelium	

The diagnosis of fungal and parasitic diseases traditionally has depended on morphologic features of the organisms and culture in the case of fungi. Serologic testing has not been widely used. Available serologic testing for fungi and parasites is limited, and the antigens for both are often cruder than their counterparts for viral and bacterial diagnosis. This factor limits specificity in a number of the procedures. A further similarity between the two can be drawn from the fact that both fungal and parasitic diseases have received more attention in recent years because of their role as opportunistic infections in patients who are immunosuppressed, and this limits the utility of serologic tests for antibody detection. Therefore, it seems appropriate to discuss immunologic factors for these two types of infections in one chapter. This chapter provides information about the immunologic aspects of these infections along with discussion of serologic testing that is available.

Parasitic Immunology

Although North Americans do not suffer greatly from parasites, parasitic infections do occur, and with the spread of acquired immunodeficiency syndrome (AIDS), several infections such as toxoplasmosis, giardiasis, and cryptosporidiosis have become more important problems. Other parasitic diseases such as malaria, schistosomiasis, and leishmaniasis are among the World Health Organization's list of the five most harmful infective diseases afflicting humans today. A further understanding of parasitic immunology will lead to better diagnosis and control of these diseases as well as add to the fundamental knowledge of the immune response itself. This section discusses the various immunologic strategies used by a host as it combats parasitic infections. Specific details about various parasites are considered separately later in the chapter, as is the diagnostic role of serologic testing methods as they relate to each parasite.

When a parasite enters a host, there are several possible results. First, there may be no infection at all because the host's innate immunity prevents the parasite from establishing an infection. In this case, the host fails to provide either the necessary physical environment or some important nutritional factor(s) needed for the parasite's survival. The host may even produce products that are toxic to the parasite.

A second outcome may be that the parasite invades the host, becomes established, and is then killed and eliminated by host defense mechanisms. These events indicate that an effective immune response has occurred. Typically, the host remains immune to reinfection for some time. This response requires antibody formation.

The third outcome is the reverse of the second. In this instance a parasite may overwhelm and kill the host. Reasons for this outcome include an organism that multiplies so rapidly that the host does not have time to mobilize its defenses, parasitic invasion of a vital organ(s), or an inadequate host immune system.

Another possible result is a long-lasting infection in which the host begins to eliminate the parasite but cannot remove it completely. In the best case, the host will control the disease for an extended period and may eventually overcome and eliminate the parasite. In the worst case, the host will succumb to the infection and die.

In yet another scenario, the host mounts a response that attacks not only the parasite but also host tissues. The effects of this inappropriate response (hypersensitivity or immune disease) on the host may be mild or severe; often the consequences for the parasite are minimal. In fact, most of the pathology associated with a parasitic infection results from the immunologic responses to the offending organism and may be more dangerous for the host than the infection itself.

Evasion of Host Defenses

Any parasite's survival depends on its ability to live in a peaceable manner with its host. If the host dies, then so does the parasite. When a parasite is recognized as a foreign entity by the host, however, the relationship becomes combative. As a host defends itself, the parasite attempts to evade the host's defense mechanisms. Parasites are very complex antigenically and have complex life cycles that involve immunologically different stages that may be found in different body locations. The net result leads to a situation in which the host may partially control the infection but not eliminate the parasite. The host continues to fight with increasingly complex responses until either the host or the parasite wins. Frequently, there is only an uneasy compromise that can be tipped in favor of either side. Many factors, some known and many others not yet known, work together to preserve the parasite's existence.

If a parasite can become sequestered within host cells, then the parasite is protected. For example, when parasites such as the tissue protozoans invade macrophages or liver cells, they are hidden from the immune system for a time because the host cannot recognize the parasite while it is inside these cells.[1] Eventually they must leave these cells and invade new ones. When they are between cells they are then vulnerable to the host's defenses.

Some parasites disguise themselves by acquiring host antigens. Schistosomes live well in unprotected blood vessels because the invading form (schistosomula) can acquire red blood cell antigens that later help to protect the adult from attack by the immune system.[2]

Other parasites possess variable antigens. The African trypanosomes evade the immune response by periodically changing their surface antigens.[3] A variant surface glycoprotein produces an unlimited group of variable antigen types. The host builds antibody, mainly IgM, to the one antigen, thereby reducing the infection. The parasite responds by changing its antigen, making the current antibody ineffective. The switching may occur very rapidly, within 5 to 6 days. The host must now make new antibody. This process of **antigen switching** can continue for long periods.

Entamoeba histolytica can shed antigens.[1] Antibody is formed, but if the antigen is not attached to the parasite, then the immune response cannot harm the offending organism.

The malaria sporozoite illustrates another defense tactic: By presenting a dominant but irrelevant antigen, the parasite deflects the immune system away from more vulnerable targets. For example, T helper (Th) 1 responses seem to be more effective against protozoa but the irrelevant response may stimulate a counterproductive Th2 response leading to harm for the host through toxic products such as nitric oxide (NO) released by activated macrophages. NO causes some of the symptoms of cerebral malaria.

Along with these specific ways used by parasites to evade the host's immune system, there are numerous nonspecific factors that interfere with the normal operation of the system as a whole. When a host eliminates a bacterial or viral infection, the immune system can shut down and rest until a new encounter occurs. Parasitic infections, however, are chronic because the host is rarely able to eliminate the source of infection, so that the immune system is forced to stay turned on. This interference often leads to immunosuppression, disruption of normal B cell and T cell functions and hypersensitivity reactions.[4] Immune complexes may form, bind complement, and activate macrophages, so that other processes are in turn stimulated with resulting problems such as the autoimmune anemia or intravascular coagulation seen in American trypanosomiasis (Chagas' disease).[5] Antigens shared by both the parasite and the host lead to autoimmune problems such as the heart and intestinal consequences seen in late stages of Chagas' disease. All of these complicated mechanisms either lead to or directly cause the pathology seen in parasitic diseases.

Immunologic Response to Parasites

The response to parasites involves the active participation of several cell types, including B and T lymphocytes, macrophages, granulocytes, and mast cells. Immunoglobulins, complement, and cytokines all help the host to overcome a parasitic infection. The immunoglobulin response includes formation of IgM, IgG, and IgA antibodies. Cell-mediated processes that help to destroy the offending organism follow antibody production. Many protozoan parasites are effectively reduced or eliminated by macrophages that have be-come activated by cytokines such as interferon-γ and migration inhibitory factor produced by sensitized T cells. Other cytokines, including interleukin-3 and granulocyte-monocyte colony-stimulating factor, act on cells of the myeloid line to cause an increase in neutrophils, eosinophils, and macrophages; thus, additional effector cells are brought in to combat the infection.

Helminth infections in particular are characterized by high levels of IgE. IgE binds to mast cells and basophils. When specific antigen–antibody combinations occur, degranulation results in the release of chemotactic factors, histamine, prostaglandins, and other mediators. One of the most important mediators released is **eosinophil chemotactic factor,** which attracts eosinophils to the infected area. Eosinophils are then able to kill worms through antibody-dependent cytotoxicity. It is believed that the ability to produce IgE evolved mainly for the purpose of dealing with parasitic infections.[6]

Although antibodies are detectable in serum and may be useful guides when diagnosing diseases caused by parasites, they have little or no correlation with the course or prognosis of the disease. Later protection from reinfection by the parasite cannot be predicted on the basis of circulating antibody levels nor can any other useful information be gained by measuring cellular responses.

Serology can, however, help identify a parasite that is present in organs or other deep tissue sites such as the brain or muscle and is not recovered in blood, urine, or feces. If a person travels to an endemic area, becomes infected with a parasite, and then returns to a nonendemic area, a positive serology test can pinpoint the time of infection. If a person who normally lives in an endemic area has a positive test, the result may only reflect a previous infection by the parasite and may not relate to the patient's current condition because antibody levels may remain elevated for years.

Serology in Protozoan Diseases

Falciparum malaria and African trypanosomiasis still produce high mortality rates despite intense efforts to control the parasites causing these diseases. Other relatively mild diseases such as amebiasis, giardiasis, and toxoplasmosis are found worldwide but have become significant problems for patients who have suppressed immune systems. Immunosuppressive drugs used to treat cancer or prevent rejection of transplanted organs, and more importantly, diseases such as AIDS, have caused these patients to be more susceptible to these infections. More recently, infections with *Cryptosporidium parvum*, *Cyclospora cayetanensis*, and several *Microsporidium* species. have become more important, especially in immunocompromised hosts. Because protozoa can live in the blood, the gastrointestinal tract, organ tissues, and macrophages, the clinical manifestations and host responses are quite varied. Several representative protozoan diseases for which serologic testing is helpful are presented here.

Toxoplasmosis

Toxoplasmosis results from infection with *Toxoplasma gondii,* a ubiquitous protozoan parasite that infects humans by ingestion of infective **cysts** (öocysts). It is thought that cysts are transferred by hand-to-mouth contact from contaminated soil or cat litter or by ingesting öocysts in raw or partially cooked pork, mutton, or beef. Transmission may also occur through blood transfusions or organ transplantation. Cats are known to be definitive hosts for this parasite, but other unknown definitive hosts must also exist because nearly 40 percent of the world's adult population is infected with this parasite.

This disease is nearly always asymptomatic or may present a mild lymphadenopathy. Rarely, the parasite may reach the central nervous system (CNS) or the eye. Invasion of the CNS can be fatal and typically only occurs in immunosuppressed patients.[7] This is one of the more common opportunistic infections seen in individuals with AIDS.

Encysted organisms can be found in any tissue. These cysts may remain viable for years, which explains why immunosuppressed patients can exhibit symptoms long after initial infection. The greatest concern, however, is the fact that *Toxoplasma* species can cross the placenta.

If the fetus is exposed during the first trimester, death is nearly always the result because of damage to the CNS. Infection during the second trimester may result in hydrocephaly, blindness, or other nervous system damage. Later infection may result in blindness or mild CNS defects. It is noteworthy that women who are exposed to this parasite before pregnancy do not transmit the infection to the fetus.

T. gondii is capable of replicating inside human macrophages. The parasite can survive indefinitely in macrophages because it is able to prevent the fusion of lysosomes with phagosomes. Normally a phagocytic cell will digest the material within the phagolysosome, but in this case digestion does not occur. The ability of macrophages to kill the parasite is greatly increased if the parasite is first exposed to antibody. Antibody-coated *Toxoplasma* organisms trigger normal phagocytosis, which ultimately kills the organism. Immunocompromised patients may have severe problems with this infection, a fact that further confirms the role played by antibody in controlling this disease.

Serologic testing plays an important role in the diagnosis of toxoplasmosis because isolation of the organism involves tissue specimens and requires a difficult and lengthy procedure. Generally, a seroconversion to an antibody-positive state, a fourfold increase in titer, or high levels of IgM antibody is considered diagnostic.

Enzyme immunoassay (EIA) tests for IgM or IgG and indirect fluorescent antibody (IFA) tests for IgG are available and should be performed when congenital toxoplasmosis is suspected. IFA testing has been widely used, but EIA appears to be more sensitive and is the method of choice.[8] Elevated titers of both antibody classes suggest that infection has occurred within the previous 3 to 9 months. Elevated IgG titers without IgM antibody suggest an older infection. Paired samples whose collection is separated by 3 weeks may be tested to confirm the presence of recent infection because with recent infection titers to both antibody classes will be rising. IgM titers thus provide important information.

Newborns with congenital toxoplasmosis will have detectable IgM antibody, and the mother's IgM titers will further support the diagnosis (Table 23–1). Specific IgA antibody assays provide even more sensitive methods for early detection and confirmation of congenital toxoplasmosis and should be performed for newborns suspected of harboring the parasite. Polymerase chain reaction (PCR) technology using amniotic fluid seems to be most useful in the diagnosis of prenatal congenital toxoplasmosis.

At the present time, there are no useful serologic procedures for diagnosing CNS infection in immunocompromised patients.[7] The reason for this is that these

TABLE 23–1. Interpretation of Toxoplasma Serologic Test Results

Titer IIF-IgG	EIA-IgM	Interpretation
<1:16	Negative	No evidence of exposure
>1:16	Negative	Infection probably acquired more than 1 year ago
=1:1024	1:4–1:256	Infection probably acquired within the past 18 months
=1:1024	=1:1024	Recent infection, probably acquired within the past 4 months
EIA = Enzyme immunoassay.		

patients do not produce detectable levels of specific antibody against the parasite.

Other Protozoa

Entamoeba histolytica, Entamoeba histolytica/dispar, Cryptosporidium parvum, Giardia lamblia, and *Trichomonas vaginalis* are all parasites that are normally identified by microscopic examination of specimen materials. Feces are tested for *E. histolytica, E. histolytica/dispar, C. parvum,* and *G. lamblia*; urine or vaginal discharge is tested for *T. vaginalis.* In each case, immunologic procedures are directed toward identifying the organism or a soluble antigen found in the specimen. Serum studies are not used at all. The identification rates for each test compare favorably with conventional identification techniques, but immunologic procedures offer an important advantage because a technologist who is not experienced in parasitology can successfully perform them. Direct fluorescent antibody (DFA) and enzyme-linked immunosorbent assay (ELISA) kits are available for these organisms. The DFA methods use monoclonal antibody labeled with fluorescein isothiocyanate against the parasite's cell wall to visualize the initial antibody-parasite complex. *Cyclospora spp.* autofluoresce is a characteristic that is exploited as a useful additional diagnostic technique for identifying this parasite in feces, but it can lead to confusion and incorrect interpretation of DFA reactions used to detect other parasites, such as *C. parvum.*

EIA methods use enzyme conjugated to either antigen or antibody, depending on the assay being performed. After the antigen–antibody reaction has occurred and excess materials have been removed, a suitable substrate is added to react with remaining enzyme. The amount of product formed is proportional to the concentration of the unknown antigen or antibody being measured. The ELISA methods capture organisms or soluble antigen by adding samples to antibody-coated wells. Subsequent reactions cause a

chromogen to change color to indicate the presence of bound antigen. More details about this procedure are given in the laboratory exercise for this chapter.

PCR techniques have been developed to identify *Naegleria fowleri, Giardia lamblia, Toxoplasma gondii,* and *Trypanosoma cruzi* but are not yet used routinely in the lab. Finally, a latex agglutination method and a deoxyribonucleic acid (DNA) probe are available for *Trichomonas vaginalis* detection. Table 23–2 lists commercially available immunodiagnostic kits and reagents. (EIA and ELISA methods are not differentiated.)

Helminth Infections

Intestinal helminth infections are relatively simple to diagnose because eggs, adult round worms, and segments of tapeworms are easily recovered from stool specimens. However, larvae or embryos of some tapeworm species can leave the host's intestine and migrate to other tissue sites. The pathology produced by these wandering parasites depends on the damage caused to the organ or tissue invaded. Because symptoms are often vague or mimic other disease processes, it is difficult to identify the parasite as the causative agent. Serodiagnostic tests can provide helpful informa-

TABLE 23–2. Available Immunodiagnostic Tests for Parasitic Diseases

Disease	Antibody Tests*	Antigen Tests Available?
Amebiasis	EIA, IHA	No
Babesiasis	IFA	No
Chagas' disease	EIA, CF	No
Cryptosporidiasis	IFA	Yes
Cysticercosis	IB, EIA	No
Echinococcosis	EIA, IHA, IB	No
Fascioliasis	EIA	No
Filariasis	EIA	No
Giardiasis	. . .	Yes
Leishmaniasis	IFA, CF	No
Malaria	IFA	No
Paragonimiasis	EIA, IB	No
Pneumocystosis	. . .	Yes
Schistosomiasis	EIA, IB	No
Strongyloidiasis	EIA	No
Toxocariasis	EIA	No
Toxoplasmosis	EIA, IFA, EIA-IgM	No
Trichinellosis	BF, EIA	No
Trichomoniasis	. . .	Yes
Trypanosoma cruzi	EIA, IFA, CF	No

Courtesy of CDC, Atlanta, GA.
EIA = Enzyme immunoassay; IHA = indirect hemagglutination; IFA = indirect immunofluorescence; CF = complement fixation; IB = immunoblot; BF = bentonite flocculation; and IgM = immunoglobulin M.

tion when investigating these problems, especially in cysticercosis and echinococcosis. Current methods include IFA tests; slide, tube, and precipitin tests; complement fixation; particle agglutination tests; and enzyme-linked immunoassays, among others. Most commercial kit systems are based on an ELISA system. DNA probes are used in immunoblot methods at the Centers for Disease Control and Prevention (CDC) in Atlanta to diagnose cysticercosis, echinococcosis, paragonimiasis, and schistosomiasis. Table 23–3 lists tests performed at the CDC. Samples for CDC processing must be sent via state laboratories because the CDC does not accept specimens sent directly by private laboratories or physicians.

Limitations of Parasitic Serology

It is as important in clinical immunology as it is in all clinical laboratory areas to find the most straightforward and economic procedure for each test method. However, it is also important to consider the specificity and sensitivity of the method when choosing a procedure. Because no proficiency testing is currently offered in the area of parasitic serology, it is very difficult to evaluate the quality of commercial products. In the United States, commercial kit manufacturers must obtain Food and Drug Administration (FDA) approval

before selling their products. The FDA only requires that a new method be equivalent to a method that has already been approved.

Researchers at the CDC have expressed concern that, over time, the quality of new test kits may drift in a negative direction because a new kit may not be quite as good as the one used for comparison but may still be approved.[10] A further problem is that individual laboratories can and do develop their own methods using antigens purchased from various sources. Because the FDA does not regulate these procedures, the quality assurance burden then belongs to the individual laboratory providing the test. Because it is often difficult to find and prepare antigens that are highly specific for these parasites, there can be a large variation in results reported by various laboratories.

Another problem affecting the choice of a procedure is timing. A procedure may detect only a certain class of antibody such as IgM; thus, the test must be performed when the patient is producing IgM, or the diagnosis may be missed. A particular antibody produced against a certain stage in a parasite's life cycle may not be recovered by a given procedure, so again timing becomes important. It must not be forgotten that related organisms produce similar antigens, which, in turn, induce the formation of cross-reacting antibodies. This problem reduces a procedure's specificity. Although all of these problems must be taken into consideration, it

TABLE 23–3. Antibody Detection Tests Offered at the Centers for Disease Control and Prevention

Disease	Organism	Test
Amebiasis	*Entamoeba histolytica*	Enzyme Immunoassay (EIA)
Babesiosis	*Babesia microti*	Immunofluorescence (IFA)
	Babesia spp. WA1	
Chagas' disease	*Trypanosoma cruzi*	IFA
Cysticercosis	Larval *Taenia solium*	Immunoblot (Blot)
Echinococcosis	*Echinococcus granulosus*	EIA, Blot
Leishmaniasis	*Leishmania braziliensis*	IFA
	L. donovani	
	L. tropica	
Malaria	*Plasmodium falciparum*	IFA
	P. malariae	
	P. ovale	
	P. vivax	
Paragonimiasis	*Paragonimus westermani*	Blot
Schistosomiasis	*Schistosoma* spp.	Fluorescent antibody staining technique (FAST-ELISA)
	S. mansoni	Blot
	S. haematobium	Blot
	S. japonicum	Blot
Strongyloidiasis	*Strongyloides stercoralis*	EIA
Toxocariasis	*Toxocara canis*	EIA
Toxoplasmosis	*Toxoplasma gondii*	IFA-IgG, EIA-IgM
Trichinosis	*Trichinella spiralis*	EIA, Bentonite flocculation

For additional information about these tests, how to submit specimens for testing, or for test results and interpretation, call the Division of Parasitic Diseases, at (770)488-4431.

should be emphasized that with a clear understanding of parasitology and the principles of immunology, useful diagnostic information can be provided for the physician.

Fungal Immunology

Fungal infections are increasing worldwide at an alarming rate. This may be in part because of improved methods of reporting these diseases. More significant, however, is the positive correlation between the incidence of fungal infections and the increased use of broad-spectrum antibiotics, use of immunosuppressive agents, organ transplants, and incidence of immunodeficiency diseases. Fungal diseases often are the first defining infection in AIDS. Many saprophytic fungi formerly dismissed as cultural contaminants, are now reported as opportunistic pathogens.[11]

Mycotic Infections

Of the many thousands of species of **fungi** that have been described, only 150 to 200 species are generally recognized as primary pathogens in humans. Those fungi that are etiologic agents of human infection are normally soil saprophytes that have been traumatically introduced into body tissues or accidentally inhaled into the lungs. These exogenous pathogens can grow at the relatively elevated temperature of the human body and can survive cellular defenses. A few endogenous organisms, for example, the yeast *Candida albicans,* also can cause infection when the host defense is deficient for only a brief period.[11]

The development of a fungal infection depends on the virulence of the fungus, the number of infecting fungi inhaled or injected into the tissue, and the immune status of the host.[11] Natural immunity to fungal infection is very high, with the normal response being both cellular and humoral. However, the humoral mechanism is of minor importance in immunity against mycotic infections because the first line of defense is provided by cellular mechanisms involving macrophages, neutrophils, and T lymphocytes. In the majority of cases, the cellular defenses of normal persons are sufficient, and infections resolve spontaneously.

Fungi are eukaryotic cells with nuclei and have rigid cell walls. Fungi, pathogenic to humans, have two fundamental structural forms, appearing either as filamentous **molds,** as **yeasts,** or sometimes in both forms. Molds are composed of **hyphae** and **conidia.** Hyphae are filamentous tubular branching structures that intertwine to form a dense mat called a **mycelium.** Conidia are asexual reproductive structures produced at the tip or along the sides of fertile hyphae. Yeasts are unicellular and reproduce asexually by budding.[12,13]

Although most fungi are monomorphic, some fungi exhibit **thermal dimorphism.** These dimorphs reproduce both as molds, at 25°C to 30°C, and as yeasts, at 35°C to 37°C. The mycelial mold form is the saprophytic state found in nature; the yeast form is the parasitic or pathogenic state found in tissue in disease, with the exception of *Coccidioides immitis,* which grows as a **spherule** at 35°C to 37°C. The thermal dimorphs are the etiologic agents of serious systemic **mycoses** that can be life threatening.[14]

The identification of the etiologic agent is critical for treatment and management of the patient when a fungal infection has been established. Because culture does not always reveal the infectious agent, immunologic procedures can provide the first presumptive evidence of the infection.[15]

Serology in Mycotic Diseases

Antibody detection, antigen detection, and the identification of fungi in patient specimens or culture are the three areas in which immunologic procedures have found major application. Serologic tests also can yield information on the effects of chemotherapy. In many cases, serologically positive test results stimulate continued efforts to isolate and identify the etiologic agent in culture.[15]

Selection of the tests to be performed depends on the etiologic agent of the mycosis. The clinician must provide the laboratory with all the pertinent information available, including the patient's symptoms, history of other past or present infections, and medical treatments that have left the patient immunocompromised or debilitated. The patient's occupation, place of residence, and record of travel also are important because some occupations expose an individual to opportunistic or pathogenic fungi that might not otherwise have been considered, and many fungi are endemic to specific geographic areas. Because serologic tests are effective at different stages of mycotic disease and because the stage of the disease may not be known, the best procedure is to use a combination of serologic tests and a variety of related antigens to identify the antibodies of the etiologic agent. Serial dilutions of serum should be made after an initial 2- to 3-week interval (of the acute phase), midway through an infection, and after recovery (the convalescent phase) to determine if and how the titer is changing. Titers of 1:32 or a fourfold or greater rise in titer are significant in making a diagnosis as long as the patient is immunocompetent.

Serodiagnostic tests are commercially available with different degrees of sensitivity and specificity for aspergillosis, blastomycosis, candidiasis, coccidioidomycosis, cryptococcosis, histoplasmosis, paracoccidioidomycosis, and sporotrichosis. Some of the tests can be performed in routine laboratories. The following discussion provides information about available serologic testing for four of these diseases.

Aspergillosis

Aspergillus species are found worldwide in soil and air, in decaying vegetation, and on stored grains (Fig. 23–1). **Aspergillosis** is an opportunistic infection predominantly caused by *Aspergillus fumigatus, A. flavus, A. niger,* and *A. terreus.* Other pathogenic species of *Aspergillus* are involved with less frequency. Typical clinical infections may be colonizing, allergic, or disseminating, depending on the pathologic findings in the host. Aspergillosis usually occurs secondary to another disease, but it can develop in apparently normal individuals as well.[11,16]

Pulmonary colonization is usually a primary condition induced by inhalation of large numbers of conidia. Allergic bronchopulmonary aspergillosis is characterized by allergic reactions to the toxins and the endotoxins of *Aspergillus* species. Allergy, asthma, or transient pulmonary infiltrates may develop when hypersensitive individuals are exposed repeatedly to large numbers of conidia.[11] Disseminating or invasive aspergillosis (IA) is usually found in immunocompromised individuals with chronic granulomatous disease.[17]

Immunodiffusion and Counterimmunoelectrophoresis Tests   Ouchterlony immunodiffusion (ID) or counterimmunoelectrophoresis (CIE) for antibodies are methods available for Aspergillosis testing. In the ID or CIE methods, the presence of one or more lines of serum precipitins is suggestive but not conclusive evidence of an active infection (Fig. 23–2). Three or more lines are associated with aspergilloma (fungus ball) or with IA if the patient is not anergic. The *Aspergillus* reference antiserum must demonstrate three or more bands with *Aspergillus* reference antigen for test results to be valid. Nonspecific banding can be caused by C-reactive protein. The immunodiffusion tests will be positive only if the patient is immunocompetent, and they are of limited value for IA cases because these patients are often anergic.[15,18]

Enzyme Immunoassay   An EIA method has been developed to detect the serum galactomannan antigen of *Aspergillus.* This test is valuable for diagnosis of immunocompromised patients with Aspergillosis, but it is not available in the United States at this time.[15]

Candidiasis

Infections with *Candida albicans* and several other *Candida* species are collectively called **candidiasis.** *Candida albicans* is regarded as the most common cause of all serious fungal diseases. It is a normal endogenous inhabitant of the alimentary tract and the mucocutaneous regions of the body, and it can become an opportunistic pathogen in debilitated and immunocompromised hosts. Systemic involvement is rare except when the yeasts are seeded into the body in large numbers through indwelling catheters, organ transplantation, the needles of drug abusers, and after prolonged therapy with antibiotics or treatment with steroids and corticosteroids.[11]

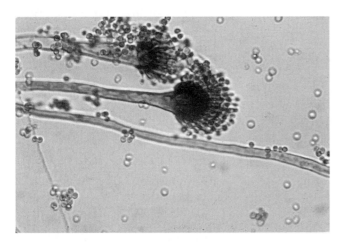

FIG. 23–1. Aspergillus fumigatus; LPCB stain × 450.

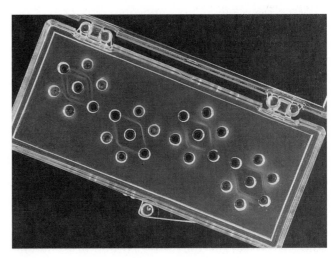

FIG. 23–2. Immunodiffusion patterns of selected fungal antibodies. (Courtesy of Immunomycologies, Norman, OK.)

Intact skin and mucous membranes are barriers to invasion of this fungus. Cellular defenses protect against mucocutaneous infection because most individuals have some antibodies to *C. albicans.* Opsonic serum factors and the ability of polymorphonuclear cells to phagocytize the yeast cells are also believed to play a part in immunity.[11] Hematogenous dissemination occurs in patients with neutropenia.

Immunodiffusion and Counterimmunoelectrophoresis Tests ID and CIE methods for antibodies give comparable results and both reliably detect antibodies in systemic candidiasis in immunocompetent hosts. A heat-stable cytoplasmic antigen is used with positive-control sera containing at least three of the seven known precipitins. Formation of one or more bands between the reagent antigen and patient's serum is considered a positive reaction. Systemic candidiasis is presumptively identified when serial dilutions of specimens show an increasing number of precipitin bands or convert from negative to positive. The patient's symptoms, direct smears and cultures should be considered to validate positive ID and CIE tests.[15]

Latex Agglutination (LA) The LA test for antibodies is quantitative, and it can be of diagnostic and prognostic value. Latex particles sensitized with a homogenate antigen of *C. albicans* are reacted with patient sera and control sera. When this screening test is positive, a serial dilution is performed and reported as the highest dilution giving a 2+ reaction. A titer of 1:4 suggests either an early infection, colonization, or a nonspecific reaction. A titer of 1:8 or greater, conversion from a negative to a positive test, or a fourfold increase in titer is presumptive evidence of invasive infection.[15]

Enzyme Immunoassay Antibody detection tests have little or no value in immunocompromised patients; therefore, tests for antigenemia must be performed for these patients. A double-antibody sandwich EIA method can be used to detect antigenemia. Concentrations greater than 2 ng/mL are presumptive evidence of active candidiasis.

Reverse Passive Agglutination Test A reverse passive LA test is also available for detection of antigenemia.[15] A recent study indicated that when a titer of 1:8 was used to indicate a positive test result, the sensitivity was 50 percent and the specificity was 73 percent.[19]

Coccidioidomycosis

Coccidioides immitis is the etiologic agent of **coccidioidomycosis.** The fungus is endemic in the southwestern United States, especially in the San Joaquin Valley in California (where it is called "valley fever") and in northern Mexico. *C. immitis* is a mold found primarily in alkaline desert soil in hot semiarid regions. Animals, especially desert rodents, have been shown to be vectors. The infectious conidia become airborne in dust storms or when disrupted during construction projects.[10,11,20] Primary pulmonary coccidioidomycosis results from inhalation of dust containing the fungus. Sixty percent of infections are asymptomatic and self-limiting in immunocompetent individuals. Hosts who are symptomatic may develop an acute primary pulmonary disease resembling the flu that resolves without treatment or that may become a chronic progressive pulmonary disease or progress to secondary infections. Hematogenous dissemination to the skin (erythema nodosum), bones, subcutaneous tissues, lymph nodes, and meninges is rare and occurs in as few a 1 percent of all cases of coccidioidomycosis.[11,20]

The antigen developed for serologic identification of circulating antibodies of *C. immitis* is coccidioidin, which is an antigen filtrate of broth cultures of mycelial growth. Serologic test methods available for coccidioidomycosis are discussed following.

Complement Fixation Complement fixation (CF) is the most widely used quantitative serodiagnostic method for identifying infections with *C. immitis*.[15] Complement-fixing antibodies of the IgG class develop in 3 to 6 months after the onset of symptoms. Titers of 1:2 to 1:4 are presumptive evidence of an early infection and should be repeated in 3 to 4 weeks. A titer of 1:16 is indicative of an active infection, particularly when accompanied by a positive ID test. Titers greater than 1:16 occur in 90 to 95 percent of patients with disseminated coccidioidomycosis. Titers parallel the severity of the mycoses.[17] Serum, cerebrospinal fluid (CSF), pleural, peritoneum, and joint fluids can be studied in this test. When CSF is positive with a titer of 1:2 or higher, it is indicative of coccidioidal meningitis 95 percent of the time. False-negative results occur in patients with solitary pulmonary lesions. Cross-reactions in patients with acute histoplasmosis will occur as false-positive reactions.[15,20]

Tube Precipitation (TP) Test Precipitating IgM antibodies appear in 1 to 3 weeks after infection in 90 percent of symptomatic patients; therefore, a positive TP test can be an early indication of a primary infection. If precipitins are formed in any dilution of this test, it is considered to be diagnostic. The precipitins disappear within 4 to 6 months in 80 to 90 percent of patients with coccidioidomycosis, even in cases with dissemination. This makes the test of little prognostic value. The TP test is, however, highly specific with very few cross-reactions.[11,15,18,20]

Immunodiffusion Agar gel double ID tests are as

sensitive as complement fixation tests and are not subject to anticomplementary reactions. The ID method is the most commonly used screening test for the diagnosis of coccidioidomycosis. When diffusion bands form in the agar gel that are continuous or identical with the reference antisera, the bands represent coccidioidin antigen and patient antibody reactions. Single bands typically indicate chronic infections, and two or more bands usually indicate active disease or dissemination. Serum dilutions can be performed for quantification of coccidioidin antibodies. This test is highly specific when reference antisera are used.[11,13,18,20]

Latex Agglutination   Latex particles sensitized with coccidioidin are reacted with inactivated patient serum in the LA method. This procedure is not recommended for testing CSF or diluted sera because many false reactions occur. The LA test is positive early in the course of the disease, but as many as 10 percent of the cases of coccidioidomycosis confirmed by culture or serology give false-negative results with an LA test. A CF test and/or an ID test should be performed for confirmation when LA screening tests are positive.[11,15,18,20]

Enzyme Immunoassay   EIA tests for IgG and IgM antibodies are available for use with serum or CSF. Positive EIA tests should be confirmed with CF or TP tests because the EIA test is not absolutely specific.[15]

Cryptococcosis

Cryptococcus neoformans is the etiologic agent of **cryptococcosis** (Fig. 23–3) The pigeon is the chief vector, and *C. neoformans* is found where pigeons roost and deposit their excreta.

Following inhalation of the yeast, cryptococcosis initially may be asymptomatic and unapparent, or it may develop as a symptomatic pulmonary infection. Encapsulation and the ability to synthesize melanin appear to be the significant virulence factors. Untreated infections with *C. neoformans* have a predilection for disseminating to the CNS and the brain. In disseminated disease, the yeast spread is hematogenous. Any organ or tissue of the body may be infected, but localization outside the lungs or brain is relatively uncommon. There is little humoral response elicited by infections with *C. neoformans* whether the patient is immunosuppressed or not. In normal patients, subclinical infection usually is resolved rapidly by growth-inhibiting substances present in body fluids.[11] Serious clinical disease is found in patients with debilitating diseases and immunosuppression; AIDS patients are the latest group with a predisposition to disseminated infections. Primary and secondary cutaneous cryptococcosis are regularly encountered clinical manifestations in immunosuppressed patients.[11,15]

Meningitis occurs in approximately two-thirds of the infections that disseminate. The predilection of the fungus for the CNS is postulated to be because of the absence of inhibitory factors in spinal fluid and the minimal phagocytic response found there.[11]

Latex Particle Agglutination (LPA) Antigen Test
When cryptococcosis is first suspected, the detection of the capsular polysaccharide antigen of *C. neoformans* in patient specimens can be made by the LPA test.[14] Inactivated serum or spinal fluid and positive and negative human reference sera are each mixed with latex particles sensitized with rabbit anticryptococcus globulin in rings on a test slide. The test is read macroscopically for agglutination. For it to be valid, the negative control must be negative and the positive control must show 2+ agglutination. Any agglutination is considered a positive test if controls are acceptable. Quantitative results can be obtained by performing a serial dilution. The titer is reported as the highest dilution showing 2+ agglutination. A titer of 1:2 suggests infection, but a titer of 1:4 or greater is evidence of an active infection. Higher titers correlate with the severity of infection. Positive titers are found in CSF in 95 percent of cases involving the CNS.

Cross-reactions may occur with rheumatoid factor (RF) and with circulating antibodies that bind with nonreactive polysaccharide in immune complexes. Treating the serum or CSF specimens with a protease that destroys RF and cleaves antibodies in the immune complexes can eliminate these reactions. Extraction of RF and circulating antibodies in serum can also be accomplished by treatment with ethylenediaminetetra-

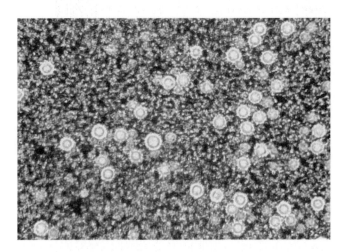

FIG. 23–3. India ink preparation; Cryptococcus neoformans × 1000. (From Kern, ME: *Medical Mycology: A Self-Instructional Text.* FA Davis, Philadelphia, 1985, p 53, with permission.)

acetic acid (EDTA) and boiling it for 5 minutes. False-positive results in spinal fluid can be eliminated simply by boiling it.[15,18]

Tube Agglutination (TA) Test   The TA test can be used as both a qualitative screening test and a semi-quantitative test. Serum or CSF from patients suspected of being infected with *C. neoformans* is inactivated to destroy complement. The serum or spinal fluid, an anti-cryptococcus positive control, and a negative control of rabbit serum are each mixed in test tubes with a Cryptococcus antigen suspension of weakly encapsulated yeast cells. The tubes are incubated and then refrigerated overnight. Reactions are read for agglutination. The positive control must read 3+ to 4+. Tests with reactions greater than the negative control are considered to be positive. The test can be made semiquantitative by performing a serial dilution and following the same procedure as that for the screening test. The titer is reported as the highest dilution showing any degree of agglutination. A titer of 1:2 or greater is suggestive of a current or recent infection with *C. neoformans.* Approximately 90 percent of patients with pulmonary cryptococcosis will demonstrate antibody titers in the TA test. As the mycosis progresses, antigens begin to appear with a decrease in antibody production. Following treatment, a decrease in antigen titers and a reappearance of antibodies indicate a good prognosis. The TA test has a specificity of 89 percent with extrameningeal infections.[15,18,21]

Enzyme-Linked Immunoassay   An EIA test is available to detect antigens of *C. neoformans* in both serum and CSF. The EIA method for antigen detection is more sensitive than the latex agglutination, but takes more time to perform.[15,18]

Indirect Fluorescent Antibody Test   Indirect immunofluorescence tests are available for the detection of antibodies to *C. neoformans.* They are most valuable when antigen tests are negative; moreover, they can be combined with antigen tests to determine the prognosis of the patient. A positive test suggests a recent or present infection with *C. neoformans* or a cross-reaction with another fungus. IFA tests have a specificity of 77 percent and a sensitivity of 50 percent. Both false-negative and false-positive results do occur.

SUMMARY

Serologic testing for parasitic and fungal diseases is less routine than for other infectious diseases because test availability is limited and diagnosis is usually made from culture and morphologic features of the organisms. However, some serologic tests are available and can be useful for detection of these diseases.

Clearly the nature of the immune response as related to parasitic infections is complex. Most parasitic diseases are usually diagnosed by other more direct methods such as fecal, blood, or urine examination, and thus serologic procedures are not frequently needed. However, clinical manifestations of several parasitic diseases such as toxoplasmosis are not always clear cut. In these cases, it may be possible to confirm the diagnosis serologically. In the United States, serum for such studies is often sent for serologic testing to a state public health reference laboratory. Occasionally, a state laboratory may send specimens to the CDC in Atlanta, Georgia. Many private laboratories also offer testing for a few parasites such as *Entamoeba histolytica, Entamoeba histolytica/dispar, Trichinella spiralis, Giardia lamblia,* and *Toxoplasma gondii. T. gondii* is also included as part of the ToRCH (Toxoplasma, rubella, cytomegalovirus, and herpes) panel, which is used to evaluate congenital and neonatal infections of newborn infants.

Testing methods used in parasitic serology cover the full range of methods available in immunology. Table 23–2 illustrates that everything from latex agglutination to countercurrent electrophoresis has been used or is currently being used to identify and quantify antibodies against parasites. New diagnostic procedures can be expected in the future, especially as DNA probe technology develops, but these tests will remain expensive for some time. In underdeveloped countries in which parasitic infections are common, high cost will limit the benefits from these procedures.

Serologic tests are useful for both the diagnosis and prognosis of patients with fungal infections. Cultural identification and/or finding the etiologic agents in direct mounts and in histopathologic preparations of clinical specimens is not always possible. Positive serologic tests are often the first suggestive evidence of mycotic infection. Tests with different degrees of sensitivity and specificity for aspergillosis, candidiasis, coccidioidomycosis, and cryptococcosis are presented in this chapter. Serodiagnostic test findings should be used in conjunction with the patient's symptoms, history, and other clinical findings. Because cross-reactions are sometimes encountered, it is recommended that a battery of tests and antigens be used to more easily interpret test results. Table 23–4 provides a summary of the mycoses presented in this chapter and the serologic tests that have proven to be useful for their diagnosis.

TABLE 23–4. Fungal Serodiagnostic Tests

Fungal Agents	Tests	Antigens	Interpretation
Aspergillus fumigatis *Aspergillus niger* *Aspergillus flavus* *Aspergillus terrus*	ID	*A. fumigatis* *A. niger* *A. flavus* *A. terrus*	One or more precipitin bands suggest an active infection; three to four bands are found in cases of aspergilloma and in invasive aspergillosis.
	RIA/EIA		Detects *Aspergillus* species antigenemia in immunodeficient patients
Candida albicans	ID	*C. albicans*	One or more precipitin bands are considered to be a positive reaction; cross-reactions are found with other *Candida* species.
	LA	*C. albicans*	Semiquantitative test with serum dilutions. Titer of 1:4 coupled with a positive ID test is presumptive evidence of invasive infection.
	EIA		Detects cell wall mannan in *Candida* antigenemia Concentrations greater than 2 ng/mL are presumptive evidence of invasive candidiasis.
Coccidioides immitis	CF	Coccidioidin, spherulin	Titers of 1:2 to 1:4 in sera are suggestive of infection; titers 1:2 or greater in CSF are indicative of CNS infection.
	TP	Coccidioidin	IgM antibodies are detected 1 to 3 weeks after the onset of symptoms.
	ID	Coccidioidin	A good screening test. A single precipitin band indicates chronic infection; two or more bands indicate active or disseminated infection.
	LA	Coccidioidin	A screening test that is positive soon after symptoms appear. It is very sensitive but not very specific.
	Exoantigen		Detects presence of cell-free antigen extracts.
Cryptococcus neoformans	LA		Uses latex particles coated with anticryptococcal antibody. Titers of 1:2 are suggestive of infection and titers of 1:8 are diagnostic. Positive titers in the CSF indicate CNS infection.
	TA	Cryptococcal antigen	Both a qualitative screening test and a semiquantitative test. Antibody titers of 1:2 or greater are presumptive evidence of infection.

ID = Immunodiffusion; RIA = radioimmunoassay; EIA = enzyme immunoassay; LA = latex agglutination; CF = complement fixation; CSF = cerebrospinal fluid; CNS = central nervous system; TP = tube precipitation; TA = tube agglutination.

Exercise: Giardia Lamblia *Disease Testing*

PRINCIPLE

The qualitative determination of *Giardia lamblia* trophozoite and cyst antigens in feces is accomplished using rabbit and mouse antisera. Giardia specific antigen (GSA 65) is a 65K MW glycoprotein produced in abundance by Giardia protozoa as they multiply in the intestinal tract. The test sample is added to a microtiter sample well. During the first incubation, GSA 65 antigens present in the stool supernate are captured by antibody bound to the well. The second anti-Giardia antibody is added. During the second incubation, this antibody "sandwiches" the antigen. After washings that remove unbound enzyme, substrate is added that develops color in the presence of the enzyme complex. Any amount of color indicates a positive reaction.

REAGENTS, MATERIALS, AND EQUIPMENT

Test kit such as ProSpect Giardia or ColorVue Giardia containing the following:

1. Test strips: microplate containing anti-Giardia antibody (eight wells per strip)
2. Test strip holder
3. Enzyme conjugate—mouse monoclonal anti-Giardia antibody with thimerosal
4. Positive control
5. Negative control
6. Substrate—tetramethylbenzidine (TMB) in buffer
7. Wash buffer 10X concentration
8. Stop solution—0.5 N hydrochloric acid
9. Specimen dilution buffer

Other materials required but not provided include the following:

Stool specimen collection containers
Wash bottle or dispenser for wash buffer
Timer that measures minutes
Distilled or deionized water

Optional materials include the following:

Microplate reader
Micropipettes
Plastic or glass disposable test tubes
Vortex mixer

SAMPLE PREPARATION

(There is no change on first part, but omit fresh or frozen stools and the paragraph below it.)

Dilution in Wells

Label one tube for each specimen. Add 0.4-mL specimen dilution buffer (SDB) to each tube. Coat one swab with specimen, and vigorously mix into SDB. Express as much fluid as possible, and discard the swab. Put a transfer pipet into the tube.

If specimen is watery or preserved, mix by shaking. No further preparation is necessary.

PROCEDURE*

Only one set of controls is needed per run.

1. Break off the required number of wells needed (number of samples plus 2 for controls) and place in a strip holder. Return the rest of the strips to the foli pouch, and reseal tightly.
2. Add four drops of the negative control to well #1 and four drops of positive control to well #2. (Use both undiluted.)
3. Add 100 µL of SDB to each of the remaining wells.
4. Add one drop of the stool specimen to each test well. Samples can be added directly or prediluted in tubes before adding to wells.
5. Incubate the microplate at room temperature (20°C to 25°C) for 60 minutes.
6. Shake out or aspirate the contents of the wells and wash.**
7. After the last wash, dump out contents, and bang on clean paper towel or aspirate.
8. Add four drops (200 µL) of enzyme conjugate to each well.
9. Incubate for 30 minutes at room temperature.
10. Decant and wash each well five times, as before.
11. Add four drops (200 µL) of color substrate to each well.
12. Incubate the microplate for 10 minutes.
13. Add one drop of stop solution to each well. Mix wells by tapping the strip holder.
14. Read reactions within 10 minutes after adding stop solution. Read manually or at 450 nm if an ELISA reader is used.

INTERPRETATION OF RESULTS

Visual

Positive: Any sample well that has yellow of at least 1+ intensity.
Negative: Colorless.

NOTE: The negative control should be colorless. However, the positive control well must be equal to or

---

*Adapted from the ProSpect Giardia Microplate Assay.

**Washings consist of filling each well with the diluted wash concentrate, shaking out the contents, and refilling the wells for a total of three times. Avoid generating bubbles in the wells during the washing steps.

greater than 2+ reaction on procedure and than the negative control for the test to be valid.

ELISA Reader

Zero the reader on air. Read the wells at 450 nm.

Positive: Absorbance reading of 0.25 and above.
Negative: Absorbance reading of less than 0.16. Tests with faint yellow color should be repeated.

COMMENTS

Giardia lamblia is a protozoan parasite that lives in the intestinal tract. Giardiasis is the most common parasitic disease in the United States and causes an estimated 100 million mild infections and 1 million severe infections each year. It is transferred from person to person through the fecal-oral ingestion of cysts. This disease is common in day-care centers and in other institutions where people are confined for extended periods. Contaminated drinking water is also a source of infection. Giardiasis has been reported in 5 to 19 percent of homosexual men. Symptoms of the acute disease include diarrhea, nausea, weight loss, malabsorption, abdominal cramps, flatulence, and anemia. Because acute, chronic, and asymptomatic infections occur and because symptoms are similar to those of many other intestine diseases, it is important to accurately diagnose the problem so that correct treatment can be given.

Diagnosis of giardiasis is frequently made by observing the parasite in fecal preparations. This method relies on an experienced technologist to correctly identify the organism. The diagnosis is often missed when an insufficient number of samples are examined because the excretion of organisms is frequently intermittent. Other more invasive methods such as sigmoidoscopy or biopsy have been used as well. The alternate approach, an ELISA method, such as the one presented earlier, offers a rapid noninvasive technique that does not require the observation and identification of an intact organism. These results suggest that immunologic procedures can play a significant role in the diagnosis of some parasitic diseases.

Review Questions

1. Compared to a host's response to the mumps virus, overcoming a parasitic infection is more difficult for the host because of which of the following characteristics of parasites?
   a. Large size
   b. Complex antigenic structures
   c. Elaborate life cycle
   d. All of the above

2. Most of the pathology associated with parasitic infections results from which of the following?
   a. Symbiotic relationships with the host
   b. Elaborate parasitic life cycles
   c. Hypersensitivity reaction to the offending organism
   d. Innate defense mechanisms of the host

3. Parasites are able to evade host defenses by which of the following means?
   a. Acquisition of host antigens
   b. Changing surface antigens
   c. Sequestering themselves within host cells
   d. All of the above

4. The chronic nature of parasitic infections is due to the host's:
   a. Inability to eliminate the infective agent
   b. Type I hypersensitivity response to the infection
   c. Ability to form a granuloma around the parasite
   d. Tendency to form circulating immune complexes

5. Clinical information provided by studying the immune response to parasitic diseases:
   a. Aids in correctly diagnosing the disease
   b. Predicts the prognosis of the disease
   c. Determines the possibility of reinfection by the parasite
   d. All of the above

6. The presence of both IgM and IgG antibody in toxoplasmosis infections suggests that the infection:
   a. Occurred more than 2 years ago
   b. Occurred less than 18 months ago
   c. Is chronic
   d. Has resolved itself

7. Soluble antigens found in feces are associated with infections by:
   a. *Trichomonas vaginalis*
   b. *Giardia lamblia*
   c. *Cryptosporidium parvum*
   d. b and c only
   e. a, b, and c

8. Which of the following are factors that have enabled saprophytic fungi to cause infections in humans?
   a. Their ability to survive the body's cellular defenses
   b. Their traumatic introduction into body tissues
   c. Use of antibiotics and immunosuppressive agents
   d. All of the above

9. When a mycosis is suspected, patient information must be acquired for all of the following *except:*
   a. Symptoms and physical examination
   b. Occupation, residence, and travel
   c. Medical treatment and medications
   d. Exercise program

10. Serodiagnosis is most important in making a rapid and presumptive diagnosis of fungal infections when:
    a. The patient is under 12 or over 50 years of age
    b. The patient has an undiagnosed acute or chronic respiratory infection
    c. Cultures of specimens are positive
    d. Histologic tissue slide preparations are positive

11. Because the stage of the mycosis is often not known, what is the best way to proceed when initiating serodiagnosis?
    a. Use a skin test in an endemic area because a positive skin test is diagnostic.
    b. Use a combination of serologic tests.
    c. Serial testing is excessive; a single test is always diagnostic.
    d. Use a single, specific antibody.

12. Serodiagnostic tests after infection has been established are most likely to be positive in which of the following cases:
    a. The patient has developed a state of anergy.
    b. The patient is immunocompromised.
    c. The patient is immunocompetent.
    d. The tests were taken before antibodies had time to develop.

13. Which is the characteristic of nonspecific cross-reactions?
    a. Occur as a result of crude unpurified antigens
    b. Occur with only one genus of fungi
    c. Do not interfere with fungal identification
    d. Tend to remain at high titer as a mycosis develops

14. Two serologic tests currently used for the diagnosis of aspergillosis and candidiasis are:
    a. Complement fixation (CF) and enzyme immunoassay (EIA)
    b. Immunodiffusion (ID) and counterimmunoelectrophoresis (CIE)
    c. Counterimmunoelectrophoresis (CIE) and complement fixation (CF)
    d. Enzyme immunoassay (EIA) and immunodiffusion (ID)

15. A 27-year-old man from Ohio, diagnosed with AIDS, developed chest pains and after a short period of time also developed severe headaches with dizziness. His hobby was raising messenger pigeons. His physician ordered a sputum culture and spinal tap, and both were positive for a yeastlike fungus. These findings are most consistent with infection by:
    a. *Candida albicans*
    b. *Coccidioides immitis*
    c. *Cryptococcus neoformans*
    d. *Histoplasma capsulatum*

16. Which of the following serologic tests detects the polysaccharide capsule antigen in serum and CSF of patients with suspected infection with *Cryptococcus neoformans?*
    a. Complement fixation (CF)
    b. Hypersensitivity skin test
    c. Latex agglutination (LA)
    d. Hemagglutination test

17. A young man from New York state was stationed at an air base in southern California. He developed flulike symptoms with chest pain and a high fever. Cultures were taken, and spherules were identified in direct preparations of his sputum. With this information, the physician could make a presumptive diagnosis of:
    a. Blastomycosis
    b. Coccidioidomycosis
    c. Cryptococcosis
    d. Histoplasmosis

18. What is the most widely used quantitative serologic test for identification of antibodies in infection with *Coccidioides immitis?*
    a. Complement fixation (CF)
    b. Latex agglutination (LA)
    c. Exoantigen test
    d. Fluorescent antibody test

References

1. Goodenough, UW: Deception by pathogens. Sci Am 79: 344–355, 1991.
2. Gryseels, B: Human resistance to *Schistosoma* infections. Parasitol Today 10:380–384, 1994.
3. Barry, JD: The relative significance of mechanisms of antigenic variation in African Trypanosomes. Parasitol Today 13:212–218, 1997.
4. Collier, L, Balows, A, and Sussman, M (eds): Topley and Wilson's Microbiology and Microbial Infections, ed. 9. Oxford University Press, New York, vol 5, pp 69–70.
5. Tarleton, RL: Pathology of American Trypanosomiasis. In Warren, KS (ed): Immunology and Molecular Biology of Parasitic Infections, ed. 3. Blackwell Scientific Publications, Boston, 1993.
6. Roitt, IM: Essential Immunology, ed. 7. Blackwell Scientific, Oxford, 1991.
7. Mariuz, P, Bosler, EM, and Luft, BJ: Toxoplasmosis in individuals with AIDS. Infect Dis Clin North Am 8:365–381, 1994.
8. Kagan, IG, and Maddison, SE: Serodiagnosis of parasitic diseases. In Rose, NR, et al (eds): Manual of Clinical Laboratory Immunology, ed. 4. American Society for Microbiology, Washington D.C., 1992, pp 529–543.
9. Heard, N, Marx-Chemla, C, and Foudrinier, F, et al: prenatal diagnosis of congenital toxoplasmosis in 261 pregnancies, Prenatal Diag 17: 1047–1054, 1997.
10. Wilson, M, and Schantz, P: Nonmorphologic diagnosis of parasitic infections. In Balows, A, Hausler, WJ, et al (eds): Manual of Clinical Microbiology, ed. 5. American Society for Microbiology, Washington, D.C., 1991, pp 717–726.
11. Rippon, JW: Medical Mycology: The Pathogenic Fungi and Pathogenic Actinomycetes, ed. 3. WB Saunders, Philadelphia, 1988.
12. Dixon, DM, Rhodes, JC, and Fromtling, RA: Taxonomy, classification, and nomenclature of fungi. In Murray, PR, Baron, EJ, Pfaller, MA, et al (eds): Manual of Clinical Microbiology, ed. 7. American Society for Microbiology, Washington, D.C., 1999, pp 1661–1667.
13. McGinnis, MR: Laboratory Handbook of Medical Mycology. Academic Press, New York, 1980.
14. Miller, LE, et al: Manual of Laboratory Immunology, ed. 2. Lea & Febiger, Philadelphia, 1991, pp 291–306.
15. Reiss, E, Kaufman, L, Kovacs, A, and Lindsley, M: Clinical immunomycology. In Rose, NR, et al: Manual of Clinical Immunology, ed. 6. American Society for Microbiology, Washington, D.C., 2002, pp 559–583.
16. Koneman, EM, et al: Mycology. In Koneman, EM, Allen, SD, Janda,

WM, et al: Color Atlas and Textbook of Diagnostic Microbiology, ed. 5. Lippincott-Raven, Philadelphia, 1997, pp 983–1070.

17. Forbes, BA, et al: Laboratory methods in basic mycology. In Forbes, BA, Sahm, DF, and Weissfeld (eds): Bailey and Scott's Diagnostic Microbiology, ed. 11. Mosby, St. Louis, MO, 1998.

18. McGinnis, MR, and Tilton, RC: Immunologic diagnosis of fungal infection. In Howard, DA, et al (eds): Clinical and Pathogenic Microbiology, ed. 2. Mosby, St. Louis, MO, 1994, pp 641–648.

19. Petri, MG, Konig, J, Moecke, HP, Gramm, HJ, et al: Epidemiology of invasive mycoses in ICU patients: A prospective multicenter study in 435 non-neutropenic patients. Paul-Ehrlich Society for Chemotherapy, Divisions of Mycology and Pneumonia Research. Intensive Care Med 23:317–325, 1997.

20. Zimmer, BL, and Pappagianis, D: Serology of coccidioidomycosis. Clin Microbiol Rev 3:247–273, 1990.

21. Package insert: Immunoscan Cryptoccal Latex Antibody Test, Baxter Healthcare. Deerfield, Ill., 1994.

22. Black, R, et al: Giardiasis in day-care center: evidence of person to person transmission. Pediatrics 60:486–491, 1977.

23. Craun, G: Waterborne Giardiasis in the United States, 1965–1984. Lancet 513–514, 1986.

24. Smith, J: Identification of fecal parasites in the Special Parasitology Survey of the College of American Pathologists. Am J Clin Pathol 72:371–373, 1979.

25. Kleeman, KJ, and Gilmour, L: Cost evaluation of an EIA screening test for *Giardia*. Am Clin Lab 26, 1992.

Glossary

Ab-toxin: Antibody to tumor-associated antigens, which are covalently linked to a toxic moiety to help destroy tumor cells.

Accelerated rejection: A form of rejection that occurs within 1 to 5 days after second exposure to tissue antigens based on reactivation of B and T cell responses.

Activation unit: The combination of complement components C1, C4b, and C2b that form the enzyme C3 convertase, whose substrate is C3.

Acute GvHD: Graft-versus-host disease, which occurs shortly after immunocompetent cells are transplanted into a recipient. It is characterized by skin rashes, diarrhea, and increased susceptibility to infection.

Acute phase response: Proteins and cells in the blood that increase rapidly in response to an infectious agent. It is considered part of natural immunity.

Acute phase reactants: Normal serum proteins that increase rapidly as a result of infection, injury, or trauma to the tissues.

Acute rejection: Rejection of tissue that takes place within days to weeks after transplantation, caused by cell-mediated immune reactions.

Acute rheumatic fever: A disease that develops as a sequel to group A streptococcal pharyngitis, characterized by the presence of antibodies that cross-react with heart tissue.

Acquired immunity: See acquired immune response.

Adaptive immune response: Host response to foreign agents that depends on T and B lymphocytes and is characterized by specificity, memory, and recognition of self versus nonself.

Adjuvant: A substance administered with an immunogen that enhances and potentiates the immune response.

Affinity: The initial force of attraction that exists between a Fab site on an antibody and one epitope or determinant site on the corresponding antigen.

Agglutination: The process by which particulate antigens such as cells aggregate to form large complexes when specific antibody is present.

Agglutination inhibition reaction: An agglutination reaction based on competition between particulate and soluble antigens for a limited number of antibody-combining sites. Lack of agglutination is a positive test result.

Agglutinin: An antibody that causes clumping or agglutination of the cells that triggered its formation.

AIDS: Acquired immunodeficiency syndrome, a disease affecting the immune system caused by human innumodeficiency virus.

Allele: A different form of a gene that codes for a slightly different form of the same product.

Alloantigen: An antigen that is found in another member of the host's species and that is capable of eliciting an immune response in the host.

Allograft: Tissue transferred from an individual of one species into another individual of the same species.

Allotype: A minor variation in amino acid sequence in a particular class of immunoglobulin molecule that is inherited in Mendelian fashion.

Alpha-fetoprotein: Glycoprotein normally found in small amounts in adults. Used as a tumor marker to indicate hepatocellular carcinoma or testicular cancer.

Alternative pathway: A means of activating complement proteins without antigen–antibody combination. This pathway is triggered by constituents of microorganisms.

Amplicon: A copy of a select portion of DNA that is obtained by the polymerase chain reaction.

Amplification: Techniques that increase either target nucleic acid or a signal probe to identify a specific nucleic acid sequence in a patient specimen.

Analyte: The substance being measured in an immunoassay.

Anaphylatoxin: A small peptide formed during complement activation that causes increased vascular permeability, contraction of smooth muscle, and release of histamine from basophils and mast cells.

Anaphylaxis: A life-threatening response to an allergen characterized by the systemic release of histamine.

Antibodies: Serum factors in the blood formed in response to foreign substance exposure. Antibodies are also known as immunoglobulins.

Antibody-dependent cell cytoxicity: The process of destroying antibody-coated target cells by natural killer cells, monocytes, macrophages, and neutrophils, which have specific receptors for immunoglobulin.

Anti-DNase B: An antibody directed against DNase B, which is secreted by group A streptococci.

Antigens: Macromolecules that are capable of eliciting formation of immunoglobulins (antibodies) or sensitized cells in an immunocompetent host.

Antigen switching: A protecting mechanism used by parasites that involves varying synthesis of surface antigens to evade an immune response by the host.

Anti-Hbe: Antibody to hepatitis B capsid antigen.

Anti-HBs: Antibody to hepatitis B surface antigen.

Antinuclear antibody (ANA): Antibody produced to different components of the nucleus during the course of several autoimmune diseases. Examples include anti-DNA, antideoxyribonucleoprotein, and antiribonuclearprotein antibodies, all of which occur in systemic lupus erythematosus.

Arthus reaction: A type III hypersensitivity reaction that occurs when an animal has a large amount of circulating antibody and is exposed to the antigen intradermally, resulting in localized deposition of immune complexes.

ASO titer: A test for the diagnosis of poststreptococcal sequelae, based on the neutralization of streptolysin O by antistreptolysin O found in patient serum.

Aspergillosis: An opportunistic fungal infection predominantly caused by *Aspergillus fumagatus.*

Ataxia-telangiectasia (AT): An autosomal recessive syndrome that results in a combined defect of both cellular and humoral immunity. The defect is in a gene responsible for recombination of immunoglobulin superfamily genes.

Atopy: An inherited tendency to respond to naturally occurring allergens; it results in the continual production of light.

Attenuated vaccine: A vaccine that uses live organisms that have been changed, through heat, aging, or chemical means, so that the organism is no longer pathogenic.

Autoantigen: One that belongs to the host and is not capable of eliciting an immune response under normal circumstances.

Autocrine: Produced by the cell that stimulates the same cell to grow.

Autograft: Tissues removed from one area of an individual's body and reintroduced in another area in the same individual.

Autoimmune disease: A condition in which damage to body organs results from the presence of autoantibodies or autoreactive cells.

Avidity: The strength with which a multivalent antibody binds a multivalent antigen.

Bence-Jones proteins: Proteins found in the urine of patients with multiple myeloma. They are now recognized as monoclonal immunoglobulin light chains.

Biohazardous: Hazards caused by infectious organisms.

Body substance isolation (BSI): A modification of Universal Precautions not limited to bloodborne pathogens that considers all body fluids and moist body substances to be potentially infectious.

Bone marrow: The largest tissue of the body, located in the long bones. Its role is the generation of hematopoietic cells.

Borrelia burgddorferi: A spirochete that is the causative agent of Lyme disease.

Branched chain DNA amplification: A technique used to detect a small amount of DNA through the use of several hybridization steps that create a branching effect with several nucleic acid probes.

Bruton's agammaglobulinemia: An X-linked recessive immunodeficiency disease that results in a lack of mature B lymphocytes and immunoglobulins of all classes.

Bystander lysis: A phenomenon that occurs in complement activation when C3b becomes deposited on host cells, making them a target for destruction by phagocytic cells.

CA-125: Antigen normally expressed in the developing fetus that can be used as an indictor of ovarian cancer.

C-kit ligand: Growth factor that affects the growth of the most primitive precursor cells in the bone marrow. Also known as stem cell factor.

C-reactive protein: A trace constituent of serum that increases rapidly following infection or trauma to the body and acts as an opsonin to enhance phagocytosis.

C1 inhibitor (C1INH): A glycoprotein that acts to dissociate C1r and C1s from C1q, thus inhibiting the first active enzyme formed in the classical complement cascade.

C4-binding protein (C4BP): A protein in the complement system that serves as a cofactor for factor 1 in the inactivation of C4b.

Calcitonin: A peptide hormone produced by the parathyroid, thyroid, and thymus glands. Used as a marker for thyroid carcinoma and endocrine neoplasma type 2A.

Candidiasis: An opportunistic fungal infection caused by *Candida albicans* and other *Candida* species.

Capture assay: An enzyme immunoassay using two antibodies: The first binds the antigen to solid phase, and the second contains the enzyme label and acts as an indicator.

Cell flow cytometry: An automated system for identifying cells based on the scattering of light as cells flow single file through a laser beam.

Cellular immunity: The theory that resistance to disease is based on cellular elements in the blood.

Centers for Disease Control and Prevention (CDC): A governmental agency of the U.S. Department of Health and Human Services that deals with control of communicable, vector-borne, and occupational diseases.

CD4 T cell: Type of lymphocyte that provides help to B cells to initiate antibody formation.

Chain of infection: A continuous link between three elements—a source, a method of transmission, and a susceptible host.

Chancre: The initial lesion that develops on the external genitalia in syphilis.

Chemical Hygiene Plan: A plan for safe use of chemicals in the laboratory that includes the following: appropriate work practices, standard operating procedures, personal protective equipment, use of fume hoods and flammables safety cabinets, employee training requirements, and medical consultation guidelines.

Chemiluminescence: The production of light energy by a chemical reaction.

Chemokines: A large family of homologous cytokines.

Chemokinesis: The migration of specific classes of leukocytes toward the source of chemokines, chemical messages.

Chemotaxin: A chemical messenger that causes migration of cells in a particular direction.

Chemotaxis: The migration of cells in the direction of a chemical messenger.

Chronic granulomatous disease (CGD): A trait inherited in either an X-linked or autosomal recessive fashion that results in a defect in the microbicidal function of neutrophils.

Chronic GvHD: Graft-versus-host disease that occurs over time when transplanted immunocompetent cells react with recipient cells. It is characterized by involvement of skin, eyes, mouth, and other mucosal surfaces.

Class I MHC (HLA) molecules: Proteins coded for by genes at three loci (A, B, C) in the major histocompatibility complex. They are expressed on all nucleated cells and are important to consider in the transplantation of tissues.

Class II MHC (HLA) molecules: Proteins coded for by the DR, DP, and DQ loci of the major hisotocompatibility complex. They are found on B cells, macrophages, activated T cells, monocytes, dendritic cells, and endothelium.

Class switching: The production of immunoglobulins other than IgM by daughter cells of antigen-exposed B lymphocytes.

Classical pathway: A means of activating complement that begins with antigen–antibody combination.

Clonal selection theory: A theory postulated to explain the specificity of antibody formation, based on the premise that each lymphocyte is genetically programmed to produce a specific type of antibody and is selected by contact with antigen.

Cloned enzyme donor immunoassay: Type of immunoassay in which an analyte is labeled with a part of an enzyme. The enzyme only becomes active if it is not bound by antibody and it attaches to an additional enzyme moiety.

Cluster designation (CD): Another term for cluster of differentiation.

Clusters of differentiation (CD): Antigenic features of leukocytes that are identified by groups of monoclonal antibody expressing common or overlapping activity.

Coagglutination: An agglutination reaction using bacteria as the inert particle to which antibody is attached.

Coccidioidomycosis: A fungal disease caused by *Coccidioides immitis* that is endemic to the southwestern United States and may be characterized by primary pulmonary infection.

Codominant: When both alleles at a particular gene locus are expressed.

Cold autoagglutinin: Antibodies that react below 30°C, typically formed in response to diseases such as *Mycoplasma* pneumonia and certain viral infections.

Colony stimulating factor (CSF): A protein in human serum that promotes monocyte differentiation.

Common variable immunodeficiency: A heterogeneous group of immunodeficiency disorders that usually appears in patients between the ages of 20 and 30 years. It is characterized by a deficiency of one or more classes of immunoglobulins.

Complement: A series of proteins that are normally present in serum and whose overall function is medication of inflammation.

Complement fixation: The uptake of complement resulting from the combination of antigen with specific antibody. This can be used to test for the presence of either antigen or antibody. Sheep red blood cells coated with hemolysin are used as indicator particles. Lysis of the sheep cells occurs if either antigen or antibody is not present.

Complement-dependent cytotoxicity (CDC): Killing of cells that results from attachment of antibody with activation of complement.

Conformational epitope: Key antigenic site that results from the folding of one chain or multiple chains, bringing certain amino acids from different segments of a linear sequence or sequences into close proximity with each other so they can be recognized together.

Congenital syphilis: The transfer of syphilis from an infected mother to the fetus during pregnancy. It results in disease or death.

Conidia: Asexual reproductive structures produced by fungi at the tip of hyphae; also known as spores.

Constant region: The carboxy-terminal segment (half of immunoglobulin light chains or three quarters of heavy chains) that consists of a polypeptide sequence found in all chains of that type.

Contact dermatitis: A delayed hypersensitivity reaction caused by T cell sensitization to low molecular weight compounds, such as nickel and rubber, that come in contact with the skin.

Cross-immunity: The phenomenon in which exposure to one infectious agent produces protection against another agent.

Cross-reactivity: A phenomenon that occurs when an antibody reacts with an antigen that is structurally similar to the original antigen that induced antibody production.

Cryoglobulins: Immunoglobulins of the IgM class that precipitate at cold temperatures, causing occlusion of blood vessels in the extremities if a patient is exposed to the cold.

Cryptococcosis: A fungal disease caused by *Cryptococcus neoformans* and characterized as a pulmonary infection that may spread to the central nervous system and the brain.

Cyst: Inactive form of a parasite that can transmit infection.

Cytokine: Chemical messenger produced by stimulated cells that affects the function or activity of other cells.

Cytolytic T cells (CTL): Lymphocytes bearing the CD8 marker whose function is to destroy foreign or virally-infected cells.

Cytomegalovirus: A virus in the herpes family that is responsible for infection ranging from a mononucleosis-like syndrome to a life-threatening illness in immunocompromised patients.

Decay-accelerating factor (DAF): A glycoprotein found on peripheral red blood cells, endothelial cells, fibroblasts, and epithelial cell surfaces that is capable of dissociating and C3 convertases formed by both the classical and alternative pathways.

Delayed hypersensitivity: An immune response in which antibody production plays a minor role. It is primarily caused by activated T cells.

Deoxyribonucleic acid (DNA): The nucleic acid whose sugar is deoxyribose. It is the primary genetic material of all cellular organisms and DNA viruses.

Diapedesis: The process by which cells are capable of moving from the circulating blood to the tissues by squeezing through the wall of a blood vessel.

DiGeorge anomaly: A congenital defect of the third and fourth pharyngeal pouches that affects thymic development, leading to a T cell deficiency. Patients are subject to recurring viral and fungal infections.

Diluent: One of the two entities needed for making a dilution. It is the medium making up the rest of the solution

Direct agglutination: An antigen–antibody reaction that occurs when antigens are naturally found on a particle.

Direct allorecognition pathway: Pathway in which recipient T cells recognize intact HLA molecules on donor cells.

Direct antiglobulin test: A technique to determine *in vivo* attachment of antibody or complement to red blood cells, using antihuman globulin to cause a visible agglutination reaction.

Direct immunofluorescent assay: A technique to identify a specific antigen using an antibody that has a fluorescent tag attached.

Dot-blot: A serologic test that uses microparticles of antigen using an antibody that has a fluorescent tag attached.

Early rejection: See accelerated rejection.

Electrophoresis: The separation of molecules in an electrical field based on differences in charge and size.

Endocrine: Internal secretion of substances such as hormones or cytokines directly into the bloodstream that cause systemic effects.

Endogenous pyrogen: A substance produced by the body that causes fever. Interleukin-1 is an example.

Endosmosis: The movement of the buffer particles during electrophoresis.

Env: A structural gene of HIV that codes for envelope proetein gp160, gp120, and gp41.

Enzyme-linked immunosorbent assay (ELISA): An immunoassay that employs an enzyme label on one of the reactants.

Eosinophil chemotactic factor: A preformed mediator released from basophils and mast cells during an allergic reaction. It is responsible for attracting eosinophils to the area.

Eosinophil chemotactic factor of anaphylaxis (ECF-A): Preformed factor in granules of mast cells that attract eosinophils to the area.

Epitope: The key portion of the immunogen against which the immune response is directed; also known as the determinant site.

Epstein-Barr virus: A DNA virus of the herpesvirus family. It is responsible for infectious mononucleosis, Burkitt's lymphoma, nasopharyngeal carcinoma, and B cell lymphomas.

Erythema chronicum migrans: A rash associated with Lyme disease. It begins as a small red papule and expands to form a large ring with a central clear area.

Exoantigen: An antigen excreted by a bacterial or fungal cell as it metabolizes.

Exocytosis: Release of hydrolytic and lysosomal enzymes from phagocytes that is triggered by complement-coated immune complexes adhering to tissue surfaces.

External defense system: Structural barriers that prevent most infectious agents from entering the body.

Fab fragment: Fragment of an immunoglobulin molecule obtained by papain cleavage that consists of a light chain and one half of a heavy chain held together by disulfide bonding. The Fab fragment represents one antigen-binding site on the immunoglobulin molecule.

F(ab)2: Fragment of an immunoglobulin molecule obtained by pepsin cleavage that consists of two light chains and two heavy chain halves held together by disulfide bonding. This piece has two antigen-binding sites.

Factor H: A control protein in the complement system. It acts as a cofactor with factor I to break down C3b formed during complement activation.

Factor I: A serine protease that cleaves C3b and C4b formed during complement activation. A different cofactor is required for each of these reactions.

Fc fragment: Fragment of an immunoglobulin molecule obtained by papain cleavage that consists of the carboxy-terminal halves of two heavy chains. These two halves are held together by disulfide bonds. This fragment spontaneously crystallizes at 4°C.

Flocculation: The formation of downy masses of precipitate that occurs over a narrow range of antigen concentration.

Flow cytometry: See cell flow cytometry.

Florescence: Results from compounds that have the ability to absorb energy from an incident light source and convert that energy into light of a longer wavelength.

Fluorescence polarization immunoassay (FPIA): An immunoassay based on the change in polarization of fluorescent light emitted from a labeled molecule when it is bound by antibody.

Fluorescent antinuclear antibody (FANA) testing: Testing for the presence of antinuclear antibodies using animal cells and an antihuman immunoglobulin with a fluorescent tag. Antinuclear antibodies can be categorized on the basis of the fluorescent staining patterns exhibited.

FTA-ABS test: Fluorescent treponemal antibody absorption test, a confirmatory test for syphilis, which detects antibodies to *Treponema pallidum* by using antihuman immunoglobulin with a fluorescent label.

Fungi: Organisms made up of eukaryotic cells with rigid walls composed of chitin, mannan, and sometimes cellulose.

Gag: A structural gene of HIV that codes for three core proteins: p15, p17, and p24.

Gel electrophoresis: Method of separating either proteins or DNA based on their size and electrical charge. Samples are placed in wells on the gel and exposed to an electrical current.

Genotype: Actual alleles, for a particular trait, that are inherited.

Germinal center: The interior of a secondary follicle where blast transformation of B cells takes place.

Glomerulonephritis: A condition that produces damage to the glomeruli of the kidney and is often triggered by an immune response.

Goodpasture's syndrome: A type of glomerulonephritis caused by antibodies to glomerular basement membrane.

Graft-versus-host response (GVHR): A condition that results from transplantation of immunocompetent cells into an immunodeficient host. The transfused cells attack the tissues of the recipient.

Granulocyte-CSF: A cytokine produced by fibroblasts and epithelial cells committed to become granulocytes.

Granulocyte-macrophage-CSF: A cytokine produced by T cells and other cell lines that stimulates an increased supply of granulocytic cells and macrophages.

Graves' disease: An autoimmune disease characterized by hyperthyroidism caused by the presence of antibody to thyroid-stimulating hormone receptors. Antigen–antibody combination results in continual release of thyroid hormones.

HAART: Highly active antiretroviral therapy, a multidrug regimen that is the standard of treatment for HIV infection.

Haplotype: A set of genes that are located close together on a chromosome and are usually inherited as a single unit.

Hapten: A simple chemical group that can bind to antibody once it is formed, but which of itself is incapable of stimulating antibody formation unless tied to a larger carrier molecule.

Hashimoto's thyroiditis: An autoimmune disease that results in hypothyroidism caused by the presence of antithyroglobulin and antimicrosomal antibodies, which progressively destroy the thyroid gland.

HbcAg: Core antigen associated with infection with hepatitis B virus.

HbeAg: Antigen associated with the capsid of hepatitis B virus.

HbsAg: The surface antigen of hepatitis B virus, the first marker to appear in hepatitis B infection.

Heavy (H) chain: One of the polypeptide units that makes up an immunoglobulin molecule. Each immunoglobulin monomer consists of two heavy chains paired with two light chains.

Hemagglutination: An antigen–antibody reaction that results in the clumping of red blood cells.

Hemagglutination inhibition reaction: A test for detecting antibodies to certain viruses, based on lack of agglutination as a result of antibody neutralizing the virus.

Hemolytic disease of the newborn (HDN): A cytoxic reaction that destroys an infant's red blood cells because of placental transfer of maternal antibodies to Rh antigens.

Hemolytic titration (Ch50) assay: An assay that measures complement activating ability by determining the amount of patient serum required to lyse 50 percent of a standardized concentration of antibody-sensitized sheep erythrocytes.

Hepatitis: Inflammation of the liver caused by radiation, exposure to chemicals, autoimmune disease, or viruses.

Hereditary angioedema: A disease characterized by swelling of the extremities, the skin, the gastrointestinal tract, and other mucosal surfaces as a result of a deficiency in the complement inhibitor C1INH.

Herpes simplex virus: A DNA virus, found as type I and type II, which causes acute infection characterized by the development of small fluid-filled vesicles on the skin or mucous membranes.

Heteroantigen: An antigen of a species different from that of the host, such as other animals, plants, or microorganisms. These are capable of stimulating an immune response in the host.

Heterophile antibody: Antibody that cross-reacts with antigens that are different from the antigen originally responsible for its production.

Heterophile antigen: An antigen that exists in unrelated plants or animals but that is either identical or closely related, so that antibody to one will cross-react with antibody to the other.

Hinge region: The flexible portion of the heavy chain of an immunoglobulin molecule that is located between the first and second constant regions. This allows the molecule to bend to let the two antigen-binding sites operate independently.

Histamine: A vasoactive amine released from mast cells and basophils during an allergic reaction.

Histocompatibility antigens: Antigens found on cells that are highly polymorphic and elicit a transplant response.

Histocompatibility tests: Laboratory testing to determine individual histocompatibility antigens on donor and recipient cells involved in a transplant.

HIV: Human immunodeficiency virus, a retrovirus that is responsible for causing AIDS. There are two types of HIV, designated HIV-1 and HIV-2.

HLA genotype: Actual alleles, for HLA antigens, that are inherited.

HLA phenotype: The expression of HLA genes that actually appear as proteins on cells.

Hodgkin's lymphoma (HL): A malignant disease that typically begins in one lymph node and is characterized by the presence of Reed-Sternberg cells, giant multinucleate cells that are usually transformed B lymphocytes.

Homogeneous enzyme immunoassay: An immunoassay in which no separation step is necessary. It is based on the principle of a decrease in enzyme activity when specific antigen–antibody combination occurs.

Host-versus-graft response (HvGR): Recognition by the host of nonself histocompatibility antigens on grafts that may result in rejection.

Human chorionic gonadotropin (hCG): A hormone secreted by the trophoblast of the developing embryo, which rapidly increases during the early stages of pregnancy and is the basis of pregnancy testing.

Humoral immunity: Protection from disease resulting from substances in the serum.

Hyaluronidase: An enzyme produced by bacteria that breaks down hyaluronic acid in connective tissue.

Hybridization: Specific binding of two single-stranded DNA segments, as in binding of a probe with a known nucleic acid sequence to an unknown piece of DNA.

Hybridoma: A cell line resulting from the fusion of myeloma cell and a plasma cell. These can be maintained in tissue culture indefinitely and produce a very specific type of antibody known as monoclonal antibody.

Hyperacute rejection: Rejection of tissue that occurs within minutes or hours following transplantation, because of antibodies, already present, to ABO and HLA antigens.

Hypersensitivity: A heightened state of immune responsiveness.

Hyphae: Filamentous tubular branching structures characteristic of some fungi.

Hyposensitization: A treatment for allergies that involves the buildup of IgG antibodies to block the effects of IgE.

Idiotype: The variable portion of light and heavy immunoglobulin chains that is unique to a particular immunoglobulin molecule. This region constitutes the antigen-binding site.

IgM anti-HBc: Antibody that is the first to appear in hepatitis B infection. It is of the IgM class and is directed against core antigen on the virus particle.

Immediate hypersensitivity: Reaction to an allergen that occurs in minutes and can be life-threatening.

Immune adherence: The ability of phagocytic cells to bind complement-coated particles.

Immunity: The condition of being resistant to infection.

Immunoblotting: A technique used to identify antibodies to complex antigens and consisting of electrophoresis of the antigen mix followed by transfer of the pattern to nitrocellulose paper for reaction with patient serum.

Immunoelectrophoresis: A semiquantitative gel precipitation technique in which protein are first separated by electrophoresis and then subjected to double diffusion with antibodies directed against the individual proteins.

Immunofixation electrophoresis: A semiquantitative gel precipitation technique similar to that of immunoelectrophoresis, except that antibody is added directly to the surface of the gel after electrophoresis has taken place.

Immunofluorescent assay (IFA): Identification of antigens on cells using an antibody with fluorescent tag.

Immunogen: Any substance that is capable of inducing an immune response.

Immunoglobulin (Ig): Glycoproteins in the serum portion of the blood that are considered part of humoral immunity.

Immunoglobulin superfamily: Proteins involved in molecular recognition or cellular adhesion whose three-dimensional shape is similar to that of immunoglobulins.

Immunology: The study of the reactions of a host when foreign substances are introduced into the body.

Immunoradiometric assay (IRMA): A radioimmunoassay that uses excess labeled antibody to determine the amount of patient antigen present.

Immunosurveillance: The mechanism by which the body rids itself of transformed or abnormal cells.

Indirect allorecognition pathway: Presentation of processed donor HLA peptides bound to HLA class II molecules to CD4+ lymphocytes. This results in antibody formation against the donor graft.

Indirect antiglobulin test: A technique to determine *in vitro* antigen–antibody combination. Antihuman globulin is used to cause a visible agglutination reaction with antibody-coated red blood cells.

Indirect immunofluorescent assay: A technique to identify antigen by using two antibodies: one that is specific to the antigen, and a second that is an antihuman immunoglobulin with a fluorescent tag.

***In situ* hybridization:** Binding of a nucleic acid probe to target DNA located in intact cells.

Inflammation: Cellular and humor mechanisms involved in the overall reaction of the body to injury or invasion by an infectious agent.

Innate immune response: See natural immunity.

Interferons: Cytokines produced by T cells and other cell lines that inhibit viral synthesis or act as immune regulators.

Interleukin-1: A cytokine produced by macrophages in response to binding by T cells. It induces production of interleukin-2 by antigen-exposed T lymphocytes, mobilizes neutrophils from the marrow, and stimulates production of acute phase reactants.

Interleukin-2: A growth factor, produced by antigen-activated T cells, that triggers proliferation of the T cells producing it.

Interleukin-3: A cytokine produced by T helper cells of both Th1 and Th2 subtypes that stimulates the proliferation of immature marrow cells that are not yet committed to a specific lineage.

Internal defense system: Defense mechanism inside the body in which both cells and soluble factors play essential parts.

Invariant chain: A protein that associates with HLA class II antigens shortly after they are synthesized to prevent interaction of their binding sites with any endogenous peptides in the endoplasmic reticulum.

Isotype: A unique amino acid sequence that is common to all immunoglobulin molecules of a given class in a given species.

Joining (J) chain: A glycoprotein with a molecular weight of 15,000 that serves to link immunoglobulin monomers together. These are only found in IgM and secretory IgA molecules.

Kappa (κ) chain: One of two types of immunoglobulin light chains that are present in approximately two thirds of all immunoglobulin molecules.

Lambda (λ) chain: One of two types of immunoglobulin light chains that are present in approximately one third of all immunoglobulin molecules.

Lancefield group: A means of classifying streptococci on the basis of differences in the cell wall carbohydrate.

Lattice formation: The combination of antibody and multivalent antigen to produce a stable network that results in a visible reaction.

Law of Mass Action: A law used to mathematically describe the equilibrium relationship between soluble reactants and insoluble products. It can be applied to antigen–antibody relationships.

Lectin pathway: A pathway for the activation of complement based on binding of mannose binding protein to constituents on bacterial cell walls.

Leukemia: A progressive malignant disease of blood-forming organs, characterized by proliferation of leukocytes and their precursors in the bone marrow.

Ligase chain reaction (LCR): A means of increasing signal probes through the use of an enzyme called a ligase, which joins two pairs of probes only after they have bound to a complementary target sequence.

Light (L) chain: Small chain in an immunoglobulin molecule that is bound to the larger chain by disulfide bonds. The two types of light chains are called kappa and lambda.

Linear epitope: Amino acids following one another on a single chain that act as a key antigenic site.

Linkage disequilibrium: When two genes are inherited together with greater frequency than would be expected.

Lipopolysaccharide (LPS): Refers to a class of bacterial lipid found in the cell walls of gram-negative bacteria, which triggers release of cytokines from white blood cells.

Low ionic strength saline: Used to enhance agglutination reactions by decreasing the surface charge on red blood cells.

Lymph node: A secondary lymphoid organ that is located along a lymphatic duct and whose purpose is to filter lymphatic fluid from the tissues and act as a site for processing of foreign antigen.

Lymphoma: Cancer of the lymphoid cells that tends to proliferate as a solid tumor.

Macrophage-monocyte-CSF: A cytokine that induces growth of hematopoietic cells destined to become monocytes and macrophages.

Mannose-binding lectin (MBL): Normally present protein in the blood that binds to mannose on bacterial cells and initiates the lectin pathway for complement activation.

Metastatic growth: The transfer of disease from one organ to another not directly connected with it.

Material Safety Data Sheet (MSDS): An MSDS contains information on physical and chemical characteristics, fire, explosion reactivity, health hazards, primary routes of entry, exposure limits and carcinogenic potential, precautions for safe handling, spill clean-up, and emergency first aid information.

Major histocompatability complex (MHC): The genes that control expression of a large group of proteins originally identified on leukocytes but now known to be found on all nucleated cells in the body. These proteins regulate the immune response and play a role in graft rejection.

Membrane attack complex: The combination of complement components C5b, C6, C7, C8, and C9 that becomes inserted into the target cell membrane, causing lysis.

Memory cell: Progeny of an antigen-activated B or T cell that is able to respond to antigen more quickly than the parent cell.

Molecular mimicry: The similarity between an infectious agent and a self-antigen that causes antibody formed in response to the former to cross-react with the latter.

Monoclonal antibody: Very specific antibody derived from a single antibody-producing cell that has been cloned or duplicated.

Monoclonal gammopathy: A clone of lymphoid cells that cause overproduction of a single immunoglobulin component, called a paraprotein.

Monoclonal immunoglobulin: See monoclonal antibody.

Mold: A filamentous growth form found in fungi.

Multiple myeloma: A malignancy of mature plasma cells that results in a monoclonal increase in an immunoglobulin component. The most common component increased is IgG.

Multiple sclerosis: An autoimmune disease in which the myelin sheath of axons becomes progressively destroyed by antibodies to myelin proteins.

Myasthenia gravis: An autoimmune disease characterized by progressive muscle weakness caused by formation of antibody to acetylcholine receptors.

Mycelium: A dense mat formed by some fungi that is made up of intertwined hyphae.

Mycoses: Diseases produced by fungus.

NASBA: Nucleic acid sequence-based amplification, a method for increasing the number of copies of RNA in viral load testing for HIV infection.

Natural immunity: The ability of the individual to resist infection by means of normally present body functions.

Negative selection: The process by which T cells that can respond to self-antigen are destroyed in the thymus.

Neoplastic cells: Cells that have gone through malignant transformation and that continue to grow without regard to normal growth signals or controls.

Nephelometry: A technique for determining the concentration of particles in a solution by measuring the light scattered at a particular angle from the incident beam as it passes through the solution.

Nephritogenic strain: A strain of group A streptococcus that is capable of inducing glomerulonephritis.

Neutrophil chemotactic factor: A preformed mediator released from mast cells and basophils during an allergic reaction whose function is to attract neutrophils to the area.

Non-Hodgkin's lymphoma (NHL): A wide range of cancers of the lymphoid tissue, of which B cell lymphomas represent the majority.

Nonsuppurative complication: An infection in which the inflammatory response is not present in the affected organ but elsewhere in the body. An example is poststreptococcal glomerulonephritis.

Northern blot: Technique for the identification of specific RNA sequences by separating short RNA molecules electrophoretically, denaturing them, transferring the pattern to a nitrocellulose membrane, and incubating with a labeled probe that is specific for the sequence of interest.

Nucleic acid probe: Short strand of DNA or RNA of a known sequence used to identify a complementary nucleic acid strand in a patient specimen.

Occupational Safety and Health Administration (OSHA): Monitors and enforces safety regulations for workers.

Oncofetal antigens: Antigens that are expressed in the developing fetus and in rapidly dividing tissue, such as that associated with tumors, but which are absent in normal adult tissue.

Oncogene: Gene that encodes a protein capable of inducing cellular transformation.

One-way MLR: A means of determining the amount of proliferation of responder CD8+ T cells to nonself antigen. Stimulator cells are treated with a DNA inhibitor so that DNA synthesis indicates proliferation of responder cells only.

Opsonins: Serum proteins that attach to a foreign substance and enhanced phagocytosis (from the Greek word "to prepare for eating").

Oxidative burst: An increase in oxygen consumption in phagocytic cells, which generate oxygen radicals used to kill engulfed microorganisms.

Ouchterlony double diffusion: A qualitative gel precipitation technique in which both antigen and antibody diffuse out from wells cut in the gel. The pattern obtained indicates whether or not antigens are identical.

p24 antigen: A core structural protein that is part of the HIV virion.

Particle-counting immunoassay (PACIA): A technique for measuring residual nonagglutinating particles in a specimen using nephelometry to determine the amount of forward light scatter. Antigen–antibody combination decreases light scatter so that the amount of patient antigen present is indirectly proportional to the amount of light scattered.

Paraprotein: A single immunoglobulin component produced by a malignant clone of lymphoid cells in lymphoproliferative diseases.

Paracrine: Secretions such as cytokines that only affect target cells in close proximity.

Paroxysmal nocturnal hemoglobinuria (PNH): A disease characterized by complement-mediated hemolysis of erythrocytes resulting from a deficiency of decay-accelerating factor on the red blood cells.

Passive agglutination: A reaction in which particles coated with antigens not normally found on their surfaces clump together because of combination with antibody.

Passive cutaneous anaphylaxis: An allergic skin reaction produced when serum containing IgE against a particular allergen is injected under the skin and that individual is later exposed to the allergen.

Passive immunity: Immunity that is dependent on injection of preformed antibodies.

Passive immunodiffusion: A precipitation reaction in a gel in which antigen–antibody combination occurs by means of diffusion.

Periarteriolar lymphoid sheath: White pulp of splenic tissue, which is made up of lymphocytes, macrophages, plasma cells, and granulocytes. It is found surrounding central arterioles.

Personal protective equipment (PPE): Items such as gowns, masks, gloves, and face shields, used to protect the body from infectious agents.

Phagocytosis: From the Greek, *phagein,* meaning "cell-eating." The engulfment of cells or particulate matter by leukocytes, macrophages, or other cells.

Phagolysosome: The structure formed by the fusion of cytoplasmic granules and a phagosome during the process of phagocytosis.

Phagosome: A vacuole formed within a phagocytic cell as pseudopodia surround a particle during the process of phagocytosis.

Plasma cell: A transformed B cell that actively secretes antibody.

Plasma cell dycrasias: Immunoproliferative diseases characterized by overproduction of a single immunoglobulin component by a clone of lymphoid cells.

Pleiotrophy: Many different actions of a single cytokine. It may affect the activities of more than one kind of cell and have more than one kind of effect on the same cell.

Pol: A structural gene of HIV, which codes for reverse transcriptase and an endonuclease.

Polymerase chain reaction (PCR): A means of amplifying tiny quantities of nucleic acid using a heat-stable polymerase enzyme and a primer that is specific for the DNA sequence desired.

Positive predictive value: The percent of all positives in a serologic test that are true positives.

Positive selection: The process of selecting immature T lymphocytes for survival on the basis of expression of high levels of CD3 and the ability to respond to self-MHC antigens.

Postexposure prophylaxis: Course of preventative treatment used following exposure to potentially infectious organisms.

Postzone phenomenon: Lack of a visible reaction in an antigen–antibody reaction caused by an excess of antigen.

Precipitation: The combination of soluble antigen with soluble antibody to produce visible insoluble complexes.

Primer: Short sequences of DNA, usually 20 to 30 nucleotides long, used to hybridize specifically to a particular target DNA to help initiate replication of the DNA.

Primary follicle: A cluster of B cells that have not yet been stimulated by antigen.

Primary response: The initial response to a foreign antigen.

Properdin: A protein that stabilized the C3 convertase generated in the alternative complement pathway.

Prostate specific antigen (PSA): An antigen associated with prostate tissue that increases greatly if prostate cancer is present.

Prozone phenomenon: Lack of a visible reaction in antigen–antibody combination caused by the presence of excess antibody. This may result in a false-negative reaction.

Purine: Nitrogenous bases adenine and guanine incorporated into DNA and RNA, which represent part of the genetic code.

Purine–nucleoside phosphorylase (PNP) deficiency: Lack of the enzyme purine nucleoside phosphorylase. The deficiency is inherited as an autosomal recessive trait. Accumulation of a purine metabolite is toxic to T cells, leading to a defect in cell-mediated immunity.

Pyrimidine: Nitrogenous bases cytosine and thymine in DNA and cytosine and uracil in RNA, which form part of the genetic code.

Pyrogenic exotoxins: Toxins given off by bacterial cells as they grow, which are responsible for production of a fever and a rash.

Qβ replicase reaction: Amplification of a detection probe made by inserting a short RNA sequence into the bacteriophage called Qβ. When the Qβ probe binds to a specific target sequence, it is increased to detectable levels by using an RNA polymerase enzyme called Qβ replicase.

Radial immunodiffusion: A single-diffusion technique in which antibody is incorporated into a gel and antigen is measured by the size of a precipitin ring formed when it diffuses out in all directions from a well cut into the gel.

Radioimmunoassay (RIA): A technique used to measure small concentrations of an analyte, using a radioactive label on one of the immunologic reactants.

RAST: Radioallergosorbent test. It measures antigen-specific IgE by means of a noncompetitive solid-phase immunoassay.

Reagin: An antibody formed during the course of syphilis that is directed against cardiolipin and not against *Treponema pallidum* itself.

Recognition unit: The complement component that consists of the C1qrs complex. This must bind to at least two Fc regions to initiate the classical complement cascade.

Respiratory burst: An increase in oxygen consumption that occurs within a phagocytic cell as it begins to engulf particulate matter.

Restriction endonuclease: Enzymes that cleave DNA at specific recognition sites that are typically 4 to 6 base pairs long.

Restriction fragment length polymorphisms (RFLPs): Variations in nucleotides within DNA that change where restriction enzymes cleave the DNA. Where mutations occur, different size pieces of DNA are obtained, resulting in an altered electrophoretic pattern.

Reverse passive agglutination: A reaction in which carrier particles coated with antibody clump together because of a combination with antigen.

Reverse transcriptase: An enzyme produced by certain RNA viruses to convert viral RNA into DNA.

Rheumatoid arthritis (RA): An autoimmune disease that affects the synovial membrane of multiple joints. It is characterized by the presence of an autoantibody called rheumatoid factor.

Rheumatoid factor (RF): An antibody of the IgM class produced by patients with rheumatoid arthritis that is directed against IgG.

Ribonucleic acid (RNA): The nucleic acid containing the sugar ribose. It is the primary genetic material of RNA viruses and plays a role in the transcribing of genetic information in cells.

RIST: Radioimmunosorbent test developed to measure total IgE.

Rocket immunoelectrophoresis: A technique used to quantify antigens on the basis of the height of a rocket-shaped precipitin band obtained when radial immunodiffusion is combined with electrophoresis.

Rosetting: A daisy pattern created by sheep red blood cells, which adhere to CD2 antigens found on T cells.

RPR test: Rapid plasma reagin test; a slide flocculation test for syphilis that detects the antibody called reagin.

Rubella virus: An RNA virus that causes German or 3-day measles.

S protein: A control protein in the complement cascade that interferes with binding of the C5b67 complex to a cell membrane, thus preventing lysis.

Sandwich immunoassays: Immunoassays based on the ability of antibody to bind with more than one antigen.

Sandwich hybridization: A nucleic acid detection method using two probes, one of which is placed on a solid support, such as a membrane or microtiter plate, to capture the target DNA. A second labeled probe, which binds to a second site on the target DNA, is added to detect specific gene sequences.

Secondary follicle: A cluster of B cells that are proliferating in response to a specific antigen.

Secretory component (SC): A protein with a molecular weight of 70,000 that is synthesized in epithelial cells and added to IgA to facilitate transport of IgA to mucosal surfaces.

Sensitization: 1. The combination of antibody with a single antigenic determinant on the surface of a cell without agglutination. 2. Induction of an immune response.

Serial dilution: A method of decreasing the strength of an antibody solution by using the same dilution factor for each step.

Seroconversion: The change of a serologic test from negative to positive as a result of the development of the measurable antibodies in response to infection or immunization.

Serology: The study of a noncellular portion of the blood known as serum.

Serotype: A means of grouping bacteria on the basis of variation in cell wall proteins identified by specific antisera.

Serum sickness: A type III hypersensitivity reaction that results from the buildup of antibodies to animal serum used in passive immunization.

Severe combined immunodeficiency (SCID): An inherited deficiency of both cell-mediated and antibody-mediated immunity. It results in death in infancy caused by overwhelming infections.

Shell vial: A small container that has a single layer of cells on the bottom and is used for culturing viruses.

Single diffusion: A precipitation reaction in which one of the reactants is incorporated in the gel, while the other diffuses out from the point of application.

Solute: One of the two entities needed for making a dilution. It is the material being diluted.

Southern blot: Technique for the identification of specific DNA sequences in which DNA is cleaved into fragments by enzymes, separated electrophoretically, denatured, transferred to a nitrocellulose membrane, and incubated with a labeled probe that is specific for the sequence of interest.

Spherule: A saclike funnel structure that is filled with endospores when mature.

Spleen: The largest secondary lymphoid organ in the body, located in the upper left quadrant of the abdomen. Its function is to filter out old cell and foreign antigens.

Standard Precautions: Guidelines describing personnel protection that should be used for the care of all patients and including handwashing, gloves, mask, eye protection, face shield, gown, patient-care equipment, environmental control, linens, taking care to prevent injuries, and patient placement.

Streptolysin O: A protein capable of lysing red and white blood cells, which is given off by some groups of streptococci as they grow.

Stringency: Conditions that affect the ability of a probe to correctly bind to a specific target DNA sequence. These include temperature, salt concentration, and concentration of formamide or urea.

Suppurative complication: A result of infection characterized by the accumulation of white cells in a localized area where the invading organism is found.

Syngraft: The transfer of tissues or organs between genetically identical individuals such as identical twins.

Systemic lupus erythematosus (SLE): A chronic inflammatory autoimmune disease characterized by the presence of antinuclear antibodies. Symptoms may include swelling of the joints, an erythematous rash, and deposition of immune complexes in the kidneys.

Tabes dorsalis: Degeneration of the lower spinal cord that occurs in neurosyphilis and is characterized by a shuffling gait caused by partial paralysis.

Tertiary syphilis: The last stage of syphilis that appears months to years after secondary infection. It is characterized by granulomatous inflammation, cardiovascular disease, and central nervous system involvement.

Thermal dimorphism: A phenomenon found in some fungi in which the organism reproduces as a mold at 25°C to 30°C and as a yeast at 35°C to 37°C.

Thymocyte: Immature lymphocyte, found in the thymus, that undergoes differentiation to become a mature T cell.

Thymus: A small, flat bilobed organ found in the thorax of humans, which serves as the site for differentiation of T cells.

Thyroid-stimulating hormone (TSH): A hormone produced by the thyroid gland that binds to specific receptors, causing thyroglobulin to be broken down into secretable T3 and T4.

Thyroid-stimulating hormone receptor antibody (Trab): An antibody that is directed against the receptor for thyroid-stimulating hormone. It is associated with Graves' disease and results in overstimulation of the thyroid gland.

Thyroid-stimulating immunoglobulin (TSI): Another name for thyroid-stimulating hormone receptor antibody.

Thyrotoxicosis: A condition caused by overproduction of thyroid hormones, as seen in Graves' disease.

Titer: A figure that represents the relative strength of an antibody. It is the reciprocal of the highest dilution in which a positive reaction occurs.

Toxoplasmosis: A parasitic disease that is usually transmitted to humans by cysts found in contaminated soil, cat litter, or improperly cooked pork.

Transcription-mediated amplification (TMA): Method of increasing target DNA through the use of two enzymes, an RNA polymerase and a reverse transcriptase, to make new strands of DNA

Transforming growth factor (TGF): A group of cytokines that regulate the immune response by inhibiting proliferation of lymphocytes and other cells to promote healing.

Transient hypogammaglobulinemia: A condition characterized by low immunoglobulin levels that occur in infants around 2 to 3 months of age. It is believed to be caused by delayed maturation of one or more components of the immune system and usually corrects itself spontaneously.

Transporters associated with antigen processing (TAP): Proteins that are responsible for the ATP-dependent transport of newly synthesized short peptides from the cytoplasm to the lumen of the endoplasmic reticulum for binding to class 1 HLA antigens.

Treponema pallidum: A spirochete that is the causative agent of syphilis.

Tumor-associated antigens: Antigens found on tumor cells that are not unique to such cells but that can still be used to distinguish them from normal cells.

Tumor infiltrating lymphocyte (TIL): Lymphocytes within a tumor mass that are able to react with antigens on tumor cells to help destroy them.

Tumor necrosis factor (TNF): A major mediator of the innate defense against gram-negative bacteria.

Turbidimetry: A technique for determining the concentration of particles in a solution based on the change in absorbance caused by the scattering of light that occurs when an incident beam is passed through the solution

Type I diabetes mellitus: A disease characterized by insufficient insulin production as a result of an autoimmune process that causes selective destruction of the beta cells of the pancreas.

Tzanck smear: A rapid method for the diagnosis of blistering disorders such as herpes simplex; performed by staining cells from a lesion and examining for the presence of multinucleated giant cells.

Universal Precautions (UP): Guidelines stating that all body fluids are capable of transmitting diseases and recommending wearing gloves, face shields, and disposing of all needles and sharp objects in puncture-resistant containers without recapping.

Vaccination: From *vacca,* the Latin word for cow; the procedure of injecting immunogenic material in the body to induce immunity.

Viral load tests: Quantitative tests for HIV nucleic acid that are used to predict disease progression and to monitor the effects of antiretroviral therapy.

Variable region: The amino-terminal region of an immunoglobulin molecule (half of a light chain or quarter of a heavy chain) that has consider variations in amino acid sequence. This part is responsible for the specificity of a particular immunoglobulin molecule.

Varicella-zoster virus: A herpes virus that is responsible for chicken pox and zoster or shingles.

Variolation: The procedure of deliberately exposing an individual to material from smallpox lesions.

VDRL test: A flocculation test for reagin antibody found in syphilis; designed by the Veneral Disease Research Laboratories.

Waldenström's macroglobulinemia: An immunoproliferative disease caused by a malignancy of lymphocytes that results in production of IgM paraproteins.

Warm autoimmune hemolytic anemia: An autoimmune disease that results in the destruction of red blood cells caused by formation of IgG antibody that reacts at 37°C.

Western blot: A confirmatory test for HIV based on separation of HIV antigens by electrophoresis followed by transfer or blotting of the antigen pattern to a supporting medium for reaction with test serum.

Wiskott-Aldrich syndrome (WAS): A rare X-linked recessive syndrome characterized by immunodeficiency, eczema, and thrombocytopenia.

Xenograft: The transfer of tissue from an individual of one species to an individual of another species, such as animal tissue transplanted to a human.

Yeast: A unicellular form of certain fungi that reproduce asexually by budding, in which the parent cell divides into two unequal parts.

Zone of equivalence: The point in an antigen–antibody reaction at which the number of multivalent sites of antigen and antibody are approximately equal, resulting in optimal precipitation.

Answers

Chapter 1

Answers to Review Questions

1. **b.**   2. **a.**   3. **c.**   4. **c.**   5. **c.**   6. **b.**   7. **a.**   8. **d.**

Chapter 2

Answers to Review Questions

1. **a.**   2. **d.**   3. **c.**   4. **c.**   5. **a.**   6. **d.**   7. **d.**   8. **b.**
9. **c.**   10. **d.**   11. **c.**   12. **b.**   13. **a.**

Answers to Case Studies

1. Although the cholesterol levels were within normal limits for both HDL and total cholesterol, recent studies indicate that an increase in CRP has been associated with a greater risk of a future heart attack. Increased fibrinogen levels are also associated with an increased risk for a future cardiovascular event, although it is not as great a risk factor as increased CRP. An increase in both of these acute phase reactants indicates an underlying chronic inflammatory process. Such a process has been found to be associated with atherosclerosis, a condition leading to damage to coronary blood vessels. Rick's wife should help him by encouraging him to follow a healthy diet and to lose weight through exercise.

2. CRP is one of the first indicators of a possible infection. If the infection were bacterial in nature, an increase in the white blood cell count should have been seen. This increase would mainly be due to recruitment of neutrophils to help fight the invading organism. If, on the other hand, an infection is due to a virus, there is typically no apparent increase in the white blood cell count. As an acute phase reactant, CRP levels increase dramatically within 24 hours, long before specific antibody can be detected. Thus, an increase in CRP supports the likelihood that an infection is present. The fact that the mono test result was indeterminate probably indicates a small amount of antibody present, but not enough for a definite positive test. Repeating the mono test in a few days will give a chance for a detectable level of antibody to be formed.

Chapter 3

Answers to Review Questions

1. **c.**   2. **a.**   3. **d.**   4. **a.**   5. **c.**   6. **b.**   7. **a.**   8. **c.**
9. **a.**   10. **b.**   11. **b.**   12. **d.**   13. **b.**   14. **a.**

Answers to Case Studies

1. The normal CD19+ cells indicate that there is not a lack of B cells, which presumably are capable of responding to antigen and producing antibody. The population that does seem to be most affected is the T cells, which carry CD3 on their surface. T helper cells are necessary for a B cell response, especially IgG. Thus, this indicates an immunodeficiency due to a low number of T cells, most likely T helper (CD4+) cells.

2. This patient has a lymphocytic leukemia that is of the B cell variety. CD19 is a pan-B cell marker. The fact that CD10 or the CALLA antigen is not present indicates that these cells are not precursors but are more highly differentiated. Knowledge of the type and stage of development of lymphocytes present aids in treatment decisions.

Chapter 4

Answers to Review Questions

1. **d.**   2. **b.**   3. **a.**   4. **c.**   5. **d.**   6. **b.**   7. **b.**   8. **d.**
9. **c.**   10. **c.**

Answers to Case Study

1.

a. The only antigens matching with the mother's type are HLA A9/B5/Cw3. Therefore, this is one haplotype, and the other set of genes inherited together (haplotype) are HLA A11/B18/Cw8.

b. The second haplotype possessed by the child matches that of the former boyfriend exactly. Therefore, the boyfriend is a likely candidate to be the father.

c. The principle of paternity testing is based on exclusion. This man cannot be excluded because he possesses all the HLA antigens inherited by the child that do not belong to the mother. While it cannot be said with absolute certainty that this man is the father, with so many alleles at each locus, the probability of someone unrelated to the child having an exact match is extremely low. Therefore, this man should be forced to pay child support.

Chapter 5

Answers to Review Questions

1. **a.** 2. **a.** 3. **d.** 4. **b.** 5. **c.** 6. **d.** 7. **a.** 8. **c.** 9. **b.**
10. **a.** 11. **c.** 12. **d.** 13. **b.** 14. **b.** 15. **c.** 16. **b.**

Answers to Case Studies

1. Presence of IgM only is an indicator of an early acute infection. IgM is the first antibody to appear, followed by IgG. In a reactivated case of mono, a small amount of IgM might be present, but IgG would also be present. The memory cells created by the first exposure to the virus would trigger production of IgG in a much shorter time. Thus, this patient is experiencing the disease for the first time.

2. Chronic respiratory infections may be due to a decrease or lack of IgA, but this is not the case here. Normal IgG and IgM levels indicate that this child is not immuno-compromised. The increase in IgE is an indicator that the cold symptoms may actually be due to allergy. This is especially evident in the springtime, when pollen is at high levels. The child should be tested for specific allergies to determine what is causing the actual symptoms. Treatment with antihistamine may help to relieve symptoms.

Chapter 6

Answers to Review Questions

1. **b.** 2. **a.** 3. **d.** 4. **c.** 5. **a.** 6. **b.** 7. **d.** 8. **b.**
9. **b.** 10. **d.** 11. **c.** 12. **d.**

Answers to Case Study

1.

a. Infection is the most common cause of immature myeloid cells. However, it is relatively rare to see cells as immature as promyelocytes and myeloblasts in this setting. One would worry about the presence of a myeloid leukemia when such immature cells are present. If the morphology of the myeloid cells is abnormal it might suggest a myelodysplastic syndrome that is developing into leukemia.

b. It is always useful, and sometimes essential, to get a clinical history to interpret a blood film. You should discuss the patient with the clinician or have the medical director of the laboratory review the medical record.

Chapter 7

Answers to Review Questions

1. **b.** 2. **c.** 3. **d.** 4. **d.** 5. **c.** 6. **a.** 7. **b.** 8. **a.**
9. **d.** 10. **a.** 11. **b.** 12. **c.** 13. **b.** 14. **d.** 15. **c.**
16. **d.**

Answers to Case Studies

1.

a. A decreased Ch_{50} indicates a problem with the classical pathway. The decreased radial hemolysis with a buffer that chelates calcium indicates a problem with the alternative pathway also.

b. Levels of C3 and C4 are normal, indicating that a deficiency of one or more of the membrane attack components is involved. While a lack of C1q or C2 cannot absolutely be ruled out, the fact that the alternative pathway is also affected is a second indicator that the common components C5–C9 are the ones involved. Since defense against encapsulated bacteria such as meningococi is reduced if there is a decrease in C5–C9, the patient's symptoms are in accord with this conclusion.

c. In order to confirm the actual deficiency, testing for the individual components C5 through C9 should be performed. Since this type of deficiency reduces the overall functioning of the complement system, patients should receive prompt therapy when signs of infection are noted.

2.

a. While the abdominal pain and vomiting could be due to a number of infectious agents, the normal white blood cell count decreases the likelihood of a bacterial infection. The accompanying swelling of the hands and legs may be an indicator of a possible inflammatory problem associated with continuous activation of the complement system. Since this has been a recurring problem, the likelihood of an immune problem is increased. The fact that total serum protein is within the normal range, it is unlikely that the deficiency is due to lack of antibody production. A decrease of one complement component would not be apparent on a total protein determination.

b. Reduced levels of both C4 and C2 could be due to inheritance of defective genes for both components. However, the probability of that is extremely rare. A more plausible explanation would be that the deficiency of both C2 and C4 is due to overconsumption rather than a lack of production.

c. A lack of C1-INH would result in overconsumption of C4 and C2. As this is the most common deficiency of the complement system, this represents a likely explanation for the symptoms, and should be determined by testing for this component.

Chapter 8

Answers to Review Questions

1. **c.**　2. **a.**　3. **a.**　4. **a.**　5. **c.**　6. **b.**　7. **d.**　8. **a.**
9. **c.**　10. **b.**　11. **c.**　12. **a.**　13. **b.**　14. **a.**

Answers to Case Study

A. All specimens should be capped.

B. Use to dry off hands and turn off faucet.

C. Both the needle and the activated protective shield must be discarded.

D. Discard all contaminated materials in biohazard containers. Use 1:10 sodium hypochlorite, stored in a plastic bottle and prepared weekly. Allow the solution to dry on the area before removing.

E. Standard Precautions require gloves and handwashing with all body fluids, not just those containing blood as specified by UP.

Chapter 9

Answers to Review Questions

1. **c.**　2. **d.**　3. **b.**　4. **d.**　5. **b.**　6. **a.**　7. **a.**　8. **b.**
9. **c.**　10. **a.**　11. **b.**　12. **d.**　13. **a.**　14. **c.**

Answers to Case Study

1.

a. The results indicate normal levels of IgG and IgM, but a decreased level of IgA. This most likely indicates a selective IgA deficiency, the most common genetic immuno-deficiency. Selective IgA deficiency occurs in approximately 1:1000 individuals.

b. A decrease in serum IgA most likely indicates a decrease in secretory IgA, the immunoglobulin that is found on mucosal surfaces. Individuals with a selective IgA deficiency are more prone to respiratory tract and gastrointestinal tract infections, since this represents the first line of defense against organisms that invade mucosal surfaces.

c. Nephelometry is a more sensitive method for measuring immunoglobulin levels. It is able to detect small quantities of immunoglobulins present. Results are obtained faster than for RID, and since the process is automated, it is not subject to human error in reading the results. Other errors that may occur in radial immunodiffusion include overfilling or underfilling of wells, nicking of wells, and inaccurate incubation time or temperature. Therefore, nephelometry has largely replaced RID for measurement of immunoglobulin levels.

Chapter 10

Answers to Review Questions

1. **b.**　2. **c.**　3. **a.**　4. **c.**　5. **a.**　6. **b.**　7. **c.**　8. **c.**
9. **b.**　10. **d.**　11. **c.**　12. **d.**

Answers to Case Study

1.

a. The positive test on an undiluted patient specimen indicates that at least 10+ IU/ml of rubella antibody is present. This indicates immunity to the virus if the patient was tested immediately after exposure to the disease.

b. The presence of antibody indicates that the patient will not likely be reinfected with the virus. Therefore, she does not have to be concerned about possible consequences for the fetus.

c. The antibodies detected are most likely due to vaccination and not the disease itself. If there is any question about how soon after exposure the patient was tested, a serum sample should be frozen. An additional specimen should be collected if any clinical symptoms appear, or after 30 days. Both specimens should be tested simultaneously using the semi-quantitative procedure. A four-fold increase in titer would indicate recent infection.

Chapter 11

Answers to Review Questions

1. **c.**　2. **a.**　3. **b.**　4. **c.**　5. **b.**　6. **c.**　7. **b.**　8. **b.**
9. **c.**　10. **b.**　11. **c.**　12. **a.**

Answers to Case Study

1.

a. A negative finding only means that no parasites were observed for that particular specimen at that particular time. It does not automatically rule out the possibility of parasites being present.

b. Capture enzyme immunoassays that are specific for parasites such as Giardia and Cryptosporidium are available. Typically solid phase such as microtiter wells is coated with specific antibody, and very small amounts of antigen can be detected. If a parasite is suspected, and traditional test results are negative, this would be the next step.

c. Capture enzyme immunoassays are very sensitive and are capable of detecting minute amounts of parasitic antigens that may be present. This is important in testing a stool culture due to the fact that large amounts of parasitic antigens may not be present at any one time. Many of these organisms such as Giardia and Cryptosporidium are extremely small and may not be easily found on a stained slide preparation.

d. In addition to the increased sensitivity, enzyme immuno-assays are simple to perform and are less time-consuming than traditional testing for parasites. Since instrumentation is usually used, the results are more easily interpreted with less subjectivity than stained smears.

Chapter 12

Answers to Review Questions

1. **d.** 2. **a.** 3. **a.** 4. **b.** 5. **d.** 6. **c.** 7. **a.** 8. **d.** 9. **a.** 10. **b.** 11. **a.** 12. **d.**

Chapter 13

Answers to Review Questions

1. **c.** 2. **b.** 3. **b.** 4. **b.** 5. **d.** 6. **a.** 7. **a.** 8. **d.** 9. **d.** 10. **c.** 11. **a.** 12. **c.**

Answers to Case Studies

1.

a. An increase in eosinophils is typically found in allergic individuals. Interleukins released by stimulated Th1 cells are involved in the recruitment of eosinophils from the bone marrow. While there are other causes of eosinophilia, such as a parasitic infection, an increased number most often indicates an allergic reaction.

b. IgE levels of greater than 333 IU are considered to be abnormally elevated if the patient is over the age of 14. In this case, the young age of the patient plus the accompanying symptoms all point to the likelihood that an allergic tendency is present.

c. Allergen-specific testing, either in the form of RAST testing or skin testing would be indicated to determine specific allergens. Skin testing is considered to be more sensitive, but *in vitro* testing is easier on the patient. In either case, specific allergens need to be identified in order for treatment to be successful.

2.

a. A positive DAT indicates that the red cells are coated with either antibody or complement components. The destruction of some red cells is the reason for the man's symptoms.

b. The most likely cause of the positive DAT is the presence of an antibody of the IgM class. It might be an anti-I, triggered by *Mycoplasma pneumoniae*. This is a cold-reacting antibody.

c. A DAT that is only positive with anti–C3d indicates that only complement products are present on the red cells. This is a further indication that the antibody is an IgM antibody, as it does not remain on the cells at 37°C but does trigger complement activation, which can cause the cell destruction.

Chapter 14

Answers to Review Questions

1. **a.** 2. **c.** 3. **d.** 4. **d.** 5. **c.** 6. **d.** 7. **c.** 8. **a.** 9. **b.** 10. **b.** 11. **a.** 12. **c.**

Answers to Case Studies

1.

a. In systemic lupus erythematosus, a low titer rheumatoid factor is often present. Conversely, a low titer of antinuclear antibodies can be found associated with rheumatoid arthritis. Thus, these two cannot be differentiated on the basis of the slide agglutination test results.

b. The decreased red cell count may be due to presence of a low level autoantibody directed against red cells, often associated with lupus.

c. A fluorescent antinuclear antibody (FANA) test is a good screening test to help distinguish between these two conditions. A homogeneous pattern or a peripheral pattern would be indicative of lupus, while a speckled pattern can sometimes be found in rheumatoid arthritis or lupus. Therefore, if a speckled pattern is obtained, more specific testing such as an immunodiffusion assay should be done. Presence of anti-Sm antibody would be diagnostic for lupus. This is what was found in this case.

2.

a. The low T4 level, enlarged thyroid gland, and presence of antithyroglobulin antibody are all indicators of Hashimoto's thyroiditis.

b. Antithyroglobulin antibodies progressively destroy thyroglobulin produced by the thyroid. Thyroglobulin is normally cleaved in the thyroid to produce secretable hormones triiodothyronine (T3) and thyroxine (T4). Presence of antithyroglobulin antibodies causes enlargement of the thyroid due to the immune response, and hypothyroidism results, characterized by tiredness and weight gain.

c. Graves' disease is also an autoimmune disease that affects the thyroid, but it is characterized by hyperthyroidism. In this disease, antibodies to thyroid-stimulating hormone receptors are produced, sending a signal to the thyroid to constantly produce T3 and T4. Symptoms include nervousness, insomnia, restlessness, and weight loss, exactly opposite to characteristics of Hashimoto's thyroiditis.

Chapter 15

Answers to Review Questions

1. **b.** 2. **c.** 3. **c.** 4. **d.** 5. **a.** 6. **d.** 7. **e.**

Chapter 16

Answers to Review Questions

1. **c.** 2. **c.** 3. **d.** 4. **b.** 5. **a.** 6. **a.** 7. **a.** 8. **d.**

Answers to Case Studies

1.

a. The constant bacterial infections coupled with laboratory results indicate an immunodeficiency disease, likely Bruton's agammaglobulinemia, or severe combined immuno-deficiency syndrome (SCIDS).

b. Both conditions are inherited as an x-linked recessive gene, which affects males almost exclusively.

c. To differentiate between the two immunodeficiency states, several types of testing are recommended. Measurement of serum IgA, IgM, and IgG levels should be performed to determine if in fact all classes of antibody are absent. Enumeration of classes of lymphocytes should also be determined by flow cytometry. In SCIDS, both T and B cell development is affected, and both lymphocyte populations would be deficient, while in Bruton's agammaglobulinemia, only B cell development is affected. Since the differential

indicates that some lymphocytes are present, this would indicate Bruton's agammaglobulinemia. Flow cytometry findings confirming the presence of T cells only confirm this diagnosis.

2.

a. The decrease in the T cell population coupled with facial abnormalities indicate Di George syndrome. The weak gamma band indicates that some antibody production is occurring, but is decreased due to low numbers of T helper cells.

b. Di George syndrome, unlike most other immuno-deficiency diseases, is due to abnormal embryonic development rather than an inherited genetic deficiency. The third and fourth pharyngeal pouches fail to develop normally, affecting development of the thymus and causing possible mental retardation and facial anomalies.

c. Treatment depends upon the severity of the T cell deficit. This condition can be treated with fetal thymus transplantation, or with thymic hormones if there is some thymic function.

Chapter 17

Answers to Review Questions

1. **b.** 2. **c.** 3. **d.** 4. **d.** 5. **b.** 6. **b.** 7. **a.** 8. **e.**

Answers to Exercise

1. Child 1 could only inherit DQ2, DR17, B8, Cw7 and A24 from the father, since these antigens do not occur in the mother. Therefore, the tentative haplotype assignments for the father are:

DQ2, DR17, B8, Cw7, A24
DQ2 or X, DR13, B8 or X, Cw7 or X, A1

The second haplotype of child 1 must be DQ1, DR1, B35, Cw4, A3. Therefore, the tentative maternal haplotypes are:

DQ1, DR1, B35, Cw4, A3
DQ1, DR13, B60, Cw3, A2

2. The following haplotypes can now be assigned to the children:

Child 1: (a) DQ2, DR17, B8, Cw7, A24
DQ1, DR1, B35, Cw4, A3
Child 2: (a) DQ2, DR17, B8, Cw7, A24
DQ1, DR13, B60, Cw3, A2
Child 3: (a\b) DQ2, DR17, B8, Cw7, A1 Cross-over between (a) locus C and (b) locus A

(d) DQ1, DR13, B60, Cw3, A2
Child 4: (b) DQ2, DR13, B8, Cw7, A1
(d) DQ1, DR13, B60, Cw3, A2 Homozygous DR13
Child 5: (b) DQ2, DR13, B8, Cw7, A1
(c) DQ1, DR1, B35, Cw4, A3

Note: Child 4 and 5 resolve the question on the (b) haplotype of whether or the DQ and B loci are null alleles (blanks, X) or were expressed DQ2 and B8. In both Child 4 and Child 5 they were expressed as DQ2 and B8.

3. There are no genotypically identical sibling donors for Child 1, the patient who is genotype (a,c).

Child 2 (a,d) is mismatched for 1 DR, 1 B, and 1 A antigen; 3 antigen mismatch if HLA-C is not included.

Child 3 (a\b,d) is mismatched for 1DR, 1 B and 2 A antigens because of the recombinant haplotype; 3 antigen mismatch.

Child 4 (b,d) is mismatched for 1 DR, 1 B, and 2A antigens because of a 2 haplotype mismatch; 3 antigen mismatch.

Child 5 (b,c) is mismatched for 1 DR and 1 A antigen because of a 1 haplotype mismatch; 2 antigen mismatch. If a sibling were to be become the organ donor, child 5 would be the best available match among these siblings.

Chapter 18

Answers to Review Questions

1. **d.**   2. **c.**   3. **d.**   4. **d.**   5. **b.**   6. **b.**   7. **d.**   8. **b.**
9. **b.**   10. **b.**   11. **d.**   12. **d.**   13. **d.**   14. **c.**   15. **a.**

Answers to Case Studies

1.
a. There is residual tumor, because the CA 15.3 levels dropped too slowly and stayed above background. She should be placed on chemotherapy.
b. The tumor is not responding to the chemotherapy, so the chemotherapy should be changed.

Adjuvant immunotherapy with anti-her2neu can be used in combination with cisplatin.
2.
a. Nonseminomatous testicular tumors.
b. Immunohistochemical analysis of a biopsy of the tumor.
c. Monitoring therapy
3.
a. These results, high serum PSA levels, high PSA velocity and low bound/free ratio indicate that the patient has a prostatic adenocarcinoma.
b. A biopsy should be performed.
c. The PSA velocity is 6.5–3.5 = 3. 3/3.5 = 86%.

Chapter 19

Answers to Review Questions

1. **c.**   2. **d.**   3. **d.**   4. **b.**   5. **d.**   6. **b.**   7. **c.**   8. **c.**
9. **d.**   10. **b.**   11. **d.**   12. **d.**   13. **c.**   14. **b.**   15. **c.**
16. **b.**   17. **b.**

Answers to Case Studies

1.
a. Almost 25 percent of individuals with Lyme disease do not exhibit the characteristic rash. Its presence is a good indicator of Lyme disease, but absence of the rash does not rule out the possibility of the disease.
b. There are a number of false positive results in EIA testing, including syphilis, other treponemal diseases, infectious mononucleosis, and autoimmune diseases such as rheumatoid arthritis. Thus, low levels of antibody might indicate one of these other diseases. However, false negative results in Lyme disease are also possible due to a low level of antibody production. Therefore, an indeterminate test neither rules out nor confirms the presence of Lyme disease.
c. If there is a history of a tick bite and patient symptoms are consistent with Lyme disease, then a confirmatory Western Blot test should be performed. The Western blot is fairly specific for Lyme disease. If 5 of 10 protein bands specific for

Borrelia burgdorferi are positive, this confirms presence of Lyme disease.
2.
a. While it is possible the mother's positive RPR test could be a false positive, it is also likely that the mother is in the latent stage of syphilis, with no obvious signs of the disease. Although syphilis is not sexually transmitted during this stage, it can be transmitted from a mother to her unborn child. Many infants do not exhibit clinical signs of the disease at birth, but if infected and untreated, a large percentage of babies develop later symptoms, including neurologic deficits such as blindness and mental retardation.
b. A positive RPR on a cord blood could be due to transplacental passage of mother's IgG antibodies. A titer should be performed on the cord blood, and a serum sample obtained from the infant in several weeks. If infection is present in the infant, the titer will remain the same or increase. An IgM capture assay could also be performed. Presence of specific antitreponemal IgM would indicate that the infant had been exposed to *Treponema pallidum,* since IgM antibodies do not cross the placenta.
c. Since there is a good chance that the infant is at risk for congenital syphilis, immediate treatment with penicillin can prevent any further neurologic consequences.

Chapter 20

Answers to Review Questions

1. **c.**   2. **d.**   3. **c.**   4. **b.**   5. **b.**   6. **b.**   7. **d.**   8. **a.**
9. **c.**   10. **a.**

Answers to Case Study

1.
a. Post-streptococcal glomerulonephritis
b. Group A *Streptococcus pyogenes*
c. Immune complexes resulting from the combination of streptococcal antigen- antibody combinations are deposited in the glomeruli of the kidney. These immune complexes stimulate an inflammatory response in the area causing tissue damage and impaired kidney function

Index

Page numbers followed by f indicate figures; t, tables.